DOCUMENTA OPHTHALMOLOGICA

PROCEEDINGS SERIES

VOL. IV

Editor

HAROLD E. HENKES

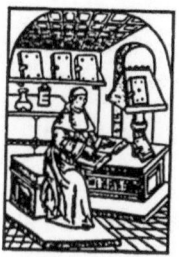

DR. W. JUNK B.V. PUBLISHERS, 1974
THE HAGUE   THE NETHERLANDS

XIth I.S.C.E.R.G. SYMPOSIUM

Edited by

E. DODT AND JEROME T. PEARLMAN

Bad Nauheim, May 1973

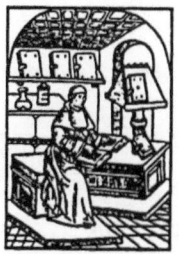

DR. W. JUNK B.V. PUBLISHERS, 1974
THE HAGUE   THE NETHERLANDS

ISBN-13: 978-90-6193-144-7   e-ISBN-13: 978-94-010-2340-5
DOI: 10.1007/978-94-010-2340-5

CONTENTS

INTRODUCTION

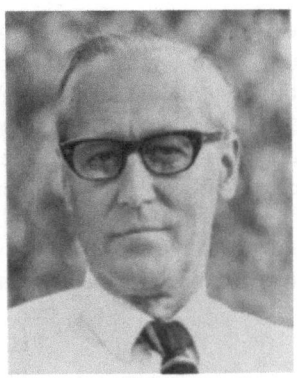

Professor GÖSTA KARPE

GÖSTA KARPE was born in Vadstena, Sweden, 1908.
His medical education started in 1927 at the Karolinska Institute in Stockholm
During his study he worked parttime in the department of physiology. KARPE
served as a resident in the ophthalmological department of Serafiner lasarettet
from 1937 till 1941. That year, the university eye clinic was transferred to the
newly built Karolinska Sjukhuset, where KARPE became assistant-head of the
out-patient department, and lecturer in ophthalmology. In 1949 he was appoin-
ted professor in ophthalmology at the Karolinska Institute and head of the
department of ophthalmology at Karolinska Sjukhuset.

KARPE received his doctor degree in 1945 upon completion of his thesis:
'The basis of clinical electroretinography'. This original work opened up a
completely new field of clinical investigation. Soon Swedish and foreign pupils
flocked into his department to study his new method, a technique at present
accepted as an indispensable tool in ophthalmic practice. Since 1945 his work
as well as that of his pupils have been devoted mainly to this field of research.
KARPE, too, showed great interest in medical organizations abroad. He acted
for many years as a member of the Board of the Scandinavian University
Hospital in Korea. His main interest however, went undoubtedly to his 'own'
Society of which he served as first president from the very beginning in 1958
till 1972.

GÖSTA KARPE has set his seal on the ISCERG right from the beginning, stressing the necessity to keep a balance between the interests of physiologists and ophthalmologists. KARPE stressed again and again the clinical character of the Society. Working with physiologists and clinicians has not always been easy, but GÖSTA was convinced that the ISCERG should perform a mediator's task between the basic scientists on the one hand, and the clinicians on the other, with the aim to bring newly-won knowledge into the ophthalmic clinic.

In the years of GÖSTA's presidency clinical electroretinography has made enormous progress and adjacent fields of clinical investigation have been opened up succesfully.

It is important that we, as a Society, stick closely to the newest developments in this field. However, KARPE's original method for recording the human ERG is still in use with satisfaction in a number of clinics. It is quite clear that there exists still a need for a simple and sound recording technique, as a routine procedure available in almost any ophthalmic clinic around the world, and it is equally clear that our society has a task in stimulating such a development. As a token of our esteem for the man who started clinical electroretinography over 30 years ago and who guided the Society for 15 years, the Board decided to dedicate the eleventh Symposium of our Society to GÖSTA KARPE.

HAROLD E. HENKES
President
International Society for
Clinical Electroretinography

THE CONCEPT 'RECEPTIVE FIELD'

RAGNAR GRANIT

(Stockholm)

Professor EBERHARDT DODT asked me to provide an Introduction to this meeting and gave me a free hand in the choice of a subject. I was very touched by his courtesy and kind loyalty in remembrance and felt that something had to be done to express my appreciation of his proposition.

The title of my Introduction ought to have been given a subtitle: how it strikes an ex-vision man when he takes a look at the labours of his successors. In general, of course, he is willing to admire the imagination and technical skill with which the subject has been developed. Progress has indeed been striking. When ultimately I seized on the concept 'receptive field' for a few remarks, this was because I have been wondering whether it has not seen its most prolific days and now could be allowed a period of rest for recovery and renewed uptake at some later date. I mean that on the whole other approaches to visual problems lately have seemed to me more rewarding.

SOME RETINAL ASPECTS

Essentially 'receptive fields' form an organized retinal matrix of excitation and inhibition modifying the responses of single ganglion cells so that both an increase or a decrease of light within the overlapping pick-up areas of a number of such cells leads to a discharge of impulses. It is tempting to regard the pick-up area of each ganglion cell as a spatial unit. The dimensions of such pick-up areas or receptive fields and their overlap with one another strikes one as having been somewhat neglected. Not until very recently (IKEDA & WRIGHT, 1972; HAMMOND, 1973) has it, for instance, become clear, that the centre of a concentric centre-surround field not only has a surround of opposite properties but that the latter also has a surround repeating the centre-properties, both in the retina and in the geniculate body of the cat. And for some time we have known of the McIlwain-effect which influences firing ganglion cells in these structures at a distance of the order of 30 to 50°, the stimulus being movement of an object at those distances.

Movement is of course a most essential parameter of visual stimulation and movement creates overlap of fields. The eyes move incessantly, the head moves, the body is in motion, objects move against a steady background etc. Then, at the next projection, the outcome of all this unavoidable scanning of the surrounding world is thrown upon *non-movable foci* for re-interpretation in order to be dispatched to further sites for re-reinterpretation. The visual centres or areas have now in the papers of COWAN and of ZEKI reached a minimal number of nine'. Since in higher mammals on- and off-centre fields with opposite surrounds are stated wholly to dominate their retinae, something of this pattern will be reflected onwards until finally it is lost in the cascading synaptic organizations and interactions. Why this particular field-pattern should be the most suitable first stage for whatever information in the end is extracted at all those nine stations seems to be an essential question of coding principles. My guess is that the answer lies hidden within the polyganglionic matrix rather than within their individual receptive fields as such.

Let me put those problems a little differently: what is being explained by the existence of a retinal organization emerging in the shape of receptive fields? The responses to light and darkness and their antagonism were known long before the organizational features of the receptive fields through KUFFLER'S paper of 1953 rose to prominence. These facts were familiar in terms of single ganglion cell or fibre responses. They explained characteristic properties of seeing as an act. I do believe that the two types of concentric fields in the retinae of higher mammals represent a significant discovery and they serve, of course, as a kind of necessary *point d'appui* of the measuring technique. But what have they added to our understanding of vision, by which I mean seeing as an act? Relatively little, I should say. However, I cannot lay claim to have followed the literature well enough to equate my own ignorance with the knowledge of the up-to-date specialists in the field. It seems to me convincing to assume that concentric fields, in order to survive in the evolution, must have betoken a significant biological asset for the organism. What is this asset? This, briefly, is my question re-formulated. It is difficult merely to consider functions which the retinae of frogs and rabbits can handle without much need for this sort of an organization.

Speaking of frogs and rabbits, it is clear that there the concept of 'receptive field' has been turned into something very different. This the experimenters have done by thinking of the field as the detector of a 'cue'. Some of these cues represent quite advanced postulates of frog psychology. Now, sensory physiology is, and always has been a science in quest of cues. A classical example is the spectral distribution of sensitivity of rhodopsin which serves as a cue for our own scotopic distribution of perceived thresholds of light. To look for 'cues' in receptive fields seems to me, therefore, a quite legitimate pursuit. The most obvious criticism of it is that the selection of the proper stimulus plays a role for the result. In slight exaggeration: if we were to stimulate with a spiral pattern we might discover spiral-pattern detectors without making any advance whatsoever towards our goal of getting hold of the principles of coding. An advantage of using retinae of frogs and rabbits, rather then the cortex of the cat would be the increased chance of finding explanations of 'cues' in terms of structure, as many retinae on the whole are better known than the cortices of cats and monkeys. A good example is BARLOW & LEVICKS's (1965) analysis of the directional sensitivity to movement of the rabbit's ganglion cells. Their

4

work followed the classical approach of physiology: to define a function, refer it to a structure, and then provide a final hypothesis in terms of operations carried out by that structure. If the 'receptive field' is brought into the final hypothesis, the interpretation presupposes (I) that the function actually requires one particular type of receptive field and (II) a notion as to how the field does it. The concepts 'cue' and 'receptive field' are not interchangeable. On the whole it seems to me that the least important element of detector philosophy has been the specific concept of 'receptive field'.

The second question (how it does it) would nowadays be discussed in terms of 'coding', my term 'cue' probably being regarded as oldfashioned. The problem itself remains the old one: what is the fraction of experience recorded by a given cell and how does it do it. Present-day techniques have allowed us to raise such questions in terms of single ganglion cells or fibres, but what, if the really significant visual cues already at the retinal level happened to be basically tied to multicellular ganglionic activity, a minimal number of overlapping receptive fields?

All functional features need not necessarily in the first instance be thought of in terms of cues. The retina shares with the motoneurones of the spinal cord and the pyramidal cells of the motor cortex the differentiation into phasic and tonic ganglion cells, the X and Y cells of ENROTH-CUGELL & ROBSON (1966). These parallels extend to conduction velocities in that the tonic X-cells have slower conduction rates than the phasic Y-cells (CLELAND, DUBIN & LEVICK, 1971; FUKADA, 1971). To be sure, the receptive fields are reported to be different in the two types of cell but this does not explain their X or Y character. The phasic cells are likely to be specialized for temporal changes such as the perception of velocity of movement.

THE GENICULO-STRIATE PATH

It is a striking and well-known fact that the centre-surround antagonism of concentric type not only is preserved at the geniculate level but actually is improved upon (HUBEL & WIESEL, 1961). At the retinal level there is no off-effect in the state of dark adaptation. This is not true for the dorsal lateral geniculate. Many other lines of evidence suggests that a new deal takes place at that level. I refer to work by JUNG, CREUTZFELDT, BAUMGARTNER, MAFFEI, FIORENTINI. The anatomists tell us that there is both convergence and divergence of optic nerve fibres on the geniculate and we have long been familiar with the presence of interneurones in that nucleus. Interpretations are available for the redistribution of on- and off-centre retinal cells to produce their geniculate namesakes. Inhibition is known in two versions, as surround inhibition, also called synergistic inhibition, which partly may be of the recurrent type, and as reciprocal inhibition (JUNG, CREUTZFELDT). The geniculate body can be influenced from the cortex and from the reticular formation. Apart from the binocular rearrangement of fibres, nothing is really understood of the *raison d'être* of all these complications. All the more remarkable does it seem that at the geniculate level of the geniculo-striate path, which is the one serving discrimination by contrast, the on/off-off/on concentric arrangement is preserved and improved upon. This suggests that such an organization is the optimal one for ensuring that small shifts in the level of illumination or retinal location produce the maximum of information obtainable from the polyganglionic retinal response to the scanning process.

Such considerations lead one to think that CAMPBELL and his many co-workers (ENROTH-CUGELL, KULIKOWSKY, MAFFEI, ROBSON and others) in their exciting work on spatial frequency-detectors and contrast may have hit upon 'des Pudels Kern', the real purpose of the concentric excitation-inhibition fields that I have been discussing. On the spatial-frequency hypothesis there would be a large number of narrow-band spatial filters tuned to different frequencies (cycles in grating per degree), each with its own contrast sensitivity. The optimal frequencies of the band-pass filters are inversely related to field diameter. In much of this work gratings of constant luminance, but variable spatial frequency, have been used, contrast being defined as $L_{max} - L_{min}$ divided by $L_{max} + L_{min}$, mean luminance being the latter sum divided by 2. Contrast sensitivity is the inverse value of contrast required for a constant criterion response. By application of FOURIER analysis the spatial-frequency hypothesis has been extended to square-wave patterns by CAMPBELL & ROBSON (1968) and by MAFFEI & FIORENTINI (1972). CAMPBELL & ROBSON have shown that the contrast sensitivity of the square-wave pattern is determined by the amplitude of its fundamental sine component and MAFFEI & FIORENTINI have synthetized a square-wave pattern from sine-wave components injected into different eyes, the way yellow is synthetized by green into one eye and red into the other.

The old sensory physiologists used to think of the eye as a synthetic and the ear as an analytic organ because a trained ear could pick up the components of a periodic sound while the eye had to be satisfied with the blended compound. But if the eye operates by a sine-wave recorder of form in spatial contrast, then their mistake was to stare their eyes out at colour instead of considering form as the more essential purpose of visual perception.

With these notions we have reached the cortex by the geniculo-striate passage and there HUBEL & WIESEL's discovery of cortical cells sensitive to orientation and direction of movement looms large. Neither response is developed at the level of the geniculate body (speaking now of cats and monkeys). The spatial-frequency hypothesis throws new light on all these problems of 'detectors'. If it be accepted, there is available a detector without the psychological definitions inspired by the frog retina, yet capable of a great deal, and there is more to come. The spatial-frequency idea is still at an early stage of development; yet some of its psychophysical consequences have already been worked out in experiments and the theory is accessible to a mathematical treatment. Single cell detector studies are at a disadvantage in both these respects, whatever the accuracy of the analysis of the structure of their receptive fields, in which much also depends upon the technical approach; witness the differences of opinion between HUBEL & WIESEL, SPINELLI & BARRETT (1969) and BISHOP with his colleagues (1971).

With two gratings produced by beam-splitting CAMPBELL & KULIKOWSKI

(1966) showed that, if one used a vertical test grating and turned its companion over it at different angles for masking purposes, the perceived contrast sensitivity depended on the orientation of the masking companion. For identical (vertical) directions of the two gratings there was a masking effect, a kind of selective adaptation to orientation, that fell off exponentially as the angle between them was increased. At 12° on either side of the vertical test, the masking was reduced by a factor of 2. BLAKEMORE & CAMPBELL (1969) have studied psychophysically the adaptation produced by a superposed contrast-grating and found this process also to possess interocular transfer. It has even been possible to demonstrate such selective adaptations by recording a smoothed-out evoked potential in man (CAMPBELL & MAFFEI, 1970). The demonstration that contrast-sensitivity produced by spatial frequencies combines with sensitivity to orientation seems to me a singularly interesting finding.

I cannot here review the many experiments inspired by the spatial-frequency hypothesis. The ones I have mentioned suggest that if there is no selective adaptation to an assumed detector property, then it is likely not to be fundamental. There is, for instance, none to width of a bar. Lines, edges and bar widths, inasmuch as they are assumed to be represented by detector cells, may indicate apparent detectors and not real ones, 'real' taken in the sense of representing primary coding. The emphasis of many recent experiments is thrown on spatial-frequency detectors of different orientations and thus on multicellular events.

This section should really be concluded with some words on the results of ablation experiments but this would carry us too far for an introduction. Let me end by quoting from DOTY's summary (1973): 'Despite these problems of definition (sc. adequate tests) it is clear that processes in nonstriate cortex are able to sustain an unexpectedly high level of vision in the absence of the striate system in certain species'.

THE SUPERIOR COLLICULUS

The receptive fields of this structure are very large; up to 70° are stated to be very common in the cat, from 2 to 90° in the monkey, all according to SPRAGUE, BERLUCCHI & RIZOLATTI (1973). The particular geometry which according to HUBEL & WIESEL is such a marked feature of their so-called 'simple cells' (quite complex, according to BISHOP and his colleagues) is absent in the colliculus which as a structure long has been held to play a role in the regulation of eye movements. In agreement with this view, the most striking property of the colliculus is that it requires a moving stimulus and to this its cells are sensitive, sometimes with, sometimes without directionality. The explanatory significance of the concept 'receptive field' seems difficult to evaluate for a size variation from 2 to 90 degrees.

Directional sensitivity we have now seen represented in the ganglion cells of the rabbit's retina, in the striate cortex of cats and monkeys and in the colliculus. Relatively large, geometrically unorganized fields occur in the merely movement -sensitive cells of the rabbit's retina, both on/off- and on-fields of

7

about 3° are in addition directionally sensitive (BARLOW, HILL & LEVICK, 1964). The large fields respond to fast, the small ones to slow movement, as seems *eo ipso* reasonable. The BARLOW-LEVICK explanation may well be valid for directional sensitivity in all three cases (rabbit retina, cortex, colliculus), but very little of the receptive-field concept is reflected in its formulation based, as it is, on a lopsided distribution of inhibition.

I have given this much time to movement and direction of movement because these responses, as well as velocity, are likely to be fundamental cues with cellular representations of their own. What then about the stationary background against which eye movements occur? Exceedingly suggestive are the observations by WURTZ (1969 a, b) on the monkey. The animal was trained to make a 20° eye movement in the horizontal direction. In its striate cortex 188 units were studied. Of them 32% continued to give an excitatory response, a burst of spikes, when the eye moved rapidly over the stimulus which was a slit of light of optimal orientation for the cell in its stationary position. A group of units, 20% in number, were inhibited by movement although they, too, had been excited by a stationary stimulus. This seems quite unexpected. The largest group, 48% of the total, did not respond to movement although the units fired to a stationary or very slowly moving test. The latter property all units seemed to share. They were distinguished merely by their response to movement. Thus it seems that by different cells ample cues are being provided for both the stationary and the moving outer world.

SUMMARY

I indicated in the beginning of this talk that my reading of papers on vision is cursory rather than systematic and so I may well have formed a wrong opinion of what is what. I have tried to motivate my impression that the concept 'receptive field' has been overplayed, extremely useful though it has been at one stage of the analysis. Much of what we want to understand and have means of furthering cannot just now be profitably furthered by sticking to 'receptive fields' as a major object of research. They represent but one aspect of the search for the biological 'hardware' explaining 'cues' by principles of coding. But, as I said, I do not exclude the possibility that the concept 'receptive field' may turn up at some later date imbued with new relevance and with an explanatory value that at the moment is scant in relation to the labour devoted to analysing vision in terms of it.

REFERENCES

BARLOW, H. B., HILL, R. M. & LEVICK, W. R. Retinal ganglion cells responding selectively to direction and speed of image motion in the rabbit. *J. Physiol. (Lond.)* 173: *377-407* (1964).

BARLOW, H. B. & LEVICK, W. R. The mechanism of directionally selective units in rabbit's retina. *J. Physiol. (Lond.)* 178: *477-504* (1965).

BISHOP, P. O., COOMBS, J. C. & HENRY, G. N. Responses to visual contours: spatio-temporal aspects of excitation in the receptive fields of single striate neurones. *J. Physiol. (Lond.)* 219: *625-657* (1971).

BLAKEMORE, C. & CAMPBELL, F. W. On the existence of neurones in the human visual system selectively sensitive to the orientation and size of retinal images. *J. Physiol. (Lond.)* 203: *237-260* (1969).

CAMPBELL, F. W. & KULIKOWSKI, J. J. Orientational selectivity of the human visual system. *J. Physiol. (Lond.)* 187: *437-445* (1966).

CAMPBELL, F. W. & MAFFEI, L. Electrophysiological evidence for the existence of orientation and size detectors in the human visual system. *J. Physiol. (Lond.)* 207: *635-652* (1970).

CAMPBELL, F. W. & ROBSON, J. G. Application of Fourier analysis to the visibility of gratings. *J. Physiol. (Lond.)* 197: *551-566* (1968).

CLELAND, B. G., DUBIN, M. W. & LEVICK, W. R. Sustained and transient neurones in the cat's retina and lateral geniculate nucleus. *J. Physiol. (Lond.)* 218: *473-496* (1971).

DOTY, R. W. Ablation of visual areas in the central nervous system. In: Handbook of Sensory Physiology. Editor: R. JUNG. VII/3, pp. 483-582. Springer-Verlag, Berlin, Heidelberg, New York (1973).

ENROTH-CUGELL, C. & ROBSON, J. G. The contrast sensitivity of retinal ganglion cells of the cat. *J. Physiol. (Lond.)* 187: *517-552* (1966).

FUKADA, Y. Receptive field organization of cat optic nerve fibers with special reference to conduction velocity. *Vision Res.* 11: *209-226* (1971).

HAMMOND, P. Contrasts in spatial organization of receptive fields at geniculate and retinal levels: centre, surround and outer surround. *J. Physiol. (Lond.)* 228: *115-117* (1973).

HUBEL, D. H. & WIESEL, T. N. Integrative action in the cat's lateral geniculate body. *J. Physiol. (Lond.)* 155: *385-398* (1961).

IKEDA, H. & WRIGHT, M. J. The outer disinhibitory surround of the retinal ganglion cell receptive field. *J. Physiol. (Lond.)* 226: *511-544* (1972).

MAFFEI, L. & FIORENTINI, A. Processes of synthesis in visual perception. *Nature (Lond.)* 240: *479-481* (1972).

SPINELLI, D. N. & BARRETT, T. W. Visual receptive field organization of single units in the cat's visual cortex. *Exp. Neurol.*, 24: *76-98* (1969).

SPRAGUE, J. M., BERLUCCHI, G. & RIZZOLATTI, G. The role of the superior colliculus and pretectum in vision and visually guided behavior. In: Handbook of Sensory Physiology. Editor: R. JUNG. VII/3, pp. 27-102. Springer-Verlag, Berlin, Heidelberg, New York (1973).

WURTZ, R. H. Response of striate cortex neurons to stimuli during rapid eye movements in the monkey. *J. Neurophysiol.* 32: *975-986* (1969a).

WURTZ, R. H. Comparison of effects of eye movements and stimulus movements on striate cortex neurons of the monkey. *J. Neurophysiol.* 32: *987-994* (1969b).

Author's address:

The Nobel Institute for Neurophysiology
Karolinska Institutet
S – 104 01 Stockholm 60

THE ROD OUTER SEGMENT, ITS PATHOLOGY AND CLINICAL IMPLICATIONS

EDGAR AUERBACH

(Jerusalem)

This is an expanded version of the ISCERG lecture given in Bad Nauheim. The author felt that it may give a clearer picture of the subject to the reader.
After much consideration, he decided not to include any figures as they are familiar to those interested in this subject.

This audience need not be convinced of the significance for vision of the scotopic mechanism in general and of the rod receptor system in particular. I have been asked to speak about normal rod function and to try to link it with abnormal function and outright pathology. The resolution of organs and tissues into their structural elements down to their molecular bases, which modern technology renders feasible, makes us aware of the existence of an amazingly wide range of malfunctions. Indeed, research during the last 10 to 15 years has given us enough information to find cases of the relationship between normal function and its failure of which I will discuss a few.

I will devote the time allotted to the very beginning of the chain of events which leads to vision and concentrate mainly on the outer segment of the rod photoreceptor. Despite its minuteness, it is of prime interest because of the interaction of the visual pigment molecules with light quanta, and of the interaction of the individual with information from the environment. What is more, this initial portion of the visual system represents a special challenge, for it combines the physical-chemical aspects of absorption with the physiological aspects of nervous excitation, membrane function and energy transfer. Indeed, it is the quantum catch in the visual pigment molecules which triggers a signal to the higher centers. These in turn learn to understand the coded messages arriving in form of nervous action potentials. As to the effect of quantum absorption, it is excitation, and excitation only, which makes the outer segments of the photoreceptors click, and it is so sensitive that the excitation of a rod receptor by only a single energy quantum suffices to send a signal to the next synaptic station (HECHT, SHLAER & PIRENNE, 1942). In the words of RUSHTON (1965), 'rods have achieved the theoretical perfection of sensitivity, for it is limited by the quantal structure of light itself'.

With the almost explosive introduction during the last two or three decades of new and sensitive techniques and methods and their continuous improvement, our understanding and appreciation of the visual processes at the ultrastructural and molecular level have increased enormously. The biochemical era is still in full swing and another era has already vigorously begun. Electron microscopy, autoradiography, microspectrophotometry and the microelectrode technique in electrophysiology unfold a new, exciting story about the working mechanisms of the visual processes starting at the photoreceptor level, a story, the details of which a few years ago could only be conjectured. The increased knowledge and new conceptions together with the better comprehension of underlying phenomena, permit the diagnosis of pathological entities which before could not even be classified, let alone understood. Present knowledge also makes a better appreciation possible of the amazing achievements of the pioneers who paved the way, and who had at their disposal comparatively very simple means. These achievements are connected with men such as SCHULTZE, CAJAL, BOLL and KÜHNE to name only a few in the last century, and LYTHGOE, GRANIT, DARTNALL, WALD and many others in the first half of this century.

In order to understand the mechanisms underlying the function of the rod outer segments, it is necessary to know that the retinal photoreceptors are not only cells which happen to obtain visual pigments to catch light quanta, but that these cells stem from the neuroepithelium of the optic cup and genuine cerebral neurons. In fact, they are first-order neurons in a chain of afferent cerebral connections which, as a result of stimulation, transmit information to the cortex of the brain. All photoreceptors known, including those in primates, are built according to a common plan. The information-carrying energy quanta belonging to the frequency octave of the visible electromagnetic spectrum, are absorbed in the molecules of the visual pigments contained in the receptor outer segment; in the rat rod outer segment at least ten million molecules are present. All visual pigments are defined as the chromophore 11-cis retinaldehyde coupled with a specific protein, opsin. Somewhat similar to a photometer, although not so simple by far, the photoreceptors are built to transduce radiant energy extremely rapidly into electrical potentials and to convey the information to the second-order neurons with which they are synaptically connected. Therefore the three properties of the photoreceptors – quantum absorption, energy transduction and impulse conduction – initiate a chain of neural events to the brain via afferent neural connections which lead to perception.

While photoreceptors display in the dark a low resting membrane potential of -20 mV to -40 mV, at light stimulation the membranes of all vertebrate photoreceptors examined hyperpolarize (TOMITA, 1965) (in contrast to depolarization of the membrane potentials which generally occurs in the nervous system including the other sensory receptors) with a a sustained and graded response induced by an extracellular current flow (PENN & HAGINS, 1969; WERBLIN & DOWLING, 1969). This processing of the information, which begins in the receptor, gradually becomes more sophisticated as the electrical impulses ascend to the higher brain centers, where they eventually lead to appropriate conscious responses.

I will confine myself, as already said, to the events in the vertebrate eye which occur at the beginning of the chain when light quanta are absorbed in the chromophores of the visual pigments which produce a cis-trans isomerization of its

12

retinyl group (HUBBARD & WALD, 1952; HUBBARD & KROPF, 1958). It was first postulated that this 11-cis isomer possesses higher free energy than the all-trans isomer due to steric hindrance. This proved wrong when HUBBARD (1966) demonstrated that the calculated difference between the two steric configurations was about eight times as much as the experimental value.

The quantum absorption eventually results in a transient change in the membrane potential of the photoreceptor, which is the first detectable neural sign. The absolute threshold, i.e. the minimum amount of energy in order just to see, is determined by the absorption of only 5 to 14 energy quanta or photons in as many molecules of the visual pigment. One quantum absorbed in one photoreceptor was shown to be sufficient to excite it after starting a series of photochemical reactions in each photoreceptor (HECHT et al., 1942). We will try in the following to explain from experimental facts as to how it appears that this molecule in the visual pigment is able to trigger an excitation. However, we cannot do this clearly since the initiating mechanism which, immediately after quantum absorption, governs the process of rhodopsin participation to impulse transmission eventually leading to visual sensations, is yet still incompletely understood.

About 10 % of the energy quanta which enter the eye at ordinary illumination are absorbed in the visual pigments; the rest is either reflected from the corneal surface (4%), or caught by stable melanin pigments of the lens, but mainly of the pigment epithelium and the uvea (HECHT et al., 1942). Those absorbed in the molecules of the visual pigment start a series of photochemical and electrical processes which stand at the beginning of the signal transmission to the brain. Depending on environmental illumination which determines the status of adaptation, a small amount of the light incident upon the retina is not absorbed in the black coating of the eye, i.e. in the pigment epithelium, but is reflected outside and can be measured. This phenomenon explains the principle of ophthalmoscopy and was utilized by WEALE (1953a, 1953b) and by RUSHTON (1952, 1953) for the in vivo measurement of the absorbance by means of reflection densitometry, a method originated by BRINDLEY & WILLMER (1952).

The 11-cis retinaldehyde (retinal) of the visual pigments is bound by a Schiff base (BALL et al., 1948, 1949; PITT et al., 1955; BOWNDS & WALD, 1965; BOWNDS, 1967; AKHTAR et al., 1965, 1967) to one of the specific retinal proteins named by WALD (1951), opsins, which are different in rods and cones (scotopins and photopsins). These are considered to be lipoproteins (KRINSKY, 1958a; POINCELOT et al., 1969) but there is also evidence that they may be glycoproteins free of lipid (HELLER, 1968, 1969). The 11-cis isomer of retinal in fact is an essential part of the visual pigments of most vertebrates, and is one of the few aldehydes which combine with opsin. It is the active form of vitamin A, which occurs in animal tissues only; it has also been synthesized. Its precursor, the provitamin A, is contained in several carotenoid pigments of green plants and yellow vegetables. They occur in several chemical forms. The most active type, predominantly found in nature, is β-carotene which is a symmetrical molecule of two β-ionone rings connected by a carbon chain. The crucial experiments to prove the essential role of carotene were performed by MOORE (1929, 1930). He administered carotene to vitamin A-deficient rats and found that their livers had stored vitamin A. In other words, carotene is the metabolic provitamin A, and when consumed by the animal body is active only after conversion to vitamin A or retinol which is primary alcohol and which occurs mainly prior to absorption in the intestinal wall (BALL et al., 1947). The ability to absorb carotenoids directly is different among vertebrates. In the rat, for instance, direct absorption of ingested carotenoids, as is the case in man, is minimal. Esterified retinol is stored in the liver but free all-trans retinol circulates in the blood. Recently, it has been suggested that the most stable ground-state geometry of the retinol chromophore has not only an 11-cis linkage but also a 12-s-cis one (HONIG & KARPLUS, 1971; GILARDI et al., 1971) The 12-s-cis linkage would explain why its spectrum is not much degraded by the sterically hindered 11-cis linkage (WALD, 1972/73).

Now, where more precisely are the visual pigment molecules located in the rod outer segments? How are they arranged in order to make maximal use of the light input? And what is the immediate consequence of a quantum catch? Rhodopsin is found in the plasma membrane of the outer segment (BLASIE, WORTHINGTON & DEWEY, 1969), but it is mainly contained in the disk membranes. More explicity, the opsins are part of the membranous structures of the rods and cones in all photoreceptors in vertebrate eyes up to the primates. As to the rods, within their membranous outer segments, built-in stacks of about a thousand double-membrane disks or flattened saccules are found. (In the frog there are even some 1800 disks.). They are perpendicular to the outer segment and fairly parallel to each other. Since studies with polarized light (SCHMIDT, 1938; DENTON, 1959; WALD, BROWN & GIBBONS, 1963) have shown that the rhodopsin molecules are orientated parallel to the disk planes, they are most likely part of the disk structure. More recent evidence has shown that most, possibly all, of the protein of the rod outer segment disk is that of rhodopsin (HALL, BOK & BACHARACH, 1969), the 11-cis retinal of which closely fits into a 'pocket' of the opsin. The conclusion that in dark adaptation not only the protein molecules of rhodopsin but also its chromophores are almost completely in the planes of the disk membranes and perpendicular to the axis of the outer segments, and therefore also to the light path, seems to be generally agreed upon and stems from observations with polarized light (WALD, BROWN & GIBBONS, 1962). It is emphasized that despite the three-dimensional configuration of the chromophore prosthetic group, the plane of the chromophore is parallel to the plane of the disk. This is necessary, for light is absorbed only when its electrical vector is parallel to the plane.

Rhodopsin in the dark, the 11-cis retinal, together with its opsin, constitute then a substantial portion of, and possibly even represent, the whole structural element of the disks within the rod outer segments. The rhodopsin within the disk membranes of the rods seems to float in an oily mixture of fatty acid chains of phospholipids (BLASIE & WORTHINGTON, 1969) which is about as viscous as olive oil (CONE, 1972).

Outer segments of rods differ from those of cones (see p. 20). While the disks in mature rods seem to be isolated from the membrane of the outer segment and from each other (COHEN, 1960, 1963, 1965, 1968; DOWLING & GIBBONS, 1961;

14

NILSSON, 1964, 1965), except for an invagination or infolding at its proximal base close to the inner segment (COHEN, 1970), those of the cones are open to the extracellular space and their membranes are continuous with one another and with the outer segment membrane (COHEN, 1968). As first found in the frog, the disks in the rod outer segment are free-floating membranous organelles with an inside (intradisk) space or cavity separate and distinct from the rods intracellular space by semipermeable membranes (GRAS & WORTHINGTON, 1969; BLAUROCK & WILKINS, 1969; HELLER, OSTWALD & BOK, 1971). These disks are electrically uncoupled and separated from the plasma membrane by 100 to 200 nm, and it is the sodium conductance of the latter which is regulated by light (PENN & HAGINS, 1972; HAGINS, 1972). We will soon discuss this question.

We do not wish to enter the problem of the biological membrane which may perhaps need revision from the classical Davson-Danielli model (see KORN, 1968). Preparations for electron miscroscopy may be assessed with caution because the somewhat rough treatment entails the possibility of artifacts (NIR & PEASE, 1973). This is avoided by the low-angle X-ray diffraction studies of cross-sections of disk membranes which were carried out in living outer segments (GRAS & WORTHINGTON, 1969; BLAUROCK & WILKINS, 1969). Moreover, FALK & FATT (1969) showed the likelihood of the difference between the membrane of the rod outer segments and the disk membranes through chemical methods by using various fixatives.

Important is the difference in structure in the outer segments of rods and cones, on the one hand, and of rod plasma membranes and disk membranes, on the other hand. In rods, after quantum absorption in the rhodopsin molecules of these free-floating and isolated disks, a special mechanism would be expected to enable the visual signal to traverse the cytoplasma and to excite the cell membrane of the outer segment across the gap between the disk membranes and outer plasma membrane. This mechanism certainly should be different from that in cones, where the disks are attached to, and continuous with, the cell membrane so that their intradisk spaces represent extensions of the extracellular ventricular space. The observation of WEALE (1968) that certain fixatives, such as formaldehyde, more rapidly alter the axis of polarization in rods than in cones, despite the cone intradisk space opening in the extracellular, seems to underscore this difference. He suggests that the permeability of the membranes of rods may differ very significantly from that of cones. The difference in rod and cone membranes is also supported by the already mentioned findings of FALK & FATT (1969), which they interpret to demonstrate a fundamental difference in the structural composition of rod and cone lamellae, the cone invaginations being more stable than the rod disks. Besides, this greater stability may be the reason for the difficulty in extracting cone visual pigments.

These differences between the two kinds of photoreceptors may also have an influence on the kinetics of the regeneration of the visual pigment; at least they may be one factor. Data from psychophysical experiments in congenital achromats recently reported by AUERBACH (1973) and AUERAACH & KRIPKE (1974) point, in addition to normal rods, to three kinds of cones but all filled with rhodopsin, yet exhibiting up to three rates of photopic kinetics in addition to the normal scotopic one.

A photoreceptor electrical response is elicited by the absorption of light quanta in the molecules of the visual pigments. However, in order to clarify what produces the response of the receptor cell, the primary photochemical processes consequent to absorption and prior to excitation have to be elucidated.

Light-induced excitation in the photoreceptor starts with the isomerization of the 11-cis chromophore to the all-trans prelumi configuration (YOSHIZAWA & KITO, 1958; YOSHIZAWA & WALD, 1963) which latter was recently given the perhaps better name of batho-pigments by YOSHIZAWA (1972), and possibly retains the 12-s-cis linkage (HONIG & KARPLUS, 1971). This isomerization of the chromophore occurs in less than 20 picoseconds (BUSCH et al., 1972) and initiates a transient change in the cell's membrane permeability and potential. The potential resulting from the photochemical change itself is the initial detectable neural signal, the early receptor potential (see below) for whose generation only the stages up to metarhodopsin II are responsible (ABRAHAMSON, 1972/1973).

As to the action of light on the visual pigment, the suggestion was originally made by FUORTES & HODGKIN (1964) and later taken up by BAYLOR & FUORTES (1970) in single cones of turtles, that on illumination rhodopsin may excite both the vertebrate and invertebrate receptor cell by releasing an internal transmitter which modulates the conduction of ions. This was substantiated in vertebrates by HAGINS, PENN & YOSHIKAMI (1970) and HAGINS (1972). Finally YOSHIKAMI & HAGINS (1971, 1972/73) proposed that calcium ions act as the internal transmitter. The authors suggested that both in the intradisk cavities of rods and in the extracellular spaces of rods and cones Ca^{++} ions are of higher concentration than in intracellular, that is extradisk, spaces of the rods. Quantum absorption by a rhodopsin molecule gives rise to an increase in Ca^{++} permeability of the membranes of disks and outer segment. This in turn increases the concentration of Ca^{++} in the intracellular space with the result that the sodium channels in the plasma outer rod membrane are blocked, preventing depolarization of the receptor membrane. The characteristic disk arrangement in the rods creates for the light a large membranous surface which is not in the path of the 'dark current', but which is light-sensitive and can trigger excitation.

The 'dark current' mentioned is a large, positive extracellular current which is believed to be carried as an influx of Na^+ ions, and flows from the inner segment inwards through the outer segment membrane (see YOSHIKAMI & HAGINS, 1972/73). Light reduces the 'dark current' by local action in the outer segment in that it seems to reduce Na^+ conductance of the plasma membrane (HAGINS, PENN & YOSHIKAMA, 1970). Simultaneously, the membrane potential of the receptor becomes hyperpolarized by the action of light (TOMITA, 1965) in that it becomes more negative inside compared to the outside. The constant current flow in the dark, therefore, decreases in the light which, together with the prevention of Na^+ flow into the outer segment, explains the hyperpolarization.

To completely understand the role of Ca^{++} ions in promoting hyperpolarization of the cell membrane consequent to light input, evidence is still missing.

16

However, indirect evidence indicates that Ca^{++} ions control, or play an important part in controlling, Na^+-permeability of the receptor membrane. The increase of the membrane resistance to Na^+ influx following illumination was suggested by TOYODA, NOSAKI & TOMITA in 1969 and shown by KORENBROT & CONE (1972) working with frogs and rats to be linear with the number of rhodopsin molecules bleached without affecting other ions. In rods, where the disks are largely isolated from the outer membrane in contrast to cones, quantum absorption opens a hole in the disk membrane and releases the intradisk Ca^{++} ions which would travel to the outer membrane where they close the Na^+-channels. Likewise, also the extracellular Ca^{++} is assumed to participate in the excitation of the rods because their outer membrane contains rhodopsin. Therefore, at illumination, the calcium released by light into the intracellular space could come either from the disk cavity or the extracellular space (YOSHI-KAMI & HAGINS, 1972/73). In the opinion of YOSHIKAMI (1972/73, discussion p. 255), the calcium source mobilized would depend on whether a light quantum is absorbed by the rhodopsin in the disk or that in the plasma membrane.

This is all very complicated, especially the dual choice of calcium ions for rod excitation, and in the general discussion of the Bochum Symposium (p. 361 f.) on the internal transmitter, it appeared to Dr. BONTING that, when the free extracellular Ca^{++} can close off the Na^+ channels as does the intradisk Ca^{++}, the latter would lose much in efficiency to trigger the rod excitation; consequently the rod would behave like a cone. He concluded that, while in principle extracellular Ca^{++} could act on the Na^+ channels of the rod outer membrane, it is not necessary and will probably not happen at low light intensities.

To summarize this important topic, the effect of Ca^{++} following illumination and the hyperpolarizing response to light appear to result from the permeability decrease of the photoreceptor membrane for sodium ions. Therefore, the primary effect of light in the excitation of the vertebrate rod is the cis-trans isomerization of the chromophore which elicits the receptor potential by transiently decreasing the permeability of the photoreceptor membrane to sodium ions (TOMITA, 1972). This is in contrast to the excitation in the rhabdomere membrane of invertebrates since their photoreceptor membranes are becoming depolarized by light. HAGINS (1965) and HAGINS & COWORKERS (1962) furnished the clearest example of the role of the visual pigment molecule after quantum absorption in in the sectioned squid photoreceptor. Initiated by the visual pigment a transient change in membrane permeability, sufficient to excite the cell, could be demonstrated over a short portion of the receptor by the inward flow of ionic current through the membrane at, or near, the illuminated area. This potential is the already mentioned initial neural signal detectable in the visual system.

A process of this kind, which seems to produce the receptor potential, is then the result of this flow of ionic membrane current. However, the a-wave of the ERG has a latency of several milliseconds. This is obviously too long to be the direct result of quantum absorption, and to represent the initial electrical result of light input. Recently, the time interval after absorption and prior to the elicitation of the a-wave could be bridged by the discovery of the early receptor potential (ERP) in the Cynemolgus monkey by Brown & Murakami (1964a), a potential which depends on the structure of the receptor and the orientation of the visual pigment. The potential is generated in the outer segment of the receptor as the direct result of a very intense light flash, is independent of ionic exchanges through membranes, and has a scarcely detectable latency which must be shorter than 0.5 μsec (Cone, 1967) which in itself makes it likely that the potential is generated near or at the region of quantum absorption in the pigment molecule, i.e. within the cell membrane (Hagins & McGaughy, 1968a, 1968b; Brown & Murakami, 1964b, 1964c; Brown, Watanabe & Murakami, 1965). This 'early receptor potential' is, therefore, a response generated by the direct action of light on the visual pigments and has been observed in vertebrate and invertebrate eyes. It consists of an initial corneo-positive component R1 and a slower corneo-negative one R2 which are directly dependent on the photochemical changes. The ERP represents the immediate consequence of quantum absorption (from a very strong gas discharge lamp) in millions of visual pigment molecules which are simultaneously activated and isomerized to the all-trans configuration producing a transient charge in them. The ERP is then a measure of the visual pigment concentration in that it is most likely generated by charge dispacements, which are produced directly by the activity of rhodopsin molecules (Cone, 1965; Arden & Ikeda, 1965). It can be recorded both directly from the retinal receptor and, like the ERG, from the outside of the eye. The ERP is, therefore, not directly related to changes in membrane permeability (Pak, 1965; Brindley & Gardner-Medvin, 1966) with their exchanges of free ions as is the case with the slower a-wave. The latter is the 'late receptor potential' (LRP) and the leading edge of Granit's P-III. This wave, in contrast to the ERP, is a graded, hyperpolarizing potential (Tomita, 1972; Werblin & Dowling, 1969), generated in the region of the cilium or the inner segment of the photoreceptor.

The ERP may be a tool to throw more light on the properties of the visual pigment molecule, including the knotty problem of how, more precisely than described, quantum absorption in the visual pigment molecules initiates an excitation of the visual pigment, a point which is not yet fully satisfactorily explained. However, the ERP was useful already for studying both the electrical and structural properties of squid photoreceptors (Hagins & McGaughy, 1968a) and the association of the pigment molecule with the cell membrane (Hagins & McGaughy, 1968b; Cone & Brown, 1967). Moreover, R1, the initial component of the biphasic ERP with practically no latency, is considered to be produced by the extremely fast, highly unstable first photochemical change, which is the isomerization and the conversion of the 11-cis rhodopsin over (hypsorhodopsin demonstrated by Yoshizawa & Horiuchi (1972) to) all-trans prelumi- (or batho-) rhodopsin to the further photochemical intermediates (R2 representing the meta I to meta II stage). The conversion to the prelumi stage, according to Wald (1972/73), is at present considered the only direct result of the action of light in the entire chain of photochemical conversions, which excites the pigment molecule to an energy level at which 11-cis retinal becomes isomerized to the all-trans configuration. Moreover, the

18

assumption that the ERP is the direct result of light absorption in visual pigment molecules, independent of ionic exchanges through membranes, is very much supported first by the fact that it can be recorded below the freezing point, and secondly from evidence in the largely rod-dominated retina of the albino rat in that it could be demonstrated that the action spectra of R1 and R2 of the ERP are equal and correspond with the absorption spectrum of rhodopsin (CONE, 1964; PAK & CONE, 1964). Moreover, retinal degenerations of the inner segments prior to the outer ones show the ERP to be unaffected in contrast to the LRP which latter disappears (ARDEN & IKEDA, 1965).

To conclude, the fact that the voltage recorded in the ERP (i.e. the amplitude) is a linear function of the stimulus intensity (i.e. of the molecules activated by the stimulus) strikingly discloses that it is a molecular response directly depending on the visual pigment, and not one elicited by ionic changes through membranes which have a longer latency and where this relationship is logarithmic.

The question arises as to the significance of the charge displacements which produce the ERP, since they appear too small by far to start off electrical signals to the receptor synapses for further afferent transmission. They may be strong enough, however, to disturb significantly neighbouring molecules in the membrane with the possible result to alter ionic permeability around the pigment molecule. Consequently, it is probable that a significant change in ionic permeability may be produced by the pigment molecule activated by light. It follows further, that the charge displacements which generate the ERP are linked to the mechanism which is responsible for the initiation of an excitatory response of a photoreceptor by the pigment molecule (CONE & PAK, 1971).

Now, in order to understand the pathology of rod deficiencies, a phenomenon stands out which is uniquely a rod phenomenon, and which was elucidated by means of the electron microscope combined with autoradiography. DROZ (1961, 1963) initiated the method in order to study the protein synthesis in the photoreceptors of rats and mice from radioactive amino acids. By injecting these labeled amino acids into the rod inner segment and labeled cis-retinal (BRIDGES & YOSHIKAMI, 1967 in ARDEN, 1969), the constant renewal of protein synthesized from the amino acids, which becomes incorporated in the disks, as well as of vitamin A, which is taken up from the circulation (YOUNG & BOK, 1970), could be shown. The constant restoration of protein led to the discovery of the continual formation of new disks at the proximal base of the rod outer segments (DROZ, 1963; YOUNG, 1967; YOUNG & BOK, 1970). In other words, the visual pigment is steadily delivered to the disks and, as mentioned, the present evidence strongly points to its being the membrane protein of these disks. The findings of HALL et al. (1969) indicate that probably all of the protein (at least 80 to 85 %) of the rod outer segment disks represents visual pigment.

Rhodopsin, as long as the disk membranes are intact within the rods, is very stable and apparently not renewed (see pp. 21, 24). The renewal rate of the disks differs among species and was found, for instance, in the frog red rods to be 36/day and to traverse the length of the outer segment in 6 to 7 weeks (HALL, BOK & BACHARACH, 1968, 1969), while in green rods it is 25/day (YOUNG & DROZ, 1968).

19

The point has to be particularly stressed, that in the adult frog a continual renewal of protein was found in the outer segments of rods as well as of cones, a phenomenon of great advantage to preserve vision, especially in view of the fact that outer segments are easily damaged. There is, however, a striking difference between rods and cones, in addition to the morphological one described before (see pp. 14 f.). While in the rod outer segment a continual formation of new membranous disks occurs as well as a continual incorporation of protein formed in the inner segment, in the cone outer segments there is no evidence of disk renewal. In these, the protein becomes diffusely distributed in the layers of the outer segments. This essential difference, as well as the one in form and size of cones and rods, may reflect different pathology (YOUNG, 1969) for which, however, no direct evidence could be found in the literature. In other words, the continual replacement of old disks by new ones is a rod phenomenon while in cones a small proportion of the protein is similarly displaced to the outer segments but no new disks are formed (YOUNG & DROZ, 1968).

The regeneration at rod outer segments was experimentally shown in monkeys by producing detachment of the retina from the pigment epithelium. As KÜHNE (1878) already knew nearly a hundred years ago rhodopsin regeneration is inhibited by retinal detachment and the rods degenerate. On reattachment, they regenerate (KROLL & MACHEMER, 1969a), a finding which could be predicted not only by surgical experience but also by the experimental data of DOWLING (1964), who demonstrated outer segment regeneration following vitamin A feeding in vitamin A-deficient rats, provided the rod inner segments and the nuclei were intact. Regeneration of cone outer segments, though slower, could also be shown after reattachment of the monkey retina (KROLL & MACHEMER, 1969b), a process whose mechanism is not yet understood.

Protein synthesis occurs, then, in the inner segment of the photoreceptor, which is responsible for the cell metabolism. Protein flows through the Golgi complex past the mitochondria through the connecting cilium (YOUNG, 1968) into the outer segment (DROZ, 1963; YOUNG & DROZ, 1968). In the latter, the protein appears first at its base, the radioactive amino acids appearing as a band across, and gradually moves towards its tip. The cilium, therefore, not only represents a path for signal transfer, but also a cytoplasmic connection between the two segments of the photoreceptor. In addition to the ciliary connection, a cytoplasmic bridge between the inner and outer segments was found in several mammals through which the cytoplasma of the inner segment comes into direct contact with the basal disks of the outer segments (RICHARDSON, 1969); this important finding has not yet been confirmed.

The pigment epithelium, important for the nutrition from the choroid of the receptor cell layer in the retina, is essential for sustaining vision. On exposure to bright light, rhodopsin is bleached and the 11-cis configuration is isomerized to alltrans which is energetically the lowest ground-state of all retinal isomers. In the further course of photochemical changes, the retinal becomes liberated, is reduced by alcohol dehydrogenase to retinol, which is vitamin A, and moves fast into the pigment epithelium. However, now rhodopsin has to be regenerated for vision to continue, and this is an energy-yielding reaction, the energy

20

coming from an unknown source. Work is done, and retinol is oxidized in the dark in the retina to retinal after, apparently in the pigment epithelium, the re-isomerization of vitamin A from trans to cis has occurred. The pigment epithelium participates in this process since it stores appreciable amounts of 11-cis vitamin A (KRINSKY, 1958b). During dark adaptation this and the newly iso-merized 11-cis iretinol re-enters the outer segment, the retinal combines with op-sin, and rhodopsin is resynthesized (WALD, 1935a, 1935b; DOWLING, 1960b). In all fairness, it has to be mentioned that KÜHNE already in 1878 (and EWALD & KÜHNE, 1878) noted the significance of the pigment epithelium for rhodopsin regeneration in that he observed that the separation of the retina from the pigment epithelium inhibits regeneration.

Moreover, the pigment epithelium has another equally important task still. The continuous disk production at the proximal end of the outer segment makes the removal of the old disks at its distal end necessary, so that the entire rod outer segment undergoes a constant renewal (YOUNG, 1967, 1971a). This pro-cess can be followed by observing the labeled amino acids gradually moving along the outer segment. The disks, therefore, move steadily to the distal end of the rod outer segment until eventually they are shed into the pigment epithelium. There is thus a continuous turnover of visual pigment, which occurs also in the dark though at a reduced rate (BRIDGES & YOSHIKAMI, 1969). The detached disks were called phagosomes by YOUNG & BOK (1959) in order to distinguish them from other cellular inclusions produced by the pigment epithelium cells them-selves. The ingested disks are phagocytized in the cytoplasma of the pigment epithelium and eventually disappear (DROZ, 1963; COHEN, 1963; YOUNG, 1967; YOUNG & BOK, 1970). The first investigators who not only observed this phe-nomenon in the human pigment epithelium but also appreciated its true signi-ficance were BAIRATI & ORZALESI (1963).

What finally happens to the phagosomes is still unclear. Acid phosphotase (by means of particles called lysosomes (APPELMANS et al., 1955)) may participate in the enzymatic digestion of the disk material, but how enzymes are delivered to the phagosomes still awaits clarification. At any rate, structures resembling lyso-somes were found in the cells of the pigment epithelium which may digest the phagosomes (NOVIKOFF, 1961) (see p. 25). Moreover, as already mentioned, the intimate relationship of the outer segments to the pigment epithelium and the presence of vitamin A are necessary for the process to continue (SPITZNAS & HOGAN, 1970).

Without vitamin A it soon comes to an end, although only less than 0.01 % of the total amount in the adult human body is present in ocular tissues and connected with retinal function (MOORE, 1964). This low vitamin A content suggests that ocular concentration is metabolically controlled and that dietary supplementation with retinol or precursors would not enhance the visual process in a normally supplied individual. In short, the continuous synthesis of outer segment membranes occurring in mature rods, but not in cones, suggests rhodopsin to be a stable protein (see p. 19) which, however, exhibits a large turnover. This is due to the event at the outer segment tip, which brings about the shedding of the disks into the pigment epithelium and is simultaneously a mechanism to preserve structure during the life-time of the individual by continuous renewal. As to cone outer segments, the renewal mechanism is not understood.

What role does the pigment epithelium play in the disk removal? There is not complete agreement on this question. YOUNG (1971b) found in the rhesus monkey that the pigment epithelium does not actively remove the disks. However, SPITZNAS & HOGAN (1970) demonstrated in the eyes of two humans that the pigment epithelium sends out slender, fringe-like microvillous projections into the potential ventricular space (COHEN, 1972) between the outer segments and broad rampart-like projections which surround their tips with a cytoplasmic sheet. The latter seems to be important to maintain the normal cohesion between the two layers. The ventricular space is in fact the residue of the fluid-filled space of the embryonic optic vesicle, and is the thin space which persists between retina and pigment epithelium. It is occupied by a homogenous mass which is comprised mainly of a complex mixture of mucopolysaccharides and proteins (FINE & ZIMMERMAN, 1963; HALL & HELLER, 1966/69; FREEMAN & WORTMAN, 1966). It is believed that vitamin A may be important for the bio-synthesis of the mucopolysaccharides (WOLF & VARANDANI, 1960). They seem to be an integral part of the retina and essential for structure and function, although there does not seem to be conclusive evidence for their physiological function. We will later discuss the pathology which may occur with their absence (p. 28).

Now, what happens when something goes wrong at either end of the rod outer segment? When either the protein carrier of the visual pigment or vitamin A or its precursor, the provitamin A, the carotenoids, are not available for some reason? This may be the result of lack of vitamin A in the food or malfunction e.g. in the gastro-intestinal tract prior to, and during, absorption of carotene in its wall which may prevent the conversion to retinol (ROELS, 1966; function e.g. in the gastro-intestinal tract prior to, and during, absorption in its wall of carotene which may prevent the conversion to retinol (ROELS, 1966; FISHER et al., 1970). It may also be due to a liver disease, such as cirrhosis, which results in malabsorption in the intestine (GOODHART, 1968) let alone the decreased storage power of the liver for vitamin A. A defect in the pigment epithelium may also occur which prevents the phagosomes from being phagocytized.

The original finding correlating the photochemical events in vision with nyctalopia due to vitamin A deficiency leads back to 1935 when GEORGE WALD (1935a, 1935b) discovered that the bleaching of rhodopsin produces retinaldehyde which in turn becomes reduced to vitamin A. However, also the much more recent experiments performed by DOWLING (1960a, 1960b, 1964) and DOWLING & WALD (1958a, 1958b, 1959) in albino rats fed with a diet lacking vitamin A, had a great impact on the whole subject of vitamin A deficiency. These authors combined biochemical and electrophysiological methods. They observed that the same relationship exists between rhodopsin content of the retina and log ERG threshold both in normal rats in the dark immediately after a strong light adaptation and in vitamin A deficient (nyctalopic) rats.

Using the ERG as an indicator of retinal function and sensitivity, they found that the log ERG threshold rose linearly with the fall in rhodopsin concentration. In other words, there is a logarithmic relationship between threshold and bleached rhodopsin, both in vitamin A-deficient rats and in normal strongly light-adapted rats. This finding confirms more accurately the densitometric one of CAMPBELL & RUSHTON (1955), who showed that rhodopsin regenerated exponentially with the same time constant as the rod branch of the dark adaptation curve. The relationship was also confirmed by RUSHTON's (1961) psychophysical measurement of dark adaptation in a human achromat. This was possible since rod function is here not masked by photopic activity and can, therefore, be followed above the normal photopic threshold, a fact which was also shown by AUERBACH & KRIPKE (1974). This logarithmic relationship was, however, criticized by WEALE (1964). The dark adaptation experiments in a human subject on a diet lacking vitamin A showed the process to be reversible (WALD, JEGHERS & ARMINIO, 1938; WALD & STEVEN, 1939). This was later shown by DOWLING & WALD (1958a) and by DOWLING (1964) in refeeding the experimental rats with vitamin A, which was, however, only successful if the rod inner segments were still intact.

These experiments are very convincing as far as rats are concerned. However, caution seems to be necessary in comparing the result with other species since rat rhodopsin is said to be atypical among mammals (WEALE, 1973; LEWIN et al., 1970; HIGHMAN & WEALE, 1973).

Regarding the protein opsin, which was long neglected, evidence was furnished by the rat experiments of DOWLING & WALD (1958a) that opsin becomes chemically unstable in the absence of retinal. This implies that the chemistry of opsin is critically connected with the effects of quantum absorption in the visual pigment and would have two consequences. Since opsin cannot be maintained in the retina in vitamin A deficiency, it follows that the rod outer segments deteriorate because of the protein being the matrix of the disk membrane.

In order to close experimentally this cycle, the effect of protein depletion on the ERG was compared with that of vitamin A deficiency in the rat (AUERBACH et al., 1964). In both deficiencies, the same relationship was observed, which in addition was identical to that found by DOWLING & WALD (1958a). The curves from the experiment with vitamin A-depleted and protein-depleted rats plotted as a function of stimulus strength were parallel to each other as well as to those obtained by DOWLING & WALD despite the different experimental approaches used by the two groups. The impaired retinal function found in protein deficiency leads also to nyctalopia and may be the consequence of the failure to form opsins. This will soon be discussed.

The data of VEEN & BEATON (1966) indicated the existence of a plasma protein carrier for vitamin A; they also discussed the participation of an albumin subfraction in the retinol transport mechanism. This was confirmed by the studies of KANAI, RAZ & GOODMAN (1968) on binding and transport of retinol to the ocular tissues. They were able to show that the transport of retinol in the plasma involves interaction with two carrier proteins. Renitol is the form in which the metabolized carotene is present in the blood, and which, after being released, interacts in the plasma with specific proteins, so-called retinol-binding proteins (RBP). These circulate in the plasma and are bound to a larger protein which is identical to the thyroxine-binding prealbumin (PA) of the human plasma. The former, the RBP, solubalize retinol and protect it during the transport to the tissues including the eyes. The isolation, purification and identification of the retinol-RBP complex and the RBP-PA complex seem essential for the mechanism responsible for the retinol transport in the plasma of the body tissues. Since the plasma retinol level is regulated only partially by the concentration of the carrier proteins, it follows that the retinol supply in the tissues is probably not solely dependent on the retinol store in the liver.

VEEN & BEATON (1966) have shown in the rat that plasma retinol levels transported from the liver are altered by protein or calorie deprivation or by both. This may result from dietary deprivation on the level of protein-bound retinol. A severe protein-calorie malnutrition in children with vitamin A deficiency was described by ARROYAVE et al. (1961). That protein deficiency impairs also carotene utlization, i.e. its absorption/conversion, was shown in the rat by MATHEWS & BEATON (1963) as well as vitamin A mobilization and transport from the liver. The mechanisms, however, of vitamin A released from liver and other tissues are as yet not completely understood as well as its transport to the various tissues including the eye.

The retina presumably receives retinol via the blood (internal carotid and ophthalmic artery) carried by the RBP-PA complex. Protein and vitamin A deficiencies often occur together in that in protein deficiency the absorption and conversion of the carotenoids, i.e. the dietary provitamin A, and the absorption of retinol may be impaired. Also impaired may be the utilization of the liver stores of esterified vitamin A (see p. 14).

There is one very practical therapeutic aspect which should be emphasized. Protein supplementation in the diet of protein deficient individuals brings about an increase in serum vitamin A, possibly through mobilization of liver stores (ARROYAVE et al., 1961; ROELS, 1966; FISHER et al., 1970). However, it also increases the overall vitamin A requirement. Protein supplementation may then result in vitamin A deficiency when low storage reserves are depleted. Simultaneous retinol supplementation is, therefore, necessary in previously malnourished individuals in order to avoid nyctalopia.

As dicussed before (p. 19 f) and shortly recapitulated, new protein reaches continually the outer segment from the inner one over the connecting cilium and is incorporated by the disks at the proximal end of the outer segment. After uniting with the chromophore group, the visual pigment is composed and is not renewed as long as it is part of the disk membrane in the outer segment. It is, therefore, intrinsically very stable as shown by radiobiochemical methods (HALL, BOK & BACHARACH, 1968, 1969). Rhodopsin is broken down when the disk is shed into the pigment epithelium.

Vitamin A deficiency is characterized ultrastructurally in that the phagosomes disappear from the pigment epithelium, and that both the rod outer segments and the pigment epithelium show signs of primary degeneration (DOWLING & WALD, 1958b). The first changes seem to occur in the disks of the outer

24

segments which swell and fragmentate and finally are absorbed. Recovery following refeeding of vitamin A, i.e. regeneration of new outer segments, is only then possible, when the inner segments are still intact. However, the cause is far from being understood (DOWLING, 1964). Disturbances in Bruch's membrane were observed which may have caused the degeneration of the pigment epithelium. This is possible in view of the task of Bruch's membrane (AMEMIYA, 1971), which is considered as the blood-ocular barrier between the choroidal blood and the retinal receptors for the two-way passage of metabolites and nutrients. However, the degeneration of the visual cells in the vitamin A deficient rats may also be due to faulty synthesis of protein and not to primary degeneration and fragmentation of the rod outer disks.

Now, what about the rod deficiencies when something goes wrong at the distal end of the outer segment? When there is a defect to phagocytize excess outer segment disks in the pigment epithelium? There are inherited retinal dystrophies known to appear without any tangible cause in rats, mice, dogs and man at some period in the life of the animal. The histology at advanced stages of these inherited degenerations as well as the ERG findings are very similar to those found in severe vitamin A deficiency. For this reason they were especially studied in order to possibly obtain an experimental model of human retintitis pigmentosa.

A great deal of work was done with dystrophic rats, especially with the RCS rats (Royal College of Surgeons). The disease is characterized by a probably late appearing progressive loss of visual receptor cell outer segments and disks, the onset of which may coincide with the beginning of their developmental period. DOWLING & SIDMAN (1962) in their integrated analysis of retinal function, chemistry and cellular structure in mutant rats, found the ERG to be normal for the first 18 days of life which was confirmed by HERRON et al.'s (1969) autoradiographic studies. Only then does the ERG gradually begin to deteriorate until extinction at the age of 2 months. DOWLING & SIDMAN's data indicate that the disease does not involve a primary defect of vitamin A or rhodopsin metabolism or synthesis of an abnormal opsin. They found histologically a hitherto unrecognized process in that there was an accumulation of disorganized extracellular material between the distal end of the rod outer segments and the pigment epithelium. It could be shown that while this extracellular material builds up, even as the rod outer segments initially increase in size, the rhodopsin content is increasing almost twice the normal amount in the 20-day-old rat. This extracellular material was later identified autoradiographically by HERRON et al. (1969) to be excess outer disks. There is, then, an imbalance between the function to produce new disks and that to eliminate or remove the discarded disks. Though new disk production continues for some time in the dystrophic rat, they are not phagocytized by the pigment epithelium.

On the other hand, inclusions resembling lysosomes are present in pigment epithelium cells of dystrophic rats particularly during the initial period of rod differentiation (DOWLING & SIDMAN, 1962) and may be involved in phagocytosis (see p. 22). The degeneration of the rods may then be initiated by the lytic enzymes originating in the pigment epithelium (BURDEN et al., 1971). In spite of this, it is also possible that retinal dystrophy in the rat is a disease of the pigment epithelium which has lost the ability to digest the phagosomes. In addition to phagocytize the accumulating phagosomes, poor nutritional supply from the choroid to the visual cells participates in their death. The same group of investigators (HERRON et al., 1971) later found evidence that disk production continues in the dystrophic rat even as the degeneration of the rod outer segment is progressing, and that the accumulation of the extracellular material, i.e. the phagosomes, between the rod inner segments and the pigment epithelium does not much decrease the availability of amino acids to the inner segment until the age of 36 days; labeled amino acid can still be seen within the degenerated extracellular disks. The authors believe these findings to suggest that in the dystrophic rat the pigment epithelium does not digest the phagosomes, and that they are removed, by an unknown mechanism by way of the inner retina. This degenerative process continues until finally the bipolar cells are adjacent to the pigment epithelium.

An important observation has been made by DOWLING. Rhodopsin, as could be shown by other means, is a very stable molecule (see p. 19), since both in vitamin A deficiency and in dystrophic rats its decline can largely be prevented when the animals are kept in the dark. This was found even in animals otherwise wholly depleted of Vitamin A and in dystrophic animals raised in the dark which had more rhodopsin than litter mates raised in the light. This supports BERSON's (1971) recent hypothesis advocating light deprivation in early retinitis pigmentosa. It is not impossible that persons afflicted with retinitis pigmentosa or nyctalopia are more sensitive to an abundance of light than normal persons (NOELL, 1965; KUWABARA & GORN, 1968), which is in accord with my personal observation.

DOWLING's observation led to an interesting speculation by HERRON et al. (1969, 1971). Because of the histological similarity of the retina in the dystrophic rat with the retina in advanced stages of human retinitis pigmentosa, they reasoned that the pathogenesis of both conditions is possibly similar. One may then be able, they speculate, to possibly slow down the rate of early clinical deterioration by slowing down the production of extracellular disks, e.g. by inducing a relative vitamin A deficiency. They argue further, that vitamin A, given in the past to 'cure' retinitis pigmentosa, may just as well have had the opposite effect. This may also be an explanation why Adaptinol (BAYER) once recommended not only in cases of night blindness but also in retinitis pigmentosa is without effect in the latter condition. We had the opportunity to observe the effect of this drug for extended periods of time in six patients suffering from retinitis pigmentosa at various stages. Whether it accelerated the disease is hard to tell but it did not seem to slow down the process.

The reasoning of HERRON et al., however, is in sharp contrast to results from the only study group to my knowledge which reports a marked improvement of advanced cases of retinitis pigmentosa by treatment with vitamin A, although the improvement reported lasted only as long as the treatment. CAMPBELL, HARRISON & TONKS (1964) measured the vitamin A and carotenoid content in the blood of a large number of subjects suffering from retinitis pigmentosa and found both clearly subnormal. In their opinion, these patients have no ability

26

to store vitamin A and, therefore, depend on their carotene to make up for their vitamin A deficiency. Since this is the only report of this kind, which to my knowledge has not been confirmed, and since it is in contrast also to my own experience, I am unable to comment.

Congenital nyctalopia is considered to be a stationary disease. However, it should be mentioned that among 95 patients suffering from congenital nyctalopia of both the Schubert-Bornschein and the Riggs type, we found nine patients whose ERG decreased in amplitude during 7 to 10 years of observation (AUERBACH, GODEL & ROWE, 1969). Of these, two showed slight fundus changes which were not present before, and which consisted of atypically pigmented peripheral foci together with slight pallor of the papilla and slightly constricted arteries. However, no other signs were noticed, such as visual field changes, etc., and in no case was ERG extinction found.

Whatever the implications of this observation, there is one syndrome, the Bassen-Kornzweig syndrome (1950), which exhibits a relationship between retinitis pigmentosa and vitamin A. Up to now twenty-five cases were reported in the literature (WOLFF et al., 1964; v. SALLMANN et al., 1969). The disease affects also the erythrocytes which are spike-shaped (acanthocytosis). Apart from typical retinitis pigmentosa and very much raised visual threshold, there are neuromuscular disturbances with ataxia and steatorrhoea (SALT et al., 1960). However, the apparent causa causans is the absence of a specific lipoprotein from the serum and, accordingly, the disease is called a-beta-lipoproteinemia. The most interesting point is that oral supplementation of vitamin A lowers the threshold, practically normalizes the ERG and brings the serum vitamin A to normal values, only to become subnormal again after discontinuation of the treatment. However, even treatment maintained over years does not seem to prevent the development of the retinal degeneration. Therefore, it seems that vitamin A deficiency, though playing a role, is not the cause of the disease. This the more so, since in the absence of beta-lipoprotein from the serum, carotenoids are also absent.

Where do we stand? True, serum vitamin A, visual threshold and ERG threshold are linked to each other as DOWLING has shown in rats. But the absence of beta-lipoprotein is not explained, and it would be just too simple to blame a genetic factor at the present stage of our knowledge.

Moreover, there is apparently no relationship to the mucopolysaccharides (mentioned on p. 22) which were demonstrated in the interstitial material between the photoreceptors (FINE & ZIMMERMAN, 1963). It is essentially the work of HALL & HELLER (1966), who furnished the evidence that the mucopolysaccharides are mainly synthesized in the myoid region of the inner segments of the visual cells and extruded into the extracellular space. Here they form a matrix of a complex mixture with proteins, the components of this matrix being unequal in different animal species. It is possible that also the pigment epithelium may contribute to its production.

Since being an integral part of the retina, the mucopolysaccharides are essential to its normal function and structural integrity in mediating and regulating the metabolite exchange between retina and choroid as well as the vitamin A exchange between retina and pigment epithelium. The physiological importance of the mucopolysaccharides in the eye, and indeed for the entire organism, is emphasized by the wide range of genetically determined physical and mental degenerations which are produced by a disturbance of their metabolism. They are classified in six pathological syndromes, since at present we have no better classification of these mucopolysaccharidoses (MPS) than that based on the clinical defect (MCKUSICK, 1969). The genetic factor is autosomal recessive in all disorders except one (MPS II, Hunter Syndrome) in which the inheritance is X-linked recessive. The immediate cause of the MPS is an excessive storage of a mucopolysaccharide in the tissues, as evidenced by an excessive urinary excretion, which may be due to a defective binding to the protein (DORFMAN, 1964). In several patients, apparently not related to any one specific MPS type, retinal degenerations were found, often presenting themselves as typical retinitis pigmentosa (LEUNG et al., 1971). Frequently, nyctalopia is found as we were able to show both by means of the ERG and by psychophysical tests carried out in two young brothers of very high IQ, typically suffering from MPS II (Hunter Syndrome) (ABRAHAM et al., 1974a), and in two young sisters suffering from MPS IV (Morquio Syndrome) (ABRAHAM et al., 1974b).

I close in a somewhat subdued vein. While our knowledge of the structural and functional aspects is fast increasing, which is largely in line with the rapid technological progress, the pathological entities (and not only those mentioned here) still resist complete understanding and full elucidation. On the other hand, we begin to become aware of possible links with human pathology such as, for example, the failure of normal co-ordination between disk production and phagocytosis found in dystrophic rats or in the vitamin A deficiencies.

The question whether we possess at present sufficient understanding of the normal conditions, that we can point to a common denominator for inherited retinal degenerations can only be answered with no. The evidence available does not permit any clear-cut conclusion. In some cases, beta-lipoprotein is absent from the serum, in others there is a defect in the metabolism of the mucopolysaccharides or a faulty binding with the protein, or there may perhaps be an enzymatic defect. There is also the positive effect of darkness and the possible hypersensitivity to light of persons suffering from retinitis pigmentosa and nyctalopia. As to the latter, damage was shown to occur to the visual cells by excessive light energy (NOELL, 1965; NOELL et al., 1966a, 1966b) which may be due to a disturbance in the exchange of metabolites and fluid across the epithelial cells (HANSSON, 1971).

REFERENCES

ABRAHAM, F. A., YATZIV, S., RUSSELL, A. & AUERBACH, E. Electrophysiological and psychophysical findings in the visual system of a family with two siblings affected by a mild type of Hunter's syndrome (MPS II). *Arch. Ophthal. 9: 181* (1974).

ABRAHAM, F. A., YATZIV, S., RUSSELL, A. & AUERBACH, E. Electrophysiological and psychophysical findings in the visual system of a family with two siblings affected by Morquio syndrome (MPS IV). *Arch. Ophthal.* in press (1974).

AKHTAR, M., BLOSSE, P. T. & DEWHURST, P. B. The active site of the visual protein, rhodopsin. *Chem. Commun. 631-632* (1967).

28

AMEMIYA, T. Vitamin A and the retina. *The E.E.N.T. Monthly* 50: *341-346* (1971).

ARDEN, G. B. The excitation of photoreceptors. In: Progress in Biophys. and Molec. Biol. (ed. J. A. V. BUTLER) 19: Pt. 2: *373-421* (1969).

ARDEN, G. B. & IKEDA, H. A new property of the early receptor potential of rat retina. *Nature (London)* 208: *1100-1101* (1965).

ARROYAVE, G., WILSON, J., MÉNDES, J., BÉHAR, M. & SCRIMSHAW, N. S. Serum and liver vitamin A and lipids in children with severe protein malnutrition. *Am. J. Clin. Nutr.* 9: *180-185* (1961).

AUERBACH, E. Electroretinographical and psychophysical studies in achromats. *2nd Internat'l Symp. on Recent Advances in Colour Vsion Deficiencies.* Edinburgh, June (1973).

AUERBACH, E., GODEL, V. & ROWE, H. An electrophysiological and psychophysical study of two forms of congenital night blindness. *Invest. Ophthal.* 8: *332-345* (1969).

AUERBACH, E., GUGGENHEIM, K., KAPLANSKY, J. & ROWE, H. Effect of protein depletion on the electric response of the retina in albino rats. *J. Physiol.* 172: *417-424* (1964).

AUERBACH, E. & KRIPKE, B. Achromatopsia with amblyopia. II. A psychophysical study of 5 cases. *Doc. Ophthal.* 37: (1974).

BAIRATI, A. & ORZALESI, N. The ultrastructure of the pigment epithelium and of the photoreceptor pigment epithelium junction in the human retina. *J. Ultrastruct. Res.* 9: *484-496* (1963).

BALL, S., COLLINS, F. D., DALVI, P. D. & MORTON, R. A. Studies in vitamin A. II. Reactions of retinene with amino compounds. *Biochem. J.* 45: *304-307* (1949).

BALL, S., GLOVER, J., GOODWIN, T. W. & MORTON, R. A. Conversion of retinene 1 to vitamin A in vivo. *Biochem. J.* 41: *14* (1947).

BALL, S., GOODWIN, T. W. & MORTON, R. A. Studies on vitamin A. 5. The preparation of retinene-vitamin A aldehyde. *Biochem. J.* 42: *516-523* (1948).

BASSEN, F. A. & KORNZWEIG, A. L. Malformation of the erythrocytes in a case of atypical retinitis pigmentosa. *Blood* 5: *381* (1950).

BERSON, E. L. Light deprivation for early retinitis pigmentosa. A hypothesis. *Arch. Ophthal.* 85: *521-529* (1971).

BAYLOR, D. A. & FUORTES, M. G. F. Electrical responses of single cones in the retina of the turtle. *J. Physiol.* 207: *77-92* (1970).

BLASIE, J. K. & WORTHINGTON, C. R. Planar liquid-like arrangement of photopigment molecules in frog retinal receptor disk membranes. *J. Molec. Biol.* 39: *417-439* (1969).

BLASIE, J. K., WORTHINGTON, C. R. & DEWEY, M. M. Molecular localization of frog retinal receptor photopigment by electron microscopy and low-angle X-ray diffraction. *J. Molec. Biol.* 39: *407-416* (1969).

BLAUROCK, A. E. & WILKINS, M. H. F. Structure of frog photoreceptor membranes. *Nature (London)* 223: *906-909* (1969).

BONTING, S. L. General Discussion Bochum Symp. August 1972. In: Biochem. and Physiol. of Visual Pigments, Springer-Verlag, p. *351-363* (ed. H. LANGER). 1973.

BOWNDS, D. Site of attachment of retinal in rhodopsin. *Nature (London)* 216: *1178-1181* (1967).

BRIDGES, C. D. B. & YOSHIKAMI, S. Personal communication to ARDEN, G. B.

BRINDLEY, G. S. & GARDNER-MEDVIN, A. R. The origin of the early receptor potential of the retina. *J. Physiol.* 182: *185-194* (1966).

BRINDLEY, G. S. & WILLMER, E. N. The reflexion of light from the macular and peripheral fundus oculi in man. *J. Physiol.* 116: *350-356* (1952).

BROWN, K. T. & MURAKAMI, M. A new receptor potential of the monkey retina with no detectable latency. *Nature (London)* 201: *626-628* (1964a).

BROWN, K. T. & MURAKAMI, M. Biphasic form of the early receptor potential of the monkey retina. *Nature (London)* 204: *239-240* (1964b).

BROWN, K. T. & MURAKAMI, M. Early receptor potential of the vertebrate retina. *Nature (London)* 204: *736-740* (1964c).

Brown, K. T., Watanabe, K. & Murakami, N. The early and late receptor potentials of monkey cones and rods. *Cold Spring Harb. Symp. Quant. Biol.* 30: *457-482* (1965).

Campbell, D. A., Harrison, R. & Tonks, E. L. Retinitis pigmentosa. Vitamin A serum levels in relation to clinical findings. *Exp. Eye Res.* 3: *412-426* (1964).

Campbell, F. W. & Rushton, W. A. H. Measurement of the scotopic pigment in the living eye. *J. Physiol.* 130: *131-147* (1955).

Cohen, A. I. The ultrastructure of the rods of the mouse retina. *Am. J. Anat.* 107: *23-48* (1960).

Cohen, A. I. Vertebrate retinal cells and their organization. *Biol. Rev.* 38: *427-459* (1963).

Cohen, A. I. New details of the ultrastructure of the outer segments and ciliary connections of the rods of human and macaque retinae. *J. Anat. (London)* 99: *595-610* (1965).

Cohen, A. I. New evidence supporting the linkage to extracellular space of outer segment saccules of frog cones but not rods. *J. Cell. Biol.* 37: *424-444* (1968).

Cohen, A. I. Further studies on the question of the patency of saccules in outer segments of vertebrate photoreceptors. *Vision Res.* 10: *445-453* (1970).

Cohen, A. I. Rods and cones. In: Hb. of Sens. Physiol., Chapter 2, Vol. VII/2: Physiol. of Photorec. Organs (ed. M.G.F. Fuortes) Springer Verl. (1972).

Cone, R. A. Early receptor potential of the vertebrate retina. *Nature (London)* 204: *736-739* (1964).

Cone, R. A. The early receptor potential of the vertebrate eye. *Cold Spring Harb. Symp. Quant. Biol.* 30: *483-491* (1965).

Cone, R. A. Early receptor potential: photoreversible charge displacement in rhodopsin. *Science* 155: *1128-1131* (1967).

Cone, R. A. Rotational diffusion of rhodopsin in the visual receptor membrane. *Nature New Biol.* 236: *39-43* (1972).

Cone, R. A. & Brown, P. K. Dependence of the early receptor potential on the orientation of rhodopsin. *Science* 156: *536* (1967).

Cone, R. A. & Pak, W. L. The early receptor potential. In: Hb. of Sens. Physiol. Chapter 12, Vol. I, pp. 345-365, Springer Verlag (1971).

Denton, E. J. The contributions of the orientated photosensitive and other molecules to the absorption of whole retina. *Proc. Roy. Soc.* B150: *78-94* (1959).

Dorfman, A. Metabolism of acid mucopolysaccharides. *Biophys. J.* 4: (suppl.) *155* (1964).

Dowling, J. E. Night blindness, dark adaptation and the electroretinogram. *Am. J. Ophthal.* 50: Pt. II, *875-887* (1960a).

Dowling, J. E. The chemistry of visual adaptation in the rat. *Nature (London)* 188: *114-118* (1960b).

Dowling, J. E. Nutritional and inherited blindness in the rat. *Exp. Eye Res.* 3: *348-356* (1964).

Dowling, J. E. & Gibbons, I. R. The effect of vitamin A deficiency on the fine structure of the retina. In: The Structure of the Eye (ed. G. Smelser) pp. *85-99* (1961).

Dowling, J. E. & Sidman, R. L. Inherited retinal dystrophy in the rat. *J. Cell Biol.* 14: *73-109* (1962).

Dowling, J. E. & Wald, G. Vitamin A deficiency and night blindness. *Proc. Nat. Acad. Sci.* 44: *648-661* (1958a).

Dowling, J. E. & Wald, G. Nutritional night blindness. *Ann. N.Y. Acad. Sci.* 74: *256-265* (1958b).

Dowling, J. E. & Wald. G. On the mechanisms of vitamin A deficiency and night blindness. Proc. 4th Internat'l Cong. Biochem., Vienna, Symp. on Vitamin Metabolism, 1958, Pergamon Press 11: 185-197 (1959).

Droz, B. Synthesis and migration of proteins in the visual cells of rats and mice. *Anat. Rec.* 139: *222* (1961).

Droz, B. Dynamic condition of proteins in the visual cells of rats and mice as shown by radioautography with labeled amino acids. *Anat. Rec.* 145: *157-167* (1963).

EWALD, E. & KÜHNE, W. Untersuchungen über den Sehpurpur. II. Entstehung der Retinafarbe. *Unters. physiol. Inst. Heidelberg* 1: *248-290* (1878).

FALK, G. & FATT, P. Distinctive properties of the lamellar and disc edge structures of the rod outer segment. *J. Ultrastruct. Res.* 28: *41-60* (1969).

FINE, B. S. & ZIMMERMAN, L. E. Observations on the rod and cone layer of the human retina; a light and electron microscopic study. *Invest. Ophthal.* 2: *446-459* (1963).

FISHER, K. D., CARR, C. J., HUFF, J. E. & HUBER, T. E. Dark adaptation and night vision. *Fed. Proc.* 29: *1605-1638* (1970).

FREEMAN, M. I. & WORTMAN, B. Mucopolysaccharides in beef retina and small cerebarl vessels. *Invest. Ophthal.* 5: *88-92* (1966).

FUORTES, M. G. F. & HODGKIN, A. L. Changes in time scale and sensitivity in the ommatidia of Limulus. *J. Physiol.* 172: *239-263* (1964).

GILARDI, R., KARLE, I. L., KARLE, J. & SPERLING, W. Crystal structure of the visual chromophores, 11-cis and all-trans retinal. *Nature (London)* 232: *187-189* (1971).

GOODHART, R. S. The Vitamins. In: Modern Nutrition in Health and Disease. Dietotherapy (ed. M. G. WOHL & R. S. GOODHART) 4th edition. Philadelphia: Lea & Febiger, 1968. p. 213.

GRAS, W. J. & WORTHINGTON, C. R. X-ray analysis of retinal photoreceptors. *Proc. Nat. Acad. Sci.* 63: *233-238* (1969).

HAGINS, W. A. Electrical signs of information flow in photoreceptors. *Cold Spring Harb. Symp. quant. Biol.* 30: *403-418* (1965).

HAGINS, W. A. The visual process: excitatory mechanisms in the primary receptor cells. *Ann. Rev. Biophys. Bioeng.* 1: *131-158* (1972).

HAGINS, W. A. & MCGAUGHY, R. E. Fast photovoltages, receptor currents, and electrical cable constants in squid photoreceptors. *Biophys. J.* 8: *A-158* (1968a).

HAGINS, W. A. & MCGAUGHY, R. E. Membrane origin of the fast photovoltage of the squid retina. *Science* 159: *213-215* (1968b).

HAGINS, W. A., PENN, R. D. & YOSHIKAMI, S. Dark current and photocurrent in retinal rods. *Biophys. J.* 10: *380-412* (1970).

HAGINS, W. A., ZOUANA, H. V. & ADAMS, R. G. Local membrane current in the outer segment of squid photoreceptors. *Nature (London)* 194: *844-846* (1962).

HALL, M. O., BOK, D. & BACHARACH, A. D. E. Visual pigment renewal in the mature frog retina. *Science* 161: *787-789* (1968).

HALL, M. O., BOK, D. & BACHARACH, A. D. E. Biosynthesis and assembly of the rod outer segment membrane system. Formation and fate of visual pigment in the frog retina. *J. Molec. Biol.* 45: *397-406* (1969).

HALL, M. O. & HELLER, J. Mucopolysaccharides of the retina. *UCLA Forum Med. Sci.* 8: *211-224* (1969). Proc. Conf. Nov. 1966.

HANSSON, H. A. A histochemical study of cellular reactions in rat retina transiently damaged by visible light. *Exp. Eye Res.* 12: *270-274* (1971).

HECHT, S., SHLAER, S. & PIRENNE, M. H. Energy, quanta and vision. *J. Gen. Physiol.* 45: *819-840* (1942).

HELLER, J. Structure of visual pigments. II. Binding of retinal and conformational changes in light exposure in bovine visual pigment 500. *Biochemistry* 7: *2914-2920* (1968).

HELLER, J. Comparative study of membrane protein. Characterization of bovine, rat and frog visual pigments 500. *Biochemistry* 8: *675-679* (1969).

HELLER, J., OSTWALD, T. J. & BOK, D. The osmotic behavior of rod photoreceptor outer segment discs. *J. Cell Biol.* 48: *633-649* (1971).

HERRON, W. L., RIEGEL, B. W., MYERS, O. E. & RUBIN, M. L. Retinal dystrophy in the rat. A pigment epithelial disease. *Invest. Ophthal.* 8: *595-604* (1969).

HERRON, W. L., RIEGEL, B. W. & RUBIN, M. L. Outer segment production and removal in the degenerating retina of the dystrophic rat. *Invest. Ophthal.* 10: *54-63* (1971).

HIGHMAN, V. N. & WEALE, R. A. Rhodopsin density and visual threshold in retinitis pigmentosa. *Am. J. Ophthal.* 75: *822-833* (1973).

HONIG, B. & KARPLUS, M. Implications of torsional potential of retinal isomers for visual excitation. *Nature (London)* 229: *558-560* (1971).

HUBBARD, R. The stereoisomerization of 11-cis retinal. *J. Biol. Chem.* 241: *1814-1818* (1966).

HUBBARD, R. & KROPF, A. The action of light on rhodopsin. *Proc. Nat. Acad. Sci.* 44: *130-139* (1958).

HUBBARD, R. & WALD, G. Cis-trans isomers of vitamin A retinene in the rhodopsin system. *J. Gen. Physiol.* 36: *269-315* (1952).

KANAI, M., RAZ, A. & GOODMAN, D. S. Retinol-binding protein: the transport protein for vitamin A in human plasma. *J. Clin. Invest.* 47: *2025-2044* (1968).

KORENBROT, J. I. & CONE, R. A. Dark ionic flux and the effects of light in isolated rod outer segments. *J. Gen. Physiol.* 60: *20-45* (1972).

KORN, E. D. Structure and function of the plasma membrane. A biochemical perspective. *J. Gen. Physiol.* 52: *257s-278s* (1968).

KRINSKY, N. I. The lipoprotein nature of rhodopsin. *Arch. Ophthal.* 60: *688-694* (1958a)

KRINSKY, N. I. The enzymatic esterification of vitamin A. *J. Biol. Chem.* 232: *881-894* (1958b).

KROLL, A. J. & MACHEMER, R. Experimental retinal detachment and reattachment in the owl monkey. V. Electron microscopy of the reattached retina. *Am. J. Ophthal.* 67: *117-130* (1969a).

KROLL, A. J. & MACHEMER, R. Experimental retinal detachment and reattachment in the Rhesus monkey: Electron microscopic comparison of rods and cones. *Am. J. Ophthal.* 68: *58-77* (1969b).

KÜHNE, W. Zur Photochemie der Netzhaut. *Unters. physiol. Inst. Heidelberg* 1: *1-14* (1878).

KUWABARA, T. & GORN, R. A. Retinal damage by visible light. An electron microscopic study. *Arch. Ophthal.* 79: *69-78* (1968).

LEWIN, D. R., THOMPSON, J. N., PITT, G. A. & HOWELL, J. M. Blindness resulting from vitamin A deficiency in albino and pigmented guinea pigs and rats. *Int. J. Vit. Res.* 40: *270* (1970).

MATHEWS, J. & BEATON, G. H. Vitamin A and carotene utilization in protein-deprived rats. *Can. J. Biochem. Physiol.* 41: *543-549* (1963).

MOORE, T. Vitamin A and carotene. I. The association of vitamin A activity with carotene in the carrot root. *Biochem. J.* 23: *803-811* (1929).

MOORE, T. Vitamin A and carotene. V. The absence of the liver oil vitamin A from carotene. VI. The conversion of carotene to vitamin A in vivo. *Biochem. J.* 24: *692-702* (1930).

MOORE, T. Systemic action of vitamin A. *Exp. Eye, Res.* 3: *305-315* (1964).

NILSSON, S. E. G. Receptor cell outer segment development and ultrastructure of the disk membranes in the retina of the tadpole (Rana pipiens). *J. Ultrastruct. Res.* 11: *581-620* (1964).

NILSSON, S. E. G. The ultrastructure of the receptor outer segment in the retina of the leopard frog (Rana pipiens). *J. Ultrastruct. Res.* 12: *207-231* (1965).

NIR, I. & PEASE, D. C. Ultrastructural aspects of discs in rod outer segments. *Exp. Eye Res.* 16: *173-182* (1973).

NOELL, W. K. Aspects of experimental and hereditary degeneration. In: Biochemistry of the Retina (ed. C. L. GRAYMORE) Suppl. of Exp. Eye Res. (1965).

NOELL, W. K., THEMANN, H., KANG, B. S. & WALKER, V. S. Functional and structural manifestations of a damaging effect of light on the retina. *Fed. Proc.* 25: *329* (1966a).

NOELL, W. K., WALKER, V. S., KANG, B. S. & BERMAN, S. Renital damage by light in rats. *Invest. Ophthal.* 5: *450-473* (1966b).

PAK, W. L. Some properties of the early receptor response in the vertebrate retina. *Cold Spring Harb. Symp. quant. Biol.* 30: *493-499* (1965).

PAK, W. L. & CONE, R. A. Isolation and identification of the initial peak of the early receptor potential. *Nature (London)* 204: *436-438* (1964).

PENN, R. D. & HAGINS, W. A. Signal transmission along retinal rods and the origin of the electroretinographic a-wave. *Nature (London)* 223: *201-205* (1969).

32

PENN, R. D. & HAGINS, W. A. Kinetics of the photocurrent of retinal rods. *Biophys. J.* 12: *1073-1094* (1972).

POINCELOT, R. P., MILLER, P. G., KIMBEL, R. L. Jr. & ABRAHAMSON, E. W. Lipid to protein chromophore transfer in the photolysis of visual pigments. *Nature (London)* 221: *256-257* (1969).

RICHARDSON, T. M. Cytoplasmic and ciliary connections between the inner and outer segments of mammalian visual receptors. *Vision Res.* 9: *727-731* (1969).

ROELS, O. A. Present knowledge of vitamin A. *Nutr. Rev.* 24: *129-132* (1966).

RUSHTON, W. A. H. Apparatus for analysing the light reflected from the eye of the cat. *J. Physiol.* 117: *47P-48P* (1952).

RUSHTON, W. A. H. The measurement of rhodopsin in the living eye. *Acta Physiol. Scand.* 29: *16-18* (1953).

RUSHTON, W. A. H. Dark-adaptation and the regeneration of rhodopsin. *J. Physiol.* 156: *166-178* (1961).

RUSHTON, W. A. H. Visual adaptation. The Ferrier lecture, 1962, *Proc. Roy. Soc.* B162: *20-46* (1965).

SCHMIDT, W. J. Polarisationsoptische Analyse eines Eiweiss-Lipoid Systems erläutert am Aussenglied der Sehzellen. *Kolloid-Z.* 85: *137-148* (1938).

SPITZNAS, M. & HOGAN, M. J. Outer segments of photoreceptors and the retinal pigment epithelium. Interrelationship in the human eye. *Arch. Ophthal.* 84: *810-819* (1970).

TOMITA, T. Electrophysiological study of the mechanism subserving color coding. *Cold Spring Harb. Symp. quant. Biol.* 30: *559-566* (1965).

TOMITA, T. Light-induced potential and resistance changes in vertebrate photoreceptors. In: Hb. Sens. Physiol. Vol. VII/2, Chapter 12. pp. 482-511, Springer Verlag 1972. (ed. M. G. F. FUORTES).

TOYODA, J., NOSAKI, H. & TOMITA, T. Light-induced resistance changes in single photoreceptors of Necturus and Gekko. *Vision Res.* 9: *453-463* (1969).

VEEN, M. J. & BEATON, G. H. Vitamin A transport in the rat. *Can. J. Physiol. Pharmacol.* 44: *521-527* (1966).

WALD, G. Vitamin A in eye tissues. *J. Gen. Physiol.* 18: *905-915* (1935a).

WALD, G. Carotenoids and the visual cycle. *J. Gen. Physiol.* 19: *351-371* (1935b).

WALD, G. The photochemical basis of rod vision. *J. Opt. Soc. Am.* 41: *949-951* (1951).

WALD, G. Visual pigments and photoreceptor physiology. In: Biochem. and Physiol. of Visual Pigments. Symp. Bochum August 1972, pp. 1-13. Springer Verlag, 1973.

WALD, G., BROWN, P. K. & GIBBONS, I. R. Visual excitation: a chemoanatomical study. *Symp. Soc. Exp. Biol.* 16: *32-57* (1962).

WALD, G., BROWN, P. K. & GIBBONS, I. R. The problem of visual excitation. *J. Opt. Soc. Am.* 53: *20-35* (1963).

WALD, G., JEGHERS, H. & ARMINIO, J. An experiment in human dietary night-blindness. *Am. J. Physiol.* 123: *732-746* (1938).

WALD, G. & STEVEN, D. An experiment in human vitamin A deficiency. *Proc. Nat. Acad. Sci.* 25: *344-349* (1939).

WEALE, R. A. The spectral reflectivity of the cat's tapetum measured in situ. *J. Physiol.* 119: *30-42* (1953a).

WEALE, R. A. Slow and rapid regeneration in the living cat's retina. *J. Physiol.* 122: *11P* (1953b).

WEALE, R. A. Relation between dark adaptation and visual pigment regeneration. *J. Opt. Soc. Am.* 54: *128-129* (1964).

WEALE, R. A. Optical activity and the fixation of rods and cones. *Nature (London)* 220: *583* (1968).

WEALE, R. A. Personal communication. (1973).

WERBLIN, F. S. & DOWLING, J. E. Organization of the retina of the mudpuppy, Necturus maculosus. II. Intracellular recording. *J. Neurophysiol.* 32: *339-355* (1969).

WOLF, G. & VARANDANI, P. T. Studies on the function of vitamin A in mucopolysaccharide biosynthesis. *Biochim. Biophys. Acta* 43: *501-512* (1960).

33

YOSHIKAMI, S. Discussion to YOSHIKAMI & HAGINS. Bochum Symp. Aug. 1972. In: Biochem. and Physiol. of Visual Pigments, p. 255. Springer Verlag (1973).

YOSHIKAMI, S. & HAGINS, W. A. Control of the dark current in vertebrate rods and cones. Bochum Symp. Aug. 1972. In: Biochem. and Physiol. of Visual Pigments, pp. 245-255, Springer Verlag (1973).

YOSHIKAMI, S. & HAGINS, W. A. Light, calcium, and the photocurrent of rods and cones Biophys. Soc. Abst. TPM-E16 (1971).

YOSHIZAWA, T. The behaviour of visual pigments at low temperatures. In: Hb. Sens. Physiol., Vol. VII/1 (ed. H. J. A. Dartnall) pp. 146-179, Springer Verlag, 1972, Chapter 5.

YOSHIZAWA, T. & HORIUCHI, S. Cited in T. YOSHIZAWA (1972).

YOUNG, R. W. The renewal of photoreceptor cell outer segments. J. Cell Biol. 33: 61-72 (1967).

YOUNG, R. W. Passage of newly formed protein through the connecting cilium of retinal rods in the frog. J. Ultrastruct. Res. 23: 462-473 (1968).

YOUNG, R. W. A difference between rods and cones in the renewal of outer segment protein. Invest. Ophthal. 8: 222-231 (1969).

YOUNG, R. W. The renewal of rod and cone outer segments in the Rhesus monkey. J. Cell Biol. 49: 303-318 (1971a).

YOUNG, R. W. Shedding of discs from rod outer segments in the Rhesus monkey. J. Ultrastruct. Res. 34: 190-203 (1971b).

YOUNG, R. W. & BOK, D. Participation of the retinal pigment epithelium in the rod outer segment renewal process. J. Cell Biol. 42: 392-403 (1969).

YOUNG, R. W. & BOK, D. Autoradiographic studies on the metabolism of the retinal pigment epithelium. Invest. Ophthal. 9: 524-536 (1970).

YOUNG, R. W. & DROZ, B. The renewal of protein in retinal rods and cones. J. Cell Biol. 39: 169-184 (1968).

Additional References

ABRAHAMSON, E. W. The kinetics of early intermediate processes in the photolysis of visual pigments. In: Biochem. and Physiol. of Visual Pigments. Symp. Bochum, August 1972, pp. 47-56, (ed. H. LANGER), Springer-Verlag, 1973.

AKHTAR, M., BLOSSE, R. T. & DEWHURST, P. B. The reduction of rhodopsin derivative. Life Science 4: 1221-1226 (1965).

APPELMANS, F., WATTIAUX, Y. & DEDUVE, C. The association of acid phosphatase with a special class of cytoplasmic granules in rat liver. Biochem. J. 59: 438-445 (1955).

BOWNDS, D. & WALD, G. Reaction of the rhodopsin chromophore with sodium borohydride. Nature (London) 205: 254-257 (1965).

BRIDGES, C. D. B. & YOSHIKAMI, S. Uptake of tritiated retinaldehyde by the visual pigment of dark adapted rats. Nature 221: 275-276 (1969).

BURDEN, E. M., YATES, C. M., READING, H. W., BITENSKY, L. & CHAYEN, J. Investigation into the structural integrity of lysosomes in the normal and dystrophic rat retina. Exp. Eye Res. 12: 159-165 (1971).

BUSCH, G. E., APPLEBURY, M. L., LAMOLA, A. A. & RENTZEPIS, P. The kinetics of prelumirhodopsin at physiological temperatures. Proc. Nat. Acad. Sci. U.S. in press.

LEUNG, L.-S. E., WEINSTEIN, G. W. & HOBSON, R. R. Further electroretinographic studies of patients with mucopolysaccharidoses. Birth Defects: Original Article Series 7: 32-40 (1971).

McKUSICK, V. A. The nosology of the mucopolysaccharidoses. Am. J. Med. 47: 730-747 (1969):

NOVIKOFF, A. B. Lysosomes and related particles. In: The Cell, Vol. 2: Cells and their Components Parts (ed. J. BRACHET & A. E. MIRSKY), Acad. Press, pp. 423-488 (1961).

PITT, G. A. J., COLLINS, F. D., MORTON, R. A. & STOK, P. Studies on rhodopsin. VIII. Retinylidenemethylamine, an indicator yellow analogue. Biochem. J. 59: 122-128. (1955).

34

SALLMANN, L. VON, GELDERMAN, A. H. & LASTER, L. Ocular histological changes in a case of a-beta-lipoproteinemia. *Doc. Ophthal.* 26: *451-460* (1969).

SALT, H. B., WOLFF, O. H., LLOYD, J. K., FOSBROOKE, A. S., CAMERON, A. H. & HUBBLE, D. V. On having no beta-lipoprotein. A syndrome comprising a-beta-lipoproteinemia, acanthocytosis and steatorrhea. *Lancet* 2: *325-329* (1960).

WOLFF, O. H., LLOYD, J. K. & TONKS, E. L. A-beta-lipoproteinemia with special reference to the visual defect. *Exp. Eye Res.* 3: *439-442* (1964).

YOSHIZAWA, T. & KITO, Y. Chemistry of the rhodopsin cycle. *Nature (London)* 182: *1604-1605* (1958).

YOSHIZAWA, T. & WALD, G. Pre-lumirhodopsin and the bleaching of visual pigments. *Nature (London)* 197: *1279-1286* (1963).

Author's address:

Vision Research Laboratory
Hadassah Medical Center &
Medical School
P.O. Box 499
Jerusalem
Israel

ON CONE DYSFUNCTIONS

R. A. WEALE

(London)

If rods and cones were to be distinguished from each other merely by the fact that they contain different types of visual pigment, the existence of rod and cone dystrophies would be hard to understand. Even their respective morphological characteristics, which give the receptors their names, aid our comprehension but little, although the very much larger surface/volume ratio of the cone may clearly involve it in problems which the compact rod does not have to face.

However, during the last few years several observations have been made which may assuage the helpless frustration one feels when reading the literature on dystrophies. In the first place, YOUNG (1970) showed that there is a significant difference between the two types of receptor as far as concerns the rate of protein turnover. Using auto-radiography he found that the rods have a turnover period of a few weeks, whereas the cones appear to be laid down once and for all. It may be noted that this makes the cones the more nearly typical non-myelinated nervous structures (VOGT & VOGT, 1946): since they are not renewed they have the time to learn. Secondly, some of the biophysical properties of rods and cones show striking differences. Fixation with glutaraldehyde and formaldehyde acts more quickly on rods than on cones (VILLERMET & WEALE, 1968; WEALE, 1971); as this is contrary to what one would expect on the basis of the relative surface/volume ratios (cf. COHEN, 1968) differences in membrane reaction or permeability have to be considered. In a number of species, systematic differences in the optical properties of rods and cones have also been noted (WEALE, l.c.): in every case the birefringence of cones is a multiple of that of rods. If the differences in protein are no greater than those postulated for the hypothetical rod-opsin and cone-opsin and if the whole of the receptor protein is due to its visual pigment content, then the differences in birefringence have to be attributed largely to differences in lipids or in structural aspects. Electron microscopy is unable as yet to throw any significant light on relevant structural differences, so that the lipid aspect may need investigating. This is not to suggest that cone dystrophies can conceivably be due to a single factor: this facile idea is clearly ruled out e.g. by the anatomical classification given by MAUMENEE & EMERY (1972). But we have no pathology worth mentioning except for the case quoted by KRILL et al. (1973), and have no lead into the aetiology of cone dystrophies other than that provided by rare unilateral cases (GOODMAN et al., 1966), of such genetic studies as may be relied upon (KRILL et al, l.c.), and a rare case of early onset (GOODMAN et al., 1963) in which deterioration in visual acuity was shown to precede one in colour vision.

Whatever down one may have on the scientific study of vision in general and of visual defects in particular, we have to arrive at decisions about how to proceed with studies of cone dysfunctions. The tentative classification shown in Fig. 1 stresses some of the problems. We note in the first place that most of the published tests on this family of diseases produce evidence of permanently degraded function. The exception to this is provided by ophthalmoscopy. In other words, the tests are obituaries. They tell us that things have gone wrong. Their only value is that they serve to diagnose the disease, and, if the diagnosis is correct, the probable end-result and a time-scale may be forecast. They offer no path to an understanding of the underlying abnormality. Secondly, a study of the mere signs and symptoms of the diseases seems to me a waste of time if we are not prepared to devise a therapy, and I fail to see how we can do that if we do not learn to control the conditions which cause the dystrophic effects. In the case of weak solar burns and incipient tobacco amblyopia, repair processes are inferred to exist because more or less normal function can be restored if the noxious stimuli are withdrawn. In laser lesions, the distinction between damaged and dead cones seems artificial (MARSHALL, priv. comm.). But even in these cases, we have no pathology, not to mention biochemistry, to help us along. It is unlikely, however, that understanding thermal shock could throw much light on atrophic problems (WEALE, l.c.).

It is questionable also whether the study of cases of stationary achromatopsia (BLACKWELL & BLACKWELL, 1961) and partial achromatopsia (SIEGEL et al., 1966) can do anymore than to define a given end-point in any particular type of dysfunction. This means also that the battery of tests used by many a conscientious investigator involves a great deal of redundancy. This is something to guard against whenever batteries are used (COMFORT, 1969; WEALE, 1970). E.g. if one suspects that, to take an example from rod dystrophies, the final threshold is two or three log units above normal, then it is a waste of time to spend half an hour with the patient in the dark and to record dark-adaptation. If, to return to cone-dystrophies, the cone system is suspect, an investigation of the visual fields is going to yield much less information than a thorough plot of incremental thresholds across various meridians of the central retinal region (HAN-

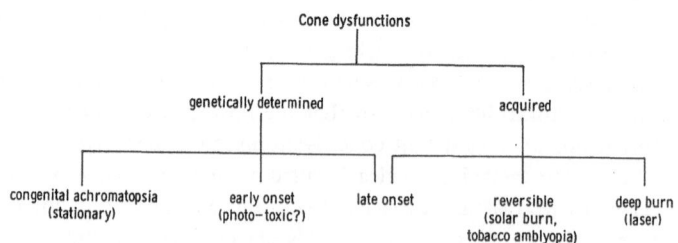

FIG. 1. Tentative classification of cone dysfunctions.

38

SEN, 1974). If the ocular media are normal and acuity is poor, a central scotoma is obligatory and need not be mapped by perimetry (BABEL & STANGOS, 1972). Conversely, the ERG and EOG provide information on different anatomical structures so that they complement, rather than duplicate, each other (STANGOS et al., 1972), and are therefore clearly useful.

This raises the question of the usefulness of the early receptor potential. There is an agreement on the basic issues. The amplitude of the potential is a measure of the number of the quanta absorbed (CONE, 1964) certainly at submaximal bleaching intensities, i.e. levels which do not entirely denude the retina of its visual pigments (ARDEN, IKEDA & SIEGEL, 1966). Moreover, if the potential is obtained from a mixed retina, the contribution of the cones is disproportionately large (GOLDSTEIN, 1968), probably because of their large surface/

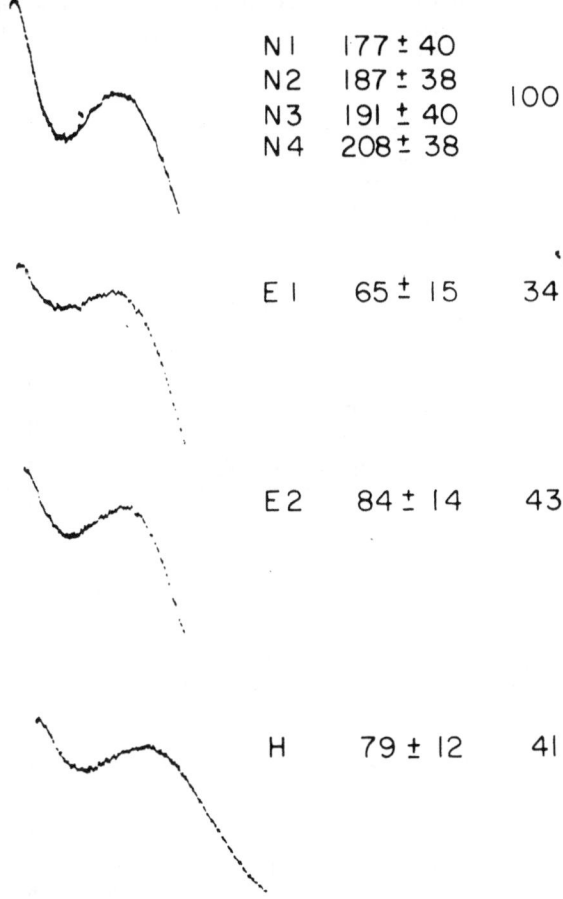

N 1	177 ± 40	
N 2	187 ± 38	
N 3	191 ± 40	100
N 4	208 ± 38	
E 1	65 ± 15	34
E 2	84 ± 14	43
H	79 ± 12	41

FIG. 2. Early receptor potentials. N1-4: normal; E1, 2: dominantly inherited 'cone degeneration'; H: autosomal recessive rod monochromatism. Amplitude in μV (original lacks calibration mark). Column on right gives the percentage of the amplitude in terms of the normal average. After GOLDSTEIN & BERSON, 1970

volume ratio (WEALE, 1969). It follows therefore, that as the ERP can be recorded from the human eye (GALLOWAY, 1967), it should provide a sensitive index of cone malfunction. GOLDSTEIN & BERSON (1970) found this to be the case (Fig. 2). In cases of familial cone dystrophy, they recorded subnormal amplitudes. They also claimed that the cone-pigments in pathological cases differ from those contained in normal retinae. The reason they advanced was based on experiments in which they measured the rate of increase of the amplitude after the eye had been exposed to an intense light (BERSON & GOLDSTEIN, 1970). Cases of retinitis pigmentosa appeared to show a faster recovery than did normal retinae. The authors' conclusion that this is a real effect is highly questionable because (a) normal retinae have a rod contribution (cf. Fig. 3) which apparently retards recovery; (b) BERSON & GOLDSTEIN compared their rates with pigment regeneration data which are slower than those obtained by other workers; (c) in some cases the error of their results amounts to 25 p.c. (cf. WEALE, 1972). It follows that while, as GOLDSTEIN & BERSON have clearly

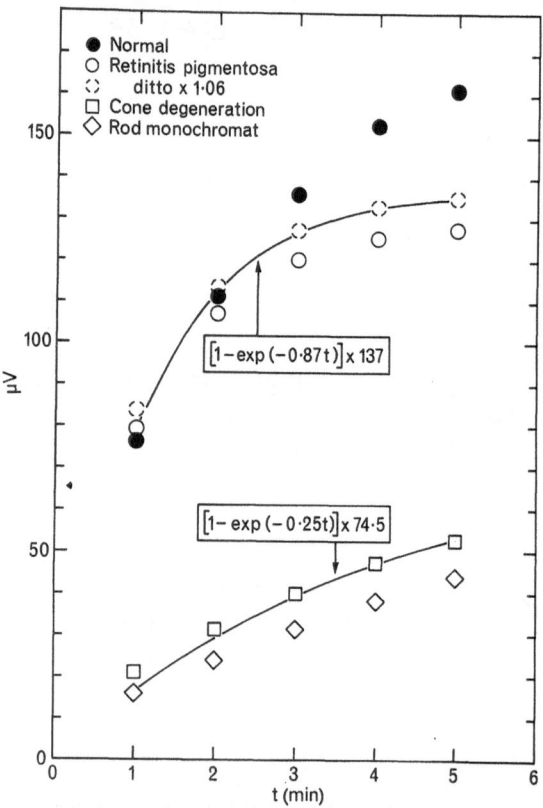

FIG. 3. Recovery of the early receptor potential compared with visual pigment regeneration curves. ERP data from BERSON & GOLDSTEIN (1970): photochemical data WEALE (1959, 1962) and RIPPS & WEALE (1969).

shown, the ERP is a useful index of the state of a retina, a refined quantitative approach has to be used with circumspection.

It seems nevertheless that, provided flash exposures do not damage the visual pathway of the neonate, the ERP may well offer at present the only monitoring device available to us to track the early progress of this body of diseases. The proviso is important. The very early onset (GOODMAN et al., 1963) has to be distinguished from that occurring after puberty (FRANÇOIS et al., 1972). It is possible that, in the early onset, we may have an example of phototoxicity (MARSHALL et al., 1972): perhaps the cones perish as a result of light exposure. It is clearly only in instances for which this can be established (and the later the onset of the disease the less likely is photo-toxicity going to be a cause) that BERSON's suggestion (1971) of partial light-deprivation for therapeutic purposes seems to merit detailed consideration.

Of course, no one has proved as yet at what level light becomes noxious. It seems that even partial light deprivation may have its drawbacks. I indicated in Fig. 1 that there may exist dystrophic processes which are normal in the sense that they may occur in all eyes. At the same time they may be distinguished – perhaps arbitrarily – from senile degenerative changes because their manifestation is comparatively mild and cannot be said to be incapacitating as far as a visual function is concerned. The sparse evidence for something worth looking into is as follows. (I) When LE GROS CLARK (1949) kept three monkeys for a month in red light, two of them showed marked degeneration in given parts of their lateral geniculate bodies. If this is due to hypo-stimulation (and the experiment needs repeating with histology extended to the retina and supplementation with electro-retinography), then the question of light deprivation becomes finely balanced. (II) The photo-chemical pigment contents of the retinal rods of cyprinids (DARTNALL et al., 1961; BRIDGES & YOSHIKAMI, (1970) vary with the photic environment, in all probability with its spectral composition (VILLER-MET & WEALE, 1972). We have to ask ourselves whether any evidence can be obtained for this occurring also in man. VERRIEST (1972) showed recently that there is no significant difference between the spectral sensitivity curve of aphakes whose average ages differed by more than thirty years. Unfortunately, the spectral range was too short in the violet part of the spectrum to enable us to decide whether this similarity extends throughout the visible part of the spectrum. A number of studies have tackled the question of long-term aphakicity from the point of view of chromaticity discrimination. E.g. Miss JANOUŠ-KOVA (1955) states that almost 25 p.c. of patients with a cataract are colour-defective also post-operatively, and LAKOWSKI (1962) reports that the colour vision of eyes of long-standing aphakia exhibit defects typical of eyes that are up to 20 years younger than normal ones of the same age as that of the aphakes. The lens may provide us with some information on changes in cone function because it acts like a yellow filter which filters the light reaching the retina for a very long time. HITCHINGS et al. (unpublished observations) examined a group of cataract patients with the Farnsworth 100-hue test on three occasions. They first tested colour vision on the good eye (which was aphakic in some of the patients): this provided the standard. They then tested the eye operated for cataract within two or three days after the operation, and again six weeks later. The preliminary results are shown in Fig. 4 and Fig. 5. The number of colour errors per sample was much greater just after the operation than just before; but six weeks later the distributive function for the operated eye was similar to that for the pre-operative control. The table in Fig. 5 gives the results for the t- and F- tests referring to the spectral regions below. E.g. there was a significant deterioration in the performance of the group tested immediately after the operation with the exception of the green and red parts of the spectrum. But, and here we come to the crunch, six weeks later the whole spectrum was normal with one signal exception: namely the short wavelength end. These data seem to indicate that post-operatively there occur changes in the colour performance of these patients which are spectrally selective. They are retarded in the blue part of the spectrum. It remains to be seen from studies extending over a period longer than six weeks post-operatively whether further improvement takes place also in the blue-sensitive cones or whether they are permanently damaged perhaps because of hypo-stimulation which has existed for years.

These data are not quoted as providing a likely clue for our understanding of the various dystrophies. But they serve to show that when the controls come to be applied they may well have to be stringent. As for the rest, one ought to repeat that we need data applying to the situation before the fait accompli. Or, if I may put it differently and quote Horace: carpe diem. This seems not only

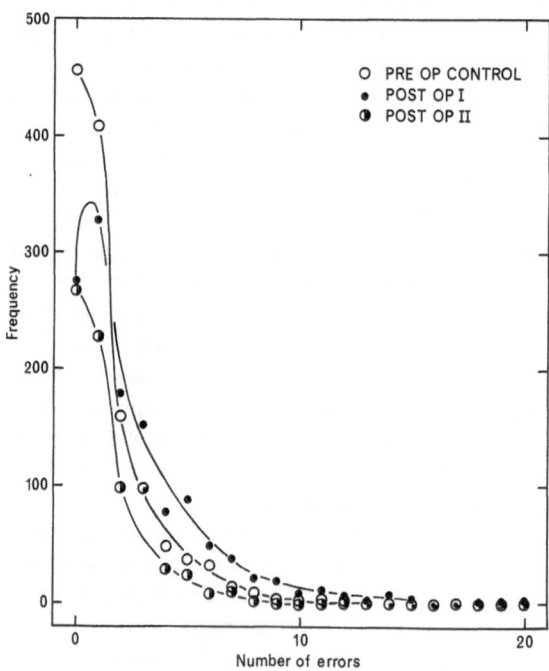

FIG. 4. Colour vision tests on aphakic patients. Frequency with which a given number of errors was made. HITCHINGS et al. (1974).

II v PRE	t	NS	<0·01	NS	NS	NS	NS	NS	NS	NS	NS
	F	NS	<0·05	<0·02	<0·001	<0·05	NS	NS	<0·02	<0·01	<0·001
PRE v I	t	<0·05	<0·01	<0·001	<0·01	<0·02	NS	<0·001	<0·01	<0·05	NS
	F	<0·01	<0·001	NS	<0·01	NS	NS	<0·01	<0·02	<0·001	<0·01

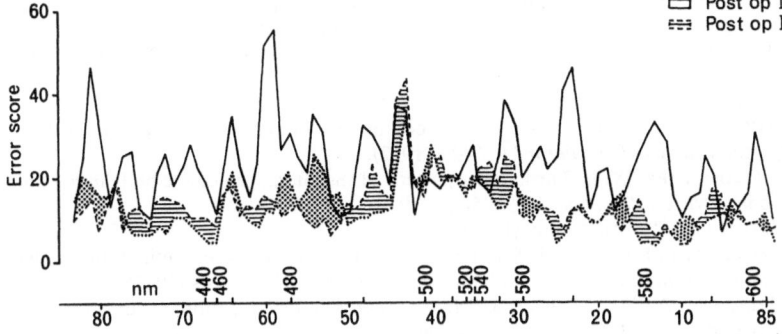

░░░ Pre op
▭ Post op I
▨ Post op II

FIG. 5. Colour vision tests on aphakic patients. Error score. The numbers at the bottom refer to tiles in the Farnsworth – 100 hue test. HITCHINGS et al. (1974).

an exhortation valuable for those studying cone-dystrophies, but strikes me also as a slogan eminently suitable for a society of clinical electro-retinographers.

REFERENCES

ARDEN, G. B., IKEDA, H. & SIEGEL, I. M. Effects of light adaptation on the early receptor potential. *Vision Res.* 6: *357-371* (1966).

BABEL, J. & STANGOS, N. Dégénérescence progressive du système photopique. *Ophthalmologica* 165: *392-395* (1972).

BERSON, E. L. Light deprivation for early retinitis pigmentosa. *Arch. Ophthal.* 85: *521-529* (1971).

BERSON, E. L. & GOLDSTEIN, E. B. Recovery of the human early receptor potential during dark-adaptation in hereditary retinal desease. *Vision Res.* 10: *219-226* (1970).

BLACKWELL, H. R. & BLACKWELL, O. M. Rod and cone receptor mechanisms in typical and atypical congenital achromatopsia. *Vision Res.* 1: *62-107* (1961).

BRIDGES, C. D. B. & YOSHIKAMI, S. The rhodopsin-porphyropsin system in freshwater fishes – 1. effects of age and photic environment. *Vision Res.* 10: *1315-1332* (1970).

COHEN, A. New evidence supporting the linkage to extracellular space of outer segment saccules of frog cones but not rods. *J. Cell Biol.* 37: *424-444* (1968).

COMFORT, A. Test-battery to measure ageing-rate in man. *Lancet* 2: *1411-1414* (1969).

CONE, R. A. Early receptor potential of the vertebrate retina. *Nature (Lond.)* 204: *736-739* (1964).

DARTNALL, H. J. A., LANDER, M. R. & MUNTZ, F. W. Progress in Photobiology (ed. B.C. CHRISTENSEN & B. BUCKMANN). Elsevier Amsterdam. *203-213* (1961).

FRANÇOIS, J., DE ROUCK, A., CAMBIE, E., & DE LAEY. J. J. Visual functions in pericentral pigmentary retinopathy. *Ophthalmologica* 165: *38-61* (1972).

GALLOWAY, N. R. Early receptor potential in the human eye. *Brit. J. Ophthal.* 51: *261-264* (1967).

43

GOLDSTEIN, E. B. Visual pigments and the early receptor potential of the isolated frog retina. *Vision Res.* 8: *953-963* (1968).

GOLDSTEIN, E. B. & BERSON, E. L. Rod and cone contribution to the human early receptor potential. *Vision Res.* 10: *207-218* (1970).

GOODMAN, G., RIPPS, H., & SIEGEL, I. M. Cone dysfunction syndromes. *Arch. Ophthal.* 70: *214-231* (1963).

GOODMAN, G., RIPPS, H., & SIEGEL, I. M. Progressive cone degeneration. In: Clinica Electroretinography *303-372* (1966).

HANSEN, E. The photoreceptors in cone dystrophies. In press.

JANUŠKOVÁ, KARLA. Barevné vidění a věk. *Cs. Oftal.* 11: *37-48.*

KRILL, A. E., DEUTMAN, A. F. & FISHMAN, M. The cone degenerations. *Doc. Ophthal.* 35: *1-80* (1973).

HITCHINGS, R. A., SILVER, JANET & WEALE, R. A. In preparation.

LAKOWSKI, R. Is the deterioration of colour discrimination with age due to lens or retinal changes? *Die Farbe* 11: *67-68* (1962).

LE GROS CLARK, W. E. The laminar pattern of the lateral geniculate body in relation to colour vision. *Doc. Ophthal.* 3: *57-64* (1949).

MARSHALL, J. Private comm. (1973).

MARSHALL, J., MELLERIO, J. & PALMER, D. A. Damage to pigeon retinae by moderate illumination from fluorescent lamps. *Exp. Eye Res.* 14: *164-169* (1972).

MAUMENEE, A. E. & EMERY, J. M. An anatomic classification of diseases of the macula. *Amer. J. Ophthal.* 74: *594-599* (1972).

SIEGEL, I. M., GRAHAM, C. H., RIPPS, H. & HSIA, Y. Analysis of photopic and scotopic function in an incomplete achromat. *J. opt. Soc. Amer.* 56: *699-704* (1966).

STANGOS, N., SPIRITUS, M. & KOROL, S. ERG et EOG dans les affections maculaires dégénératives. *Ophthalmologica* 165: *396-397* (1972).

VERRIEST, G. The relative spectral luminous efficiency in different age groups of aphakic eyes. *Die Farbe* 21: *17-25* (1972).

VILLERMET, GABRIELLE M. & WEALE, R. A. Optical activity and the fixation of rods and cones. *Nature (Lond.)* 220: *583* (1968).

VILLERMET, GABRIELLE M. & WEALE, R. A. Age, the crystalline lens of the rudd and visual pigments. *Nature (Lond.)* 238: *345-346* (1972).

VOGT, C. & VOGT, O. Ageing of nerve cells. *Nature (Lond.)* 158: *304* (1946).

WEALE, R. A. Report on the symposium on the biochemistry of the retina, by Bonting, S. L. & Daemen, F. J. M. *Exp. Eye Res.* 8: *258* (1969).

WEALE, R. A. The eye and measurement of ageing-rate. *Lancet* (1). *147*: (1970).

WEALE, R. A. On the birefringence of rods and cones. *Pflügers Arch. ges. Physiol.* 329: *244-257* (1971).

WEALE, R. A. Cone pigment regeneration, retinitis pigmentosa and light deprivation. *Vision Res.* 12: *747-748* (1972).

YOUNG, R. W. An hypothesis to account for a basic distinction between rods and cones. *Vision Res.* 11: *1-5* (1971).

Author's address:

Institute of Ophthalmology
Dept. of Visual Science
Universi.y of London
London, WC1H 9QS

ELECTRORETINOGRAPHY OF CONE DYSFUNCTION
WITH MONOCHROMATIC LIGHT.

M. CORDELLA & L. PROSPERI

(Parma)

The possibility of showing electrophysiologically the involvement of the photopic system is demonstrated from the results obtained from dynamic ERG using coloured filters, mainly with Wratten red-orange (WK 26) or red (WK 92) filters, by means of flickering, by means of O.P., and also using static ERG with high intensity white stimuli in the presence of a background light to saturate the rod ERG.

GOODMAN and al. (1963) used the flicker ERG on 47 patients suffering from achromatopsia, and they found the photopic response to be absent. With this method, the same authors (1966) were able to diagnose a progressive cone degeneration in a case which was considered until then to be a case of severe macular degeneration. KRILL (1966-1970) found that the photopic response to single red stimuli during dark adaptation was more sensitive than the reaction to flickering (absence of b wave also when the flicker fusion was subnormal). O.P. were absent in only 2 cases of 13 people studied. AUERBACH & ROWE (1966) observed that, apart from the absence of photopic response to flickering, the dynamic ERG has a characteristic behaviour: after the first minute of dark adaptation (D.A.) the a-wave is subnormal, the b_1 wave disappears, while the b_2 wave increases with the same latency of the b_1 wave of normal people subjected to the same conditions. After a period of D.A., varing from 15 to 30 minutes, the latency increases to a maximum corresponding to the scotopic wave of the normal ERG. These observations were confirmed by KRILL (1970).

KELSEY (1969) and KELSEY & ARDEN (1972) did not observed change of the ERG in cases of rod-monochromatism, using white stimuli after 10 minutes of D.A., while they observed characteristic alteration to flickering. The flicker fusion is notably reduced and the b-wave becomes rounded before fusion. This aspect is never observed in macular degeneration, even in young patients.

RUEDEMANN (1969) thinks that, apart from the flickering and apart from the response to white stimuli during L.A. and D.A., the ERG obtained with red stimuli gives important diagnostic criteria in the evaluation of the photopic system.

BERSON, GOURAS & GUNKEL (1968) were able to separate the cone response from the rod response using the flicker ERG and static ERG with high intensity white stimuli in the presence of background light to saturate the rod ERG. The results obtained permitted the authors to conclude that in cone dysfunction scotopic response and ERG are normal, while in cone-rod dysfunction scotopic ERG is not normal and EOG is reduced. According to these authors, the malfunction of the cones would not affect the capacity of the rod to D.A., which is contrary to the conclusions of ELENIUS & HECK (1958), AUERBACH & ROWE (1966), and KRILL (1970). The reverse reaction, that is the inhibition of the photopic system by the scotopic system was sustained by ALFIERI & SOLE (1968) in a study of the retinal function using A.E.R.G. with monochromatic stimuli.

We have had the opportunity to study three cases of cone dysfunction, and we were able to compare the response obtained by dynamic ERG with the response obtained in the same subjects, using monochromatic stimuli at the end of D.A.

SUBJECTS

Case No. 1-C.G.C. aged 7, male. No consanguinity between the parents. Two brothers, aged 8 and 6, are in good health, one (case No. 2) is affected by cone dysfunction. A father's cousin is suffering from pigmentary retinopathy.
Since early childhood patient has suffered from photophobia and alternating intermittent divergent squint.
R.E.V.: 20/200
L.E.V.: 20/100
The objectivity of both eyes is normal. Achromatopsia is revealed by Ishihara tests and Panel D-15.
Case No. 2 – C.M., aged 5, male. Brother of C.G.C.. He, too, suffers from photophobia and alternating intermittent divergent squint. We were not able to determine his visual acuity.
The objectivity of both eyes is normal. Achromatopsia is revealed by Ishihara tests and Panel D-15.
Case No. 3 – R.S., aged 9, male. No consanguinity between the parents. Two sisters with normal visual function. For one year he noticed a reduction of visual acuity.
R.E.V.: 20/60
L.E.V.: 20/60
The macular region shows alterations similar to those of Stargardt's disease. Achromatopsia is revealed by Ishihara tests and Panel D-15.

METHODS

Electrodes: for recording the dynamic ERG Burian-Allen electrodes were used. *Stimuli*: the light stimulus was obtained from a Vescovini photostimulator (model 481). The duration of the stimuli was about 10 millisecond. The light source was at the centre of a hemispheric bowl, which could be illuminated by diffused lighting for preadaptation. The intensity of the illumination used for the preadaptation was of 1500 Lux, which correspond to 300 Lux at the subject's eye, after diffusion. The intensity of the stimulus was 3 joules. A Wratten

46

red filter (WK 92) with a 646 nm. wavelength, 36% transmittance was used for the dynamic ERG. For monochromatic stimuli we used a red Schott interference filter (wavelength 654 nm, 36% transmittance) and a blue Schott interference filter (wavelength 445 nm, 52% transmittance).

Recording: a DC-AC Vescovini preamplifier (model 381), time constant 0,3 sec., was used for recording ERG. The output response from the preamplifier was fed into an average Signal Analyzer (Hewlett-Packard model 5480 A). For the dynamic ERG the average of 32 readings was taken after 1, 5, 10 and 15 minutes of DA. An equal number (32) of readings were averaged after 18 and 20 minutes of DA for the examination, respectively with red and blue monochromatic interference filters. After computing, the readings were transcribed by means of an x – y plotter. All the recordings were made with maximum mydriasis. All the cases were subjected to light preadaptation before recording the dynamic ERG.

RESULTS

Dynamic ERG

In all 3 cases examined, we observed that immediately after the beginning of dark adaptation there was an absence of the b_1 wave, which did not appear during the whole examination. The b_2 wave commenced to appear, as with normal subjects, after 5 minutes of DA and reached the maximum after 15 minutes of DA. The latency and the latency-to-peak of the a-wave were almost double that of normal subjects. A delay in the latency was observed also in the b_2 wave. No significant delays of the latency to peak period were observed, except at the 5th minute of DA (Table 1).

An overall reduction of the ERG amplitude was observed in all the cases examined. (Table 2).

ERG recording by monochromatic stimulus

The ERG recording after 18 minutes of DA using red monochromatic stimuli (intensity 3 joules) is characterised in normal subjects by two peaks, one negative and one positive. The negative peak is similar in latency and latency-to-peak to the a-wave recording in dynamic ERG found using a WK 92 filter.

The positive peak has a similar latency period, while the latency-to-peak is slightly reduced in comparison to that of the b_2 wave of the dynamic ERG.

In patients suffering from cone dysfunction, both the a and b_2 waves have a latency and a latency-to-peak markedly prolonged in comparison to normal subjects (Table 3).

With blue monochromatic interference filters (nm. 444, intensity 3 joules) we observed slight differences of the latency, and a significant delay of the latency-to-peak between normal and affected subjects. (Table 4)

A reduction in the amplitude of both peaks was observed also in the recordings obtained with red and blue monochromatic interference filters (Table 5).

DYNAMIC ERG
LATENCY and LATENCY to PEAK

NORMAL

D.A. time	a wave		b₁ wave		b₂ wave	
	laten.	l. to p.	laten.	l. to p.	laten.	l. to p.
1'	8 ms	20ms	32ms	40ms	//	//
5'	8 ms	20ms	32ms	40ms	50ms	58ms
10'	8 ms	20ms	32ms	40ms	50ms	100ms
15'	8 ms	20ms	32ms	40ms	50ms	108ms

CONE DYSFUNCTION

D.A. time	a wave		b₁ wave		b₂ wave	
	laten.	l. to p.	laten.	l. to p.	laten.	l. to p.
1'	16ms	50ms	//	//	//	//
5'	16ms	50ms	//	//	64ms	96ms
10'	16ms	50ms	//	//	64ms	96ms
15'	16ms	50ms	//	//	64ms	96ms

COMMENT

The dynamic ERG alone can reveal or confirm the diagnosis of cone dysfunction.

We can also confirm, by our three cases, that the scotopic system can be involved in cases of cone dysfunction, a fact which has already been observed by other authors. Nevertheless, the use of monochromatic interference filters gives us the opportunity to evaluate this.

Indeed, the reduction of the amplitude of the ERG, and the behaviour of latency period and of the latency-to-peak, particularly evident in the recording obtained with red and blue monochromatic stimuli, supports the notion that by using monochromatic stimuli it is possible to diagnose a cone dysfunction and distinguish between a pure cone and a cone-rod dysfunction.

Normal							
R.R.							
OD							
OS							
Case 1							
C.G.C.							
OD							
OS							
Case 2							
C.M.							
OD							
OS							
Case 3							
R.S.							
OD							
OS							
D.A. TIME	1'	5'	10'	15'	18'	20'	
STIMULI	DYNAMIC E.R.G.: Red filter W.K. 92 λ=646.2 n.m. Intensity: 3 joules				Monochromatic Red filter λ=654 n.m. Intensity: 3 joules	Monochromatic Blue filter λ=445 n.m. Intensity: 3 joules	

200 µV
100 ms

49

LATENCY and LATENCY to PEAK ERG ELICITED by MONOCHROMATIC RED STIMULUS (λ=654 nm. T.Max.=36%)

NORMAL

D. A. time	a wave		b₁wave		b₂wave	
	laten.	l. to p.	laten.	l.to p.	laten.	l.to p.
18'	8ms	20ms	//	//	50ms	88ms

CONE DYSFUNCTION

D. A. time	a wave		b₁wave		b₂wave	
	laten.	l.to p.	laten.	l.to p.	laten.	l.to p.
18'	20ms	50ms	//	//	88ms	104ms

LATENCY and LATENCY to PEAK ERG ELICITED by MONOCHROMATIC BLUE STIMULUS (λ=445 nm. T.Max. = 52%)

NORMAL

D. A. time	a wave		b wave	
	laten.	l. to p.	laten.	l.to p.
20'	8ms	16ms	24ms	32ms

CONE DYSFUNCTION

D. A. time	a wave		b wave	
	laten.	l. to p.	laten.	l.to p.
20'	13ms	24ms	30ms	60ms

AMPLITUDE of ERG
ELICITED by MONOCHROMATIC
RED and BLUE STIMULI

NORMAL

a wave	b2 wave
30 μV	165 μV

a wave	b wave
72 μV	330 μV

CONE DYSFUNCTION

a wave	b2 wave
15 μV	120 μV

a wave	b wave
47 μV	130 μV

RED λ=654nm   BLUE λ=445nm

REFERENCES

ALFIERI, R. & SOLE, P. Quelques aspects électrorétinographiques des phénomènes d'inhibition entre les systèmes scotopique et photopique. C.R. Soc. Biol. 160: 317 (1966).

ARDEN, G. B. & BANKES, J. L. K. Foveal electroretinogram as a clinical test. Brit. J. Ophthal. 59: 740 (1966).

AUERBACH, E. & ROWE, H. Electroretinogram and occipital response in congenital hemeralopia and rod-monochromatism. Clinical Electroretinography, Proc. of the Third Int. Symp., Illinois, 1964, p. 281, Pergamon Press, London (1966).

BERSON, E. L., GOURAS, P. & GUNKEL, R. D. Progressive cone degeneration dominantly inherited. Arch. Ophthal. 80: 77 (1968).

BERSON, E. L., GOURAS, P. & GUNKEL, R. D. Rod responses in retinitis pigmentosa dominantly inherited. Arch. Ophthal. 80: 58 (1968).

ELENIUS, V. & HECK, J. Relation of size of electroretinogram to rhodopsin concentration in normal human being and one totally colour blind. Nature 180: 810 (1957).

GOODMANN, G., RIPPS, H. & SIEGEL, I.M. Cone dysfunction syndromes. Arch. Ophthal. (Chicago) 77: 726 (1963).

GOODMANN, G., RIPPS, H. & SIEGEL, I. M. Progressive cone degeneration. Clinical Electroretinography, Proc. of the Third Int. Symp., Illinois, 1964, p. 363 Pergamon Press, London (1966).

GOURAS, P. Electroretinography: some basic principles. Invest. Ophthal. 9: 557 (1970).

KELSEY, J. H. Electrophysiological tests of visual function. Int. Ophthal. Clin. 9: 883 (1969).

KELSEY, J. H. & ARDEN, G. B. Acquired cone dysfunction. Brit. J. Ophthal. 56: 812 (1972).

KRILL, A. E. The electroretinogram in congenital color vision defects. The clinical value of electroretinography, ISCERG Symp. Ghent 1966, p. 205, Karger Ed., Basel/New York (1968).

51

KRILL, A. E. ERG and EOG: Clinical applications. *Invest. Ophthal.* 9: *600* (1970).
RUEDEMANN, A. D. JR. The electroretinogram in degenerative-diseases. *Int. Ophthal. Clin.* 9: *1005* (1969).
STEINMETZ, R. D., OGLE, K. N., RUCKER, C. W. Some physiological considerations of hereditary macular degeneration. *Amer. J. Ophthal.* 42: *304* (1956).

Author's address:

University Eye Clinic
Parma
Italy

ERG RECOVERY IN ROD- AND CONE DYSFUNCTION

P. HEILIG, A. THALER, G. GORDESCH & R. G. FREY

(Vienna)

In clinical electroretinography the extreme expression of rod- or cone dysfunction is found in the complete form of congenital total color blindness and in Schubert-Bornschein's form of congenital night blindness. The ERG traces of both anomalies represent models for the analysis of rod- and cone function or dysfunction. Comparative studies of these conditions, first performed by GOODMAN & BORNSCHEIN, can enable investigators to gain a deeper insight into electrophysiology and patho-physiology of the eye.

METHODS

ERG recovery curves of 20 normal subjects, 10 achromats and one hemeralope were recorded within 30 minutes after light adaptation of 35000 td lasting 10 minutes. The method of examination (HEILIG & THALER) and the results of clinical examination of the achromats (FREY, HEILIG & THALER) and those of the hemeralope (HEILIG, THALER & BORNSCHEIN) have been described in detail.* ERG recovery curves of the overall positive and negative waves were evaluated by means of regression analysis.

Polynomal equations $x = a_0 + a_1 t + a_2 t^2 \ldots + a_7 t^7$ are fitted by a stepwise regression procedure (BENNETT & FRANKLIN), and for test purposes the assumptions of ordinary regression analysis (normal distribution, independence and constant variance of the error term (cp. also CHRISTENSEN) are made unless nonparametric methods (Chebyshev inequality etc.) are sufficient.**

A regression equation permits one to reproduce the experimental data. Moreover, it shows the typical features of the course of ERG recovery. The comparison of the regression equations allows one to compare the different characteristics of ERG recovery curves.

---

* The term *achromat* is used only for the complete form of congenital total color blindness and the term *hemeralope* is used only for congenital night blindness of Schubert-Bornschein's type in this paper.
** A useful program is provided by IBM Application Program System/360-Scientific Subroutine Package.

1.) positive wave of normal subjects and achromats

1st to 30th minute

$$x_N = 39,04 + 24,26\ t - 0,00039\ t^4 \qquad R = 0,809$$
$$\qquad (1,02) \qquad (0,00004)$$
$$x_A = 41,40 + 16,33\ t - 0,00022\ t^4 \qquad R = 0,789$$
$$\qquad (1,06) \qquad (0,00004)$$

x_N overall amplitudes of the ERG of normal subjects
x_A overall amplitudes of the ERG of achromats
t   time of ERG recovery in darkness
R multiple correlation coefficient

The standard deviation of the regression coefficient is set in parentheses under the regression coefficient.

Considering the global course of ERG recovery, the slope (the first derivative with respect to time) as well as the amplitudes are significantly higher in normal subjects than in achromats.

In the sequel the ERG recovery curves were divided in sections and compared separately.

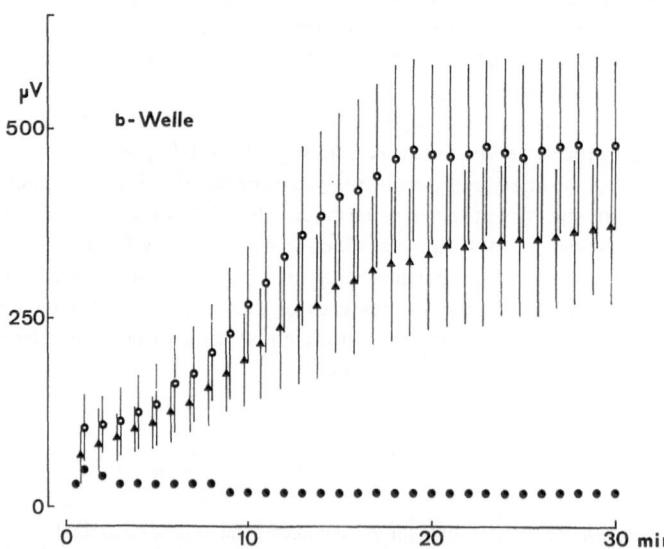

FIG. 1. Mean and standard deviation of the overall amplitude of the positive wave of 20 normal subjects (○), 10 achromats (▲), and 1 hemeralope (●) during ERG recovery. Grass intensity 4.

1st to 5th minute

$$x_N = 101,44 + 1,51\,t \qquad R = 0,279$$
$$(0,55)$$
$$x_A = 64,58 + 9,53\,t \qquad R = 0,384$$
$$(3,31)$$

In this section the slope of the recovery curve of normal subjects is less steep than that of achromats. In the 5th minute the difference between the amplitudes of both groups becomes a minimum.

6th to 15th minute

$$x_N = 147,94 + 23,87\,t \qquad R = 0,714$$
$$(1,43)$$
$$x_A = 117,44 + 15,85\,t \qquad R = 0,661$$
$$(1,48)$$

In this part of the recovery curve the rise of amplitudes in normal subjects is about 50% higher than that of achromats. Compared to the first section, there is a significant difference between the slopes of curves in normal subjects, whereas in the course of ERG recovery in achromats no break can be shown.

16th to 20th minute

The maximal difference between the amplitudes of both groups is attained towards the end of this interval.

21st to 30th minute

The courses of both groups show no significant deviation from a parallel to the t-axis.

2.) negative wave of normal subjects and achromats (fig. 2)

1st to 30th minute

$$x_N = 67,40 + 17,65\,t - 0,3712\,t^2 \qquad R = 0,570$$
$$(1,65) \qquad (0,05)$$
$$x_A = 41,65 + 13,47\,t - 0,2885\,t^2 \qquad R = 0,691$$
$$(1,27) \qquad (0,04)$$

The slope of the global course of ERG recovery as well as the amplitudes are higher in normal subjects than in achromats.

1st to 5th minute

$$x_N = 77,55 + 12,85\,t \qquad R = 0,437$$
$$(2,67)$$
$$x_A = 40,30 + 11,90\,t \qquad R = 0,344$$
$$(4,70)$$

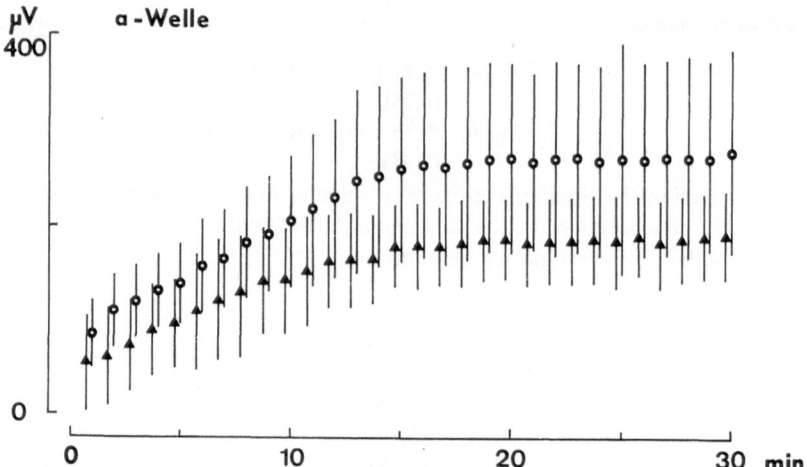

FIG. 2. Mean and standard deviation of the overall amplitude of the negative wave of 20 normal subjects (○) and 10 achromats (▲) during ERG recovery. Grass intensity 4.

In this part of recovery the slope as well as the amplitudes are higher in normal subjects.

6th to 15th minute

$$x_N = 115,4 + 12,86 \, t \qquad R = 0,502$$
$$(1,58)$$
$$x_A = 84,53 + 9,25 \, t \qquad R = 0,461$$
$$(1,80)$$

Compared with the first section of ERG recovery, neither a change in the slope of the curve of normal subjects nor in that of achromats can be proved; that means, there is no recognizable break in the course.

16th to 20th minute

Judging by the diagram, the steady state is attained within this interval. Calculations reveal a minimal increase.

21st to 30th minute

No deviation from a parallel to the t-axis can be proved for the course of recovery in both groups.

3.) positive wave of the hemeralope

The recovery takes the characteristic course of an increase during the first minute followed by a decrease, and attains its steady state before the 10th minute.

56

4.) negative wave of the hemeralope

The course of recovery does not differ from that of normal subjects.

5.) curve of the difference between the positive wave in the ERG of normal subjects and that of achromats compared with the ERG recovery curve of the hemeralope's positive wave.

$$x_D = 5,33 + 7,06 \ t - 0,00001 \ t^5 \qquad R = 0,956$$
$$(0,47)$$

x_D overall amplitudes of the ERG of normal subjects minus those of achromats.

Apart from the first to the fourth minute the curve of difference is higher than the amplitudes of the hemeralope's positive wave.

DISCUSSION

The basis for the validity of the following considerations is the assumption, that the normal electroretinogram represents the result of the summation of the potentials of rods and cones, whereas one of both components is lacking in the examined anomalous electroretinograms. If this is true, under the experimental conditions used, the ERG amplitudes of the achromat must be smaller than those of the normal subject. The difference, roughly resembling a normal photopic potential, should be comparable with the hemeralope's ERG amplitudes.

Statistical analysis of the achromat's ERG and the normal ERG support the first part of the above stated assumption and show that this is true during the whole course of recovery of the positive as well as the negative wave of ERG. These findings affirm a statement of GOURAS: 'In this abnormality, nature seems to have simply substracted the cone contribution from the normal ERG.'

However, the addition of the potentials of the achromate and those of the hemeralope does not result in normal ERG amplitudes. The positive potential of the hemeralope is smaller than the difference curve between the ERG amplitudes of normal subjects and those of achromats. Theoretically, the values of the difference curve could be higher due to an impaired rod contribution to the achromat's positive potential. This assumption appears to be very unlikely, since no symptom indicates insufficiency of the rod system in achromat. On the other hand, in congenital night blindness a series of photopic abnormalities (KRILL & MARTIN) is consistent with the hypothesis of a defect in the wiring diagram of the cone system. This defect could also account for the amplitude reduction of the x-wave of the hemeralope. From the normal appearance of the hemeralope's a-wave during ERG recovery and in the dark adapted state an intact receptor might be inferred. In contrast to the achromat's ERG, which is characterized by a simple lack of the cone contribution, the pattern of the lesion in the hemeralope's ERG is of a more complex nature.[*]

[*] This simplified working hypothesis neglects other influences upon ERG amplitudes, e.g. oscillatory potentials, latency differences, neural interaction, etc.

ABSTRACT

In the complete form of congenital total color blindness positive as well as negative overall amplitudes are smaller than those of normal ERG. By methods of regression analysis this was proved to be correct during ERG recovery as well as in the dark adapted state. Furthermore, it is shown that the positive potential in Schubert-Bornschein's form of congenital night blindness appears to be smaller than the normal x-wave. This result supports the assumption of a defect in the wiring diagram of the cone system in congenital night blindness.

REFERENCES

BENNETT, C. A. & FRANKLIN, N. L. Statistical analysis in chemistry and the chemical industry. John Wiley & Sons. Appendix 6A (1954).

CHRISTENSEN, L. R. Simultaneous statistical inference in a normal multiple linear regression model. *JASA* 68: *457-461* (1973).

FREY, R. G., HEILIG, P. & THALER, A. Die Dunkeladaptation der Achromaten. *Albrecht v. Graefes Arch. Ophthal.* 186: *55-65* (1973).

GOODMAN, G. & BORNSCHEIN, H. Comparative electroretinographic studies in congenital night blindness and total colour blindness. *Arch. Ophth.* 58: *174-182* (1957).

GOURAS, P. Electroretinography: Some basic principles. *Invest. Ophthal.* 9: *557-569* (1970).

HEILIG, P. & THALER, A. Minimum duration of dark adaptation in clinical ERG. ISCERG Symp. Pisa 1970. In: Wirth, A.: Symposium on electroretinography. Pacini/Pisa.

HEILIG, P., THALER, A. & BORNSCHEIN, H. Slow potentials of ERG in hemeralopia congenita. Xth ISCERG Symp. Los Angeles 1972. Doc. Ophthal. Proc. Series 2: 219-224. W. Junk/The Hague (1973).

KRILL, A. E. & MARTIN, D. Photopic abnormalities in congenital stationary night blindness. *Invest. Ophthal.* 10: *625-636* (1971).

SCHUBERT, G. & BORNSCHEIN, H. Beitrag zur Analyse des menschlichen Elektroretinogramms. *Ophthalmologica*, 123: *396-413* (1952).

Author's address:

IInd Eye Department
and
Computer Center of the
University of Vienna
Vienna
Austria

DIFFERENTIATION OF CONE AND ROD RESPONSE IN THE HUMAN ERG BY MEANS OF COLOUR FREQUENCY CHARACTERISTICS.

A. C. KOOIJMAN, L. P. M. BOS & L. TE STRAKE

(Groningen)

ABSTRACT

Vector retinography gives on line both phase and amplitude of the-ERG response on a flickering stimulus. With the described method it is possible to obtain:
1. with the right choice of the stimulus frequency separated responses of rods and cones.
2. in 1,5 minutes a colour sensitivity curve of the responding receptor system.
3. simple shaped colour sensitivity curves, which enables everyone to recognize the difference between cone and rod response.

In clinical ERG measurements one prefers to measure the separate responses of rods and cones to judge their functional condition. Methods to obtain this are based on the differences between the sensitivity characteristics of cones and rods.

The most important differences in this context are:
1. The rod system is sensitive to much lower light intensities than the cone system (GOURAS & GUNKEL, 1964; WALD 1945)
2. The colour sensitivities of rods and cones differ very much (PADMOS & NORREN, 1971; WALD, 1945)
3. The maximum flicker fusion frequency of rods is about 20 cps. This is much lower than the maximum flicker fusion frequency of cones, which is about 50–80 cps (GOURAS & GUNKEL, 1964; KARPE, 1958; SOKOL & RIGGS, 1971; STERNHEIM & CAVONIUS, 1972)

These differences have been shown to exist both in psycho-physical and in electroretinographic experiments. ERG flash response measurements, which are based on the first two differences need an extended legend to prevent exchange with each other (GOURAS, 1970).

Measurement of the maximum flicker fusion frequency at various intensities gives an easily recognizable result, but is a very time consuming procedure (KARPE, 1958; ZETTERSTRÖM, 1964) If there is a primary interest in the amplitude and not in the form of the response, it is possible to measure ERG responses with the use of a lock-in voltmeter (PADMOS & NORREN, 1972) Separation of rod and cone response can be obtained by stimulating the retina with various flicker frequencies. Identification of the rod and cone response is possible if we measure the colour sensitivity curve of the response mechanism.

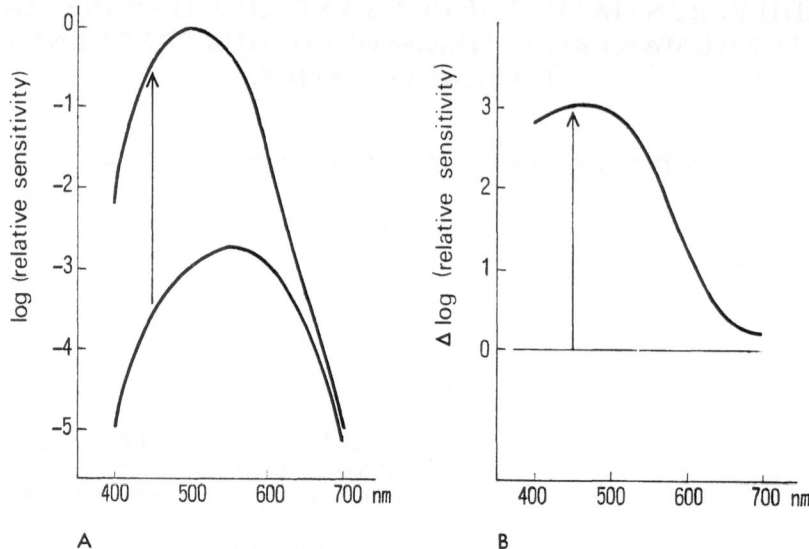

FIG. 1. A. General psychophysical curves of cones and rods. B. The logarithmic difference between the rod sensitivity and the cone sensitivity.

Recognition is facilitated by recording only the difference of the colour sensitivity with Wald's extra foveal cone sensitivity (Fig. 1).

METHOD

The eye is stimulated over a 50 degree field. The light source is a tungsten lamp.
The monochromatic colour of the stimulus is controlled by a motor driven
linear interference wedge. The wavelength depends on the area where the light
passes through the wedge. During a recording, the stimulus colour changes in
1,5 minutes from blue to red and in 1,5 minutes all the way back. The current of
the lamp is controlled by the position of the colour wedge in the lightpath in
such a way that the energy of the monochromatic stimulus is the inverse of
Wald's extra foveal cone sensitivity curve (WALD, 1945). A subject with normal
colour vision sees all the colours with equal luminosity. The energy of the light
has been measured with a thermopile (Hewlett Packard model 8334A) in
combination with a radiant flux meter (Hewlett Packard model 8330A) or a
lock-in amplifier system (Brookdeal model 467, 411, 422).

A supplementary control of the light stimulus intensity is possible with a
servo driven neutral density wedge. It contains two circular Agfa-Gevaert
wedges with a collective span of 5 density units. The frequency of the stimulus
is controlled by a rotating sectored disc, which chops the light stimulus. The
ERG is recorded with a 100 diopters contact glass with two built-in silver electrodes. After preamplification, the signal is fed into a double lock-in amplifier
system (Brookdeal model 467, 411, 422) or into an averager (CAT 400 C).

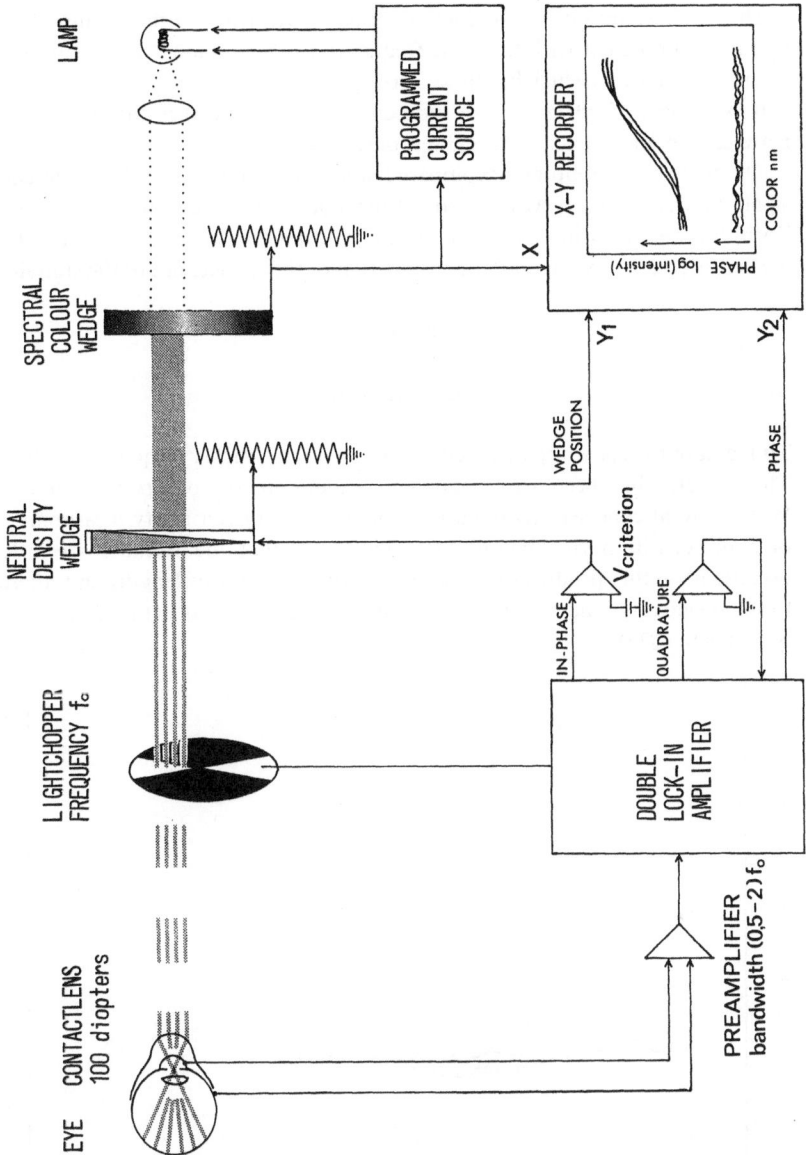

FIG. 2. Block diagram of the stimulating and measuring system. Stimulus frequency is controlled by a rotating sectored disc. Colour depends on the position of the interference wedge in the lightpath. During an experiment the colour changes in 1.5 minutes from blue to red and in 1.5 minutes all the way back. The current of the lamp is controlled by the position of the colour wedge in such a way that the spectral energy curve of the stimulus is the inverse of Wald's extrafoveal cone sensitivity curve. The amplitude of the ERG is compared with a preset criterion voltage and the difference signal serves to control the motor driven neutral density wedge. Position of the grey wedge and phase shift between stimulus and response are recorded on an x-y-recorder as a function of the wavelength of the stimulus.

61

The in-phase output of the lock-in system gives us the r.m.s. value of the response component with the same frequency as the stimulus. The quadrature output gives a value which has to be zero.

If it deviates from zero, the difference serves to correct the phase shift between reference signal and ERG response.

The response amplitude is compared with a criterion value. The difference signal between them serves to control the motor driven neutral density wedge. Both, the wedge position which is linear with the density, and the phase shift are recorded on an x-y recorder as a function of the wavelength of the stimulus.

RESULTS

Cone response

To measure the cone response, selectively, we used a flicker frequency of 30 hz. The stimulus has been made equally luminous at all colours according to Wald's foveal cone sensitivity curve. An ERG colour sensitivity measurement of a subject with normal colour vision gives a straight line on the x-y-recorder because his retina produces a criterion response at all wavelengths and, there-fore, no signal is generated to shift the neutral density wedge (Fig. 3) (PADMOS & NORREN, 1972).

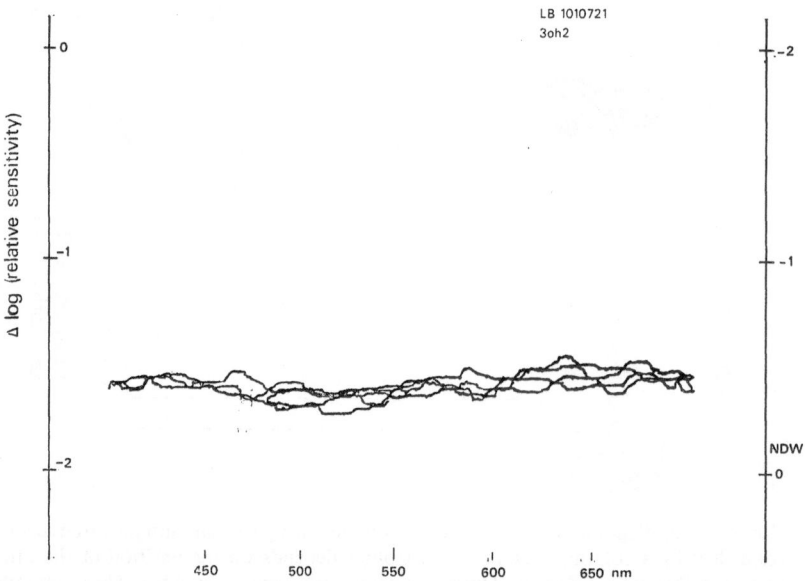

FIG. 3. Colour sensitivity measurement of the cones. The retina is stimulated with a 30 hz flickering light. This figure shows a recording of the position of the neutral density wedge. The grey wedge has hardly shifted because the stimulus has been made nearly equal luminous for cones at all wavelenghts. The programmed equal luminosity stimulus has not yet been adjusted perfectly to Wald's extra foveal cone curve, there-fore, some corrections have still to be made on this recording. The criterion response amplitude was set at 2.8 μVpp.

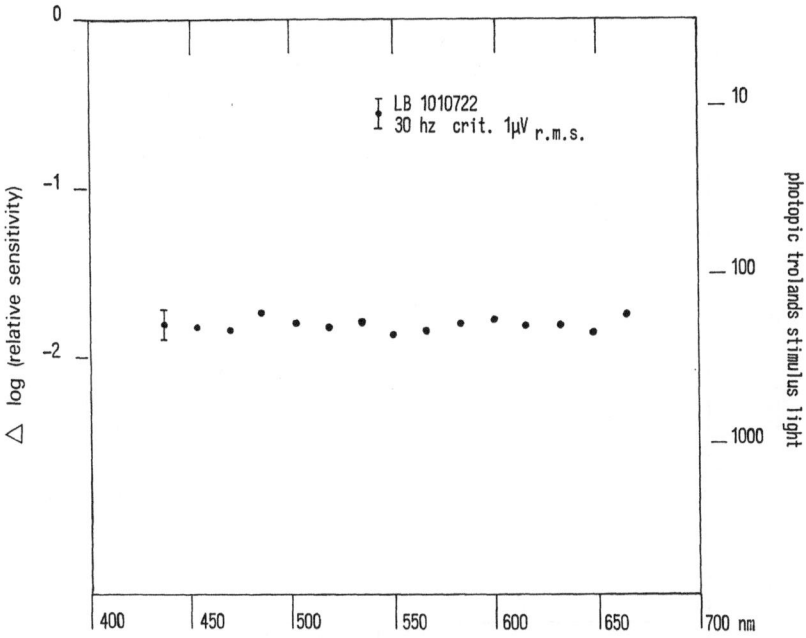

FIG. 4. Colour sensitivity measurement of the cones. Data points from the recording in Figure 3 are corrected for the deviations between the stimulus and Wald's 8° curve. A straight horizontal response line means a colour sensitivity which is identical to Wald's 8° curve.

If the recorded line is curved, it means that the subject has a sensitivity curve which differs from the standard cone sensitivity. The curve in Fig. 3 is nearly straight. Since the programmed equal luminosity stimulus has not yet been adjusted perfectly to Wald's extra foveal cone curve, we still have to make some corrections on the recording (Fig. 4) .The corrected data points are situated on a straight line. This method shows how much a subject's colour sensitivity differs from the normal cone sensitivity. Now it is, of course, very attractive to measure a colour blind person. The most conspicuous results are to be expected in a protanope (Fig. 5). The stimulus frequency is maintained at 30 hz. The dispersion between the data points is larger than in the former recording. The reason for this is that we used a lower response criterion, which was 0.6 μV, and, in addition, the subject was unexperienced. The data points give the difference between the sensitivity of the protanope subject and Wald's extra foveal cone sensitivity. In this figure we obtain the best fit with the curve which represents the difference between the psychophysical sensitivity of a protanope and the foveal cone sensitivity. I think this was to be expected, because the psychophysical colourblind sensitivity curves are measured with small foveal stimulus fields.

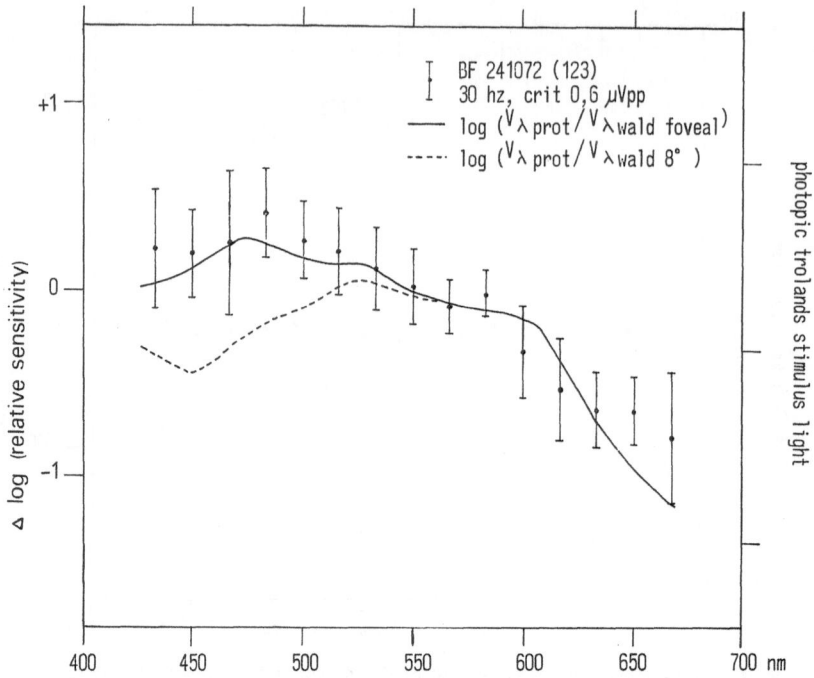

FIG. 5. Colour sensitivity measurement of a protanope. Stimulus frequency 30 hz and criterion response 0.6 μV. The measured data points are determined electroretinographically and indicate the difference between the colour sensitivity of the protanope and Wald's extrafoveal curve. The curves are the differences between the protanope colour sensitivity from Pitt (1935) with Wald's extra-foveal sensitivity (dashed) and with Wald's foveal sensitivity (drawn).

Rod response

Now we go back to our primary goal to separate the cone and rod response. To stimulate the rods we have to use a lower flicker frequency. The result of a measurement with a 4 hz stimulus is given in Fig. 6. The response amplitude was about 15 μV. Our data points fit well with the difference curve of cones and rods.

Can we be sure we only measured the response of the rod system? To check this, we have measured on an averager the response form on a 5 hz stimulus. We only did it at wavelengths of 450 and 650 nm (Fig. 7 a & b.). The subject had been dark adapted before measurement. At 450 nm the response form is nearly sine shaped and there is no change in the shape at higher amplitudes. At 650 nm at low amplitudes the response is identical to the response to blue light, but at higher amplitudes we see an extra component. That the slower sine shaped component is the rod response, and the faster component the cone response, we can conclude from these recordings and, in addition, from the recordings in Fig. 7c in which the slow component vanishes if the stimulus is

64

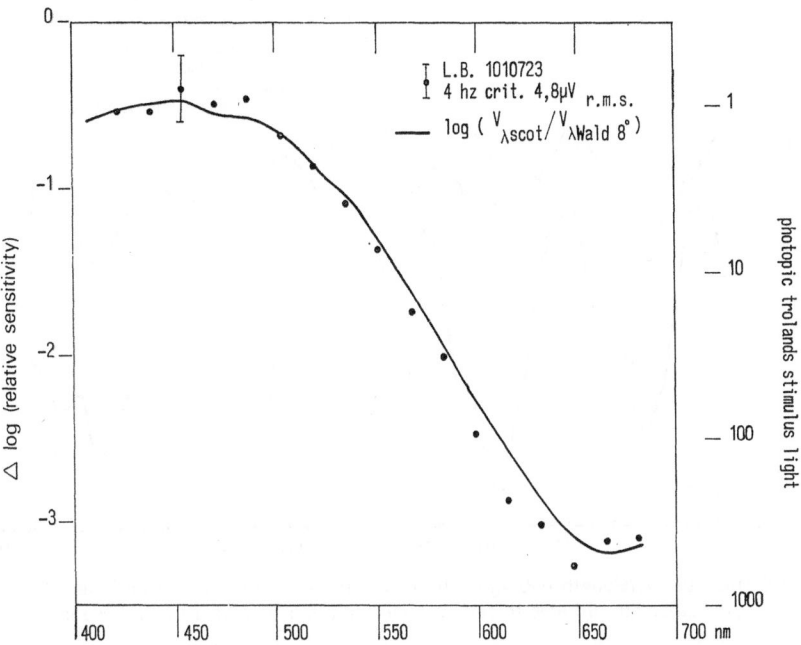

FIG. 6. Colour sensitivity measurements of the rods. Stimulus frequency 4hz, criterion response amplitude 14 μV. Data points are the average of 4 recordings and indicate the measured difference between rod sensitivity and Wald's extra foveal cone sensitivity. Drawn curve is the difference between C.I.E. rod sensitivity and Wald's extra foveal cone sensitivity.

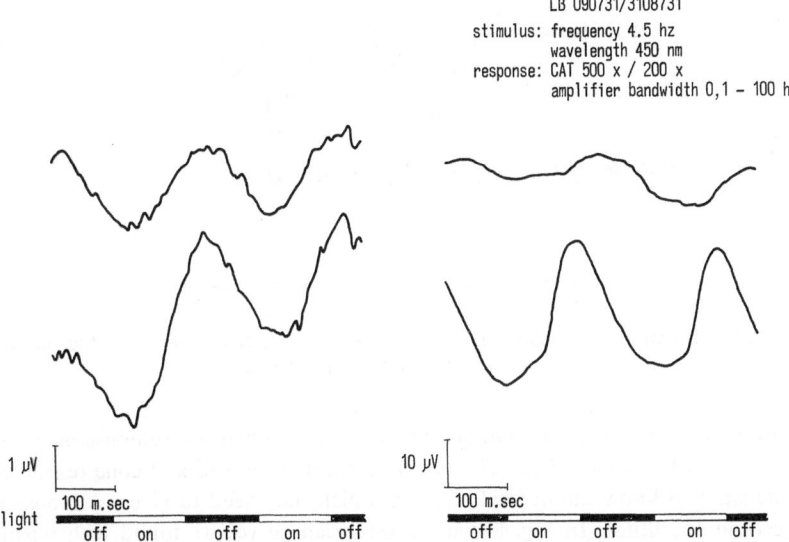

FIG. 7. Waveform of the ERG response on a 4 hz stimulus. (a) Stimulus wavelenght 450 nm. The waveform is at all recorded response amplitudes sine shaped.

65

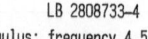

LB 2808733–4
stimulus: frequency 4,5 hz
wavelenght 650 nm
response: CAT 200 x
amplifier bandwidth 0,1 – 100 hz

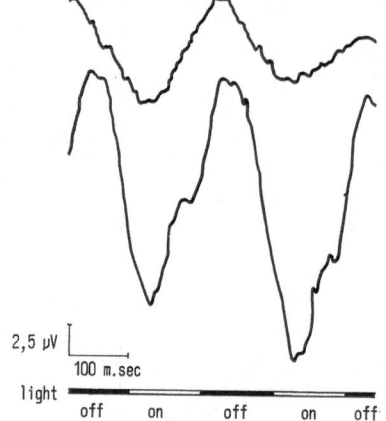

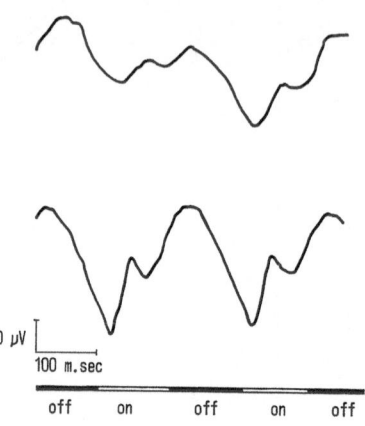

2,5 µV

100 m.sec

light

off   on   off   on   off

10 µV

100 m.sec

off   on   off   on   off

(b) Stimulus wavelength 650 nm. The waveform is at low amplitudes sine shaped. At higher am-plitudes there is a faster component added to the response.

LB 1207731
stimulus: frequency 4,5 hz
wavelength 650 nm
response: CAT 250 x
amplifier bandwidth 0,1 – 1000 hz

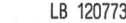

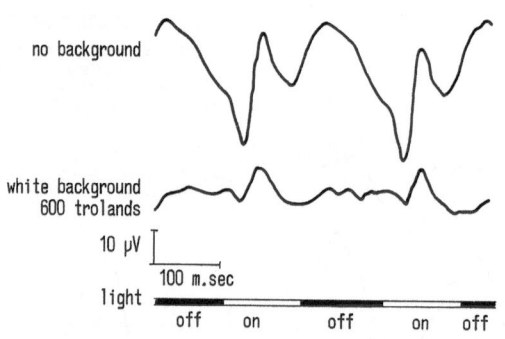

no background

white background
600 trolands

10 µV

100 m.sec

light

off   on   off   on   off

(c) Stimulus wavelength 650 nm. Slow sine shaped response vanishes if the stimulus is given on a white background.

given on a white background. So, we see there is only a rod response on a 5 hz stimulus of low intensity. After having separated the rod and cone responses, we want to know the normal stimulus which they need to give a response of certain amplitude. In Fig. 8 you see the mean curves we found with normal subjects. The subjects had been dark adapted before the measurement.

The response amplitude was about 1,5 µV. In this figure it is striking that the

66

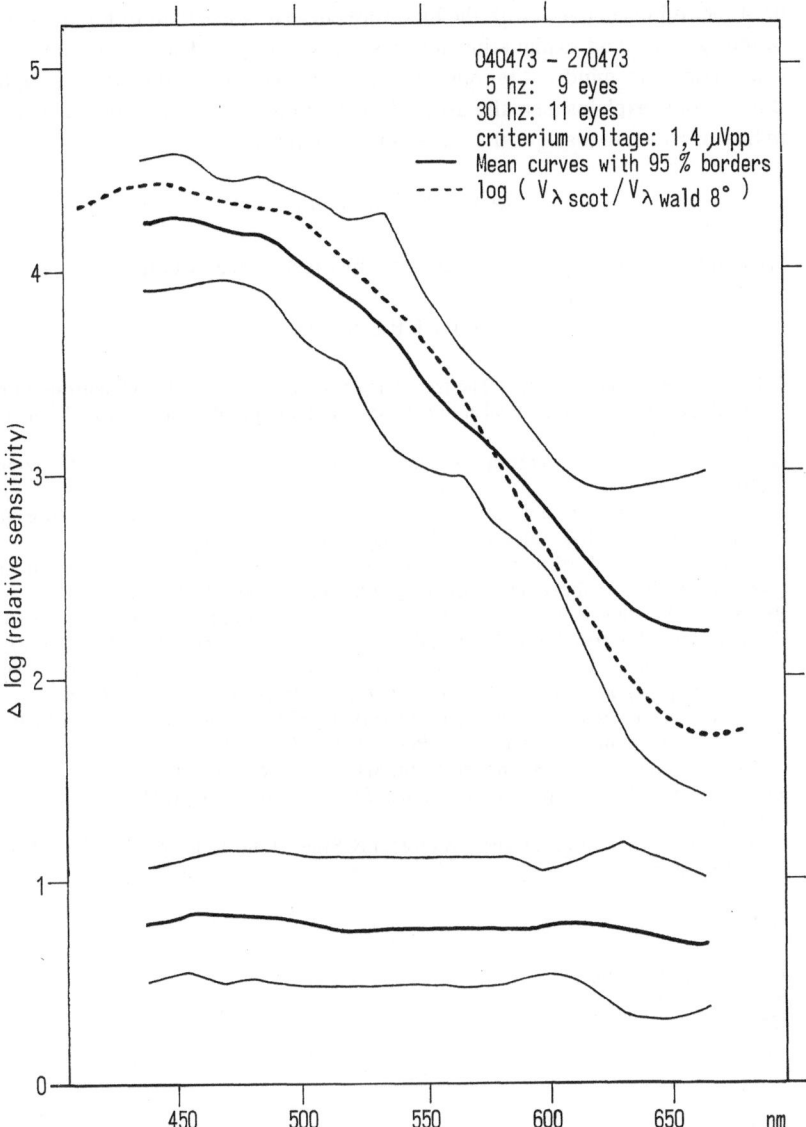

FIG. 8. Mean colour sensitivity curves with 95% probability borders at stimulus frequencies of 30 hz and 5 hz. Subjects had been dark adapted during 20 minutes before the measurements. The criterion response amplitude was 1.4 μV. The curves indicate the difference between measured sensitivity and Wald's extra foveal sensitivity. Dashed curve is the difference between the C.I.E. rod sensitivity and Wald's extra foveal cone sensitivity.

fit of the rod mean curve with the literature curve is worse than in Figure 6. We cannot give a good explanation for this difference, yet. The first explanation which comes to mind is the influence of the bandwidth of the stimulus light. But this only explains a small part of the deviation. Further investigations have to be performed to teach us the cause of the difference.

ACKNOWLEDGEMENTS

We thank Mr. ROZE and Mr DAMHOF for their technical assistance.

REFERENCES

GOURAS, P. & R. D. GUNKEL. The frequency response of normal, rod achromat and nyctalope ERGs to sinusoidal monochromatic light stimulation. *Doc. Ophthal.* 18: *137-150* (1964).

GOURAS, P. Electroretinography: Some basic principles. *Invest. Ophthalm.* 9: *557-569* (1970).

KARPE, G. Flicker Electroretinography. A standardized method of examination for clinical purposes. *Acta Belgica* 18: *Conc. Ophthal.*, 607 (1958).

PADMOS, P. & D. V. NORREN. Cone spectral sensivity and chromatic adaption as revealed by human flicker electroretinography. *Vision Res.* 11: *27-42* (1971).

PADMOS, P. & NORREN, D. V. The vector voltmeter as a tool to measure electroretinogram spectral sensitivity and dark adaption. *Invest. Ophthalm.* 11: *783-788* (1972).

SOKOL, S. & RIGGS, L. A. Electrical and psychophysical responses of the human visual system to periodic variation of luminance. *Invest. Ophthalm.* 10: *171-180* (1971).

STERNHEIM, C. E. & CAVONIUS, C. R. Sensitivity of the human ERG and VECP to sinusoidally modulated light. *Vision Res.* 12: *1685-1695* (1972).

WALD, G. Human vision and the spectrum. *Science* 101: *653-658* (1945).

ZETTERSRÖM, B. Some experience of clinical flicker electroretinography. *Doc. Ophthal.* 18: *315-329* (1964).

PITT, F. G. H. In: Colour Science, Wyszecki & Stiles, John Wiley & Sons, New York, p. 408 (1935).

Author's address:

Dept. of Ophthalmology
State University
Groningen
The Netherlands

CONE DARK ADAPTATION: COMPARISON OF PSYCHOPHYSICS AND VECTOR-RETINOGRAPHY*

DIRK V. NORREN

(Soesterberg)

Dark adaptation of the cones has, till now, mainly been measured with psychophysical techniques. It yielded a curve in which the recovery of visual sensitivity was plotted against time after offset of a bleaching background. With the introduction of the vector-voltmeter method (PADMOS & NORREN, 1972) it became possible to measure the recovery of sensitivity with electroretinography. Before that, only the recovery of the response to a fixed stimulus could be measured. Although retinography has to cope with technical difficulties as the limited time a subject can wear a contactglass and the unwanted noise because of eyemovements and blinks, the new ERG method has certain advantages above the classical psychophysical technique. First, it is an objective method. Recording under general anaesthesia is possible so that measurement of new categories of subjects, such as babies, small children and mentally retarded subjects, become possible. Research on animals is also greatly facilitated, compared to animal psychophysics. Second, the ERG method is fast. In the first minute, especially, the recording is far more accurate than what an unexperienced subject perform with the psychophysical method. Finally, the ERG method can be made completely automatic: no actions of personnel required during the measurement itself.

We now need to establish the exact relationship between the results of the psychophysical techniques and the ERG method.

In the psychophysical literature on cone dark adaptation mostly a small foveal stimulus was used, flashing on and off with a frequency around 1 Hz. The ERG method requires a wide field to obtain recordable responses, and a high stimulus frequency to suppress the rod responses and to obtain a better signal to noise ratio. We, therefore, use both methods to study the influence of several parameters: the stimulus field width, the stimulus frequency and, in order to sort out the contribution of the different cone systems, the colour of stimulus and background.

A further question is: what is the clinical significance of cone dark adaptation curves? Till now clinical adaptometry did not concentrate upon the cone branch. Therefore, this question remains largely unanswered.

One early finding is that the drug Halothane has severe influence on cone pigment regeneration (NORREN & PADMOS, 1973).

* A detailed account of this study is submitted to Vision Research.

The vector voltmeter method was described by PADMOS & NORREN (1972). Briefly, the measuring beam is chopped with a sectored disk at a fixed frequency. The ERG is signal led to the vector-voltmeter where the amplitude of the signal at the chopping frequency and phase relative to the phase of the input are derived. These values are displayed on an inkwriter. In addition, the amplitude signal is led to a neutral density wedge control box. At the control box a pre-set criterion voltage is selected and the difference signal between this and the ERG amplitude is fed to the wedge drive-motor. As a consequence, the wedge is moved so as to maintain a constant ERG amplitude. The wedge position is recorded on the ink-writer.

The light source for both the stimulus and the background beam was a Xenon-arc (Osram, XBO 450 W) powered from a light-current stabilized power supply (Heinzinger). The measuring beam passed through a Schott interference filter (15 nm bandwidth) of 577 or 456 nm, the background beam through Agfa neutral density filters and eventually a yellow (Jena OG 550) colour filter. The measuring beam subtended 45°, the background 70°, and both were seen in Maxwellian view. For the psychophysical experiments the neutral density wedge in the stimulus beam was set to move, with a constant speed, in the direction of high transmission. When the subject pressed a button the direction of rotation was reversed. He could, therefore, continually adjust the intensity of the stimulus such that the flicker was just visible. Three subjects were used with normal colour vision. A dental impression and a brow rest provided their head fixation. For the ERG experiments they wore a scleral contact lens with Ag-AgCl electrodes.

RESULTS

In all cases the dark adaptation curves obtained could be reasonably fitted with an exponential function. This made it possible to characterize the curves by one parameter, the time constant (time to reach the 1/e value).

1. Psychophysics

The small foveal field (1.3°), low frequency stimulus condition yielded time constants of about 90 sec. With increasing stimulus frequency no systematic change in time constant was found. With a large stimulus field (45°) the time constants were significantly shorter. The values ranged from 40–70 sec. Fig. 1 provides an example. Again, changing the stimulus frequency did not systematically influence the results. With large field stimuli the response is mainly determined by the extra-foveal cones. Thus, do extra foveal cones recover faster than foveal ones? Most probably, since with a 2 degree stimulus field, presented extra-foveally, equally fast recovery times were found as with large field stimuli.

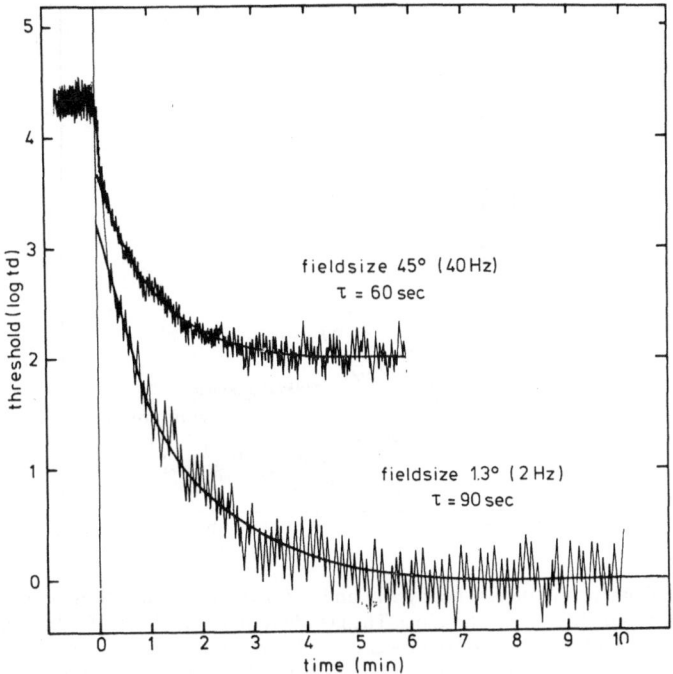

FIG. 1. Psychophysical dark adaptation of the red, green cones after bleaching during two minutes with a 10^6 td yellow light. The lower curve was recorded with a 1.3° stimulus of 577 nm, flickering with a frequency of 2 Hz. The background was 5°. The upper curve was taken with a 45 degree stimulus, flickering at 40 Hz. The background was 70° in that case.

2. Vector-retinography

Only a large field stimulus (45°) and high frequency flicker was used. Stimulus frequencies of 25 and 40 Hz did not yield significantly different time constants, but the results of the 40 Hz condition showed better reproduceability and lower error. Fig. 2 shows an example of recovery curves determined with the ERG and the psychophysical method.

3. Different cone systems

All results mentioned hitherto apply to the combined response of the red and green sensitive cone systems since a yellow stimulus was used and a yellow bleaching light. The blue sensitive cone system was measured with a blue stimulus together with a strong yellow background to suppress the response of the long wavelength systems. So, after all cone systems had been bleached by a white background, a yellow filter was inserted in the background beam. From that moment on only, the blue cones could recover. The results obtained in this condition were significantly different from the red, green cone results, in that

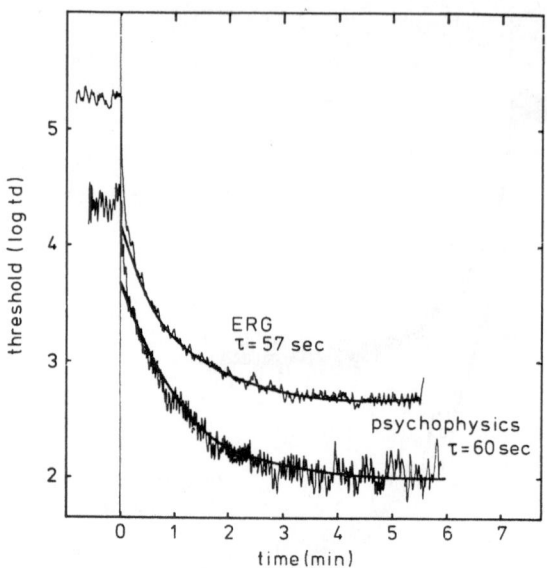

FIG. 2. Comparison of psychophysical and ERG results for identical stimulus conditions (45°, 40 Hz, 577 nm stimulus). The preadaptation was 10^6 td of yellow light given during 2 minutes. In case of the ERG curve the response criterion was 2 μV. For the psychophysical curve just visible flicker was the criterion.

the recovery required considerably more time. In the psychophysical experiments a time constant of about 140 sec was found for the foveal stimuli and 120 sec for the extra foveal ones.

With the ERG method great difficulties were met. The strong yellow background causes a lot of noise, probably because of avoidance reactions. Moreover, the blue cone response shows an early saturation so that only very low response criteria could be used. Another problem is that the blue cone system has a low high frequency response. We had, therefore, to work with a much lower stimulus frequency (8 Hz) than in case of the red, green system. However, the results obtained on one subject confirmed the psychophysical findings: a long time constant was found. Fig. 3 gives examples of a psychophysical and an ERG curve.

CONCLUSIONS

The aim of this study was to compare dark adaptation curves obtained with two different techniques: psychophysics and vector-retinography. The experiments showed that identical results can be obtained provided the experimental circumstances are the same. With a wide field and high frequency stimulus both methods yield dark adaptation curves with a time constant of about 65 sec. With small field foveal stimuli the recovery takes more time: time constants of

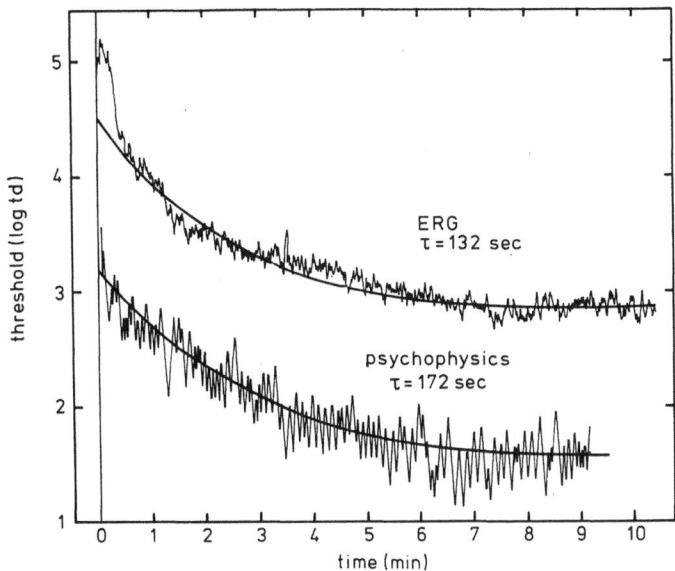

FIG. 3. Recovery of the isolated blue cone system recorded with both the psycho physical and the ERG method. First, a 2 min white (10^6td) bleach was given; at t = 0 a yellow filter was inserted into the background beam. The stimulus frequency was 8 Hz. The response criterion 1 μV. Stimulus field width 45°, background 70°. For clarity reasons the ERG curve was shifted 1 log unit upwards.

about 90 sec were found. In a condition in which only the blue cone system contributes to the response all time constants are much longer: 140 sec for foveal stimuli, 130 sec for extra foveal ones. Thus the measuring method has no influence, but the experimental conditions determine the time course of dark adaptation.

REFERENCES

PADMOS, P. & NORREN, D. V. The vector-voltmeter as a tool to measure electroretinogram spectral sensitivity and dark adaptation. *Invest. Ophthalmol.* 11: *783-788* (1972).
NORREN, D. V. & PADMOS, P. Halothane retards dark adaptation Proceedings XIth ISCERG symposium, This volume: *00-00* (1974).

Author's address:

Institute for Perception
Kampweg 5
Soesterberg
The Netherlands

ANALYSIS AND SYNTHESIS OF THE SCOTOPIC E.R.G. (RABBIT)

J. M. THIJSSEN, W. M. VAN DEN MUNCKHOF & W. M. BRAAKHUIS

(Nijmegen)

INTRODUCTION

The electroretinogram has been measured for diagnostic purposes already for several decades. The analysis is generally restricted to the characterization of the response to stimulation of the eye by short duration light flashes. This characterization generally includes the measurement of peak amplitudes and culmination times. The introduction of computer-assisted analyzing methods, e.g. by POTTS and co-workers (1971, 1972) although very useful, has not resulted in an essentially new approach, since they only use the computer to determine the above mentioned parameters of the E.R.G.

The purpose of our study is to try and find a method of analysis that will yield the parameters of the constituent processes of the E.R.G. and then to synthetize the response to various kinds of stimuli. This cannot be done without prior knowledge of the number of processes involved and of some of the characteristics of the separate responses. This can be illustrated in the following way: the responses of the processes may summate with opposite sign, or with differing latencies, thus resulting in a rather complex overall response; e.g. when two responses both containing a single maximum are summed with opposite sign a response may result with a negative and a positive maximum and two zero crossings. The maxima are governed by the first derivative of the responses and only indirectly by the maxima of the original responses.

We have taken the classical scheme of GRANIT (1933), as shown in Fig. 1, as a working hypothesis for the analysis of the E.R.G. signal. The scheme that has been recently presented by RODIECK (1972), although it is very important, is not essentially different from GRANIT's approach. So the problem of the number of processes may be considered to be solved. The next problem, the identification of the processes with the various types of cells in the retina, will be discussed below.

The experiments in this study were done with rabbits, because of the predominance of rods in their retinas and also because of the simple experimental arrangement which allowed us to work without general aneasthesia. Qualitative extrapolation to the human E.R.G. will be possible, but exact human data will have to be obtained from a separate study on the human E.R.G.

75

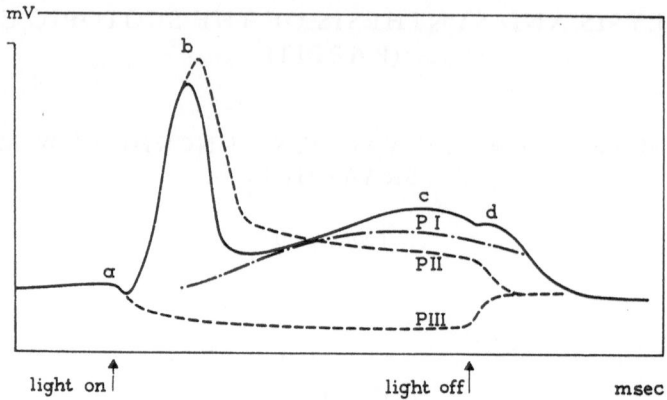

FIG. 1. The three component scheme of GRANIT for the electroretinographic response to a long duration flash. (GRANIT, 1933).

METHODS

Preparation of the animal

The experiments have been performed with rabbits without general anaesthesia. The body of the animal is tightly fixed with bandages to a small plank, and the head is pressed upon a metal bow. The eye muscles are relaxed by a retro-bulbar injection of 2% xylocain solution. The eye lids are paralyzed by intra-muscular depots of the same anaesthetic. Additionally, both corneas are locally anaesthetized by novesine (0.2%) and the pupils are dilated artificially (mydria-ticum, Roche).

EQUIPMENT

Both eyes of the animal are covered with a scleral contact lens (HENKES – VAN BALEN, infant lens), containing a chloralized silver wire. Electrical contact of the wire with the cornea is ensured by filling the lens with saline solution or with methocel (R). The electrodes within the two lenses are the active electrode and the reference electrode, and are connected with a direct coupled amplifier (band-width DC to 220 Hz). The grounding electrode is connected to one of the ear lobes. The amplifier is reset to zero-level automatically by the trigger pulse of the optical stimulator. This is very useful when one wants to average many responses with an averaging computer. We use a Data Retrieval Computer (Nuclear Chicago) for analog to digital conversion and for averaging. The 400 data registers of this DRC are read on papertape and transferred to a digital computer system (PDP-9, Digital Equipment Corp.) for further analysis.

76

The stimulator consists of an unfocussed cathode ray tube (CRT) with a very fast phosphor (Ferranti, type CL 64) and a lens that projects the light spot on a diffusing screen, subtending 90° visual angle. One scleral contact lens has a pupil of 8 mm diameter, the other (reference) is completely obscured. The CRT is driven by a current stabilized device that yields a light output proportional to the input voltage over a 50 dB range. This device can be driven by a function generator, so any kind of time pattern, e.g. pulse, square, sine, etc. can be generated. In this study we have used 10 msec. pulses exclusively.

THE THREE PROCESSES MODEL

The scheme of GRANIT (1933) displays the responses of the three constituent processes to stimulation with a relatively long duration flash. The responses to a short flash or light pulse, will be different. For a particular kind of mechanism, i.e. a linear system, the pulse response equals the first derivative of the response to a long duration flash. When the pulse duration is smaller than a particular critical value (Bloch's time in psychophysics), i.e. t_B, the response wil be independent of the flash duration, provided that the energy is kept constant. This time (t_B) has been determined by TROELSTRA (1964) for the human scotopic E.R.G. and equals 20 msec. So stimulus durations shorter than 20 msec are equivalent to the theoretical Dirac-pulse of infinitely short duration (or impulse).

The P III process of the scheme of Granit is mostly identified with the response of the receptor cells (c.f. BROWN, 1968, and RODIECK, 1972). HAGINS et al. (1970) described the extracellularly intraretinally measured impulse response of the receptor cells (albino rat) by a function:

$$f(t) = a\ t\ exp(-bt) \qquad (1)$$

where
a = gain factor
b = cut-off frequency (sec^{-1})

It is reasonable to assume that the scotopic response of the rabbit photo-receptors is very similar to the response in the rat retina. Additional evidence for the kind of impulse response as given in equation (1) can be found in the literature. BAYLOR et al. (1970) investigated the response of cones in the Turtle, SPEKREYSE & NORTON (1970) the S-potential of the goldfish retina, STARK (1968) the abdominal ganglion response of the Crayfish. The results of these authors can be summarized in a general formula describing the impulse response of the receptor cells:

$$F(t) = a\ (t-t_1)^c\ exp\{-b\ (t-t_1)\} \qquad (2)$$

a = gain factor	c = constant
b = cut-off frequency (sec^{-1})	t_1 = latency time

The value of c, found by the above mentioned authors, is equal to at least 1. The consequence of this property will be discussed below.

We have extrapolated equation (2) to the impulse response of the rabbit photo-receptors and moreover, since no alternative could be found, also to the impulse response of the processes P II and P I.

In terms of system analysis, the impulse response given by equation 2 characterizes a linear system of the order $(c + 1)$. Although it is not very logical to take the three processes, i.e. three systems, in parallel, we have continued with the scheme of GRANIT and have not assumed that any a priori relation between the three systems is known.

Equation (2) contains four parameters, so with three processes in parallel twelve parameters have to be estimated. The E.R.G. impulse response is defined H(t), then from equation 2:

$$H(t) = \sum_{i=1}^{3} a_i (t-t_{1i})^{c_i} \exp\{-b_i (t-t_{1i})\} \tag{3}$$

To fit equation (3) to the experimentally determined E.R.G. impulse response is a very elaborate procedure, even for a computer. But as follows from the experimental results, particular properties of the dependency of the parameters on the stimulus intensity may permit a simpler and therefore less time consuming fitting procedure.

EXPERIMENTAL RESULTS

The results of the analysis of the responses at a relatively high scotopic adaptation level are shown in Fig. 2. In the left part of the figure the E.R.G. impulse response is shown (dotted curve) and the best fitting impulse responses of the processes P I to P III; the number at the vertical axis represents the maximum value of the E.R.G. in micro volts. In the upper inset the relative error of estimate is presented. This error (E) is the sum of the squared deviations divided by the sum of the squared values of the experimental curve. So, if the experimental data points are given by Y_j, and the data points from the fitting procedure by $\tilde{Y}_j$, then the error is given by:

$$E = \frac{\sum_{j=1}^{m} (Y_j-\tilde{Y}_j)^2}{\sum_{j=1}^{m} (Y_j)^2} \times 100\% \tag{4}$$

The fitting procedure is continued until the error is smaller than 10%, or until the parameters are estimated with an accuracy better than 5%. In the lower inset the impulse response of the three processes is characterized in two ways: by the time and amplitude data, and by the parameters of equation 3. In the right part of Fig. 2 the accuracy of the fitting procedure can be judged, the dotted curve is again the experimental curve.

78

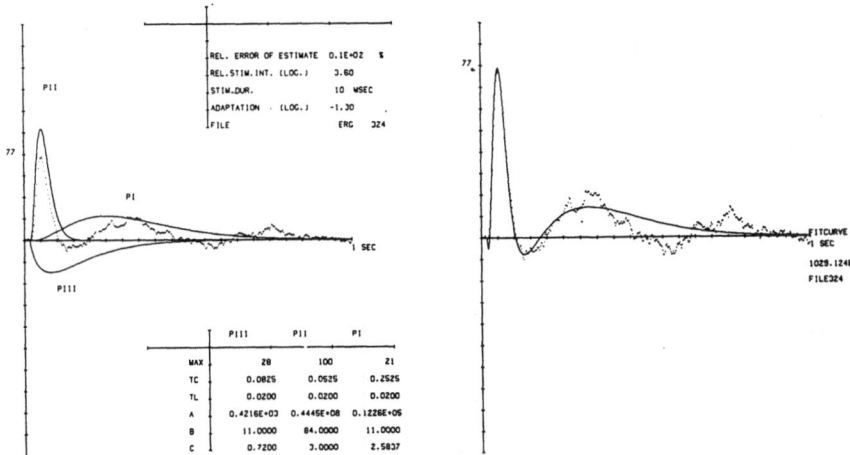

FIG. 2. Analysis of the E.R.G. response to a short flash at scotopic light adaptation. *Left*: Results of the three component analysis. The measured E.R.G. is represented by the dotted curve. Upper inset: stimulation conditions. Lower inset: Max = maximum value, TC = culmination time of max., TL = latency time, A = gain factor, B = cut-off frequency, C = power (see equations 2 and 3). *Right*: E.R.G.: dotted curve, the curve obtained by the fit procedure has been drawn.

The fitting procedure is fairly specifically carried out by the computer program for E.R.G. responses as shown in Fig. 2, containing two maxima (b-wave, and c-wave) and one, or two minima (a-wave, and a minimum between the b- and c-waves). With a dark adapted retina the response to a short light flash has a much simpler shape. In which case it is, therefore, not possible to find a unique set of parameters yielding a fit with an accuracy better than e.g. 5 %. We decided to investigate which parameters of each of the processes are independent of the adaptation level. The result is illustrated with Fig. 3, in which two impulse responses with a dark adapted retina are presented. It appears that the parameter c, i.e. the power of the time in equation 3, remains constant, whereas the gain factor (a) and the cut-off frequency (b) have to be adjusted by the computer program. A minor adjustment of the latency time is also necessary.

As can be expected, the maximum value of the b-wave, will depend on the flash intensity in such a way that it will be analogous to the relationship between the maximum value of the P II process and the flash intensity. This can be judged from Fig. 4 since both curves display approximately a proportionality.

The dependency of the parameters b and c on the flash intensity is shown in Fig. 5 and Fig. 6 again for a series of responses to light flashes at a dark adapted retina. No systematic relationship is apparent from these figures.

In conclusion: the E.R.G. registered with a scotopic light adaptation can be fitted to equation (3). With dark adaptation the time constants $(1/b_i)$ and the gain factors (a_i) have to be changed, but the power (c_i) remains constant to a first approximation. Changing the flash intensity means a different set of gain factors (a_i) to a first approximation.

79

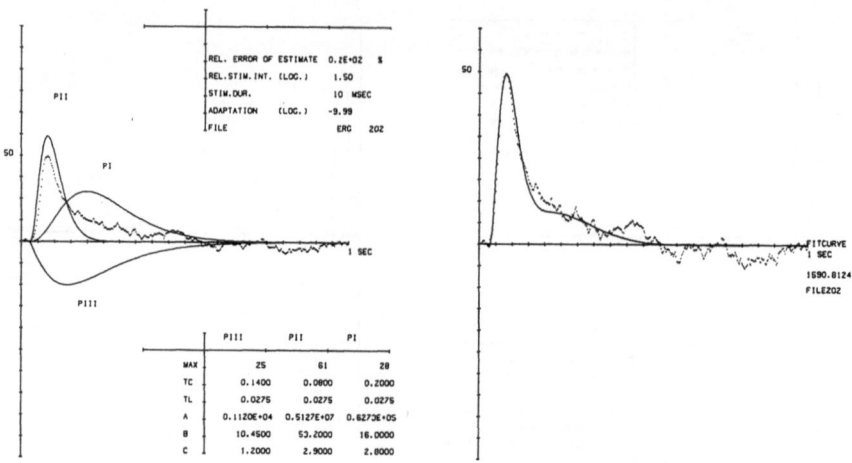

	PIII	PII	PI
MAX	25	61	28
TC	0.1400	0.0800	0.2000
TL	0.0275	0.0275	0.0275
A	0.1120E+04	0.5127E+07	0.6273E+05
B	10.4500	53.2000	16.0000
C	1.2000	2.9000	2.8000

FIG. 3. E.R.G. responses to a flash at a dark adapted retina. Upper part: low intensity flash, 1.5 relative log units. Lower part: high intensity flash, 2.1 relative log units.

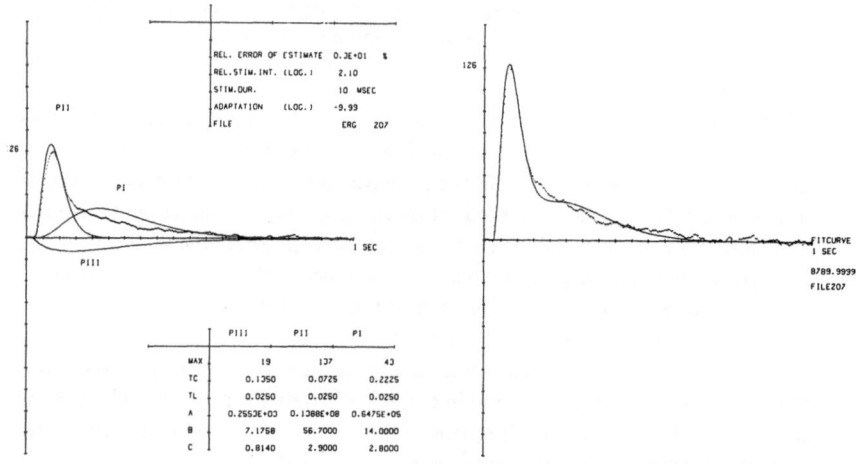

	PIII	PII	PI
MAX	19	137	43
TC	0.1350	0.0725	0.2225
TL	0.0250	0.0250	0.0250
A	0.2553E+03	0.1388E+08	0.6475E+05
B	7.1758	56.7000	14.0000
C	0.8140	2.9000	2.8000

DISCUSSION

The P I component of GRANIT's scheme is generated by the pigment epithelial cells (c.f. NOELL, 1954; BROWN, 1968; SCHMIDT & STEINBERG, 1971). The P II component has been ascribed until recently to the bipolar cells, but MILLER & DOWLING (1972) have shown that the Müller cells are most probably the generators of the E.R.G. b-wave. For this reason the P II component is only an indirect indication of the bipolar cell activity. The DC-component, which is ascribed to a different mechanism in the inner nuclear layer (c.f. BROWN, 1968) may be also present in the P II component evoked by flash stimulation. In our analysis no evidence has been found for the presence of separate b-wave and DC-component. The P III component is generated in the receptor cell layer of

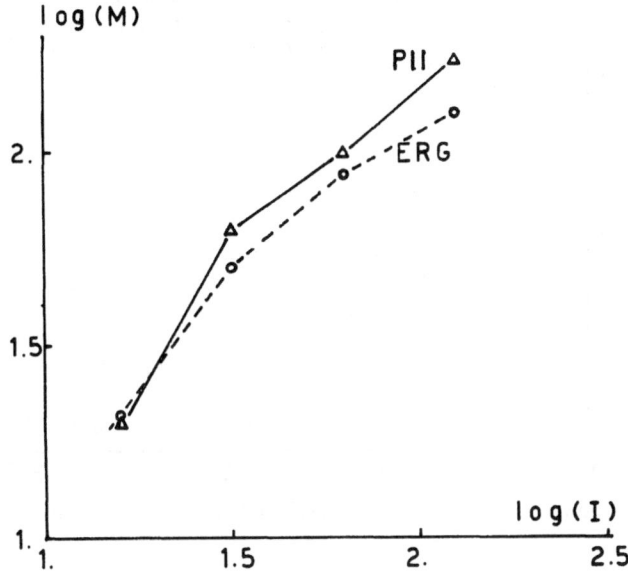

FIG. 4. The maximum value of the b-wave of the E.R.G. and the maximum of P II v. flash intensity; dark adaptation. Both axes are logarithmic, so a proportionality is present to a good approximation.

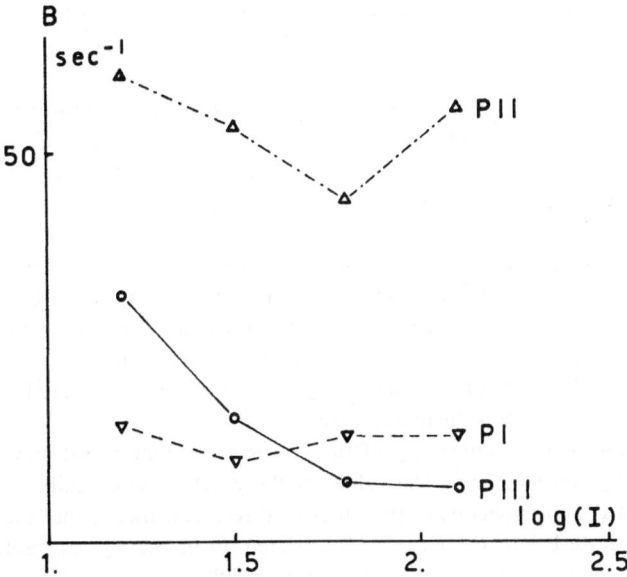

FIG. 5. The cut-off frequency (inverse of time constant) B v. log flash intensity; dark adaptation.

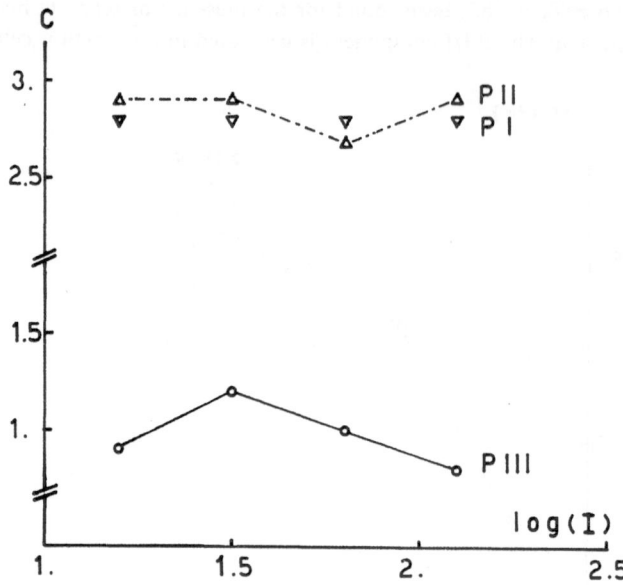

FIG. 6. The power C (or c) of equations (2) and (3) v. log flash intensity; dark adaptation.

the retina (c.f. BROWN, 1968, DOWLING, 1970, RODIECK, 1972). Since the early receptor potential can be only evoked with very high light intensities (TOMITA, 1970) and the proximal P III will not contribute very much to the E.R.G. (OGDEN, 1973) it can be concluded that the P III component is generated by the receptor cells.

It is therefore acceptable to make the statement that, if the three components of GRANIT's scheme can be isolated by an adequate curve fit procedure, valuable information can be obtained concerning the activity of the receptor cells, the bipolar cells (indirectly) and the pigment epithelial cells.

The quality of the fit procedure depends both on the signal to noise ratio of the measurement and on the uniqueness of the estimated parameters, given a reasonable choice of the function to be fitted. The signal to noise ratio can be increased by averaging techniques. The parameter estimation appears to be unambiguous only when the E.R.G. displays several maxima and minima. This may indicate that the fitting strategy we have employed has to be improved, which will be subject of further research.

The approximate constancy of the power c in equation (3) may have very interesting consequences. The value for the P III is about unity; and for the P II and P I components, of the order of three. This means that the processes that generate P I to P III can be 'translated' in physically realizable systems. These systems can be described by a linear differential equation of the order $(c + 1)$, and the systems are very much suited for hardware, or analog computer simulation. So the E.R.G. response to other kinds of stimulation can then be synthetized. Moreover, the results become more or less understandable now, because constancy of the power c means that the systems generating the P I and P III processes remain invariant, except for static adaptation effects on the gain factor and the time constants. Dynamic adaptation effects that will occur with e.g. long duration flash stimulation, have also to be studied separately. These points will be explored in the near future. The clinical significance of the analysis will depend on the outcome of the above mentioned additional research but the results obtained up to now represent an encouraging start. We will present the results of an investigation by the linear system analysis approach in a separate paper (THIJSSEN et al., 1973)

REFERENCES

BAYLOR, D. A., FUORTES, M. G. F. & O'BRYAN, P. M. Receptive fields of cones in the retina of the Turtle. *J. Physiol.* 214: *265* (1971).
BROWN, K. T. The electroretinogram: its components and their origins. *Vis. Res.* 8: *633* (1968).
DOWLING, J. E. Organization of vertebrate retinas. *Invest. Ophthalmol.* 9: *655* (1970).
GRANIT, R. The components of the retinal action potential in mammals and their relation to the discharge in the optic nerve. *J. Physiol.* 77: *207* (1933).
HAGINS, W. A., PENN, R. D. & YOSHIKAMA, S. Dark current and photocurrent in retinal rods. *Biophys. J.* 10: *380* (1970).
MILLER, R. F. & DOWLING, J. E. A relationship between Müller cell slow potentials and the E.R.G b-wave. P.p. 85-100 in: Proceedings of the VIIIth Symposium of ISCERG. A. Wirth, ed. Pacini, Pisa (1972).
NOËLL, W. K. The origin of the electroretinogram. *Amer. J. Ophthalmol.* 38: *78* (1954).
OGDEN, T. E. The proximal negative response of the primate retina. *Vis. Res.* 13: *797* (1973).
POTTS, A. M., BUFFUM, D. & BENNET, S. E. Computer-assisted analysis of the electroretinogram. P.p. 340-354 in: Proceedings of the VIIth Symposium of ISCERG. D. Basar, and Bengisu, eds. Univ. of Istanbul, Istanbul (1971).
POTTS, A. M., INOUE, J., BUFFUM, D. & FRITZ, K. J. The morphology of the human E.R.G. P.p. 170-181 in: Proceedings of the VIIIth Symposium of ISCERG. A. Wirth, ed. Pacini, Pisa (1972).
RODIECK, R. W. Components of the electroretinogram – a reappraisal. *Vis. Res.* 12: *773* (1972).
SCHMIDT, R. & STEINBERG, R. H. Rod dependent intracellular responses to light recorded from the pigment epithelium of the cat retina. *J. Physiol.* 127: *71* (1971).
SPEKREIJSE, H. & NORTON, A. L. The dynamical characteristics of color coded S-potentials. *J. Gen. Physiol.* 56: *1* (1970).
STARK, L. Neurological control systems. New York, Plenum (1968).
THIJSSEN, J. M., MUNCKHOF, W. M. VAN DEN & VENDRIK, A. J. H. In preparation.
TOMITA, A. Electrical activity of vertebrate photoreceptors. *Quart. Rev. Biophys.* 3: *179* (1970).
TROELSTRA, A. Non-linear systems analysis in electroretinography. Institute for Perception RVO-TNO. Soesterberg (1964).

Author's address:
Dept. of Ophthalmology
University of Nijmegen
Nijmegen
The Netherlands

THE FUNCTIONAL EXAMINATION OF THE HUMAN PHOTOPIC VISUAL SYSTEM WITH THE AID OF PSYCHOPHYSICAL FLICKER THRESHOLDS AND ERG FLICKER RESPONSES

J. J. MEYER*, S. KOROL**, G. OWENS**, R. GRAMONI* & P. REY*

(Geneva)

ABSTRACT

This paper deals with the use of flicker fusion thresholds, as plotted by De Lange, and averaged flicker ERG recorded with conventional clinical equipment. Different methods are developed to quantify the morphological changes of the ERG responses and express them in empirical attenuation curves. The objective and subjective results are discussed in point of view of the De Lange model.

The pathological results compared to the mean thresholds and limits in normal subjects show that when at least two values, a low frequency one and a high frequency one are established, both tests are sensitive in comparison to ordinary clinical methods.

The results suggest that for a direct comparison of the objective and the perceptive method, the low frequency range is the most informative.

In many clinical situations, the determination of the macular function as distinguished from the function of larger regions is of great importance. To evaluate the importance of a visual field loss as well to determine its retinal or retrobulbar origin, the ophthalmologist has to compare perceptual responses with objective responses such as ERG and VER, both being obtained under different conditions of stimulation (BABEL et al., 1969; KOROL, 1973).

It seems reasonable therefore to use intermittent light as a stimulus to elicit both objective and subjective responses in order to stimulate the same visual mechanism. (STERNHEIM & CAVONIUS, 1972). Intermittent light, presented at different frequencies from one or two Hz to fusion frequency, also enhances photopic conditions when in combination with background illumination (HENKES, 1964). Furthermore, when the responses to intermittent light are expressed in terms of attenuation characteristics, according to the De Lange model, we are able to compare threshold responses with supraliminar ones, as well as responses obtained with different stimulus wave forms (DE LANGE, 1958a; VAN DER TWEEL & VERDUYN LUNEL, 1965; FIORENTINI & MAFFEI, 1970). The supraliminar ERG responses however are often difficult to interpret since they tend to have a complex wave form changing with the stimulation conditions.

This paper develops methods allowing the comparison of averaged flicker ERG responses with subjective thresholds. The former were obtained with conventional clinical equipment after preadaptation and in the presence of different background illuminations. In the case of the latter we have measured the minimum depth of modulation required to detect flicker at different frequencies of an intermittent light presented on a 1° test area surrounded by a steady background (De Lange curves (DE LANGE, 1958a)).

a. De Lange curves (psychophysical flicker thresholds)

An intermittent test object of less than 1° visual angle with an illuminated background was the stimulus. The adaptation level of the undilated eye was kept constant by the background illumination at a distance of 50 cm.

The light source was either a modified TV tube which produced a sinusoïdal light, the modulation depth of which could be varied nearly from 0 to 100% (DENIER VAN DER GON et al., 1958) or a stroboscope (Strobotac Type 1531 A,

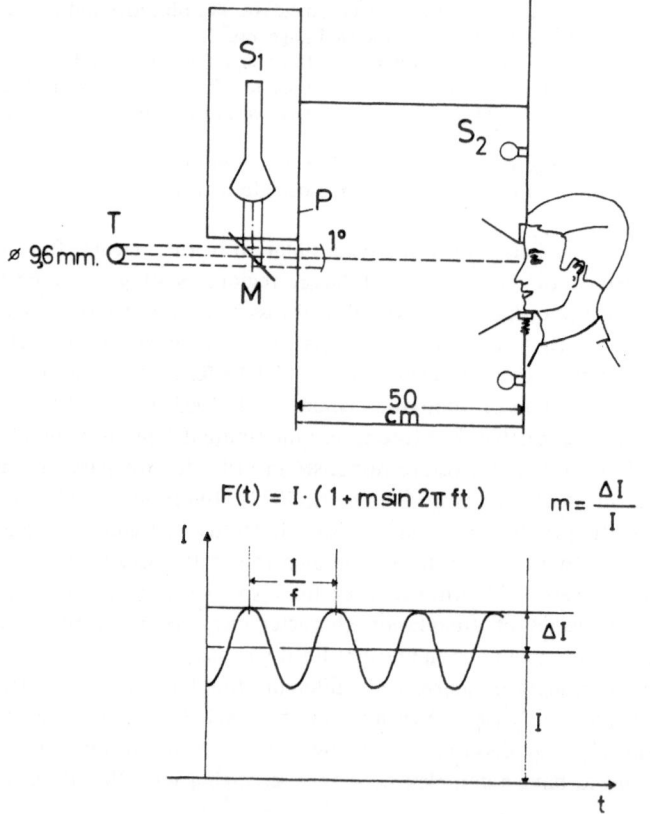

FIG. 1. Experimental apparatus for the determination of psychophysical flicker thresholds. S1: light source. S2: background light. M: mirror. T: test object of 1° visual angle. P: front panel. The lower part of the figure is the temporal course of the sinusoïdally modulated stimulus.

86

General Radio Co.), the peak amplitude of which could be reduced by neutral filters. (Fig. 1)

Fusion thresholds were determined by successive approximations (REY & REY, 1964) and expressed either as modulation percent or in transmittance values and were plotted versus frequency on a double log. scale. (Fig. 2)

40 normal subjects from 20 to 40 years of age were examined in the following 5 conditions of stimulation. 79 patients (or 130 eyes) aged 19–70 with retro-bulbar and retinal lesions were examined in the reference condition as described below.

1. The reference condition (REF) in which the brightness of the stimulus and background were equal to 170 cd/m2 (= 100%);
2. The condition of reduced stimulus (RS) in which the mean intensity of the stimulus was reduced and the background maintained at 100%, producing a local adaptation change;
3. The condition of reduced background (RB) in which the stimulus brightness was maintained at 100%;
4. The condition of concomitant reduction (CR) in which both stimulus and background were proportionately reduced.
5. The reference condition with eccentric fixation (EF).

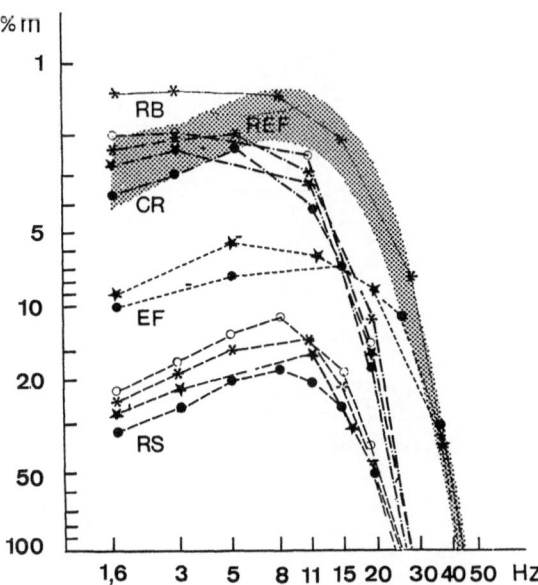

FIG. 2. De Lange curves established in normal subjects with different conditions of stimulation: REF, reference condition (shaded area: standard deviation of 40 values) RS, stimulus reduction, individual curves; RB, reduction of background, individual curves; CR, concomitant reduction, individual curves; EF, eccentric fixation and reference condition. On the abscissa, frequencies in Hz, log scale; on the ordinate, modulation amplitude in %, log scale.

b. Flicker ERG attenuation curves

The light source was a Grass stimulator in an indirectly illuminated wall, 60 cm in front of the subject. The pupil was dilated with a mydraticum Roche (1 %) and a scleral contact lens was used for electrical pickup. After light adaptation for 3 min. with a bright light of 2000 lux, the flicker ERG was recorded for a set of frequencies from one Hz to 80 Hz, depending on intensity of stimulation. The ERG responses were amplified with an AC Tektronix preamplifier type FM 122, with low and high frequency cut-offs at 0,8 and 250 Hz and displayed on a dual beam Tektronix oscilloscope type A 502; 64 responses were averaged with a Biomac 1000 averager (Data Laboratories). (Fig. 3). The ERGs were transformed into digital values for Fourier analysis.

The different amplitudes measured on the b-wave or the computed values of Fourier components were plotted as arbitrary values versus frequency on a

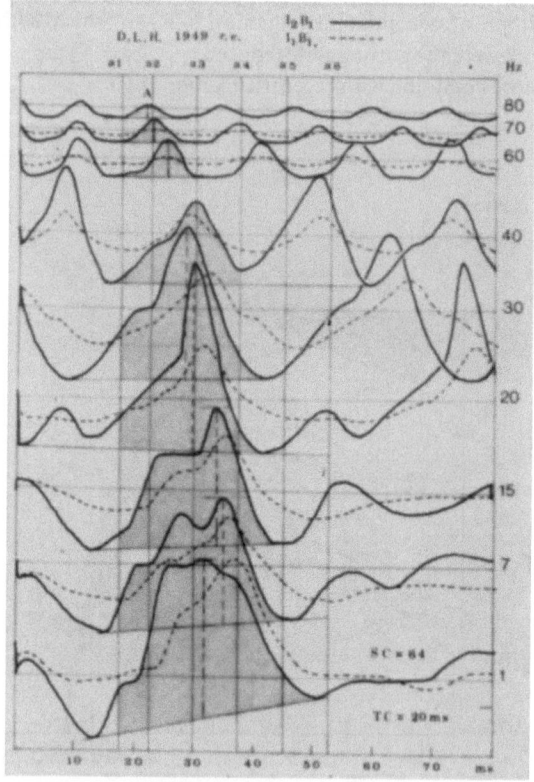

FIG. 3. Averaged flicker ERG in one subject, recorded at different frequencies in two conditions of stimulation. For each frequency, the shaded area shows the part of the response analysed with different methods. A, b-wave amplitude. a1, a2, a3, a4, a5 and a6 latencies at which the amplitude of the b-wave was measured. I_1, I_2, two different stimulation intensities. B_1, one of two different adaptation conditions. ms: time in ms. Hz: frequency stimulation in Hz.

double log. scale, according to linear system analysis methods. 10 normal subjects were examined in three different stimulation conditions. The intensity was provided with a constant background in the first 2 conditions ($I_1 B_1$; $I_2 B_1$). The background and stimulus were both increased in the third condition ($I_2 B_2$). A set of 10 pathological cases with macular or peripheral retinal lesions was examined in the $I_2 B_2$ condition.

SUBJECTIVE RESULTS

The De Lange curves established in normal subjects showed the following behaviour: (Fig. 2).
1. The low frequency thresholds were changed markedly with a change in background illumination or the fixation point.
   In Fig. 2, compare conditions REF, RB and EF, or conditions RS and CR.
2. All thresholds were enhanced with a change of stimulus intensity.
3. High frequency thresholds were elevated in the case of a concomitant reduction (CR) of background intensity and stimulus intensity.
   The results confirm the main properties of the De Lange characteristics as observed by KELLY (1964) and LEVINSON (1964): a non-linear low frequency region influenced by adaptation and spatial configuration of the stimulus changes progressively into a linear high frequency region where the fundamental component of any kind of stimulus is the most significant.
4. We could observe the same tendencies when we used a flash stimulus instead of the sinusoidal one. In this case, the characteristic curves were obtained by plotting the transmittance percent of neutral filters versus frequency, the filter being placed between the stimulator and the test area. With such a stimulus, the mean energy to the eye per unit of time changes with the frequency. We observed that intensity change has little effect on the main adaptation.

The pathological curves established by flashes or sinusoidal light showed the following relevant facts: (Fig. 4, Fig. 5)
1. All pathological cases gave anomalous curves, even when other tests were normal (for example kinetic perimetry);
2. The anomalous curves were not clearly related to specific pathology.
   For example we could observe similar curves for different pathologies.
3. Most of the curves, like the normal ones, were of three types:
   those with increased thresholds mainly in the high frequency region,
   those with increased thresholds mainly in the low frequency region, and
   those with increased thresholds for all frequencies.
4. The typical behaviour of the curves provides the possibility of expressing the temporal characteristics by means of only two thresholds represented by one point in a correlation diagram. (Fig. 5).
5. The test is sensitive to the extension of a visual field loss.

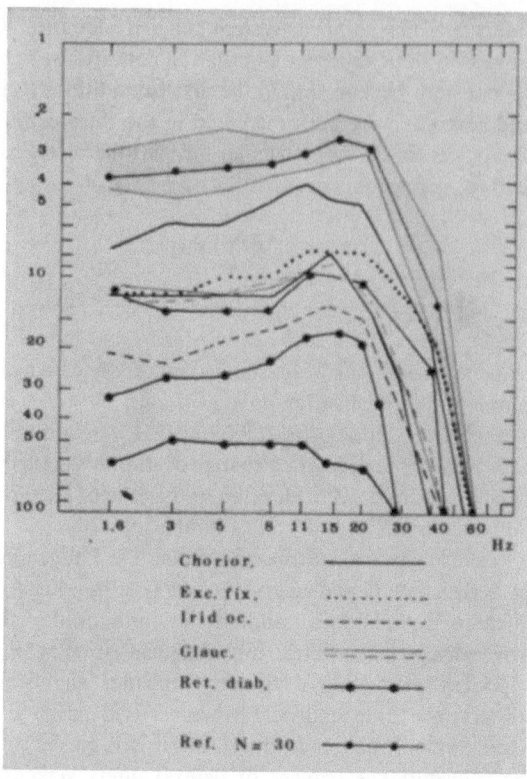

FIG. 4. De Lange characteristics obtained with stroboscopic flashes. Abscissa: frequencies in Hz, log scale. Ordinate: transmittance percent of neutral filters, log scale. Shaded area: reference condition, mean and standard deviation of 30 values. Individual curves: patients with visual pathology. (Chorioretinitis, iridocyclitis with pupillary seclusion, glaucoma, diabetic retinopathy). Exc. fix.: eccentric fixation

FLICKER ERG RESULTS

Theoretically, a sinusoidal light would be ideal. But many works concerning the ERG (VAN DER TWEEL & VERDUYN LUNEL, 1965; FIORENTINI & MAFFEI, 1970) show a linear behaviour for small signals and high frequency stimulation. According to the De Lange model, it is sensible to use a flash stimulus as we have seen in the case of perceptive results. The main advantage of a low frequency flash stimulus is that it evokes a polyphasic response which shows the activity of different retinal structures. As already mentioned, the mean energy received by the eye per time unit changes with the frequency. In the case of large diffuse eye illumination we can suppose a relative important change of the adaptation state. One can test this adaptation state by comparing averaged one Hz ERG before and after the flicker experiment.

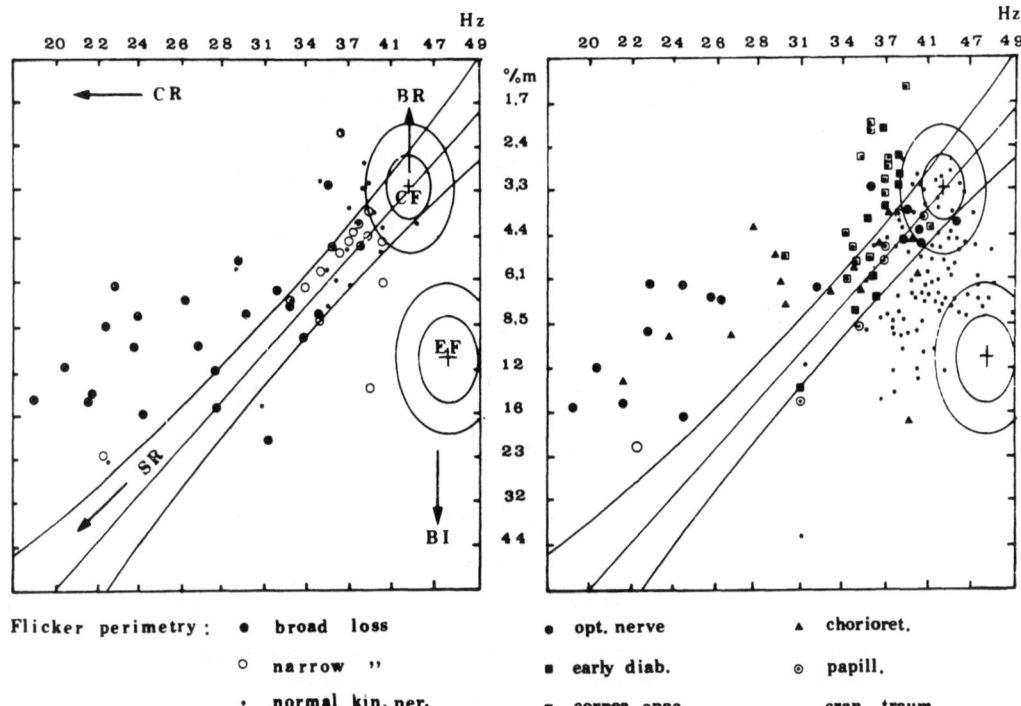

Flicker perimetry:
● broad loss
○ narrow ,,
. normal kin. per.

● opt. nerve
■ early diab.
▣ cornea opac.

▲ chorioret.
◎ papill.
. cran. traum.

FIG. 5. Correlation between threshold modulation amplitude at 5 Hz and critical fusion frequency as measured with 100% modulation. Abscissa: Critical fusion frequency in Hz. Ordinate: Modulation percent at 5 Hz. The scales were arranged in order to obtain a straight line for the RS conditions (Babel at al. (1). Labelled areas: correlation locus for normal subjects examined in different conditions (Cf fig. 2). CR, concomitant reduction. SR, stimulus reduction. BR, background reduction. BI, background increase. CF, reference condition with central fixation. EF, reference condition with eccentric fixation. The different symbols represent pathological cases. Left: perimetry results. Right: diagnosis: opt. nerve optic neuritis, early diab. early diabetes, cornea opac. corneal opacities, chorioret. chorioretinitis, cran. trauma cranial trauma, normal kin. per. normal kinetic perimetry.

a. Results in normal subjects

1. When expressed in equivalent sinusoidal stimuli the amplitude of the first component of the ERG is attenuated in the same way as the amplitude of its b-wave. In both cases an adaptation change affects essentially the low-frequency region, whereas an intensity change of the flashes gives a vertical translation of the whole curve. (Fig. 6)
2. The general form of the first component attenuation curve is that of a low-pass filter as it is in the case of the De Lange curve, but the slope is less steep than observed by others (STERNHEIM & CAVONIUS, 1972).

These results indicate a similar behaviour as with subjective flash responses.

91

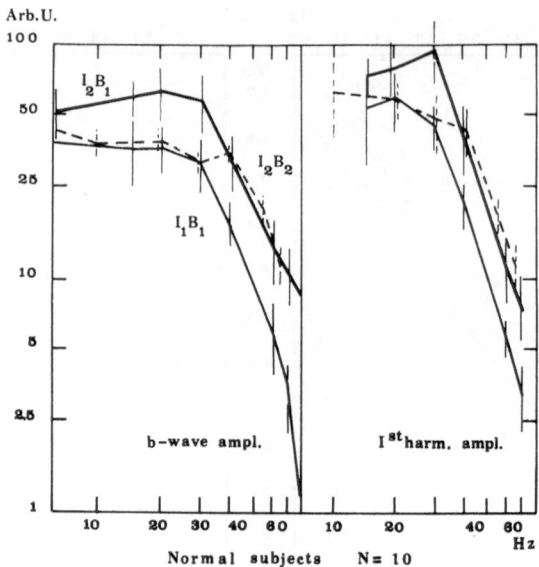

FIG. 6. b-wave amplitude and first harmonic attenuation curves. Abscissa: frequency in Hz, log scale. Ordinate: arbitrary units, log scale. Mean and standard deviation for 10 normal subjects examined in three different conditions. I_1, I_2, two different intensities. B_1, B_2, two different adaptation conditions. Left: attenuation of the b-wave amplitude, right: attenuation of the first harmonic component of the ERG.

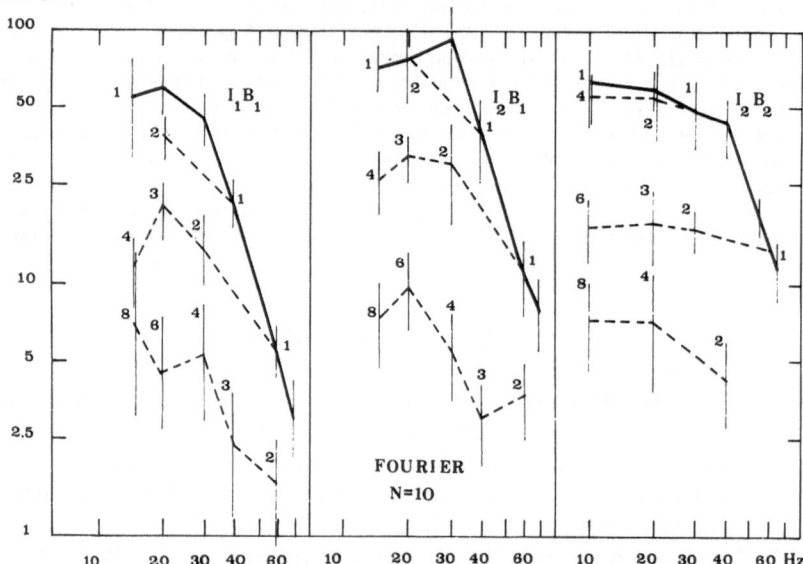

FIG. 7. Linearity test (see text). Continuous line: first harmonic attenuation as in fig. 6. Broken line: attenuation of harmonic components. Upper curves, attenuation of the 2nd harmonic of the 20 Hz ERG; middle curves, attenuation of the 4th harmonic of the 15 Hz or the 6th of the 10 Hz ERG; lower curves, attenuation of the 8th harmonic of the 15 Hz ERG or the 8th harmonic of the 10 Hz ERG. Numbers refer to the ERG harmonic analysed for stimulation frequency. Abscissa: frequencies in Hz, log scale. Ordinate: arbitrary units, log scale.

When the individual responses are considered in detail, we notice that the responses may show important irregularities in shape and latency even in the high frequency region and that a simple phase-amplitude relation does not exist (FRICKER, 1969). Also the form change of the response must be considered with the Fourier analysis of the other harmonics.

For these reasons we have developed two other methods of analysis. First, we employed the following linearity test (Fig. 7). In cases where we approach linearity in the high frequency region, and only the first harmonic is reduced, the other harmonics should remain unchanged until their corresponding frequencies become equivalent to the stimulus frequency. For example, starting with a flash response of 10 Hz, we can calculate the amplitude of the 4th, 6th, 8th and 12th harmonic. We then observe the change of amplitude of these components for higher stimulation frequencies: the 4th harmonic of the 10 Hz response compared to the second of the 20 Hz response and to the first of the 40 Hz response. The same observation is made for other harmonics. In the case of linearity these different corresponding harmonics should remain unchanged with a frequency stimulation change. According to this criterion we see that this condition is nearly fulfilled for the condition I_2B_2.

Secondly, we used a method to describe form changes (Fig. 8). To quantify the form and latency variations of the flicker ERG we measured the amplitude of the b-wave at different latencies from a base line joining the negative waves.

The results of these two methods show that the corresponding attenuation curves undergo relevant changes by changing the stimulus intensity and back-

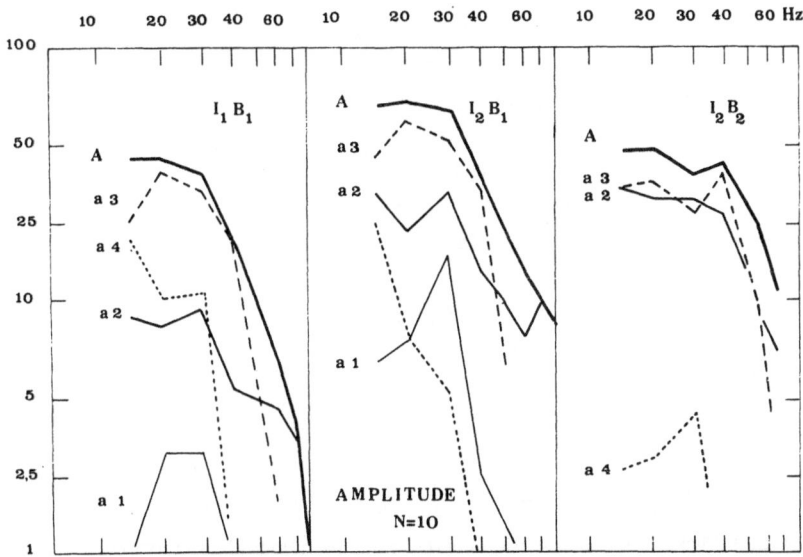

FIG. 8. Method to quantify shape and latency changes of the flicker ERG. A, b-wave attenuation. a1, a2, a3, a4, attenuation curves corresponding to the amplitudes of the b-wave measured at the different times figuring on the fig. 3. Abscissa: frequencies in Hz, log scale. Ordinate: arbitrary units, log scale.

ground intensity relations. For example in the stimulation condition $I_2 B_2$, the relative position of the curves indicates little change in the ERG form.

b. Pathological cases

For examining retinal diseases we have applied both methods of analysis of the flicker ERG recorded in the $I_2 B_2$ condition. This condition was choosen for ease of analysis regarding adaptation and linearity.

For each pathological eye the different attenuation curves were compared with the corresponding normal values established for ten normal eyes. Our findings are illustrated by the four cases presented in Fig. 9:

1. The b-wave amplitude shows the same amplitude behaviour as the amplitude of the Fourier first harmonic.
2. Only one part of the curve may lie outside the shaded area and either the high frequency region (case L. M.), the low frequency region (case M. M.

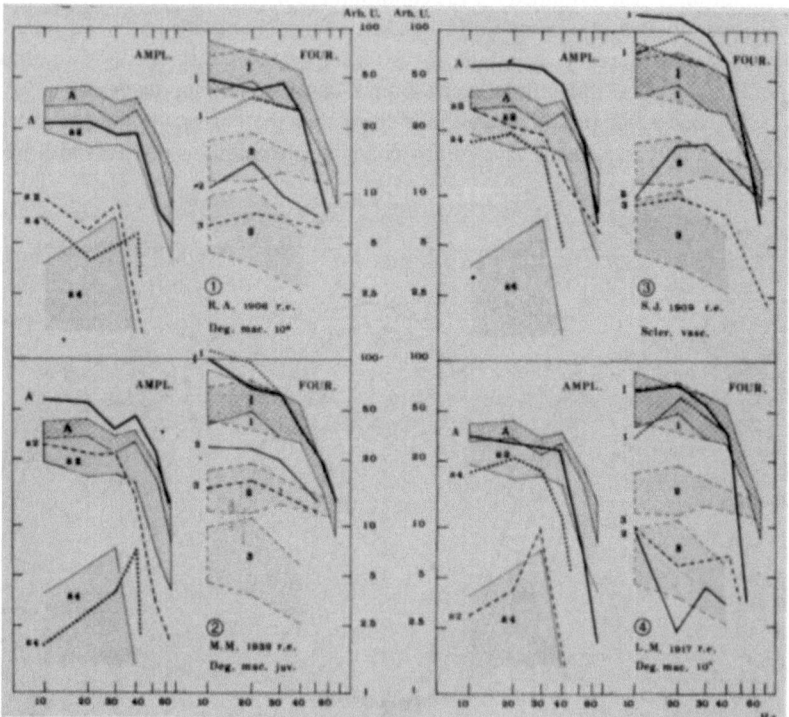

FIG. 9. Flicker ERG attenuation curves. Four pathological cases (vascular sclerosis, macular degeneration, juvenile macular degeneration). For each case: left, method for evaluating the attenuation and morphological changes of the flicker ERG. right, linearity test based on the Fourier component analysis of the flicker ERG. Shaded area: standard deviation for 10 normal subjects examined in a reference condition (I_2, B_2). Abscissa: frequencies in Hz, log scale. Ordinate: arbitrary units, log scale.

and S. J.) or the whole curve may be outside the normal value region (case (R.A.).

3. When the b-wave curve (A) and the first harmonic amplitude curve (I) are anomalous, the other components (amplitudes at different times, a2, a4, or other harmonics 1, 2, 3) lie also outside the corresponding reference values.

4. In some cases, these components may even have different anomalous positions; whereas the A and I curves are of the same type (compare case M. M. with case S. J.)

DISCUSSION

The subjective results suggest two conclusions:
- first, the fact that every De Lange curve can be represented by two thresholds is useful clinically, where tests must often be brief.
- Secondly, the test is very sensitive in detecting the gravity and the extension of a macular or perimacular visual field loss but does not permit one to determine whether it is retinal or retrobulbar origin (in contradiction with BREUKINK's opinion (BUCKSER, 1967)). To distinguish between these only the flicker ERG can help assuming that the method is sensitive enough.

When we consider the ERG responses, the conclusion is the following: the results show that b-wave amplitude or its corresponding first harmonic component give approximately the same information. To make the test more discriminative, we must consider the high- and low frequency b-wave form changes. This suggests that the recording method must not be too greatly simplified and that the b-wave form changes of the flicker averaged ERG have a significance for detecting retinal functional changes. When the b-wave amplitude measurement or first harmonic component calculation is the only possibility, we must observe at least, the same for the De Lange curves, the relation between a high frequency response and a low frequency response, i.e. one between 5 and 10 Hz, the other between 40 and 60 Hz.

The comparison of objective and subjective test is not so difficult as expected when:

1. from a theoretical point of view, we would expect that high frequency responses should be observed; on one hand we have seen that both objective and subjective responses are approximatively linear in this frequency range; on the other hand we could expect that a high frequency stimulus would help to isolate the fast macular retinal mechanisms.

2. Several macular pathological cases showed that only the high frequency region of the De Lange curves is abnormal; the faster mechanisms stimulated with the high frequency flicker ERG may be situated in the perimacular region.

3. Hypernormal responses for the low frequency region could be observed in the cases of normal high frequency flicker ERG.

These facts indicate paradoxically that a comparison between flicker ERG and the De Lange curve should be done in a nonlinear low frequency range of stimulation.

The important changes of the low frequency flicker ERG would be indirectly produced in the perimacular region by a lateral effect originating in the macular region. This hypothesis (RATLIFF et al., 1967) of important lateral effect between the macular and perimacular region would be confirmed by the fact that the low frequency region of the De Lange curve could give information about the extension of a macular or a perimacular visual field loss. In this case altered perimacular mechanisms influence the macular region. This particular behaviour lends support to a multiple channel system mechanism of different brightness units (PANTLE, 1971; BREUKINK & TEN DOESSCHATE, 1964; MEYER, 1972), the mutual influences of which would build up the polymorphic aspect of the ERG and the corresponding temporal transfer function.

Our final conclusion is that the De Lange curve and the flicker ERG attenuation curve established with conventional equipment are useful diagnostic devices for clinical application.

REFERENCES

BABEL, J., REY, P., STANGOS, N., MEYER, J. J. & GUGGENHEIM, P. The functional examination of the macular and perimacular region with the aid of flicker-fusion thresholds. *Doc. Ophthal.* 26: *248-256* (1969).

BREUKINK, E. W. & TEN DOESSCHATE, J. Attenuation curves of the human eye under normal and pathological conditions. *Ophthalmologica* 146: *143-164* (1964).

BUCKSER, S. Sub-wave nature of the albino rat electroretinogram. *Curr. Mod. Biol.* 1: *259-274* (1967).

DE LANGE, H. Research into the dynamic nature of the human fovea-cortex system with intermittent and modulated light. I. Attenuation characteristics with white and colored light. *J. Opt. Soc. Amer.* 48: *777-784* (1958a).

DENIER VAN DER GON, J. J., STRADKEE, J. & VAN DER TWEEL, L. H. A source for modulated light. *Phys. Med. Biol.* 3: *164-173* (1958).

FIORENTINI, A. & MAFFEI, L. Transfer characteristics of excitation and inhibition in the human visual system. *J. Neurophysiol.* 33: *285-292* (1970).

FRICKER, S. J. The clinical significance of ERG. Time-delay determination by means of a phase-sensitive detector system. Proc. ISCERG Symp., D. Basar Publ., Istanbul (1969).

HENKES, H. Recent advances in flicker-electroretinography. *Doc. Ophthal.* 18: *307* (1964).

KELLY, D. H. Sine waves and flicker fusion. *Doc. Ophthal.* 18: *16-35* (1964).

KOROL, S. Les potentiels évoqués visuels (P.E.V.). Etude clinique et expérimentale. Thèse n° 3294, Université de Genève (1973).

LEVINSON, J. Non linear and spatial effects in the perception of flicker. *Doc. Ophthal.* 18: *36-55* (1964).

MEYER, J.-J. Exploration de la fonction visuelle à l'aide de la lumière intermittente: courbes d'atténuation perceptive et électrorétinogramme de papillotement. Thèse n° 1574, Université de Genève (1972).

PANTLE, A. Flicker adaptation. I. Effect on visual sensitivity to temporal fluctuations of light intensity. *Vis. Res.* 11: *943-952* (1971).

RATLIFF, F., KNIGHT, B. W., TOYODA, J. & HARTLINE, H. K. Enhancement of flicker by lateral inhibition. *Science* 158: *392-393* (1967).

REY, P. & REY, J. P. Fréquence de fusion optique subjective. Comparaison de trois méthodes de mesure avant et après le travail. *Le travail humain*, 26: *135-145* (1964).

Sternheim, C. E. & Cavonius, C. R. Sensitivity of the human ERG and VECP to sinusoidally modulated light. *Vis. Res.* 12: *1685-1695* (1972).

van der Tweel, L. H. & Verduyn Lunel, H. F. E. Human visual responses to sinusoidally modulated light. *Electroenceph. Clin. Neurophysiol.* 18: *587-598* (1965).

Authors' addresses:

J.-J. Meyer
R. Gramoni
P. Rey
Institut de médecine
sociale et préventive
Université de Genève
Genève
Suisse

S. Korol
G. Owens
Clinique Universitaire
d'Ophtalmologie
Université de Genève
Genève
Suisse

PROGRESSIVE GENERALIZED CONE DYSFUNCTION

J. FRANÇOIS, A. DE ROUCK, G. VERRIEST, J. J. DE LAEY
& E. CAMBIE

(Ghent)

The mainly electro-retinographical concept 'cone dysfunction', as described by SLOAN & BROWN (1962), GOODMAN et al. (1963, 1966), BERSON et al. (1968), KRILL et al., (1970, 1973), BABEL & STANGOS (1972, 1973), includes a wide group of clinical pictures.

We have selected 17 cases of progressive cone dystrophies, which will be later described in extenso, but we should like to discuss here some aspects of these dystrophies, and particularly the ERG-EOG correlations.

The selection of these cases was made by means of the ERG modifications. The photopic ERG was either absent or reduced in such a way that the ERG picture was characteristic.

Most of our cases, however, showed also some scotopic involvement, such as a subnormal dark adaptation curve or a subnormal scotopic ERG.

Four cases only could be considered as pure cone dystrophies. Their age, at the time of the first examination, ranged from 7 to 18 years. The fundus was either normal or showed only minimal macular changes such as a slight pigmentary disturbance.

According to the state of the scotopic ERG, we could classify all our cases of cone dystrophy in 3 groups (Fig. 1).

Group I. – In the first group the scotopic ERG was normal. The amplitude curves of the a and b waves after dark adaptation were normal, but the ERG showed some time modifications, characteristic for cone dystrophies, and a modification of the a_1/a_2 relationship, which was most evident in low-flicker.

The photopic response after light adaptation was either completely absent or very reduced. In the latter case, we found either a reduction of the b wave amplitude with apparently normal oscillatory potentials or a global reduction of the photopic complex (b wave and oscillatory potentials).

The a wave was generally subnormal, although in one case within normal limits.

The time characteristics of the photopic ERG were mostly modified, the peak time of the a and b waves being increased.

The EOG was normal. The mean value of the L/D ratio was 210, that is to say the mean-value obtained in 40 normal people.

Ophthalmoscopic examination showed either a normal fundus or a slight macular pigmentation. In one case, there was a pigmentary disturbance of the retinal periphery.

99

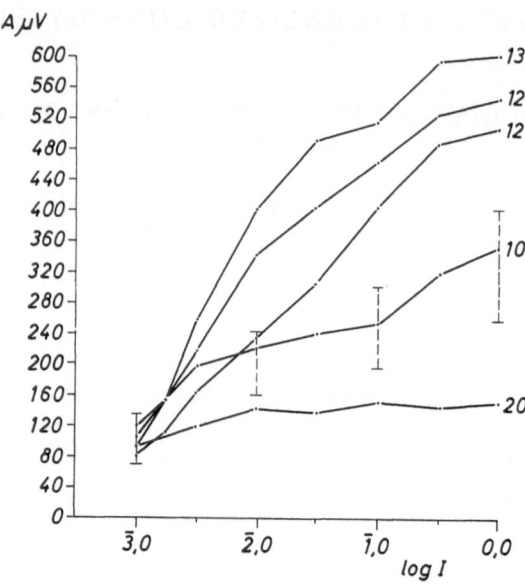

Fig. 1. Amplitude curves of the scotopic *b* wave in cases of cone dysfunction, compared to the normal mean and ± 2 S curves.

The dark adaptation curves showed a typical modification of the photopic segment with displacement of the Kohlrausch kink. In some cases the scotopic threshold, too, was not within normal limits.

We found familial cases. Among these, a brother and a sister, aged respectively 7 and 17 years and showing an albinotic fundus, had both a definitely supernormal ERG. The amplitude of, the *a* and *b* waves were beyond normal values. The duration of the *b* wave was also increased. The photopic ERG, although reduced, was still present in the younger brother and apparently absent in the older sister, but summation evidenced a negative response with increased peak time (Fig. 2). The scotopic threshold of the dark adaptation curve was raised, and this was not seen in the younger brother.

Group II. – This group was characterized by a flattening of the *b* wave amplitude curve. Responses to dim stimulations were within normal limits, but responses to bright flashes remained below normal values. The amplitude of the *a* wave was also subnormal. Time modifications of the ERG were similar to these of the first group. On the whole, this type of ERG resembled this observed in congenital monochromatism. The photopic ERG, although severely reduced, could in some cases still be present. In one case, we obtained even a photopic response of 35 μV (*b* wave).

The EOG in these cases were either normal or subnormal. The mean L/D ration was 165 (instead of 210 in normal people): Fig. 3.

The scotopic threshold of the dark adaptation curve was always normal.

Ophthalmoscopic examination showed very different pictures. In one case, the

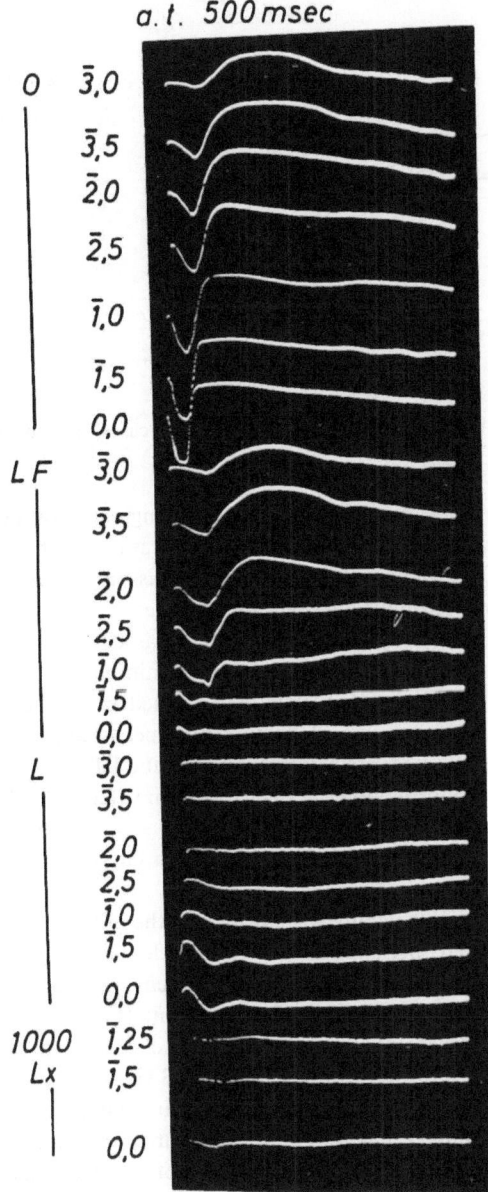

Fig. 2. ERG recordings of a case of group I (with supranormal amplitude of the scotopic *b* wave). O = darkness, LE = low flicker responses in darkness, L = adaptation to a light of 300 lux. Relative intensity of the stimulus in log. units. CAT computer. Summation of 5 responses in darkness, of 25 responses in light.

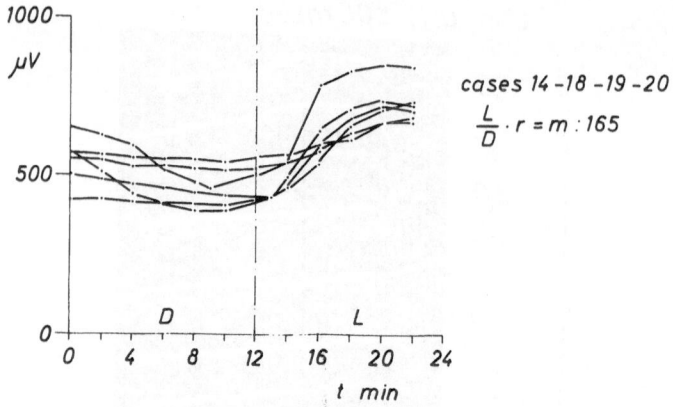

Fig. 3. Amplitude curves of the EOG in cases of group II.

fundus was completely normal and fluorescein angiography revealed no ano-maly. In other cases, we found macular degenerations with or without peri-pheral pigment disturbances. In 3 cases there was an interesting appearance, namely a macular dystrophy with snail slime reflexes.

Group III. – In this group, the scotopic ERG was definitely pathologic. The amplitude curve of the *b* wave was reduced for all stimulus intensities.

The photopic ERG was completely extinguished in all these cases. In one case only, a photopic response of about 10 µV persisted. This case could be considered as a border line case between group II and III.

The EOG was subnormal in each case, the mean value of the L/D ratio being 124 (Fig. 4).

The scotopic threshold of the dark adaptation curve was either normal or raised.

In one case the fundus picture was normal. In the other cases various fundus lesions were observed: peripapillary choroidal sclerosis, macular degeneration with snail slime reflex or with peripheral involvement, and, in 3 cases, a pig-mentary dystrophy of the inferior half of the retina (Fig. 5). Similar cases have been published by BERSON et al. (1968) and by THALER et al. (1972).

One of the patients of this group, a woman, 33 years of age and showing the characteristic ERG of a progressive cone dysfunction, had a younger sister, who had been examined 7 years before. At that time, the ERG was normal (photopic and scotopic), so that the diagnosis of localized macular degenera-tion was made. This patient could be examined again.

At the present time, the two sisters, aged respectively 33 and 20 years, show very similar fundus pictures and retinal functions. They both have a macular degeneration with choroidal sclerosis and fundus flavimaculatus of the pos-terior pole.

The colour vision is severely disturbed (red-green dyschromatopsia, type I). There is a central scotoma of about 20° (V/4). The dark adaptation curve shows a raised scotopic threshold at $\overline{3},4$, the younger at $\overline{4},0$.

102

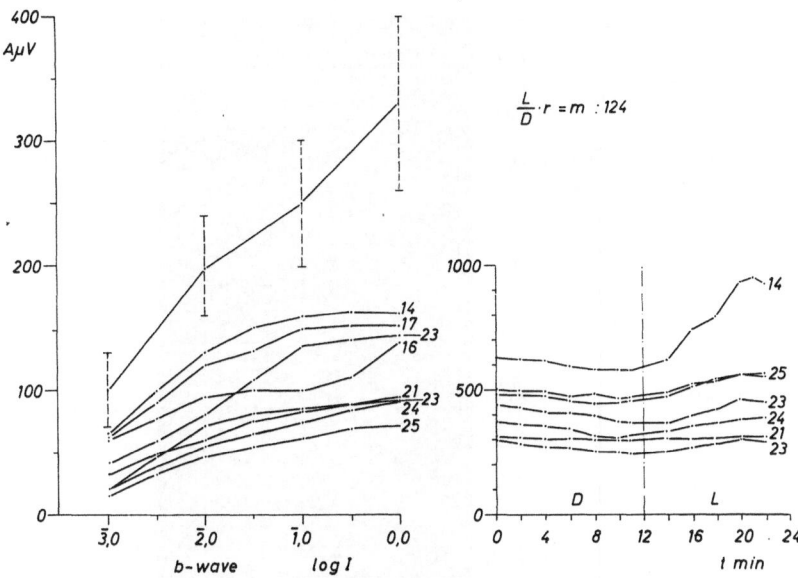

Fig. 4. At the left, amplitude curves of the scotopic *b* waves in cases of cone-rod dysfunction (group III). At the right, amplitude curves of the EOG and mean L/D ratio of group III.

But the ERG recordings are very dissimilar. The older sister has a typical cone dystrophy. The photopic ERG is absent. The scotopic ERG is subnormal, the maximal *b* wave having an amplitude of about 100 μV. The EOG is completely flat.

The younger sister, who had previously a normal ERG, shows now a very pathologic ERG, but with parallel involvement of both systems. The photopic ERG is present and has a maximal amplitude of 35 μV. The scotopic *b* wave has a maximal amplitude of 90 μV. The ratio photopic *b* wave/scotopic *b* wave is about 0,39 (in normal people, this ratio usually lies between 0,12 and 0,35).

CONCLUSIONS

1. The electro-physiological concept of cone dysfunction does not correspond to a clinical entity, but includes several distinct dystrophies.
2. There is a good correlation between the EOG modification and the behaviour of the scotopic ERG.
3. In familial cases, the electrodiagnostic tests may be very dissimilar in the affected members.

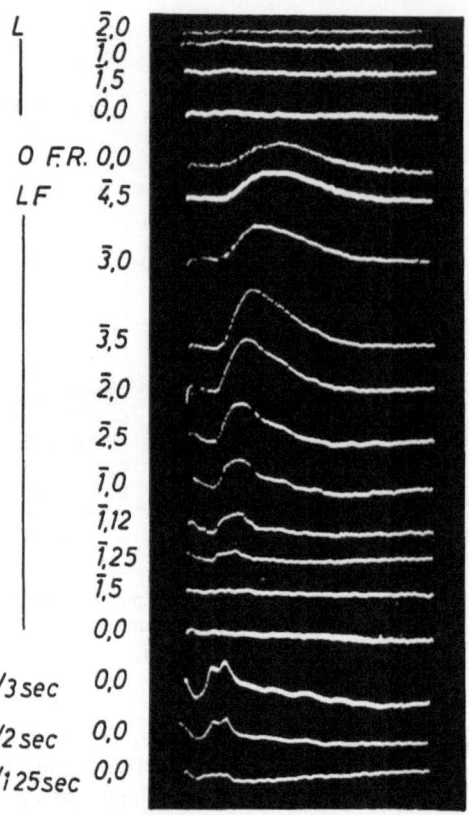

Fig. 5. ERG recording of a case with segmental pigmentary retinopathy and cone dysfunction. L = light-adapted state, O = dark adapted state, FR = red filter, LF = low flicker response (1,5 c/s). CAT computer. Analysis time 250 msec.

REFERENCES

Babel, J. & Stangos, M. Dégénérescence progressive du système photopique. *Ophthalmologica* 165: *392-395* (1972).

Babel, J. & Stangos, M. Progressive degeneration of the photopic system. *Amer. J. Ophthal.* 75: *511-525* (1973).

Berson, E. L., Gouras, P. & Gunkel, R. D. Progressive cone-rod degeneration. *Arch. Ophthal. Chicago* 80: *68-75* (1968).

Berson, E. L., Gouras, P. & Gunkel, R. D. Progressive cone degeneration, dominantly inherited. *Arch. Ophthal., Chicago* 80: *77-83* (1968).

Goodman, G., Ripps, H. & Siegel, I. M. Cone dysfunction syndromes. *Arch. Ophthal., Chicago* 70: *214-231* (1963).

Goodman, G., Ripps, H. & Siegel, I. M. Progressive cone degeneration. In: Burian, H. M. & Jacobson, J. H., Ed.: Clinical electroretinography. Pergamon Press, Oxford, 363-372 (1966).

Krill, A. E. The electroretinogram and electrooculogram: clinical applications. *Invest. Ophthal.* 9: *600-619* (1970).

KRILL, A. E., DEUTMAN, A. F. & FISHMANN, M. The cone dystrophies. *Doc. Ophthal.* 35: *1-80* (1973).
SLOAN, L. L. & BROWN, D. J. Progressive retinal degeneration with selective involvement of the cone mechanism. *Amer. J. Ophthal.* 54: *629-641* (1962).
THALER, A., HEILIG, P. & SLEZAK, H. Kombination einer angeborenen Achromatopsia mit Sektorformigen Degeneratio Pigmentosa Retinae. *Graefes Arch. Klin. Exp. Ophthal.* 183: *310-316* (1972).

Author's address:

Ophthalmological Clinic
University of Ghent, De Pintelaan 135
B 9000 Ghent
Belgium

105

ABSENT CONE FUNCTION (A SURVEY OF CLINICAL CASES)

A. PINCKERS & J. M. THIJSSEN

(Nijmegen)

INTRODUCTION

In the course of an investigation concerning congenital achromatopsia, a number of patients characterized by the absence of cone function were selected from among approximately 1000 ERG's; the findings were then compared with data from the literature.

TECHNIQUE (FIG. 1).

ERG: Photostimulation was applied with a Van Gogh stimulator SV-1B with a Xenon flash tube, mounted on an adaptometer sphere of the Goldmann-Weekers type (cf. THIJSSEN, PINCKERS & OTTO, in preparation), stimulation intensities 0.1-0.2-0.4-0.8 Joule, respectively; red filter (Kodak-Wratten No. 92) blue filter (Kodak-Wratten No. 47B). Electrodes: AgAgCl (Beckmann type 650414); the field of stimulation was 15°, the field of adaptation was Ganzfeld.

Registration:
a. mesopic conditions 0.1-0.2-0.4-0.8 Joule
b. blue and red mesopic 0.8 Joule
c. flicker frequency 20-44-54 per second, 0.2 Joule
d. 5 minutes, 2500 lux, followed by red 0.8 Joule
e. 12 minutes D.A., white light 0.2 Joule
f. blue and red 0.2 Joule.

Colour vision examination: Lighting 6 Philips' fluorescent lamps colour 57; Illumination at 1 meter, 1750 lux. Tests: AOHRR, Farnsworth Panel D-15, Farnsworth 100 Hue, anomaloscope Nagel Model II.

Since, in the course of studying presumed congenital achromatopsia (PINCKERS, 1972) it was found that in the absence of cone function, rod function varied, the ERG recordings were subdivided into 5 categories, corresponding to the degree of rod dysfunction (Table 2).

As in category I, a reduced cone response in 30% of the cases had to be attributed to media opacity, this category again was subdivided into two sub-

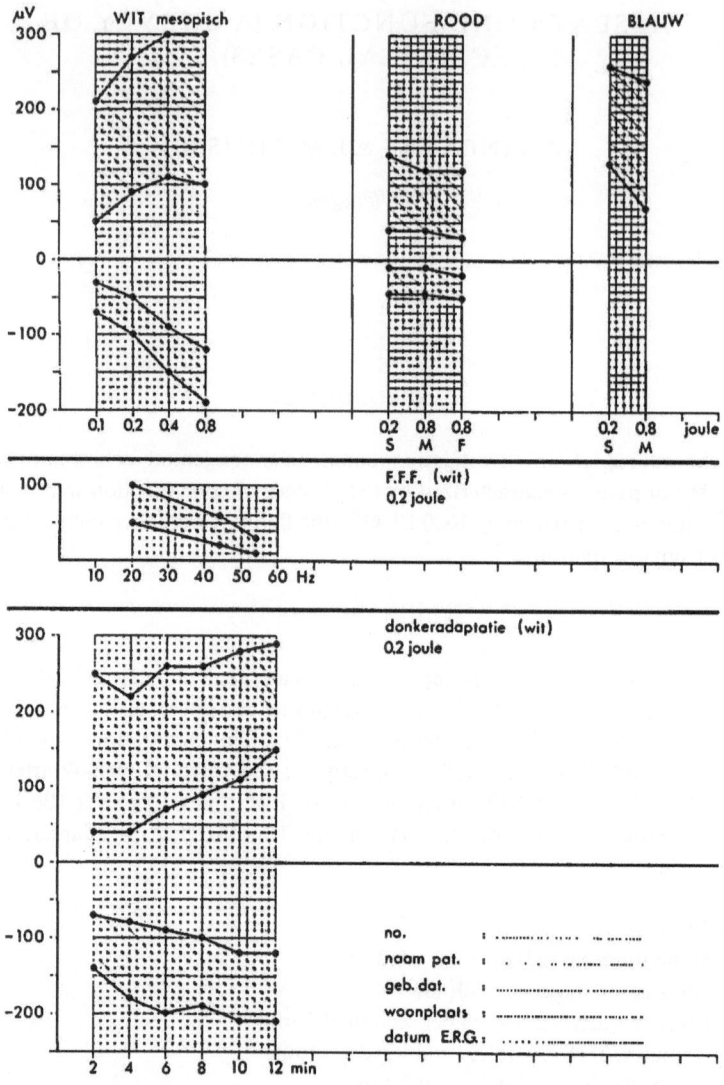

groups; although group IA was the more numerous, this group was excluded from the remainder of the investigation for the reason mentioned; this, however, does not imply that category IA might not include cases of genuine cone dysfunction.

The third table shows that the patient material is divided equally over the 5 remaining groups. GOODMAN et al. (1963) have listed the following criteria of cone dysfunction:

1. absence of photopic flicker ERG;
2. subnormal visual acuity;
3. defective color vision.

108

TABLE 2
Cone dysfunction; division of ERG in categories, expressing the various degrees of rod function

	Photopic CFF (white)	Red stimulus	Mesopic (blue, white)	D. A. (white)	Skotopic (blue)	
category I A	±	±	+	+	+	Legends: +: normal response
I B	0	0	+	+	+	±: partly diminished response
II	0	0	±	+	+	—: definitely diminished response
III	0	0	—	+	+	0: absent response
IV	0	0	—	±	±	
V	0	0	—	—	—	

TABLE 3

Absent cone function. Diagnosis and ERG categories

Diagnosis	category I B	category II	category III	category IV	category V	TOTAL
cong. achromatopsia	7	11	12	4	4	38
juv. macula deg.	7	0	2	5	6	20
nystagmus	2	3	2	0	1	8
myopia	2	1	0	3	2	8
myopia (no RG-defect)	0	2	1	0	6	9
coloboma chorioideae	0	0	0	2	0	2
nivaquin-intoxication	0	1	0	0	0	1
ablatio operata	0	0	0	1	1	2
arteriolar occlusion	0	0	0	1	0	1
perforatio bulbi	0	0	0	0	1	1
siderosis oculi	0	0	0	0	1	1
TOTAL	18	18	17	16	22	91

Also, these authors report nystagmus and photophobia as being present in a fairly large proportion of the cases. In our investigation we have adopted the criterion of an absence of a photopic flicker ERG combined with absence of a red response; all patients showed a subnormal visual acuity; colour vision was not, however, always defective; this last-mentioned point will be further discussed below.

Nystagmus was encountered in 70% of the cases and photophobia in 63%; 62% of the patients were found to have an error of refraction indicating myopia.

Table 3 shows that in presumed congenital achromatopsia, rod function is often reduced (viz. categories II through V); a 3 years' follow-up of 6 patients revealed progressive impairment of the rod function in 3 of them. This shows that congenital achromatopsia is not necessarily exclusively concerned with cone dysfunction, and also that congenital achromatopsia is not necessarily a stationary process.

Color vision was markedly defective in 90 % of the patients; and examination with the anomaloscope revealed a distinct decrease of the red-sensitivity; in 10 %, on the other hand, we only found a reduced blue-yellow sensitivity or normal color vision; it was interesting to note that these 9 patients were all myopic (Table 4).

Any discussion of myopia must always be a delicate matter. We are familiar with refraction myopia and degenerative myopia; the latter form is often encountered in combination with heredo-degenerative diseases. Myopia has been seen to occur in the x-linked form of congenital achromatopsia (SPIVEY, 1964; FRANÇOIS, 1966). VOGT (1924) described a dominant heredity with the combination of myopia, nystagmus and amblyopia. MCGREGOR (1946) one with a combination of myopia and nystagmus. Accordingly, it is not surprising that we encountered myopia in 62 % of our patients.

JAYLE et al. (1959) assert that the ERG alterations in myopia concern the photopic component in the first place. If color vision is defective, this usually means that there exists an acquired blue-yellow disorder, although a mild red-green disorder may also be present (FRANÇOIS et al., 1957).

In our material there were 9 myopic patients with an absence of cone function as demonstrated by electroretinography; on investigation of the color vision, however, this absence of cone function was not associated with a marked reduction of the sensitivity to red. On the basis of the ERG findings, these patients are to be classified in the myopic group with an abnormal ERG and with predominant cone dysfunction (JAYLE et al., 1965); on the basis of examination of the color vision alone, this diagnosis would not have been made. It is

TABLE 4
Absent cone function, myopia; colour vision normal or only blueyellow defect.

Patient	Myopia	Nystag-mus	Photo-phobia	AOHRR	Panel D-15	FM 100 Hue	Anoma-loscope	Eye
II-715	−4	−	−	strong tritan		BT+		ODS
II-719	−7	−	−	strong tritan	C/T	BT		ODS
III-2222	−9	−	−	Normal	Normal	Normal	Q=1,0	OD
	−11	−	−	strong tritan medium tetartan	C//T	BT	Q=0,77	OS
V-797	−6,5	−	−	Normal		Normal		ODS
V-1171	−7,5	+	−	Normal	Normal	Normal		ODS
V-1747	−2,5	−	−	Normal	Normal	Normal	Q=1,0	OD
	−2,5	−	−	Normal	Normal	BT	Q=1,0	OS
V-2239	−2,5	−	+	Normal	2 ME	BT	Q=0,91	OD
	−3,0	−	±	Normal	Normal	BT	Q=0,91	OS
V-2271	−7	−	−	Normal	2 ME		Q=1,0	ODS
V-2346	−3,5	−	−	Normal	Normal		Q=1,0	ODS

to be regretted that GOODMAN et al. (1963) in their discussion of cone dysfunction syndromes make no mention of the refraction, so that we cannot compare our 9 patients with their cases, as GOODMAN also, reported that in certain cases color vision was found to be defective to only a slight degree. In 5 of our 9 patients we did also an electro-oculography examination; in one case there was a subnormal Lp/Dt-ratio, the remaining 4 patients had a normal standing potential and normal Lp/Dt-ratio.

It may be concluded from our analysis that as a rule, an electroretinographically demonstrated absent cone function may be associated with a markedly defective color vision. In presumed congenital achromatopsia there may also be a reduced rod function, which occasionally is found to be progressive. As the diagnostic groups are distributed approximately equally over the ERG categories, we even feel justified in making the general statement that cone dysfunction is often associated with some degree of rod dysfunction.

There exists a form of myopia in which the color vision remains surprisingly normal, notwithstanding an electroretinographically absent cone function; accordingly in such cases the macular area is relatively well-preserved, although the visual acuity is reduced.

REFERENCES

FRANÇOIS, J. & VERRIEST, G. Les dyschromatopsies acquises. *Ann. Oculist.* 190: *844-849* (1957).

FRANÇOIS, J., VERRIEST, G., MATTON-VAN LEUVEN, M. TH., DE ROUCK, A. & MANAVIAN, D. Atypical achromatopsia of sex-linked recessive inheritance. *Am. J. Ophthal.* 61: *1101-1108* (1966).

GOODMAN, F., RIPPS, H. & SIEGEL, J. M. Cone dysfunction syndromes. *Arch. Opth.* (*Chicago*) 70: *214-231* (1963).

JAYLE, G. E. & BOYER, R. L. Les donées de l'électro-rétinographie dynamique dans la myopie. Symposium Luhacovice, *Acta Fac. Med. Univ. Brunesis* 4: *263-272* (1959).

JAYLE, G. E., BOYER, R. L. & SARACCO, J. B. L'électrorétinographie. Masson et Cie., tôme II, 929-969 (1965).

McGREGOR, I. S. Pedigree of nystagmus, myopia and congenital eye defects with mental deficiency. *Ann. Eugenics* 13: *135-140* (1946).

PINCKERS, A. Achromatopsie congénitale. *Ann. Oculist.* 205: *821-834* (1972).

SPIVEY, B. E., PEARLMAN, J. T. & BURIAN, H. M. Electroretinographic findings (including flicker) in carrier of congenital x-linked achromatopsia. *Doc. Ophthal.* 18: *367-375* (1964).

VOGT, A. Zur Genese der sphärischen Refraktionen. *Ber. Deutsch. Ophth. Ges. Heidelberg* 44: *67-71* (1924).

Author's address:

Dept. of Ophthalmology
University of Nijmegen
Nijmegen

CONE DYSTROPHY WITH DOMINANT INHERITANCE
PART 1: CLINICAL CASE HISTORIES

JEROME T. PEARLMAN, W. GEOFFREY OWEN, DAVID
W. BROUNLEY & JOSEPH J. SHEPPARD

(Los Angeles and Santa Monica)

ABSTRACT

Nine patients with acquired cone dystrophy inherited as an autosomal dominant trait are reported in a family pedigree spanning four generations. Preliminary color vision testing included the usual AO H-R-R and Ishihara pseudoisochromatic plates. In addition, dark adaptometry and electroretinography was performed. ERGs with flicker fusion determinatives confirmed the functional photopic defect. Fluorescein angiography was performed in selected cases.

None of the patients examined showed grossly demonstrable nystagmus or ophthalmoscopically visible pigmentary maculopathy. Fluorescein studies suggested the presence of a subtle deterioration of the retinal pigment epithelium, resembling a faint 'bull's eye' pattern.

Characteristic of this pedigree was the onset of color vision difficulty in early teen years with steady progression towards achromacy by the fourth or fifth decade of life.

INTRODUCTION

Color vision abnormalities were found in nine members of a single family having cone dystrophy with minimally demonstrable maculopathy or optic nerve disease. The disorder, inherited as an autosomal dominant trait, appears some years after birth and follows a slowly progressive course. The color vision defects gradually increase in severity, and produce serious impairments of the color sense resembling clinical achromatopsia.

Achromatopsia or total color blindness is a rare clinical disorder that usually has some familial aspects; several varieties are known. The congenital variety appears to be inherited as an autosomal recessive or X-linked recessive trait. (1-5) Other late appearing forms of achromatopsia are symptomatic of cone dysfunction syndromes, (6-11) usually with some evidence of macular degeneration or optic nerve disease, and at least one variety is inherited as an autosomal dominant trait.

The clinical features of the family described in this study are compared to other pedigrees in which cone dysfunction is an inherited feature.

This study was supported by USPHS Research Grant EY-00331, from the National Institutes of Health, and Postdoctoral Research Fellowship (DR. OWEN) 1 F02 EY 50, 414-01 from the National Institutes of Health, U.S. Public Health Service.

Reprint requests to JEROME T. PEARLMAN, M.D., Jules Stein Eye Institute, UCLA School of Medicine, Los Angeles, CA 90024.

In addition to routine ophthalmic evaluation with visual fields, dark-adaptation testing and electroretinography were performed. Visual acuity was measured with a highly directional Snellen projection screen. In the patient's direction, the luminance with the room light out measured 56 foot candles. With the room lights turned on, a veiling luminance of 9 foot candles was added across the screen.

Dark-adaptation studies were performed using the Goldmann-Weekers adaptometer, using a two-degree test object flickering on and off at one-second dark and light intervals. Each test was conducted in the standard manner with pupils dilated by tropicamide 1% and phenylephrine hydrochloride 10% viscous ophthalmic solutions. The patients were exposed to preadapting illumination of 18 lux (2800 abs) for five minutes. Each test lasted for a total of 45 minutes.

ERG studies were made in the routine manner of our laboratory. Following dark-adaptation testing, patients with pupils still dilated were required to dark adapt for an additional 45 minutes. Burian-Allen contact lens electrodes were then inserted under red light illumination, following the instillation of proparacaine hydrochloride 0.05% ophthalmic solution for corneal anesthesia. Single and multiple flash responses were recorded with white light of 20 msec duration. Stimulus flashes were delivered to dark-adapted eyes placed in Maxwellian view, via optical fibers from a tungsten lamp, using a Hartline shutter and a series of neutral density filters to vary stimulus intensity. Threshold responses were measured, beginning with subthreshold stimuli in single flashes. Approximately 30 seconds were allowed to elapse before presenting the next flash. As the stimulus intensity was increased, the interval between single flashes was lengthened to approximately one minute to insure the maintenance of the dark-adapted state. Multiple flash (flicker) studies were made at the conclusion of each testing session to determine critical flicker fusion values.

Each of the nine affected members of the family was tested for color discrimination using these standard screening tests:
1. Ishihara pseudoisochromatic plates*
2. Hardy-Rand-Rittler pseudoisochromatic plates**

These tests were administered in the usual manner under Macbeth illuminant C.

CASE REPORTS

The O. family was introduced to us by the propositus (III-1). Four generations of the family were found to be involved (Fig. 1). There was no history of consanguinity. Sixteen descendents of the presumed first affected members were examined. Special color vision tests were performed on nine of these, and are reported in detail in Part II of this article.

* Kanehara Shuppan Co., Ltd., Tokyo, Japan
** American Optical Company, Buffalo, New York

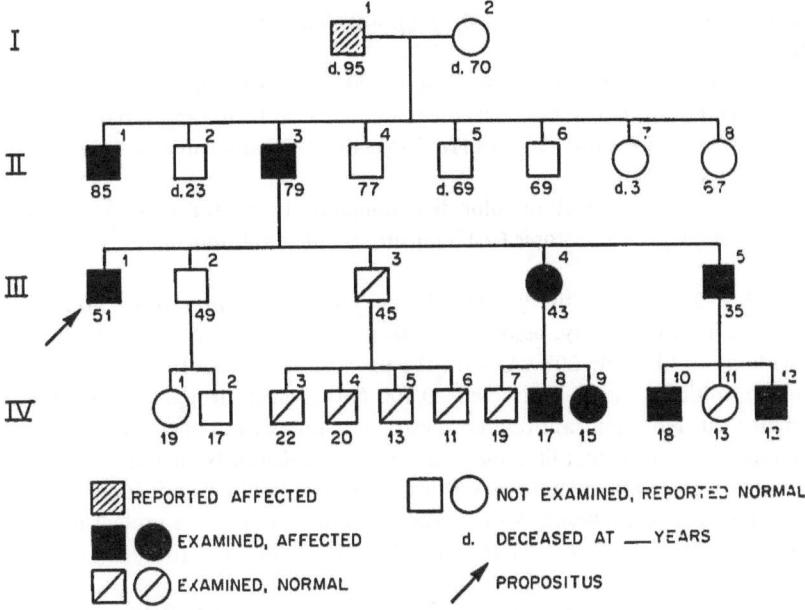

I

II

III

IV

REPORTED AFFECTED

EXAMINED, AFFECTED

EXAMINED, NORMAL

NOT EXAMINED, REPORTED NORMAL

d. DECEASED AT ___YEARS

PROPOSITUS

Fig. 1. Pedigree of family with acquired cone dystrophy, inherited as an autosomal dominant trait. Circles signify females; squares signify males.

Case 1, III-I (W.O.) – This 51-year-old man, the propositus, was first seen at the Long Beach Veterans Administration Hospital (Long Beach, California) with a history of decreased visual acuity since the age of 24 years. Several years after the onset of this symptom, the patient began to note difficulty with color vision. Photophobia had been present much of the patient's life, increasing in severity with the onset of symptoms. For years he had avoided bright lights, preferring dimly lighted rooms. During the day, the patient wore sunglasses. He felt that his vision improved at night. Visual acuity in each eye was 20/100 with room lights out; with lights turned on, the acuity dropped to finger-counting ability at five feet. No improvement could be obtained with corrective lenses. There was no nystagmus noted grossly (i.e. without slit-lamp magnification). Fundus examination revealed absent foveal reflexes, but were thought to be otherwise normal. Visual field tests (tangent screen, 1-mm white test object at 1 m) showed a three-degree scotoma, O.U. Kodachrome fundus photographs of this patient revealed a subtle pigmentary macular abnormality in both eyes. A partial, faint 'bull's eye' pattern formed an incomplete circle around the fovea. No convincing macular abnormality could be seen with fluorescein angiography, even when examined under magnification. A minimal hyperfluorescence was thought to be present on some of the photos.

The patient was unable to answer correctly any of the AO H-R-R pseudoisochromatic plates. This test was repeated on three different occasions. He was able to answer the first plate of the Ishihara series, which required no color discrimination ability. He was unable, however, to answer the first four plates

115

of the AO H-R-R- series. Each of these tests was performed under Macbeth illuminant C.

The dark-adaptation test showed an elevated cone threshold, but a normal rod development. Single ERG responses were normal with respect to threshold, but showed a CFF value of 16-18 Hz. Subjective CFF uniformly measured 9-10 Hz at all wavelengths.

The patient's total lack of color discrimination, his central scotoma, photophobia, and typically scotopic CFF indicate complete achromacy.

Case 2, II-3 (R.O.) – This 79-year-old man, father of the propositus, noticed a decrease in visual acuity, associated with poor color vision and photophobia beginning in his early 20's. As with the propositus, he saw better under dim light conditions. Visual acuity was 20/100 O.U., which dropped to 20/200 in bright light. No significant refractive error was present in either eye. No gross nystagmus was evident. Slit-lamp examination revealed early nuclear sclerosis in each lens and peripheral anterior cortical spoking. Fundus examination showed only absent foveal reflexes. A four-degree central scotoma was present in each visual field, using a 2-mm white test object at 1-m distance from the tangent screen.

The patient missed all of the screening series on the AO H-R-R plates and showed severe impairment in both the red-green and blue-yellow portions of the diagnostic series. His Ishihara responses were typical of a person with total color blindness.

Dark adaptometry revealed a slowed cone onset with a normal rod onset and final threshold.

The ERG responses to single flashes showed a normal threshold value, but the electroretinographic CFF was no greater than 12 Hz, indicating an impairment of the photopic system.

This patient's severe red-green and blue-yellow color vision impairment, decreased visual acuity with central scotomata, photophobia and scotopic CFF indicate complete achromacy. Other special tests were not performed because of the patient's age and the advanced state of his disorder.

Case 3, II-1 (F.O.) – This 85-year-old man, paternal uncle of the propositus, was examined by one of the authors (D.W.B.) at the patient's home in El Cerrito, California. He first noticed the onset of decreased vision and color vision problems with photophobia between the ages of 25 and 30 years. A further sudden decrease in vision occurred at 81 years, following a mild cerebral vascular accident. With the Rosenbaum pocket vision screener, the visual acuity of the right eye was 20/200 and that of the left eye was 20/400. Visual fields were grossly intact by confrontation. Ophthalmoscopic examination was within normal limits through undilated pupils. The patient was unable to answer correctly any of the AO H-R-R or Ishihara pseudoisochromatic test plates. Dark adaptation, ERG testing, and other color vision tests could not be obtained, because the patient was unable to travel to UCLA Medical Center.

116

Case 4, III-4 (B.O.P.) – This 43-year-old woman, sister of the propositus, first noticed difficulty with vision at the age of 10 years and began to experience color vision problems at the age of 15 years. She has noted unusual sensitivity to light most of her life.

Visual acuity was 20/70 O.U. in a dimly illuminated room. This was reduced to 20/200 O.U. with room lights on. Corrective lenses, consisting of + 0.50 sphere, O.U. did not improve her vision. There was no grossly visible nystagmus. Ophthalmoscopic examination was normal. Tangent screen fields revealed a 2- to 3-degree central scotoma in each eye with a 1-mm white test object at one meter.

The Kodachrome photographs of the patient's right eye showed a central cherry-like spot in the macula with a very faint circle of finely altered pigmentary changes surrounding the central foveal area. These changes were best seen on projection. The fluorescein photographs from this patient showed very mild hyperfluorescence in a ring-like pattern, suggesting, once again, very minimal change in the pigment epithelial layer of the retina. These changes are admittedly very faint, and could be easily overlooked.

The patient made errors on both AO H-R-R and Ishihara pseudoisochromatic test plates. She missed all of the symbols in the AO H-R-R screening series and scored a medium red-green defect (deutan type) and a medium blue-yellow defect (tritan type) in the diagnostic series.

Dark adaptometry with a 2-degree test field showed a mild slowing of cone onset and a normal rod component. The electroretinogram was normal for single flashes, with the objective CFF limited to 18 Hz. Subjective CFF was similar at wavelengths below 450 nm, but otherwise a normal CFF was found at all other wavelengths.

Case 5, IV-8 (J.P.) – This 17-year-old male, nephew of the propositus, was first examined in 1968. He is the son of an affected female member of the family (III-4). Initially, he was judged to be normal. His vision was 20/20 in each eye, and there were no fundus abnormalities.

He scored all correct answers on the AO H-R-R- screening series and the Ishihara plates.

A dark-adaptation test performed four years ago was thought to be normal. No ERG was performed.

In 1971, a repetition of the AO H-R-R- series showed a mild, but consistent red-green color vision defect. The Ishihara test was still completely normal.

Although two years older than his affected sister, this patient shows a reduced form of the same red-green defect. He clearly warrants further observation and repeated testing in the future.

Case 6, IV-9, (C.P.) – This 15-year-old female, niece of the propositus, is the daughter of affected family member, III-4.

At the time of her initial examination she complained of photophobia and decreased vision of approximately one-year duration. Her acuity measured 20/25 in each eye under dim illumination. Under bright light testing, her acuity diminished to 20/80 in each eye. No grossly visible nystagmus was present. Slit-lamp and fundus examination was normal bilaterally. No central scotomas were demonstrated by tangent screen field (April 1968). The initial AO H-R-R test revealed screening errors in both red-green and blue-yellow series. In the diagnostic series she had a mild red-green defect (unclassified) and a questionable blue-yellow defect. The Ishihara series had only three errors: Plates 7, 8, and 12.

Dark adaptometry revealed a mild slowing of cone onset with a normal rod onset and a normal rod curve and final threshold.

The ERG was remarkable only for the absence of a photopic flicker response. Her CFF, as measured by ERG response, was no greater than 10 Hz.

This patient therefore was thought to have a general protan/deutan defect somewhat different from the defect shown by her affected first cousins (IV-10, IV-12).

Case 7, III-5 (H.O.) – This 38-year-old man, a younger brother of the propositus, first experienced decreased visual acuity and color vision problems at age 25 years. He stated that he would 'squint' his eyes in bright lights to improve his vision and that he could function better at night or in dimly lighted rooms. His visual acuity measured 20/60 O.U. wearing corrective lenses in the trial frame: OD = −1.25 sph + 0.75 × 45°; OS = −1.50 sph + 0.75 × 30°. Fundus examination revealed the absence of foveal reflexes. Tangent screen fields demonstrated a two-degree central scotoma in each eye with a 1-mm white test object at one meter. No significant change in visual acuity was elicited when the level of room illumination was changed.

Fluorescein angiography revealed a faint hyperfluorescence in the foveal region of the right macula which, while barely noticeable except upon magnification, suggested some ring-like involvement of the retinal pigment epithelium. Kodachrome films of the macula were similar to those of the propositus, with the incomplete 'bull's eye' ring surrounding a homogeneous, almost central cherry-red spot-like area (Fig. 2), as described by BABEL & STANGOS (15).

Dark adaptation testing with a two-degree test field once again showed mild slowing of cone onset with a perfectly normal rod component and final dark-adapted threshold.

The ERG showed a normal response threshold to single flashes and the anticipated absence of photopic flicker: The objective CFF measured 15 Hz.

This patient did poorly on repeated testing with the Ishihara pseudoisochromatic plates, giving responses consistent with achromacy. However, with the AO H-R-R test Plates 1 and 7 were correctly answered on repeated trials.

Case 8, IV-10 (G.O.) – This 18-year-old man, nephew of the propositus and son of affected family member, III-5, had 20/20 vision in each eye when first examined in 1968. Slit-lamp and fundus examinations were normal. No previous history of photophobia or nystagmus was elicited, nor was any visual field defect found. This patient was thought to be normal until color vision testing revealed the following: He missed all of the screening plates in the red-green

118

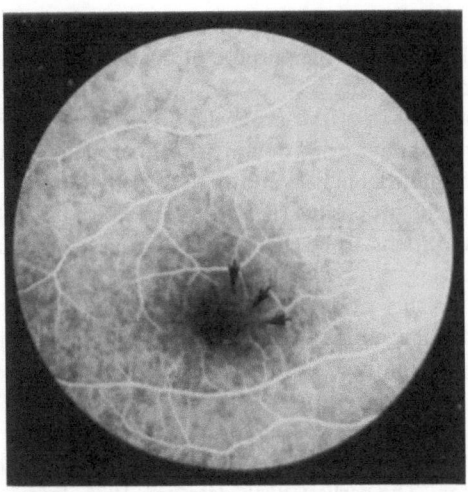

Fig. 2. Fluorescein angiogram (arterio-venous phase) of patient H.O. (III-5), showing incomplete 'bull's eye' ring of depigmentation around the fovea of the right eye.

series while correctly identifying the figures in the blue-yellow series. The diagnostic series revealed a moderate red-green defect of the deutan type. This showed slow progression over a three year period. The Ishihara test revealed a marked derangement of red-green function with responses resembling those of a person with total color blindness.

The dark-adaptation test was judged to be normal with respect to both cone and rod portions. The ERG was normal for single flashes, but showed an absence of photopic flicker. Maximum objective CFF was 12 Hz.

Case 9, IV-12 (R.O.) – The patient is a 12-year-old boy, nephew of the propositus and son of affected family member III-5. Furthermore, he is the stepbrother of the patient described in Case 8 (IV-10). Both boys have the same father, but different mothers.

This boy never had any eye difficulty or complaints related to central acuity, photophobia, or color sense. His refractive error was minimal. Vision measured 20/20 in each eye. No grossly visible nystagmus was noted. Slit-lamp and fundus features were entirely normal.

AO H-R-R- and Ishihara pseudoisochromatic plates have consistently shown a strong red-green defect over a three-year period. The former test specifies this as a deutan type of defect. No abnormality of blue-yellow color sense was found on AO H-R-R- plates.

Dark-adaptation testing was interpreted as normal, as was the electroretinogram. Objective CFF measured 18 Hz.

Other Family Members – R.C.O., 1-1, the grandfather of the propositus, was not alive at the time of this study, but his family reports that he had problems similar to known affected persons. He is reported to have suffered the onset of

119

'snow blindness' between the ages of 20 and 25 years with light sensitivity and decreased visual acuity. For the purpose of this study he is presumed to be an affected member.

R.O., III-3, a brother of the propositus, and three of his children (IV-4, IV-5, IV-6) were examined and found to be normal. A fourth son of R.O. (IV-3) was not examined, but he is known to be symptom free.

One nephew of the propositus (R.P., IV-7) and one niece (S.O., IV-11) were also examined and found to be clinically normal. Each gave normal responses to all color tests.

One younger brother of the propositus (E.O., III-2) and his two children (IV-1, IV-2) were not examined, but were thought to be normal by other family members. This group of three persons could not be tested because of geographic location.

While four generations have been discussed in this paper, birth and death dates are known for nine additional ancestors, extending the pedigree back another generation. The earliest birth date was 1835. Information concerning color vision problems in this group is totally lacking.

DISCUSSION

Familial reports of proven cone dystrophy are scarce, and as a result, the pattern of inheritance is still uncertain. We feel, therefore, that the present report is of some significance. The pedigree is large, covering as it does four generations. Furthermore, the autosomal dominant nature of the inheritance of this disease is quite clear.

Autosomal dominant inheritance is a relatively uncommon mode, though it does seem to be a feature of a number of acquired diseases of the eye including dominant optic nerve atrophy (13), vitelliform macular dystrophy (14) as well as congenital tritanopia and tritanomaly and cone dystrophies similar to that reported here (6, 8, 11).

A principal symptom of the disease shown by our patients is a serious disturbance of their ability to discriminate color. This symptom is common to all cone dystrophic syndromes (6-11, 13). The onset of the symptoms some years after birth and the relentlessly progressive nature leading toward eventual achromatopsia, indicates that our patients suffer from a cone dystrophy.

The progressive nature of the color vision defect in this family is especially meaningful, since one patient, (IV-8), developed the first symptoms of his disease during the course of this study. When first tested, he was color normal. On later testing after a four year interval, a red-green deficiency was shown. In terms of gathering further information about this disease, this patient will be of considerable interest for years to come.

Studies in which a similar progressive loss of color vision was found include those of SLOAN & BROWN (6); GOODMAN, RIPPS & SIEGEL (7); BERSON, GOURAS & GUNKEL (8); STRAUB & SCHMIDT (9); and KRILL & DEUTMAN (11). With the exception of BERSON, GOURAS & GUNKEL (8), these authors generally report evidence of nystagmus and some kind of polymorphic macular degeneration

120

with concomitant loss of the foveal reflex. Our patients most closely resemble those of BERSON, GOURAS & GUNKEL (8), where there was no clinical nystagmus and only minimally visible evidence of macular disease. While it is possible that nystagmus and marked macular pigmentary abnormalities may reveal themselves at a later date, it is significant that they are not yet observed in our oldest, most markedly affected patients, II-1 and II-3.

Certain of the patients described by GOODMAN, RIPPS & SIEGEL (7), patient 1 of group 1 and patients 33 and 40 of group II, also exhibited a cone dystrophy marked by a lack of nystagmus and of macular degeneration. It should be pointed out, however, that these cases were not genetically related to each other and that no statement was made concerning the mode of inheritance. Furthermore, since they were unrelated, one cannot conclude that they were suffering from a common disease, though the symptoms in each case were similar. By contrast, all patients in this report can be traced to a common ancestor. It is likely, therefore, that the pedigree provides the pattern of inheritance of a single type of cone dystrophy.

ACKNOWLEDGMENT

The authors gratefully acknowledge the expert and gracious technical assistance of Mrs. NOLA J. ALLSTON.

REFERENCES

1. WAARDENBURG, P. J., FRANCESCHETTI, A. & KLEIN, D. Genetics and Ophthalmology, vol. 2. Springfield, Ill., Charles C. Thomas p. 1703 (1963).
2. FRANÇOIS, J., VERRIEST, G., MATTON-VAN LEUVEN, M. TH., DE ROUCK, A. & MANAVIAN, D. Atypical achromatopsia of sex-linked inheritance. Am. J. Ophth. 1101 (1966).
3. SPIVEY, B. E. The X-linked recessive inheritance of atypical monochromatism. Arch. Ophth. 74: 327 (1965).
4. SPIVEY, B. E., PEARLMAN, J. T. & BURIAN, H. M. Electroretinographic findings (including flicker) in carriers of congenital X-linked achromatopsia. Doc. Ophthal. 18: 367 (1964).
5. EARLL, J. M., SPIVEY, B. E. & MATTEI, I. R. Atypical congenital monochromatism. Arch. Intern. Med. 118: 491 (1966).
6. SLOAN, L. L. & BROWN, D. J. Progressive retinal degeneration with selective involvement of the cone mechanism. Am. J. Ophth. 54: 629 (1962).
7. GOODMAN, G., RIPPS, H. & SIEGEL, I. M. Cone dysfunction syndromes. Arch. Ophth. 70: 214 (1963).
8. BERSON, E., GOURAS, P. & GUNKEL, R. D. Progressive cone degeneration, dominantly inherited. Arch. Ophth. 80: 77 (1968).
9. STRAUB, W. & SCHMIDT, B. Electrophysiological investigations in a family with central retinopathy. In: BASAR, D. & BENGISU, U., (Eds.): Symposium of Electroretinography. Istanbul, Faculty of Medicine, University of Istanbul (1971).
10. STEINMETZ, R. D., OGLE, K. N. & RUCKER, C. W. Some physiologic considerations of hereditary macular degeneration. Am. J. Ophth. 42: 304 (1956).
11. KRILL, A. E. & DEUTMAN, A. F. Dominant macular degenerations: the cone dystrophies. Am. J. Ophth. (to be published).
12. WRIGHT, W. D. Researches in normal and defective color vision. London, Kimpton (1947).

121

13. KRILL, A. E. & FISHMAN, G. A. Acquired color vision defects. *Tr. Am. Acad. Ophth. Otolaryng.* 75: *1095* (1971).
14. KRILL, A. E., MORSE, B. A., POTTS, A. M. & KLIEN, B. A. Hereditary vitelliruptive macular degeneration. *Am. J. Ophth.* 61: *1405* (1966).
15. BABEL, J. & STANGOS, N. Progressive degeneration of the photopic system. *Am. J. Ophth.* 75: *511* (1973).

Authors' addresses:

JEROME T. PEARLMAN
W. GEOFFREY OWEN
DAVID W. BROUNLEY
Dept. of Ophthalmology
Visual Physiology Laboratory
Jules Stein Eye Institute
UCLA school of Medicine
Los Angeles Ca 90024

JOSEPH J. SHEPPARD
Rand Corporation
Santa Monica
California

CONE DYSTROPHY WITH DOMINANT INHERITANCE
PART II: SPECIAL COLOR VISION TESTS

JEROME T. PEARLMAN, W. GEOFFREY OWEN,
DAVID W. BROUNLEY, & JOSEPH J. SHEPPARD

(Los Angeles and Santa Monica)

ABSTRACT

Of the patients examined during this phase of the study, all but one (J.P. [IV-8]) showed clear evidence of reduced color discrimination. The data for J.P. suggest that his color discrimination is just within normal limits.

There was no clear pattern by which the dystrophy progressed. Patients of similar age who obtained similar 100-Hue test scores often possessed different types of defect. Among the younger patients there was no clear correlation between patient's age and the severity of his defect.

Patients who showed gross disturbance of color discrimination appeared to have normal thresholds for their π_4 and π_5 functions. This may suggest a post-receptoral site for the red-green discrimination defect.

There was evidence, both from the data and by verbal report that, under some conditions, luminances which appeared only moderately bright to a normal observer appeared 'glaring' to our patients. It is believed that this 'glare' may contribute to the patient's inability to discriminate some colors under normal illumination levels.

INTRODUCTION

In the second phase of this study there were two principal objectives. The first of these was to establish whether or not the dystrophy possessed by those members of the family described in the preceding report proceeded according to some recognizable pattern. In order to meet this objective we evaluated the color discrimination of each individual by two methods which were considerably more sensitive than the standard diagnostic test plates of Ishihara or AO H-R-R. In addition, we measured the relative spectral sensitivity curve of each patient and compared it with averaged data from six normal subjects measured under identical conditions. Stiles π mechanism determinations were also made.

This study was supported by USPHS Research Grant EY-00331, from the National Institutes of Health, and Postdoctoral Research Fellowship (DR. OWEN) 1 F02 EY 50, 414-01 from the National Institutes of Health, U.S. Public Health Service.

Reprint requests to JEROME T. PEARLMAN, M.D., Jules Stein Eye Institute, UCLA School of Medicine, Los Angeles, CA 90024

MATERIALS AND METHODS

Apparatus

The apparatus used in this phase of the study included a two beam photostimulator of our own design. A variety of stimulus configurations could be produced using either beam separately or both beams simultaneously. These could be superimposed at will upon a background field. The wavelength and intensity of each beam and the background could be controlled independently. The stimulus and the background were viewed in Maxwellian view and appeared to be at infinity. The head of the subject was located by means of a dental bite plate and forehead rest.

Calibration of the apparatus was carried out with the aid of an Epply laboratory thermopile and a Keithley model 148 nanovoltmeter.

Color discrimination tests

Two color vision tests were administered. The first of these was the standard Farnsworth-Munsell 100-hue test. This test which is widely used and will not be described in detail here, was administered under a Macbeth lamp whose spectral energy distribution approximated C.I.E. illuminant C.

Since the eighty-five colored chips of which the Farnsworth-Munsell test is comprised are desaturated, a second method of evaluation, using highly saturated colors, was also used. These were produced with the aid of narrow bandwidth interference filters (half-bandwidth less than 8 nm) and an Ebert grating monochrometer (Jarrell-Ash). The method adopted involved the measurement of the wavelength discrimination step at a number of wavelengths throughout the spectrum. The technique for doing this has been fully described by WRIGHT (1). Our only departure from his schema was in our choice of a 7° circular, bipartite field, seen in Maxwellian view.

Determination of spectral sensitivity

This was carried out using an incremental threshold technique. The test stimulus consisted of a circular field subtending 7° superimposed on a white background, subtending 31° at the center of the subject's pupil. The retinal illumination produced by the background was 200 photopic trolands. The subject was asked to adjust a subliminal stimulus first to the point where it became just visible and then to the point where it became once more just visible. The luminance of the stimulus in the latter condition was taken to be the threshold of the stimulus. The average of ten such discriminations was taken for each wavelength tested. The stimulus was flashed once every 2 seconds and had a duration of 100 msec. The inverse of the increment threshold of the stimulus was plotted as a function of stimulus wavelength.

124

Measurements of threshold vs radiance curves (Stiles π-mechanisms)

A monochromatic, 14° stimulus, consisting of a set of vertical bars, each 1° wide, separated from its neighbors by 1°, was chosen for this experiment. The choice of such a configuration was influenced by two considerations. One of them was that such a large stimulus was sure to stimulate the great majority of cones which are concentrated within 7° of the center of the fovea. When dealing with patients who exhibit a central scotoma, this becomes important. The barred pattern provides points of high contrast all over this area which aid in the detection of stimuli. A second consideration was logistical. Since the members of the family were only available for a brief period of time and since it was necessary to use such a stimulus for another test to be administered during that time, it was decided that this configuration should be used in both cases.

The stimulus was exposed once every 2 seconds with a duration of 100 msec. The threshold was determined by the same criterion as described in the previous section. Thresholds were determined against a monochromatic background whose radiance was varied over a 5 log unit range. The data were plotted and interpreted in the manner described by STILES (2).

RESULTS

Farnsworth-Munsell 100-Hue Test

This test was attempted by patient W.O. (III-1) but he was unable to make any judgements which he felt were meaningful and was allowed to give up. Patient H.O. (III-5), the younger brother of W.O. scored 897 errors in this test. There was, needless to say, no recognizable axis to his charted data, though there was an indication of residual discrimination in the region of 575 nm. His elder son, G.O. (IV-10) scored 198 errors along axes running through points 18 and 54. H.O.'s younger son, R.O. (IV-12) scored 294 errors along similar axes though in his case the axes were less well defined. We interpreted both G.O.'s and R.O.'s data to be characteristic of a predominantly deutan defect of moderate severity.

B.O.P. (III-4) scored 445 errors. Loss of discrimination was evident in all regions of the chart, though the principal errors were grouped along axes through points 2 and 44. This indicates a strong tritan component to a general color vision disturbance. Her moderately good performance in the general region of points 20 and 64 is consistent with this interpretation.

B.O.P.'s daughter, C.P. (IV-9) scored 349 errors with a principal error axis through points 27 and 70. A strong protan defect is suggested. J.P. (IV-8, the son of B.O.P.) scored 94 errors which is just within normal limits for this test.

Wavelength discrimination

The wavelength discrimination data obtained for six observers is represented in Figs. 1a and 1b. H.O (III-5) made observations but his discrimination was everywhere so poor that it could not be repeated satisfactorily in graphical form. It will be seen (Fig. 1B) that H.O.'s sons G.O. (IV-10) and R.O. (IV-12) both exhibit a reduction of wavelength discrimination in the green-red region of the spectrum, though the extent of G.O.'s defect is clearly greater than that of his younger brother. This is consistent with the results of the Farnsworth-Munsell 100-Hue test for the yellow region of the spectrum, despite the apparent anomaly of R.O.'s higher error score in that test.

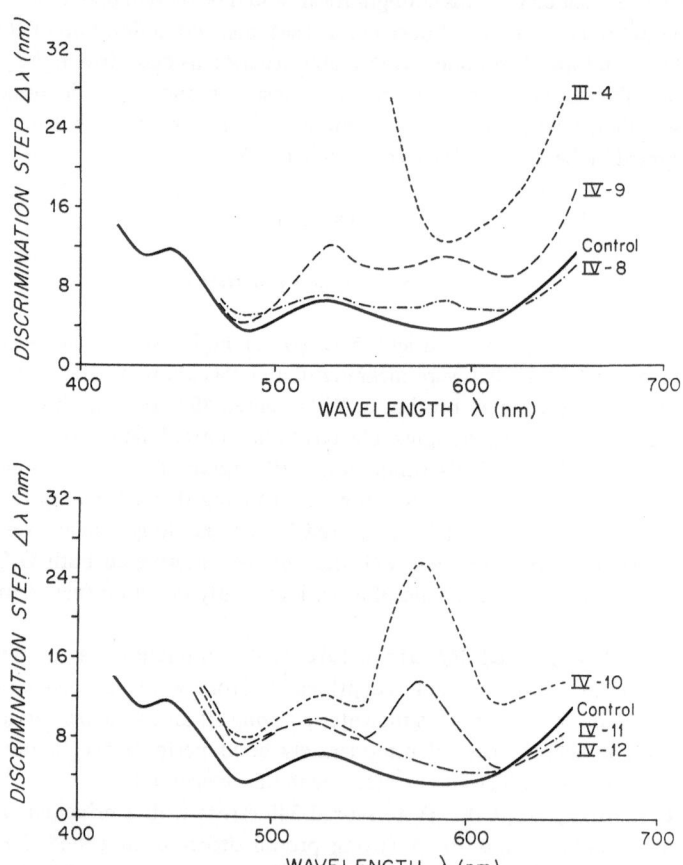

Fig. 1. Wavelength discrimination data obtained for six patients, a) B.O.P. (III-4); J.P. (IV-8); C.P. (IV-9); G.O. (IV-10); S.O. (IV-11) and R.O. (IV-12). The solid line is the averaged data of six normal trichromats. The size of the discrimination step for the normal is longer than one usually sees, though this is not unusual when untrained observers are used. Observer S.O. (IV-11) was judged normal in this and other color discrimination tests and hence did not take part in later tests.

B.O.P. (III-4) has a region of best wavelength discrimination in the green-red region of the spectrum, a feature consistent with the pronounced tritan component in her disorder which was diagnosed from her 100-Hue test data (Fig. 1A). Her daughter C.P. (IV-9) shows a general discrimination loss in the green-red region of the spectrum while her son's discrimination (J.P., IV-8) is within normal limits for the technique as applied here.

Relative spectral sensitivity

The relative spectral sensitivity of six patients are plotted in Fig. 2A and 2B. A control curve, which is the mean for six normal subjects measured under identical conditions, is shown for comparison. All curves are plotted on the same axes.

It is clear that the shapes of the curves of five of the six patients were significantly different from the normal, the exception being J.P. (IV-8). In all cases there was a general reduction in sensitivity throughout the spectrum. There is an interesting correlation between the extent of this sensitivity loss of any given patient and his error score on the 100-Hue test. In general, the greater the error score, the greater the overall sensitivity loss.

The exception to this is patient R.O. (IV-12). His data in this case, however, are probably less reliable than the others since he expressed discomfort throughout the session, becoming increasingly less cooperative as the session progressed.

The difference was taken between the curves for each patient and that of the normal. The difference curves generally bore little resemblance to the spectral efficiency curves of any of the fundamental color mechanisms. This may have been due to the fact that our patients were untrained observers. However, there is a correlation between the peak wavelengths of the difference curves and that of the mechanism diagnosed as defective by color discrimination testing. It was found that in the case of G.O. (IV-10) the difference was greatest in the region of 535 nm which is consistent with a deutan type of defect. C.P. (IV-9) had a maximal sensitivity loss near 580 nm which is consistent with her protan defect. R.O. (IV-12) showed a peak sensitivity loss near 535 nm which is consistent with his deutan effect, though this finding should be treated with reservation for the reasons given above. B.O.P. (III-4) showed a marked sensitivity loss in the blue region of the spectrum and a secondary loss close to 540, suggestive of a deutan/tritan defect. J.P.'s (IV-8) curve was similar to the normal, though of generally reduced sensitivity.

The Stiles π-mechanisms – t.v.r. curves

Figure 3 shows the major π-mechanism curves derived from the averaged data of six normal observers. In all cases these curves represent the variation of sensitivity of the various mechanisms as a function of the stimulus wavelength λ.

It may be noted that the π_0 (rod curve) appears much lower on the ordinate axis than is usual. This is because a 14° foveally fixated test stimulus, as used here, stimulates, a higher proportion of cones relative to rods than the smaller, peripherally viewed stimulus used by Stiles.

127

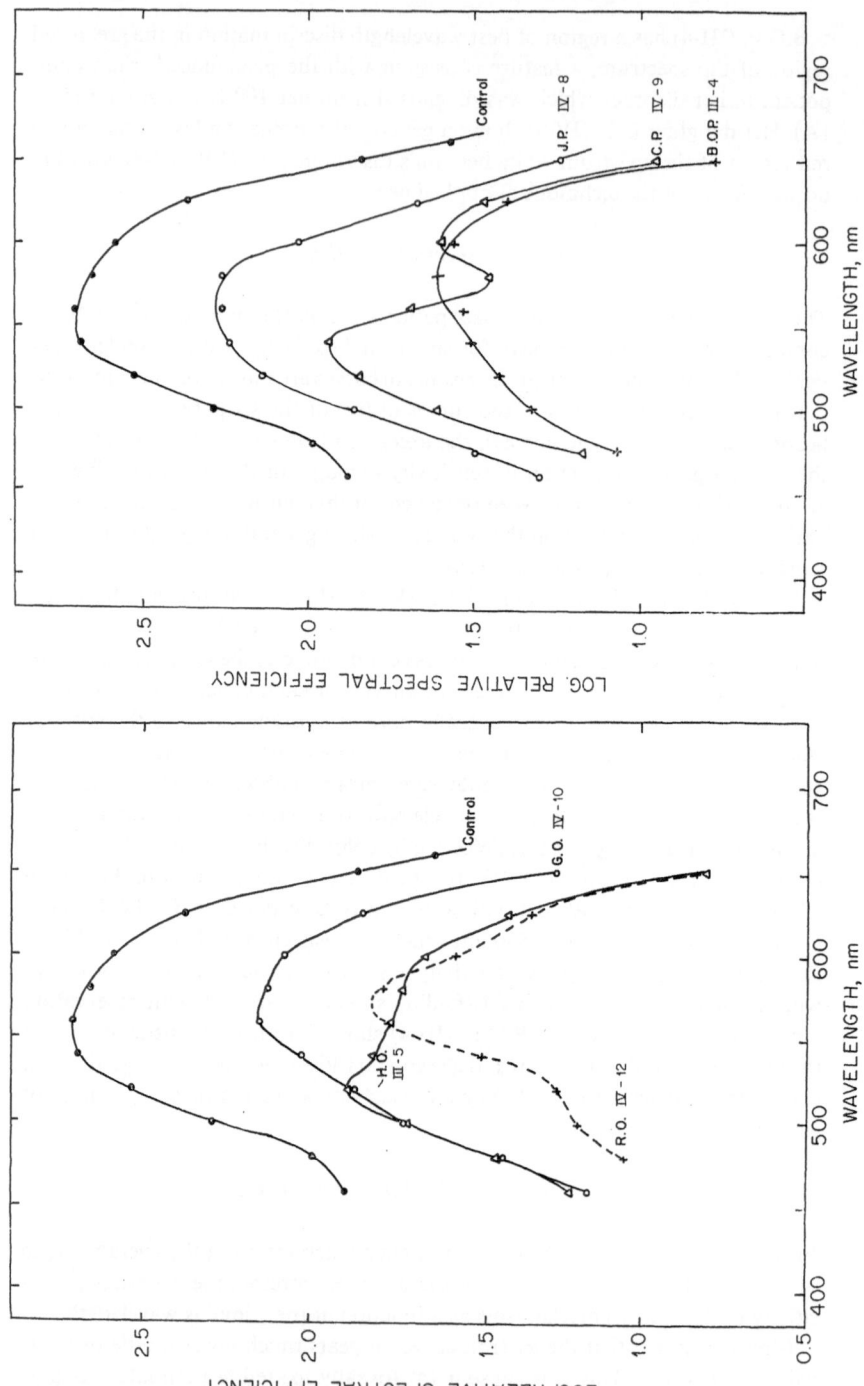

Fig. 2A, 2B. Relative spectral sensitivity (V_λ) is determined by an incremental threshold technique against a white background of luminance 200 photopic trolands. The
control curve, shown for comparison is drawn through means of the data of six normal
trichromats. The curve for R.O. is broken for reasons given in the text.

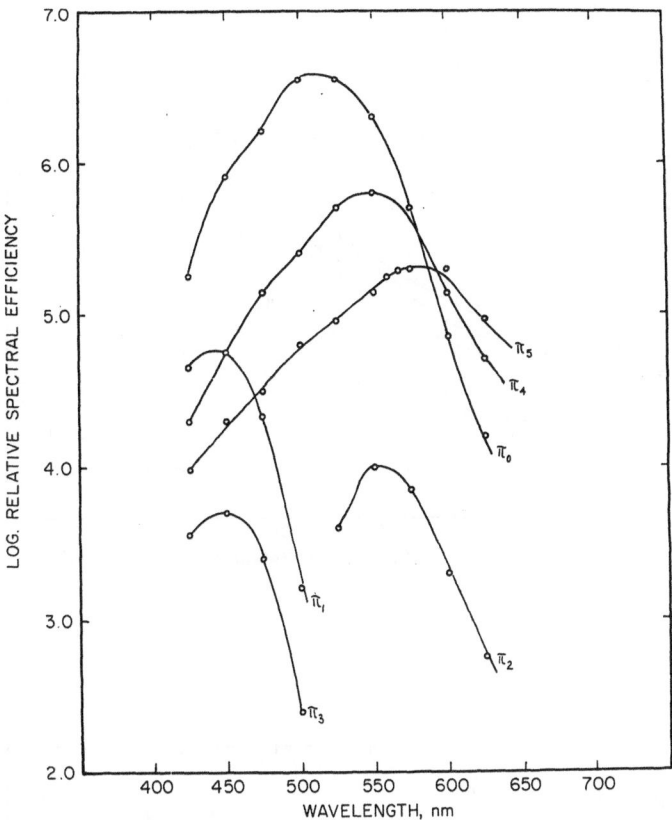

Fig. 3. The Stiles π mechanisms determined from the averaged data of six normal trichromats. The technique of measurement is described in the materials and methods section.

Figures 4A and 4B illustrate the thresholds vs field radiance (t.v.r.) curves measured for six members of the family using a test stimulus of wavelength 547 nm and a background of wavelength 501 nm. A normal curve (average of 6 observers) displaced downward by 0.5 log units, is shown for comparison. The most striking feature is that the three limbs seen in the normal curve are also clearly seen in the curves of patients B.O.P. (III-4), C.P. (IV-9), J.P. (IV-8), G.O. (IV-10) and R.O. (IV-12). The curve of H.O. (III-5) appears to consist of only a single limb which suggests a significantly lower sensitivity of his π_4 (green) and π_5 (red) mechanisms relative to the normal.

Figs 5A and 5B represent the t.v.r. curves measured with a test stimulus of wavelength 450 nm viewed against a 547 nm background. The normal curve (6 observers) is shown for comparison. It has not been displaced on either axis. During the measurement of these curves each of the patients expressed increasing discomfort due to glare as the background was raised in intensity. One patient, B.O.P. (III-4), completed the observations only with great difficulty

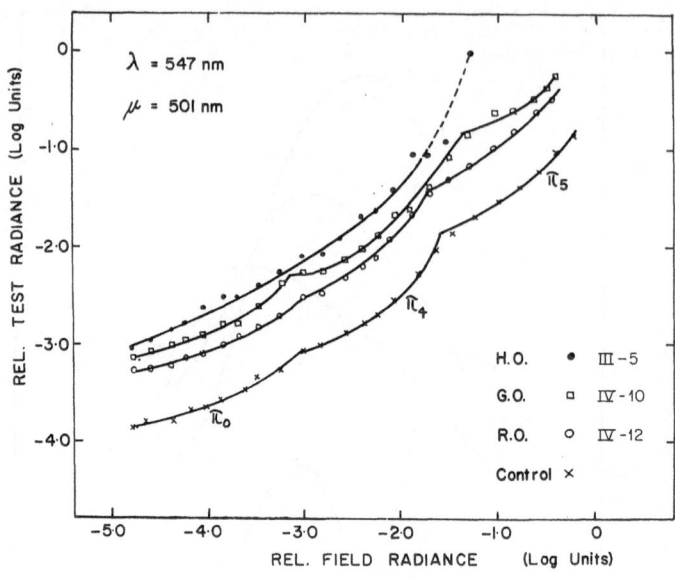

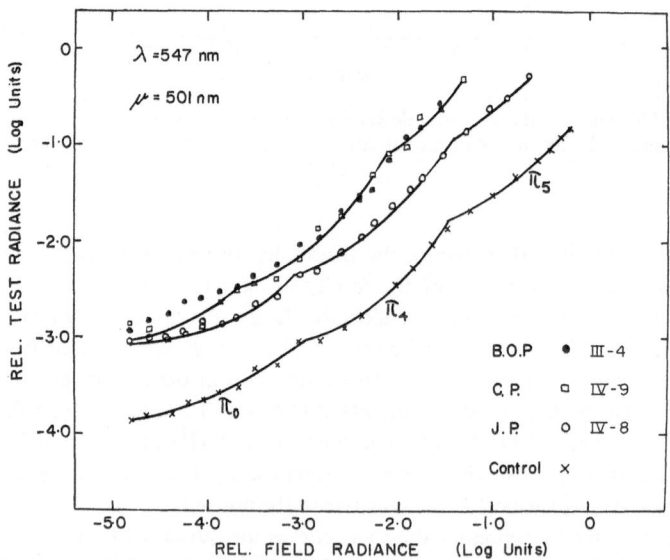

Figs. 4A, 4B. Threshold versus radiance (t.v.r.) curves measured using a stimulus of wavelength $\lambda = 547$ nm viewed against a background of wavelength $\mu = 501$ nm. The normal curve, shown for comparison, has been lowered on the ordinate scale by 0,5 log units for the sake of clarity.

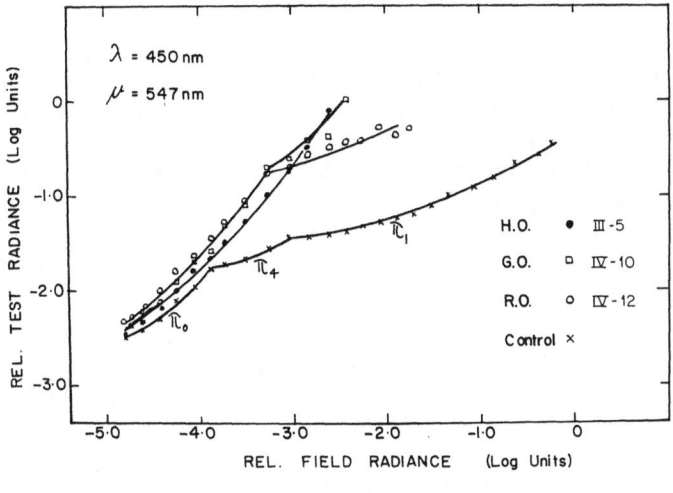

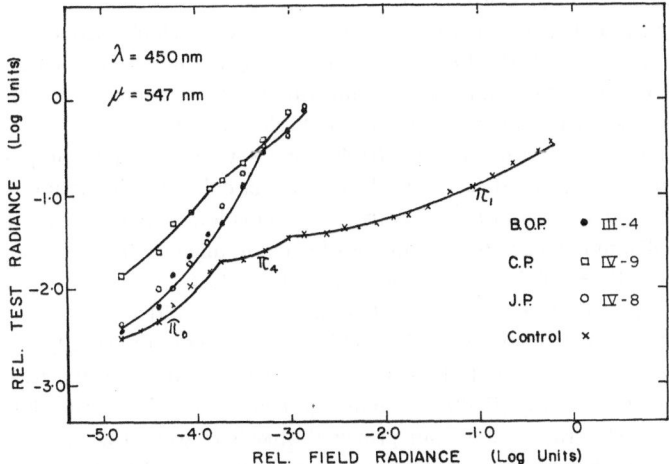

Figs. 5A, 5B. Threshold versus radiance (t.v.r.) curves measured using a stimulus of wavelength $\lambda = 476$ nm viewed against a background of wavelength $\mu = 547$ nm.

after several requests had been made to terminate the session. Others continually doubted that they would be able to complete the session.

It will be seen that the patients' curves generally possess only two limbs, unlike the normal curve which possesses three. It is not possible to say whether the upper limb is due to π_1 (blue) or π_4 (green). It appears, however, that the threshold of both these mechanisms is markedly elevated when compared with the normal. The significance of this will be discussed in the following section. The curve of H.O. (III-5), again, consists only of a single limb (π_0) indicating reduced π_1 and π_4 sensitivity.

131

There is a consistency between the results of the various tests which enables us to feel confident in our diagnosis both of the type of color vision defect and of its severity for any given patient.

W.O. (III-1), the propositus, was clearly the most severely affected patient taking part in this phase of the study. He was unable to demonstrate any color discrimination in any of the tests in which he took part. His pronounced photophobia, poor visual acuity and 3° central scotoma coupled with his total lack of color discrimination are indicative of total achromacy.

H.O. (III-5), the younger brother of W.O., also has characteristics which are consistent with achromacy, though in his case the diagnosis is less clear cut. His marked photophobia, 2° central scotoma and reduced visual acuity are indications of impaired photopic function. His t.v.r. curves showed that his π_1, π_4 and π_5 mechanisms are all of reduced sensitivity. His relative spectral sensitivity curve peaks close to 500 nm suggesting predominantly rod function at photopic levels. However, there was some indication of residual color discrimination near 575 nm in the Farnsworth-Munsell data. The shape of his relative spectral sensitivity curve was such as to suggest the presence of a long wavelength mechanism. This possibility is further strengthened by the fact that whereas his subjective C.F.F. for 475 nm and 526 nm stimuli was 11 and 14 Hz, respectively, that for an equal luminance 624 nm stimulus it was 23 Hz.

H.O.'s younger sister, B.O.P. (III-4) is less severely affected and possesses a predominantly tritan defect as evidenced by her color discrimination data. Her subjective C.F.F. as measured with wavelengths longer than 500 nm was 32-38 Hz. A 426 nm and a 450 nm stimulus of equal luminance, however, produced a C.F.F. of 17 Hz. This is consistent with a tritan defect.

H.O.'s sons both possess deutan defects though the younger son R.O. (IV-12) is more severely affected than his elder brother G.O. (IV-10).

B.O.P.'s daughter, C.P. (IV-9) possesses a pronounced protan defect while her elder brother J.P. (IV-8) is diagnosed as being just within normal limits.

As stated earlier, one of our principal objectives was to determine whether or not the progressive loss of color discrimination, so clearly evident in these patients, follows any recognizable pattern. It seems to be clear from the above diagnoses that there is not a recognizable pattern.

While we feel confident in classifying the various types of defect possessed by each family member examined, we feel much less confident in ascribing the defects to the same causes as apply to classical congenital color vision abnormalities.

One of the more puzzling features of the data is that all patients tested, with the exception of H.O. (III-5) appear to have normal π_4 and π_5 threshold at 550 nm as is evident in Figs. 4A and 4B. This is in spite of the fact that some patients (e.g., R.O. (IV-12) and C.P. (IV-9)) have markedly reduced color discrimination in the red/green region. This raises the possibility that the red/green defect possessed by these patients may not be due to a loss of either π_4 or π_5. Two possible explanations come to mind. One is that the fundamental mechanisms of these patients are different from those of the normal in terms of their spectral sensitivity.

The measurement of the spectral sensitivities of the π_1, π_4 and π_5 mechanisms involves a protracted series of observations by each patient. Our patients were unable to give up the time required for these measurements. We cannot, therefore, rule out the possibility that one or another of the mechanisms may have an abnormal spectral sensitivity. If this were so, it would imply that the visual pigment undergoes a steady change as the dystrophy progresses.

A second, and we believe more likely, explanation depends on the characteristics of the π mechanisms as defined by STILES (2). The theory of the π mechanisms requires that the incremental threshold of any one mechanism as determined by the two-color threshold technique, be independent of the activity of the others. BOYNTON, IKEDA & Stiles (3) have tested this independence and found that under some conditions it is not true. However, over a moderate range of background intensities, such as was employed in the present study, the effects of interdependence are probably small.

Assuming the independence of the π mechanisms under our conditions of measurement we have a simple interpretation of our data, since each limb of the t.v.r. curve would then be due to the activity of an isolated π mechanism. We can note that all the patients we tested, with the exception of H.O. (III-5), had normal thresholds for π_4 and π_5 (Fig. 4) under these conditions.

The discrimination of colors, however, requires that the output signals of the green sensitive mechanism (π_4) and red sensitive mechanism (π_5) be compared in some way. This must be effected by feeding these signals into a discrimination unit located at some point central to the photoreceptors in the neural chain. The work of DE VALOIS (4) suggests that in primates the lateral geniculate nucleus might be the locus of this discrimination unit.

The color discrimination of all our patients, with the possible exception of J.P. (IV-8), is disturbed. In addition, the relative spectral sensitivities of all our patients, again with the exception of J.P., show significant irregularities in shape when compared with the normal. The relative spectral sensitivity curve represents a combination (though not necessarily a linear combination), of the relative sensitivities of the three fundamental color mechanisms.

The implication of these findings is that when the signals from the color mechanisms are combined in some way, either for the purpose of making a color discrimination or a conventional brightness discrimination, the results are abnormal. Only when no combination occurs (under the conditions of measurement of the π mechanisms), do we see a normal response. This further suggests that the color discrimination loss suffered by our patients is due, not to any gradual impairment of the cones themselves, but to a developing abnormality at the site of mixing of the various signals. This site as noted above may be in the lateral geniculate nucleus.

Patient J.P. (IV-8) differs from other members of the family only in as much as his affliction is in its very early stages. Patient H.O. (III-5) however showed evidence of grossly abnormal π_4 and π_5 mechanisms as well as seriously impaired color discrimination. This may indicate that when the dystrophy reaches an advanced stage, degeneration may occur at loci prior to the discrimination unit in the visual pathway, leading to a total loss of function in the individual mechanisms. Such an explanation would be consistent both with H.O.'s central scotoma and his lack of significant maculopathy.

HONG (5) found evidence to indicate that, in his patients, the red-green discrimination losses were probably due to a post retinal lesion, whereas blue-yellow discrimination losses were retinal in origin. Our conclusions concerning the red-sensitive and green-sensitive mechanism are in agreement with those of HONG. We cannot, however, either confirm or deny HONG's proposal concerning the blue-yellow defect.

It will be seen (Fig. 5) that all patients exhibited an elevated π_1 threshold at 475 nm as compared with the normal. Under these circumstances, however, they all complained that, as the intensity of the background was raised, it became increasingly 'glaring'. This was the most common subjective description though the words 'dazzling', 'uncomfortable', 'difficult', and 'very bright' were also used. In view of this, it is not clear whether the elevation of π_1 threshold was due to a functional deficiency of that mechanism or to the contrast reduction that would result from glare. The fact that the π_4 threshold was also elevated under these same conditions suggests that glare may have been an important factor. Whether the cause of the glare is directly associated with the dystrophy or is a seperate phenomenon we cannot say.

The possibility that 'glare' may be a component in the subjective loss of color discrimination of our patients is of especial interest because it raises the possibility that by finding a method of controlling the glare, it may be possible to improve, at least slightly, the color discrimination of our patients. This line of thinking by one of us (J.T.P.) led to a clinical experiment, the results of which are summarized in the Appendix.

Finally, we are well aware that evaluation of patients' color matching using an anomaloscope would have greatly aided us in drawing conclusions. It is hoped that we will be able to obtain this data at a future date. It will also be of interest to study the development of color discrimination losses in the younger patients, particularly J. P. (IV-8) who had been judged normal on earlier visits to our laboratory, but who is now showing signs of the onset of a color discrimination loss.

APPENDIX – PART II

Because the sensation of glare seemed to be such a disabling factor to those family members with most advanced stages of this disorder, a trial application of 1 % Pilocarpine was made to determine the possibly beneficial effects of miosis on visual acuity. The drug was given to the propositus (III-1), his brother (III-5) and his sister (III-4). All three reported some initial improvement in visual acuity and in one instance an increase in color sense. B.O.P. (III-4) said she noted that a neighbor's roses were 'red'. The propositus noted a diminution of acuity after several weeks' trial, and he subsequently discontinued the drug. His brother, H.O. (III-5), still uses 1 % Pilocarpine occasionally, while B.O.P.

now uses 2% Pilocarpine routinely, feeling the relief from glare is substantial, even if the acuity is not significantly improved in terms of Snellen testing.

REFERENCES

1. WRIGHT, W. D. Researches in normal and defective color vision. London, Kimpton (1947).
2. STILES, W. S. A modified Helmholtz line-element in brightness-color space. *Proc. Phys. Soc.* 58: *41-65* (1946).
3. BOYNTON, R. M., IKEDA, M. & STILES, W. S. Interactions among chromatic mechanisms as inferred from positive and negative increment thresholds. *Vision Res.* 4: *87-117* (1964).
4. DE VALOIS, R. Analysis and coding of color vision in the primate visual system. *Cold Spr. Harb. Symp.* 30: *567-579* (1965).
5. HONG, S. Types of acquired color vision defects. *Arch. Ophthal. (Chicago)* 58: *505-509* (1957).

Authors' addresses:

JEROME T. PEARLMAN
W. GEOFFREY OWEN
DAVID W. BROUNLEY
Dept. of Ophthalmology
Visual Physiology Laboratory
Jules Stein Eye Institute
UCLA School of Medicine
Los Angeles Ca 90024

JOSEPH J. SHEPPARD
RAND Corporation
Santa Monica
California

ON PROGRESSIVE CONE DYSTROPHY*

J. G. H. SCHMIDT, H. PAULMANN & M. DEOM

(*Cologne*)

Over the past two decades various tests of visual function have led to increasing precision in the differentiation of hereditary macular diseases.

In developing our diagnostic methods we are primarily interested in knowing whether the macular dystrophy originates from a tapeto-retinal degeneration, as is often the case. The prognosis of this group is less favourable than others since we find, as a rule, more rapid destruction of retinal function. We must also expect a gradual diminution of the visual field. This is especially important with respect to educational guidance counselling (SCHMIDT & DEOM).

Furthermore, we are interested in whether an isolated disease of the cones is present or whether we can expect damage of the entire posterior eye pole. Undoubtedly, many cases in the past were repeatedly classified as juvenile macular degeneration of Stargardt's type when, in fact, they were cases of progressive cone dystrophy. Diagnosing a case as progressive cone dystrophy is not always easy, especially during the initial stage of the disease (SCHMIDT & MÄURER).

At this point, I would like to describe the cases of several of our patients.

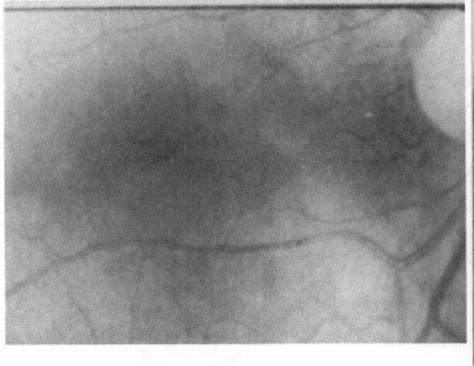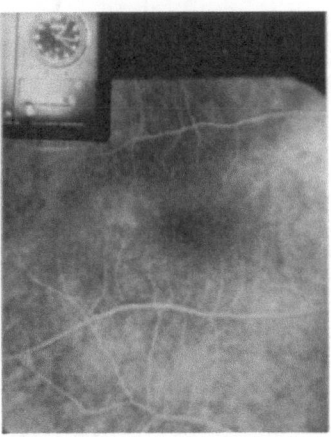

Fig. 1a

* This research was supported by Deutsche Forschungsgemeinschaft, Bonn/Bad Godesberg.

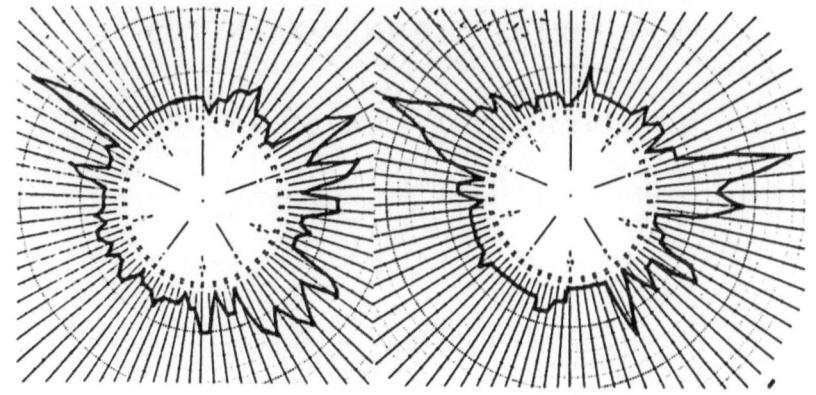

Fig. 1b

Plot of actual luminance of yellow brightness
settings in anomaloscope for various red–green
mixtures

for patient Sch.————┐
              ThD.————┤cone degeneration
              W.D.------┘
              A.H.————▲ STARGARDT'S disease

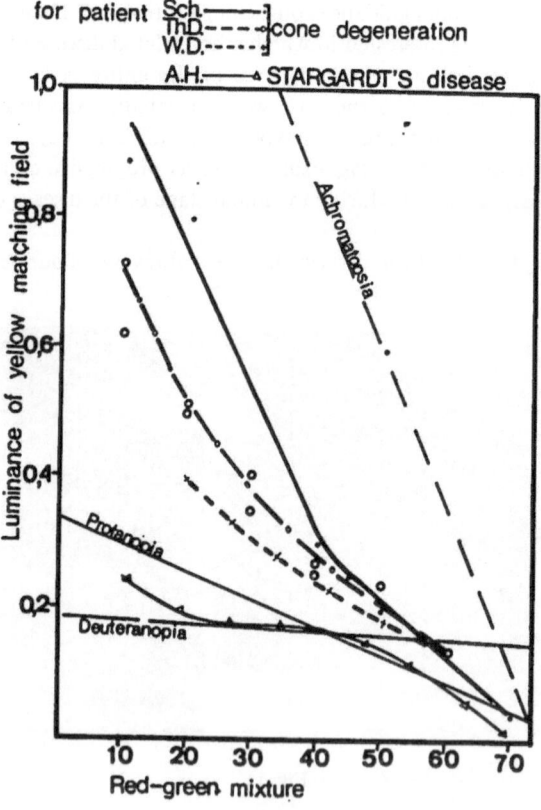

Fig. 1c

Case 1: 14-years old boy. – The mother noticed, even before the boy entered school, that he always mixed up the colors of crayons.

In the summer of 1972 the boy complained of a sudden reduction of vision in both eyes and increasing photophobia. On October 23, 1972, the boy's visual acuity measured 0,7. Approximately three months later, at the University of Cologne Eye Clinic his visual acuity was found to be 0,2. Since the ophthalmos-

Fig. 1d

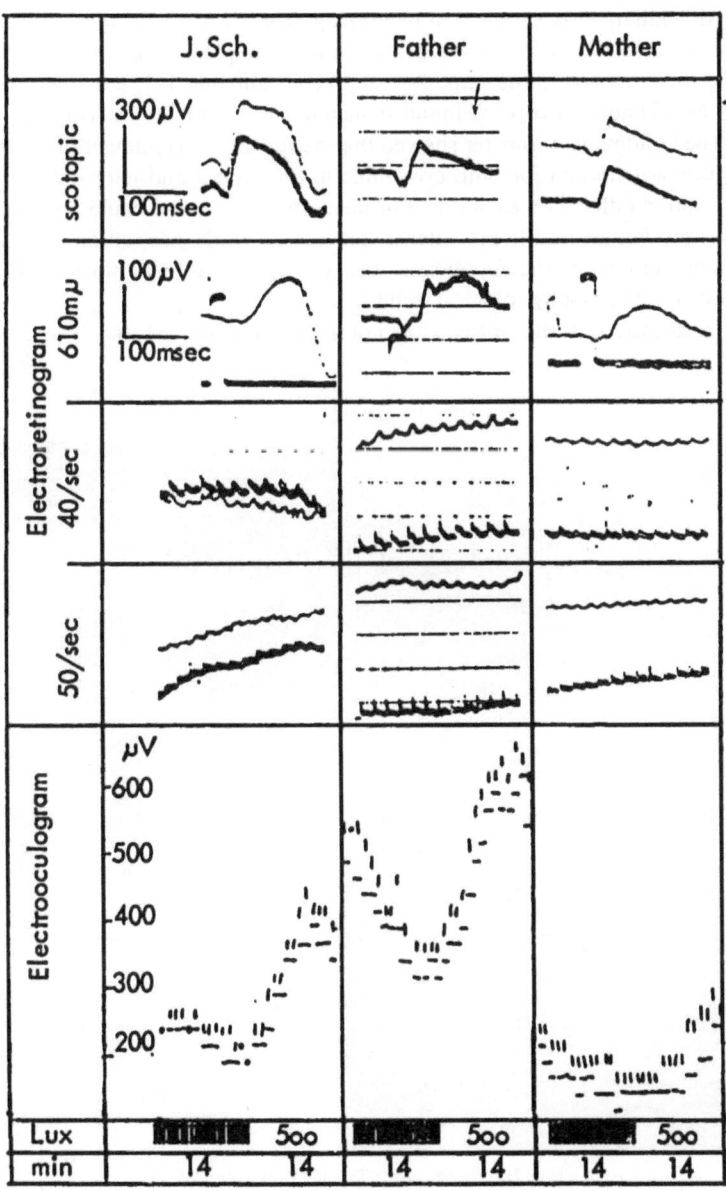

copic findings were not striking, we at first considered possibly malingering (Fig. 1a).

We learned from his mother that her brother had been night blind and red-green color blind, as well as very musical. The boy we examined demonstrated good perceptive ability and was also, according to his mother, very musical.

Six weeks later, the fundus examination revealed the first changes in the foveolar region in the form of numerous very fine pigment clumps. However, at this time we could not see any pigment in the foveolar region (Fig. 1a).

All Ishihara charts were read incorrectly. The Farnsworth-Munsell '100 hue' test revealed a combination of protan- and deutan-axis (Fig. 1b). The number of errors was nearly the same for each eye (right side 167, left side 165). On the Nagel anomaloscope we found an incomplete achromatopsia (Fig. 1c).

The Goldmann perimeter showed that peripheral perception of small moving objects was normal for both eyes while in the central and paracentral region, perception differed on each side. For instance, the right eye could not recognize even the largest and most intense red mark. Dark adaptation of the rod system, tested on the Goldmann-Weekers apparatus, was normal. Fig. 1d shows the electro-physiological results.

In the top row is the scotopic ERG of the boy and his parents.

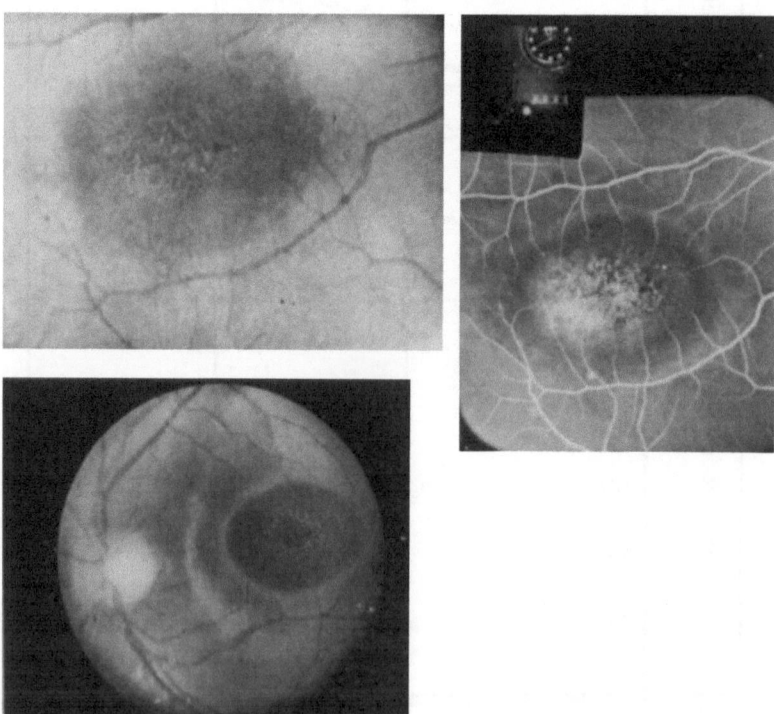

Fig. 2a. Upper row: Th. D. Left side: W. D.

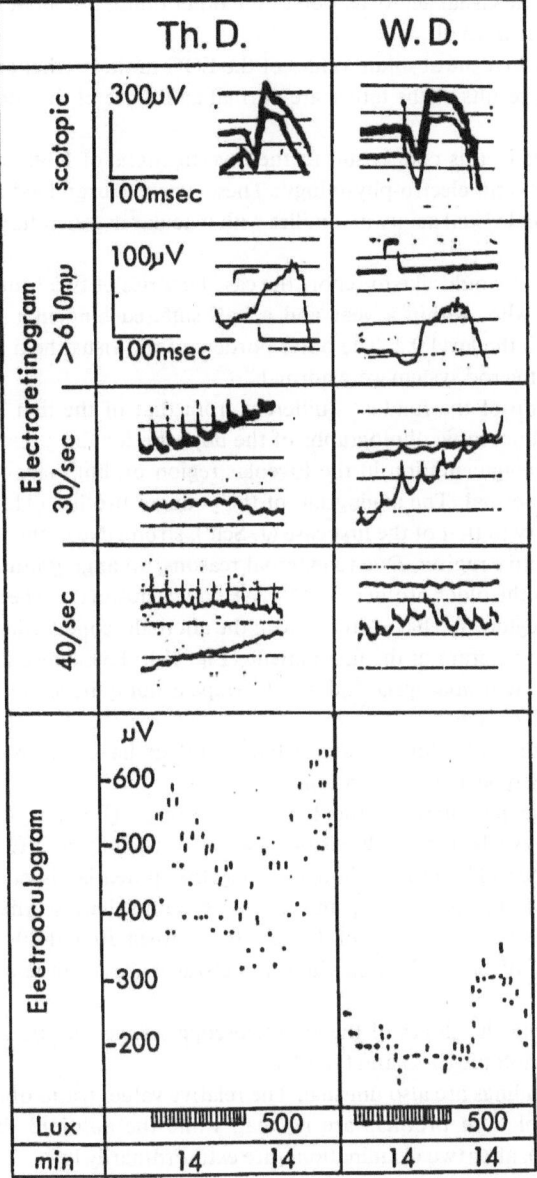

	Th. D.	W. D.
Electroretinogram scotopic	300μV ⌐ 100msec	
Electroretinogram >610mμ	100μV ⌐ 100msec	
Electroretinogram 30/sec		
Electroretinogram 40/sec		
Electrooculogram	μV -600 -500 -400 -300 -200	
Lux	▆▆▆ 500	▆▆▆ 500
min	14 14	14 14

Fig. 2b

There are no recognisable differences. We find clear differences, however, in the photopic ERG. In the case of the boy the wavelet corresponding to the x-wave (b-photopic) is missing. In the case of the father there is a clear wavelet, and in the case of the mother the wavelet is small. Also, examination of the flicker fusion frequency (FFF) shows noticeable differences between the parents

141

and the boy. The visual acuity as well as the other ophthalmological findings of the parents were normal.

It is striking that the absolute values of the EOG in the mother are pathological. The EOG results of the father are normal and those of the son are borderline values.

Let me refer in this connection to the investigations of KRILL & FRANCOIS on color vision and electro-physiology: These workers examined family members with normal visual acuity in families with macular degeneration.

Cases 2 and 3. I would like to report the case histories of two brothers (14 and 11 years old) who, within a year and a half suffered binocular reduction of visual acuity to the level 0,2. The outer borders of the visual field and the dark adaptation of the rod system were normal.

The condition of the fundus is different from that of the first case. Fig. 2a shows ophthalmoscopic photographs of the boys. Beside fine pigmentation, we find distinct depigmentation in the foveolar region on both sides. The rest of the fundus is normal. The angiogram of the younger brother (Th. D.) demonstrates, contrary to that of the first case (J. Sch.), strong dye in the ophthalmoscopically defective region. Due to external reasons, an angiogram could not be carried out on the older brother (W.D.). We could, however, expect to find dye in the foveal region. We have already seen the anomaloscope settings of the two brothers in the diagram of the first patient (Fig. 1b). These results also indicate incomplete achromatopsia. Indeed, the slope is not quite as steep as that of the first patient (J. Sch.).

Moreover, the slopes in the case of both brothers have shown constant differences during repeated examinations.

The scotopic potentials in the ERG are normal. (Fig. 2b). The photopic investigation reveals just barely visible x-waves, especially in the case of the younger brother (Th. D.). Although a negative potential is still present, a separation into the so-called a_1 and a_2-waves cannot be discerned. Also, the FFF is pathological. The FFF of Th. D. lies between 30 and 40 cycles/sec. in contrast to the older brother, in whom the disturbances were less severe, with 40 cycl./sec.

One can see that the slopes of the anomaloscope settings are parallel with the values of the photopic ERG and the FFF.

The EOG findings are also unusual. The relative values (ratio of light peak to dark trough) of both brothers are normal, while the absolute values of one brother (W.D.), after two examinations, are extraordinarily low.

At this point, I would like to mention the data of a fourth patient (SCHMIDT) whose ERG findings are essentially the same as those of the previous patients: the scotopic potentials are normal, while in the photopic ERG the x-wave is missing. The settings on the anomaloscope are very similar to those of an achromat.

However, the EOG findings differ from those of the first three patients. The rise upon illumination is completely missing in this case. The normal scotopic

142

ERG and the flat EOG lead one to assume a fundus flavimaculatus. The posterior poles of both eyes show flecks with a soft contour that have a tendency to confluence, tending to conform this diagnosis. We are dealing, therefore, with a fundus flavimaculatus with an achromatopsia.

DISCUSSION

I have so far reported findings on three patients whose ophthalmoscopic and angiographic findings correspond to Stargardt's disease; their functional peculiarities, however, rule out this type of macular dystrophy.

The first negative wave of the photopic ERG is missing in our patients, as well as the b-wave with short latency time, which corresponds to the x-wave. The question arises whether one or more electrical potential generators are missing. Possibly the chain of communication is interrupted in only one place. We could surmise that damage of the first negative wave cancels the trigger function for the x-wave. According to the investigations of several authors the negative potentials, especially those with short latency time, are connected with the photoreceptors.

The normal state of the peripheral visual field, dark adaptation, and the scotopic ERG indicate normal function of the rod system. These results and the highly pathological finding on the anomaloscope indicate specific damage of the cone system. The first case with especially rapid progression shows a normal angiogram whereas visual acuity and color vision are already highly disturbed. Only with the less advanced cases 2 and 3 do we find the disturbed functions and dye in the foveal region as an expression of damage of the pigment epithelium.

A distinction between the cases reported and Stargardt's disease which is suggested by the clinical function tests is borne out by the electro-physiological criteria. Accordingly, one would consider our cases as not involving the receptor-pigment epithelium complex as a whole, but rather a selective impairment of the cone system.

ACKNOWLEDGMENT

I am grateful to Mrs. MARLIES MÄURER for her excellent technical assistence. Mrs. ILSE FISCHER and Miss ANGELA PETERS provided the photographs.

REFERENCES

DEUTMAN, A. F. The hereditary dystrophies of the posterior pole of the eye. Van Gorcum & Comp. N.V. – Dr. H. J. PRAKKE & H. M. G. PRAKKE: Assen, The Netherlands (1971).
FRANÇOIS, J. Heredity in ophthalmology. St Louis, The C.V. Mosby Comp. (1961).
KRILL, A. E. & A. SCHNEIDERMAN. A hue discrimination defect in so-called normal carriers of color vision defects. *Invest. Ophthal.* 3: *445-450* (1964).
SCHMIDT, J. G. H. & M. DEOM. Stargardt'sche Makuladegeneration oder Makulatyp

der diffusen tapeto-retinalen Degeneration? *Ber. Dtsch. Ophthal. Ges. (Hamburg)* 72: *235-242* (1972).

SCHMIDT, J. G. H. & M. MÄURER. On the differentiation of heredo-macular degenerations. 2nd South African Intern. Ophthal. Symposium, Johannesburg (1973).

SCHMIDT, J. G. H. in preparation.

Author's address:

University of Cologne
Eye Clinic
5000 Cologne 41
W. Germany

MONOCHROMATIC ERGS IN A CASE OF PROGRESSIVE CONE DYSTROPHY.

MINORU YOKOYAMA, KENJI UI & TERUYA YOSHIDA

(Tsu, Japan)

ABSTRACT

A 32-year-old man with progressive cone dystrophy was subjected to ERG recording and psychophysical testing. Under mesopic conditions the scanning over 16 monochromatic flashes produced a series of b-waves in which the maximum response occurred at 500 nm, and no response in the range above 660 nm. The attenuation of the b-waves with increasing background illumination occurred more rapidly in the patient's eye than normal. Under photopic conditions repeated time-locked scanning permitted the recording of a series of minimal b_p-waves in which the maximum was at 540 nm and was 10 μV or less in amplitude. Psychophysical testing with the same 16 monochromatic flashes showed that a central island of the visual field, i.e. the island of residual pure cones, showed peak spectral sensitivity at 560 nm, but away from this island the peak was found to be shifted to near 500 nm with some eccentric fixation.

The clinical entity of progressive cone dystrophy (degeneration) has recently been established, predicated on the fact that there exist progressive and generalized dystrophic changes in the cone system as contrasted to a normal rod system. The electroretinogram (ERG) is of importance not only to the clinical diagnosis, but also to the analysis of normally remaining rod function and declining cone function. There are several reports (BABEL & STANGOS, 1973; BERSON et al., 1968; GOODMAN et al., 1963; KELSEY & ARDEN, 1972; KRILL & DEUTMAN, 1972; SLOAN & BROWN, 1962) on detailed findings of the ERG in the disease. However, as pointed out by BERSON (1968), in many cases the cone responses are too small for quantitative studies at different wavelengths.

We had an opportunity to study the disorder in a typical case. The patient exhibited considerable photopic response to monochromatic flashes that were balanced on a quantum basis. The same stimulating system was also used for psychophysical testing. The purpose of this report is to present the spectral response of the patient's eye under mesopic and photopic conditions, and the spectral sensitivity in several portions of degenerating retina.

MATERIALS AND METHODS

The principal subject presented a typical case of progressive cone dystrophy. Two other cases were also examined: a 41-year-old man with dominant pro-

145

gressive foveal dystrophy and a 43-year-old woman with cone-rod deficiency.

The stimulating and recording apparatus described in a previous paper (YOKOYAMA et al., 1973) from this laboratory were employed in this study, but some additional devices were used here to perform the scanning for averaging the photopic responses (b_p-waves). The principal new instrument was a time-locked address divider which could supply a limited number of addresses of the computer for each limited part of a series of spectral responses, the peak-to-peak rising phase of the b_p-waves.

Monochromatic light flashes were delivered to the subject's eye through a diffusing glass placed just before the cornea. The light source was a 500 W xenon arc (1,500 cd, 25,000 sb and 6,000°K). A disc with 16 color filters was placed in front of the collimating lens. It was rotated by a motor at various speeds, providing appropriate stimulus intervals under given levels of visual adaptation. A series of neutral filters placed in the main beam reduced the intensity of the flashes. The stimulating light flashes through all the filters were adjusted to equal quantum balance. The background illumination was provided by another light source consisting of a tungsten lamp the output of which could be varied from 1.6 to 5×10^4 trolands of retinal illumination. Red, green or blue light was also available through wide band filters when required.

The subject was placed in a supine position inside an electrically shielded room. Local anesthesia of the cornea and conjunctiva was induced with 0.4 per cent Benoxinate. A contact lens was fitted to the cornea and fixed by suction. The contact lens had an opaque diffusing glass on its front surface, giving completely diffuse illumination to the retinal area, 120° of arc. The signals from the contact lens were amplified with a R-C coupling amplifier (AVB-1 Nihon Koden, Tokyo), or were averaged by a computer (ATAC-401). The relative energies and duration of the flashes were recorded using a photodiode (PD3L, NEC).

CASE REPORT

A 32-year-old man, was first seen in January, 1971. He had noticed a gradual decrease in color discrimination about 7 years ago. For 3 years he also noticed some decrease in vision with slight photophobia, but he has had no other neurological symptoms. Family history will be described elsewhere. (YOKOYAMA et al., in press).

The visual acuity of the patient when first seen was 0.5 (n.c.) in the O.D. and 0.3 (n.c.) in the O.S. The visual fields showed central scotomas which differed in size under mesopic and photopic conditions (Fig. 1). The peripheral fields on the Goldmann perimeter were full with V/4 and I/4 white test object. The patient had no color vision when tested with the T.M.C. plates, Okuma plates and H-R-R plates. The results with the Farnsworth D-15 panel suggested a type of tritan deficiency but this was not definite. The dark-adaptation curve revealed some biphasic nature as described by SLOAN & BROWN (1962). The threshold was slightly elevated in the early phase, whereas the final threshold was almost normal (Fig. 1). There was no nystagmus and extraocular movements were full.

146

Central scotomas

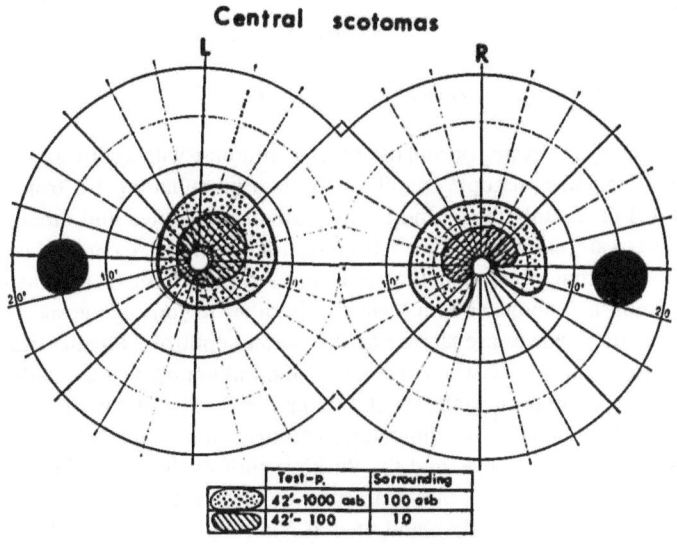

	Test-p.	Sorrounding
::::::	42'-1000 asb	100 asb
\\\\\\	42'- 100	1 0

Dark-adaptation curve

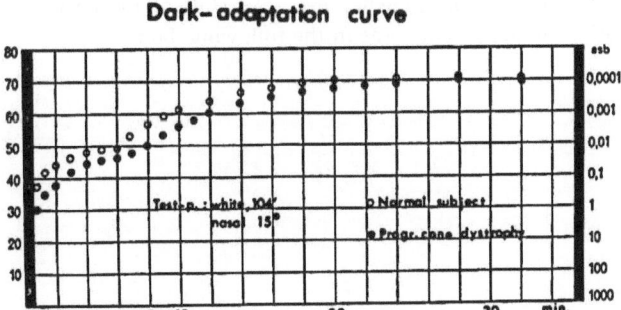

Fig. 1. Top figures are the central scotomas (January 1971). Note considerable difference between scotomas under photopic and mesopic condition of surrounding. Bottom curves are obtained also with Tübinger perimeter (February 1971).

Anterior segments were normal. Ophthalmoscopy revealed normal optic discs, vessels, and peripheral retina in both eyes. The macular area showed slight bilateral mottling of the pigment epithelium, but no 'beaten bronze' like reflexes as Stargardt's disease. On fluorescein angiography parafoveal (right eye) or ring-shaped (left eye) hyperfluorescent areas were noted in both macular lesions. These corresponded to the regions of the mesopic central scotomas (hatched areas in Fig. 1).

On follow-up, the patient's vision decreased to 0.3 (n.c.) in O.D. and 0.06 (n.c.) in O.S. after two years. The latter change may be ascribed to expansion of the central scotoma and to loss of a small central island of the visual field (Fig. 7).

147

1. Scotopic component

A normal subject's response and the patient's response with a conventional ERG ink recorder under mesopic conditions (retinal illumination, 1.6 trolands) are shown in Fig. 2. Only the a- and b-waves are demonstrated and other parts of the traces were eliminated by vertical sectioning of the recording paper. In the region of longer wavelengths the b-waves were extremely attenuated and mostly abolished above 660 nm, whereas in other regions of the spectrum the heights of the b-waves are similar to the normal controls. Further differences between them appeared when the background illumination was gradually increased to the photopic state, as shown in Fig. 3. The attenuation of the b-waves with increasing retinal illumination occurred more rapidly in the patient's eye than in the normal eye, and the Purkinje shift of the peak of the response curves could not be seen in the former, at least with such a conventional method, while it was clearly manifested at relatively low levels of the photopic state (335 trd.) in the latter. This may be simply because of the weakness of photopic response of the patient's eye. The shift of the peak could then be found with averaging technics as in the following data.

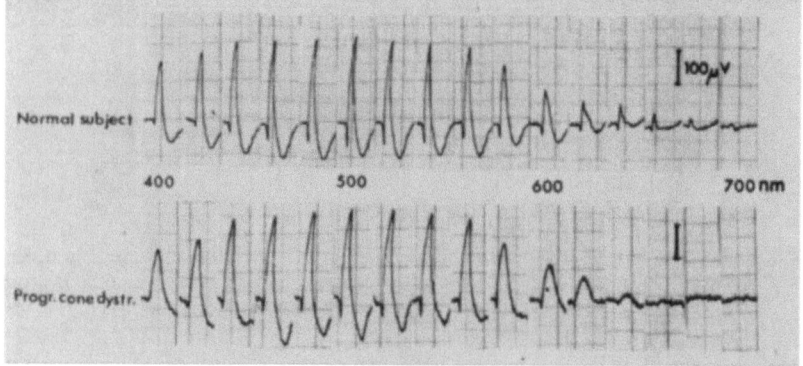

Fig. 2. Monochromatic ERGs under mesopic conditions (February 1971). For ease of comparison the recording paper was sectioned and rearranged in a series of vertical strips corresponding to only the necessary part, i.e. a- and b-waves. The responses were absent in the red-end region of the lower trace. Log flash intensity: –0.6, Flash intervals: 1.25 sec. Visual adaptation: 1.6 trd.

2. Photopic component

Under photopic conditions three types of observations were made: 1) Summation of repeated scans over 16 monochromatic flashes. 2) Averaging of each response to 3 Hz flicker of each monochromatic flash. 3) Averaging of the responses to high frequency flicker (40 Hz). Figure 4 shows the results with the

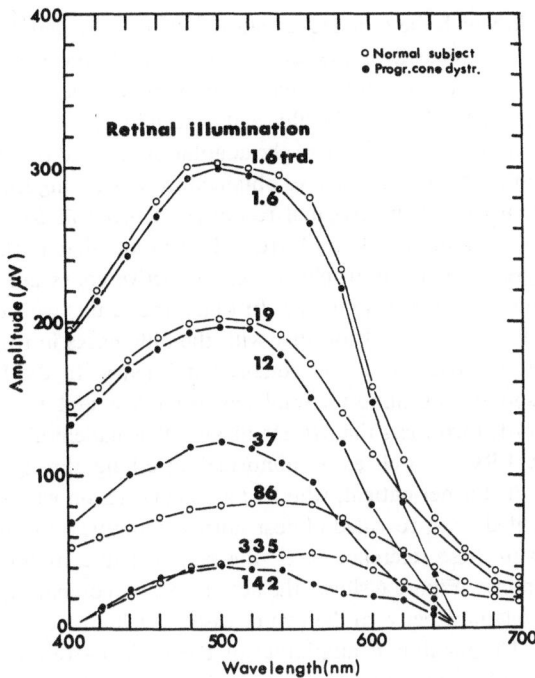

Fig. 3. The effects of gradual increase in background illumination (March 1971). With increasing retinal illumination the b-waves of the patient were more rapidly reduced than the normal control. Purkinje shift occurred at about 335 trd. in the normal response, but no shift was seen in the patient. Log flash intensity: –0.3, Flash interval: 1.25 sec.

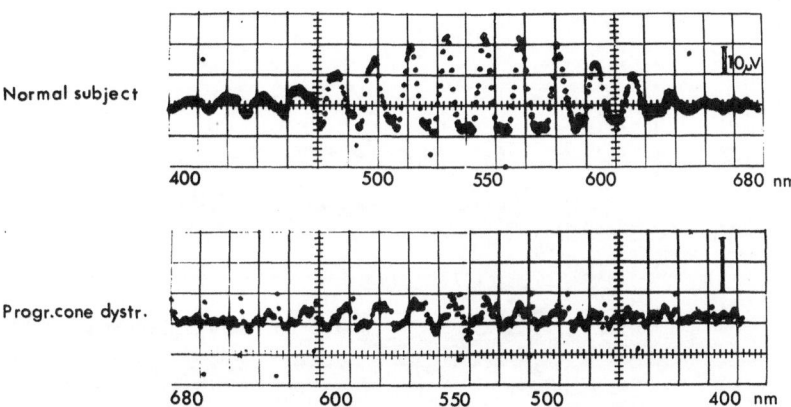

Fig. 4. Photopic b-waves with time-locked scanning (August 1973). The scanning can be repeated from the blue-end as in top trace or from the red-end as in bottom trace. Note the difference in bars for 10 μV. Log flash intensity: –0.3, Flash interval: 0.5 sec. Visual adaptation: White light, 3×10^3 trd.

149

first method in which the time-locked address divider was employed to pick up only the b-waves instead of the selective sections of the recording paper as shown in Fig. 2. One scan could be made with various time durations and could be started from the red end or the blue end as seen in each case in Fig. 4. All the conditions concerning the stimuli or the adaptation were adjusted so as to avoid any distortion of the response curves obtained from scanning from either direction. It is apparent that the maximal response occurred at 540 nm under the given photopic conditions (3×10^3 trd.). This means that Purkinje shift does occur in progressive cone dystrophy as long as active cones are still remaining and generating a detectable potential. In Fig. 5 the results with the second and third methods are illustrated together with the differences in responsiveness in progressive foveal dystrophy and cone-rod deficiency. In the latter case, the photopic response has almost completely been lost and the pure b_s-waves could be recorded with less than 10 Hz flicker. This patient also had a subnormal scotopic ERG as well as a subnormal threshold throughout the dark-adaptation. The former patient, who had a macular lesion with beaten-bronze-like depigmented area, revealed almost normal scotopic and photopic ERGs. Compared with these reference cases, the patient had a minimal but distinct photopic response. Figure 6 shows the action spectra comparing more detailed quantitative relations between the two diseases which are quite similar in clinical features. The maximum amplitude of the patient's response, which was slightly above 10μV, was unchanged throughout two years of follow-up.

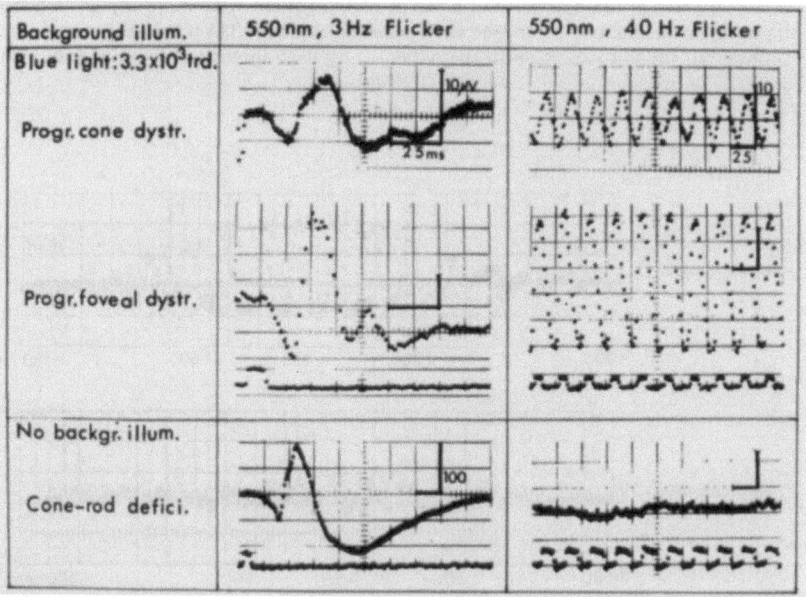

Fig. 5. Comparison with the reference cases (June 1973). In a case of cone-rod deficiency the ERG was recordable only in a dark room, and no response was recorded with the flicker above 10 Hz. In bottom records bars for amplitude and time are quite different from the others. Log flash intensity: –0.2.

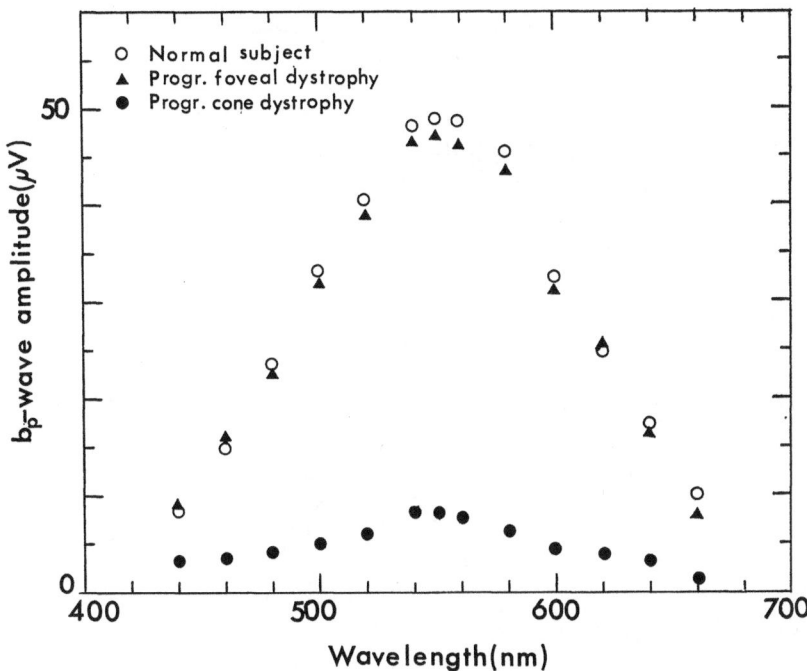

Fig. 6. Plot of photopic b-waves against wavelengths (August 1973). Each plot is an average from three scans as shown in Fig. 4. Bottom plots from progressive cone dystrophy are minimal in amplitude, but the peak reveals clearly the nature of the cone system.

3. Psychophysical test on the spectral sensitivity

The monochromatic flashes used for ERG recording were also used to determine the spectral sensitivity of the patient. The test field, 1° in diameter, was exposed in 50 msec. flashes under scotopic conditions (0.001 asb). As mentioned above, both eyes showed some changes in vision and visual fields two years later. The findings of the latter are illustrated in Fig. 7. The results were as follows: A) The foveola of the right eye, which is a central island of the residual retina, showed the maximum sensitivity at around 560 nm. B) An extrafoveal point (15° nasal) of the right eye had nearly normal sensitivity, and was most sensitive at 500 nm. C) A parafoveal point of the left eye, which had already lost a small central field area by that time, showed rod type sensitivity with the peak near 600 or 520 nm. When the patient was asked to look at something with the left eye, he usually used this parafoveal point, which is included in the photopic scotoma but not in scotopic one.

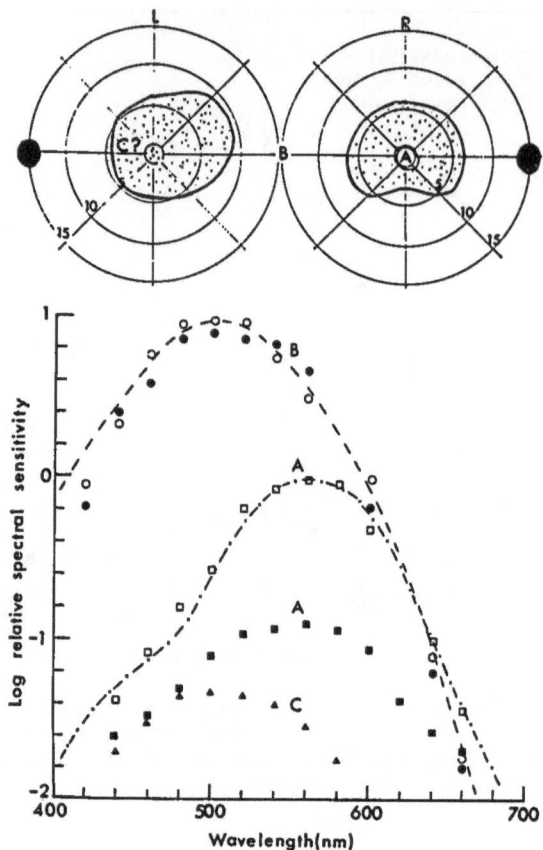

Fig. 7. Psychophysical test in different portion of the retina (June 1973). For simplicity, only the photopic scotomas are shown (top). At that time the central island of the visual field was lost in the left eye in which an eccentric fixation (C?) was used. Curves are Wald's peripheral rod sensitivity (— — —) and foveal cone sensitivity (.—.—.). All measurements were done under the visual adaptation of 0.001 asb. The monochromatic test flashes were in equal quantum balance.

COMMENT

This study reports the spectral response pattern and the spectral sensitivity in eyes with progressive cone dystrophy. The ERGs with conventional recording revealed almost a pure form of rod response without Purkinje shift even under considerable level of light adaptation up to 142 trd. However, averaged data under higher adaptation intensity clearly showed a minimal cone response of 10μV or less, showing peak response at 540 to 550 nm.

The ERG data may be indispensable to diagnosis or follow-up of this kind of retinal degeneration. With respect to this, KELSEY & ARDEN (1972) stated that the main diagnostic feature is the loss of the photopic elements of the ERG.

152

GOODMAN & RIPPS (1963) also showed clinical values of the ERG, in particular photopic flicker ERG above 25 Hz. BERSON, GOURAS, & GUNKEL (1968) pointed out the selective loss of the cone a-wave in their patients with progressive cone degeneration. BABEL & STANGOS (1973) reported on abnormal latency of the a-wave. According to these results, comparison of photopic and scotopic ERGs, high frequency flicker ERG, detailed findings of the a- and b-waves, and stimulation with red light may be the key-notes for the examination on the disease. The diagnosis for our patient was at first 'neuritis retrobulbaris', then changed to 'Stargardt's disease' after fluorescein angiography, and finally corrected to 'progressive cone dystrophy' according to the ERG findings.

Because of the progressive nature of the disease, all the findings change from year to year. In our patient, both eyes differed in phase from the time of the first examination: the right eye was always preceded by the left eye in the course of progression. The central island of the visual fields. i.e. pure cone vision, was lost during these two years in only the left eye, and the vision was reduced from 0.3 to 0.06. Thus we could test simultaneously two eyes in different phases of the condition. Psychophysical testing showed that the peak of the spectral sensitivity was at 560 nm in the right eye and around 500 nm in the left. This indicated that as long as cone function remains the maximum sensitivity in the fovea may always be near 560 nm and may not shift towards the shorter wave lengths less than 540 nm. The findings in the ERG, because of its mass nature, are not necessarily in agreement with the results of psychophysical tests. However, it seems also that as long as the cones are generating some recordable potential, the peak in the action spectra always occurs in the region from 540 to 560 nm and does not shift more to the blue side. This is an opinion, however, from our experience with only one case.

It is not the purpose of this report to describe all clinical features other than the spectral response or sensitivity. Other findings will be described in a following paper. (YOKOYAMA et. al., in press)

SUMMARY

A 32-year-old man with progressive cone dystrophy was subjected to ERG recording and psychophysical testing. The results obtained were as follows:
1) Under a mesopic condition (1.6 trd.) scanning over 16 monochromatic flashes produced a series of b-waves in which the maximum response occurred at 500 nm, with no response in the range above 660 nm. The attenuation of the b-waves with increasing background illumination occurred more rapidly in the patient's eye than in the normal control.
2) Under photopic conditions (3×10^3 trd.) repeated time-locked scanning permitted the recording of a series of minimal b_p-waves in which the maximum was at 540 nm and was 10μV or less in amplitude.
3) Psychophysical testing with the same 16 monochromatic flashes showed that a central island of the visual field, i.e. the remaining pure cone response, had maximum spectral sensitivity at 560 nm, but when this island was lost the peak was found to be shifted to near 500 nm with some eccentric fixation.

REFERENCES

BABEL, J. & STANGOS, N. Progressive degeneration of the photopic system. *Am. J. Ophth.* 75: *511-525* (1973).

BERSON, E. L., GOURAS, P. & GUNKEL, R. D. Progressive cone degeneration dominantly inherited. *Arch. Ophth.* 80: *77-83* (1968).

DEUTMAN, A.F. The hereditary dystrophies of the posterior pole of the eye. Springfield, Charles C. Thomas (1971).

GOODMAN, G., RIPPS, H. & SIEGEL, I. Cone dysfunction syndrome. *Arch. Ophth.* 70: *214-231* (1963).

KELSEY, J. H. & ARDEN, G. B. Acquired cone dysfunction. *Brit. J. Ophth.* 56: *812-816* (1972).

KRILL, A. E. & DEUTMAN, A. F. Dominant macular degenerations, the cone dystrophies *Amer. J. Ophth.* 73: *352-369* (1972).

OHBA, N. Progressive cone dystrophy. *Jap. J. Ophth.* 17 in press (1973).

SLOAN, L. L. & BROWN, D. J. Progressive retinal degeneration with selective involvement of the cone mechanism. *Amer. J. Ophth.* 54: *629-641* (1962).

YOKOYAMA, M., YOSHIDA, F. & UI, K. Spectral responses in the human electroretinogram and their clinical significance. *Jap. J. Ophth.* 17: *113-124* (1973).

YOKOYAMA, M., UI, K. & YOSHIDA, T. The spectral response in the retina with progressive cone dystrophy. *Jap. J. Clin. Ophth.* 28 in press.

Authors' address:

Dept. of Ophthalmology
Mie University
School of Medicine
TSU
Japan

HALOTHANE RETARDS DARK ADAPTATION

DIRK V. NORREN & PIETER PADMOS

(Soesterberg)

In our studies on cone dark adaptation in human subjects and macaque monkeys a light pentobarbital (Nembutal) anaesthesia is routinely used for the monkeys. With this anaesthesia the time constants (1/e values) were somewhat longer than the values found with (unanaesthetized) human subjects. To find out, first whether this is an effect of the Nembutal anaesthesia and second whether, perhaps, Halothane anaesthesia would be different in this respect, we compared both drugs in identical experimental conditions. Moreover, a muscle relaxant was used to follow the dark adaptation under very light anaesthesia. We found, much to our surprise, that Halothane has dramatic effects on the time course of dark adaptation.

Bromochlorotrifluoroethane (Halothane, Fluothane) is an inhalation anaesthetic widely used in human surgery. Concerning experiments on the visual system the use of the drug was reported to be advantageous in birds in leaving the electroretinogram unaffected (NYE, 1968). Recently, WHITTEN & BROWN (1973) described the advantages of Halothane anaesthesia with rhesus monkeys.

In our experiments it first seemed that Halothane simply slowed down the speed of recovery, but the situation appeared to be more complicated. The first dark adaptation curve measured in a series of repeated bleaching and recovery experiments showed very little or no retardation, but at the second and following curves progressive retardation of the recovery process was observed. The time constant of dark adaptation thus also depends on the recent bleaching history.

METHODS

Anaesthesia

First, a 5 mg/kg intravenous injection of the ultra short-acting sodium methohexital (Brietal, Lilly, Indianapolis) was given in order to permit intubation. After intubation, an initial dose of 30 μg/kg of the muscle relaxant pancuroniumbromide (Pavulon, Organon, Oss) was given, followed by a continuous injection of 30 μg/kg/hr. The animal was artificially respirated at 25 strokes/min with an Infant Respirator (Loosco, Amsterdam) with a mixture of 70% O_2

and 30% N_2O. This gas mixture was given during the whole course of the experiment and used a basic anaesthetic. To suppress salivation an injection of 0.1 mg/kg atropine sulfate was given and repeated several hours later. The Halothane percentage in the inspired air was controlled by a vaporiser (Vapor, Dräger, Lübeck) with an accuracy better than 0.05% Halothane. The CO_2 level of the expired air was monitored with a Capnograph (Godart-Statham, de Bilt) and maintained between 4.5 and 5.5% by means of adjusting the stroke volume (between 22 and 35 ml). The heart rate was monitored continuously. Arterial blood pressure of the upper arm was measured with the indirect auscultatory technique. The temperature of the monkey was kept at about 37.5°C.

Optics and electronics

The animal's sensitivity to light stimuli was measured with the help of vector-retinography (PADMOS & NORREN, 1972).

Briefly, the measuring beam is chopped with a sectored disk (40 Hz in these experiments in order to isolate cone function). The ERG signal is led to the vector-voltmeter where the amplitude of the signal at the chopping frequency and phase relative to the phase of the input are derived. The amplitude signal is led to a neutral density wedge control box. At the control box a pre-set criterion voltage is selected (2 µV in this case) and the difference signal between this and the ERG amplitude was fed to the wedge drive motor. As a consequence, the wedge is moved so as to maintain 2 µV ERG amplitude. The wedge position is recorded on the ink writer. Bleaching and measuring beam were both yellow (filter Jena OG550 and Schott DAL 577 nm, respectively), so we recorded only the response of the combined red and green sensitive pigments. The adaptation and stimulus were seen in Maxwellian view of 70° and 45°, respectively.

RESULTS

The lower part of Fig 1 shows a dark adaptation curve while the animal received only the N_2O anaesthesia. The time constants found in this condition compared well with the value obtained with unaesthetized human subjects (NORREN, 1974). The upper curve of Fig. 2 was recorded while the animal breathed 1.5% Halothane. The speed of recovery has decreased enormously. In both cases the preadaptation was 10^6 td presented during 10 minutes. With intermediate percentages of Halothane the speed of recovery was in between the values showed here.

Fig. 2 depicts the effect of repeated bleaching and recovery from a short 10^6 td bleach. In this case the Halothane level was 0.2%. Every 5 minutes a 10 sec bleach was given. Through the pen writer curves smooth curves were drawn by eye and all these curves were placed at the same beginning point viz. the offset of the bleaching light. The first recorded curve has a time course that is comparable to the no Halothane condition. With every bleach the re-

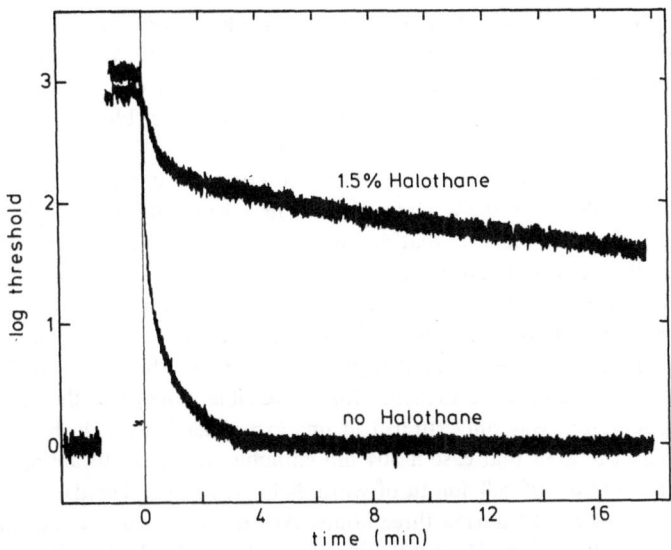

Fig. 1. Cone dark adaptation of a macaque monkey with and without Halothane anaesthesia. The sensitivity level recorded before the bleaching light was switched on, is indicated by the zero level on the vertical axis. The bottom curve represents the condition without anaesthesia. The upper curve is recorded with 1.5% Halothane anaesthesia. Both stimulus and adaptation were presented in Maxwellian view (45° and 70°, respectively). The stimulus was yellow (577 nm) and flickered with a frequency of 40 Hz in order to isolate the cone function. The preadaptation of 5.9 log td yellow light was presented during 10 minutes before zero time. The response criterion was kept at 2 μV by means of the vector voltmeter system.

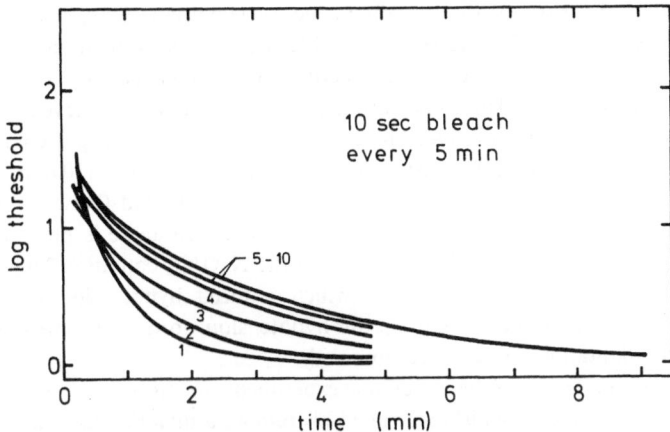

Fig. 2. Effect of repeated bleaches (10 sec) on the time course of dark adaptation measured under Halothane anaesthesia (0.2%). The speed of the first recovery is almost normal, the next bleach given after 5 minutes is followed by a markedly retarded dark adaptation. After the seventh 10 sec bleach given (with 5 minute intervals) the time constant does not increase anymore. The bleaching intensity was 5.9 log td. Though the actual recordings a smooth curve was drawn by eye. The time axis is given with reference to the time of offset of the bleach.

157

covery becomes slower, till after about seven bleaches a final state is reached in which the speed of recovery does not increase anymore. With longer bleaching times fewer steps are needed to reach the final recovery speed. For instance, with 0.2% Halothane in the inspired air, one 8 min. bleach brings the recovery to a speed that does not change anymore.

However, if we let the animal remain in complete darkness for some time (e.g. 40 minutes with 0.2% Halothane), a new 10 sec bleach is followed by a recovery that is as fast as that at the beginning of the experiment. In other words, the speed of recovery recovers in the dark. The dark period required for complete recovery depends on the Halothane percentage.

Finally, all retarding effects of Halothane, even if the animal had breathed it for 5 to 6 hours, disappeared within 3 to 4 hours after offset of the Halothane. Thus, we have no evidence for irreversible damage to the retina. Rod dark adaptation was only studied in one experiment in which the Halothane level was 1.5%. In that case a 504 nm stimulus was used, flickering at 8 Hz. A preadaptation of 5.8 log td of white light was given. The dark adaptation curve was measured during three hours. At the end of that period, the sensitivity was still rising and had still not reached the (dark adapted) level observed at the beginning of the experiment. It thus seems likely that both rod and cone darkadaptation are affected.

In another experiment Nembutal was injected (30 mg/kg) intraveneously at some moment during the N_2O/O_2 condition. The time constant was seen to increase, but the extent was very small compared to the Halothane effects.

DISCUSSION

Regarding the cause of the retarding effect of Halothane on dark adaptation, nothing definite can be said yet. A possible effect of the combination of Halothane and N_2O was excluded by experiments in which Halothane was combined with only O_2. The same slow dark adaptation was observed. Further, Halothane is known to reduce blood pressure. With very low percentages like 0.2, however, the blood pressure level remains normal ($>$ 150 mm Hg, systolic) and only after some hours shows a tendency to fall (between 100 and 150 mm Hg). Another indication that blood pressure alone is not the determining factor was obtained by injecting in the N_2O/O_2 condition 2 mg/kg/min trimethaphan camsylate (Arfonad), which induced hypotension (bloodpressure, systolic 100-120 mm). During this hypotension normal to somewhat slower dark adaptation curves were observed.

The interpretation of the Halothane experiments might best be given in terms of a store and the replenishment of 11-cis retinal, a material necessary for the regeneration of bleached pigment (RUSHTON, 1972). Briefly, the hypothesis is that the only effect of Halothane is the retardation of the replenishment of 11-cis, while the store of this material, remains intact. The first recovery after a short bleach can rely upon the stock but after further bleaches this stock is decreased. If we suppose, with RUSHTON (1972), that the time constant is inversely proportional to the concentration of 11-cis the time constant will necessarily become longer. Finally, when after many bleaches an equilibrium is reached, the time constant is determined by the replenishment speed. During a long dark period the stock is replenished again so that a fast recovery is possible once more.

Since the whole problem of the influence of the supply of 11-cis retinal is an intriguing and controversial point (ALPERN, MAASEIDVAAG & OHBA, 1971), a further study of the effect of Halothane may quite well prove to be a key to better understanding of retinal chemistry.

REFERENCES

ALPERN, M., MAASEIDVAAG, F. & OHBA, N. The kinetics of visual pigments in man. *Vision Res.* 11 : *539-549* (1971).

NORREN, D. V. Cone dark adaptation: Comparison of psychophysics and vector-retinography. Proceedings XIth ISCERG Symposium. This volume 69-73 (1974).

NYE, P. W. An examination of the electro-retinogram of the pigeon in response to stimuli of different intensity and wavelength and following intense chromatic adaptation. *Vis. Res.* 8 : *679-696* (1968).

PADMOS, P. & NORREN, D. V. The vector voltmeter as a tool to measure electroretinogram spectral sensitivity and dark adaptation. *Invest. Ophthalmol.* 11 : *783-788* (1972).

RUSHTON, W. A. H. Visual pigments in man. In: Handbook of Sensory Physiology ed. H. J. A. DARTNALL. Springer, Berlin (1972).

WHITTEN, D. N. & BROWN, K. T. The time courses of late receptor potentials from monkey cones and rods. *Vision Res.* 13 : *107-135* (1973).

Authors' address:

Institute for Perception
Kampweg 5
Soesterberg
The Netherlands

159

ELECTROPHYSIOLOGICAL TESTS IN CONGENITAL STATIONARY NIGHT-BLINDNESS WITH REGARD TO THE DIFFERENT TYPES OF INHERITANCE*

F. PONTE, G. LODATO & M. LAURICELLA

(Palermo)

ABSTRACT

The authors performed electrophysiological tests in genetically different forms of congenital stationary night-blindness: dominant autosomal, recessive autosomal and sex-linked recessive.

The ERG is always altered because scotopic responses are absent and photopic ones are normal; on the other hand, it is possible to discern two electro-oculographic groups of congenital night-blindness: one with normal EOG, the other with abnormal EOG. These types of EOG changes are independent from the patterns of genetic transmission.

These results are briefly discussed in relation to the present knowledge of the origin of the electro-oculogram.

The pattern of hereditary transmission of stationary night-blindness may display a variable behaviour. It may follow the law of autosomal recessive inheritance in some familiar groups, whereas, in other cases, it may appear as an autosomal dominant or as a sex-linked trait.

It is interesting that there are no clinical or electroretinographic differences among hereditary forms of congenital night-blindness while various electro-oculographic patterns may be noted. All genetic types show normal eyegrounds, normal day-light visual fields, absence of rod dark adaptation, lack of progression and from the electroretinographic point of view, absence or very serious reduction of the scotopic component of the ERG; on the contrary, the electro-oculogram (EOG) may be found normal or abnormal (for references, see KRILL & MARTIN, 1971). Therefore, in congenital stationary night-blindness it seems that there is no definite or constant correlation between ERG and EOG behaviour.

Clinical and nosological problems posed by the study of genetic types of night-blindness appear to be in no way resolved and remain therefore, open to wide discussion.

Recently, in 9 subjects affected by congenital night-blindness and in 2 subjects with Oguchi's disease, FRANÇOIS et al. (1971) found that EOG was normal in dominant inheritance types and abnormal in recessive inheritance types of

*This paper has been supported by a Grant of the Consiglio Nazionale delle Ricerche (Grant No. 71.01915.04).

congenital night-blindness as well as in Oguchi's disease. Consequently, they think that the electro-oculographic examination combined with other clinical tests may enable one to recognize the genetic forms of this affection.

The present report concerns 6 subjects affected by congenital stationary night-blindness of various forms of inheritance belonging to three families. Clinical and electrophysiological tests that we have studied, provide additional information concerning the relationship between the types of inheritance and ERG and EOG behaviour.

METHODS

Two of our patients belong to a family with autosomal dominant inheritance (see pedigree in Fig. 1); three patients belong to a family with recessive X-linked inheritance (see pedigree in Fig. 2). The last one is a sporadic case, probably with recessive autosomal inheritance (see pedigree Fig. 3). In the family with X-linked inheritance two of the three patients affected by night-blindness were also affected by red-green defect.

All patients had a history of severe congenital night-blindness; four of them were followed for two to four years with no evidence of progression of symptoms in any of the evaluated parameters.

The EOG was carried out on all patients; the technique of testing and the normal data obtained by this method are reported elsewhere (PONTE & LAURI-CELLA, 1971). According to ARDEN et al. (1962) recordings are carried out at 1-minute intervals for a period of 12 minutes in the dark followed by a period of 12 minutes in strong illumination (1000 lux intensity, measured at the forehead of the subject) from a 300-Watt bulb.

The EOG was recorded from each eye by an EEG apparatus (Schwarzer, model E 546) with time constant 0.3 sec and paper speed of 2.5 cm/sec. In evaluating the record, the average amplitude of each test period was measured and the ratio of the maximum light-adapted to minimum dark-adapted response was considered. In our series of 96 normal eyes (PONTE & LAURICELLA, 1971) an average value for the LP/DT ratio (light-peak/dark-trough) of 184.26 with a standard deviation of 24.27 has been found. Therefore, ratios less than 136 are considered as definitely abnormal.

The ERG was carried out in the usual way with corneal electrodes of Burian-Allen, EEG apparatus (Schwarzer, model E 546) with time constant 1 sec and a Schwarzer xenon stroboscope with the bulb placed at a distance of 30 cm from the patient's forehead. The duration of single flash was 10 μsec. The brightest light stimulus was obtained by using the maximum intensity setting on the instrument (energy 1.5 Joule/flash). Dimmer light stimuli were obtained by using minimum intensity setting on the instrument (energy 0.5 Joule/flash) and by interposing in front of the lamp a series of four-inch square neutral density filters, each differing by 0.6 log step. Control of eye position was obtained by a red fixation bulb placed upon the center of the lamp.

Subjects were previously light-adapted for five minutes to room illumination obtained by a 40 Watt, 220 Volt tungsten filament bulb illuminating a plastic diffuser in the ceiling.

Single flash photopic responses were obtained with the highest intensity light-stimulus and the room lights on. Single flash scotopic responses were obtained with dimmer intensity of stimulus in total darkness. A flicker-ERG at 30 flash/sec frequency was obtained with energy stimuli of 1.5 Joule/flash.

Dark adaptation test was carried out with Goldmann-Weekers adaptometer; colour discrimination tests were carried out with Ishihara's plates, Panel D 15, Farnsworth 100 Hue tests and Nagel anomaloscope.

CLINICAL OBSERVATIONS

1. V/1 (Family pedigree shown in Fig. 1) – Par. Antonino, aged 20 (Table 1). Both eyes: visual acuity, 10/10; media, clear; fundus oculi, normal; visual fields, slightly constricted with objects I/4 and I/2 of Goldmann's perimeter; dark adaptation, monophasic curve with final threshold of $10^{4.4}$ Log Units; chromatic discrimination, normal by the Ishihara and Panel D 15 tests; ERG, scotopic response, absent; photopic response, present and normal; EOG, subnormal LP/DT ratio in both eyes (RE = 128; LE = 129).
Diagnosis = dominant autosomal night-blindness with subnormal EOG.

2. III/1 (Family pedigree shown in Fig. 1) – Par. Bernardo, aged 55 (Table 1), father of Par. Antonino (IV/1). Visual acuity: RE, 10/10 with −0.50 sph.

TABLE 1

Case	Age	Sex	Visual acuity RE	LE	Fundus oculi	ERG scotopic	photopic	EOG RE LE (*)	Dark Adap. (**)	Inheritance (***)
1	20	M	10/10	10/10	normal	absent	normal	128 129	$10^{4.4}$	AD
2	55	M	10/10 with glasses	6/10 with glasses	normal	absent	normal	165 171	$10^{4.4}$	AD
3†	8	M	6/10 with glasses	1/10	myopic	absent	normal	133 128	10^5	RX
4	12	M	4/10 with glasses	6/10 with glasses	myopic	absent	normal	158 159	10^5	RX
5†	36	M	10/10 with glasses	9/10 with glasses	myopic	absent	normal	189 155	10^5	RX
6	26	M	10/10	10/10	normal	absent	normal	115 120	10^5	AR

(*)   LP/DT ratio
(**) Log units of final thresholds
(***) AD = Autosomal Dominant; AR = Autosomal Recessive; RX = X-linked Recessive
†   Also affected by protan defect

—1.50 cyl. ax. 170°; LE, 6/10 with —1.50 sph. —1.50 cyl. ax. 60°. Both eyes: media clear; fundus oculi, normal; chromatic discrimination, normal by the Ishihara and Panel D 15 tests; dark adaptation, monophasic curve with final threshold of $10^{4.4}$ Log Units; ERG, scotopic response, absent; photopic response, present and normal; EOG, normal LP/DT ratio in both eyes (RE = 165; LE = 171).

Diagnosis = dominant autosomal night-blindness with normal EOG.

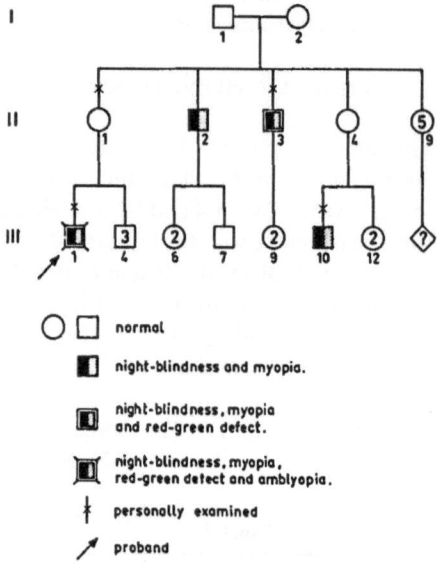

Fig. 1. Pedigree of family Par. (Congenital night-blindness with autosomal dominant inheritance).

3. III/1 (Family pedigree shown in Fig. 2) – Puc. Salvatore, aged 8 (Table 1). Sent to us from the Orthoptic Department where he had been examined for an esotropia in the left eye. Now nystagmus is noted in left eye; the angle of squint is variable from 2° looking up to 15° looking down, with vertical deviation of 10°. Visual acuity, RE = 6/10 with sph. —1, LE = 1/10 not improved by glasses; media, clear; fundus oculi, RE: the disk is pale in lower external quarter; LE: the disk is pale in external half; in both eyes: sclerosis of choroid, macular reflex evident with thin dark brown pigment deposits; in peripheral fundus, thin 'pepper and salt' pigment deposits; visual field, slightly constricted with objects I/4, I/3 and I/2 of Goldmann's perimeter. Dark adaptation, monophasic curve with final threshold of 10^5 Log Units. Chromatic test: protan red-green defect by Ishihara, Panel D 15, Farnsworth 100 Hue tests and Nagel anomaloscope. ERG: scotopic response, absent; photopic response, present and normal. EOG: sub-normal in both eyes (RE = 133; LE = 128).

Diagnosis = X-linked congenital night-blindness with myopia, red-green defect and sub-normal EOG.

164

4. III/10 (Family pedigree shown in Fig. 2) – Sca. Stefano, aged 12 (Table I),
cousin of Puc. Salvatore (III/1). Has worn glasses since the age of 7. Visual
acuity, RE: 4/10 with sph. −8; LE: 6/10 with sph. −7.50. Both eyes: media,
clear; fundus oculi, myopic. Dark adaptation, monophasic curve with final
threshold of 10^5Log Units. Chromatic test, normal by Ishihara, Panel D 15
and Nagel anomaloscope tests. ERG, scotopic response, absent; photopic
response, present and normal. EOG, normal in both eyes (RE = 158; LE
= 159).

Diagnosis = X-linked night-blindness with myopia and normal EOG.

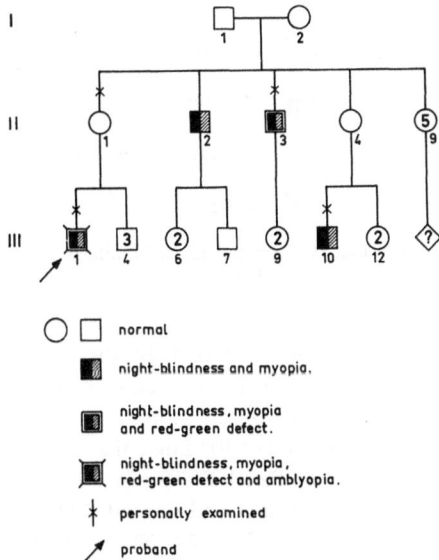

Fig. 2. Pedigree of family Puc. (Congenital night-blindness with recessive X-linked
inheritance).

5. II/3 (Family pedigree shown in Fig. 2) – Spa. Agostino, aged 36 (Table I),
uncle of Puc. Salvatore (III/1). Visual acuity, RE: 10/10 with −6 sph. −0.50
cyl. 110°; LE: 9/10 with −5.50 sph. −0.50 cyl. ax. 110°. Both eyes: media,
clear; fundus oculi, myopic with slight choroidal sclerosis in the posterior
part. Dark adaptation, monophasic curve with final threshold of 10^5 Log
Units. Chromatic test, protan red-green defect by Ishihara, Panel D 15,
Farnsworth 100 Hue tests and Nagel anomaloscope. ERG, scotopic response, absent; photopic response, present and normal. EOG, normal
LP/DT ratio in both eyes (RE = 189; LE = 155).

*Diagnosis = X-linked congenital night-blindness with myopia, red-green defect and
normal EOG.*

6. II/2 (Family pedigree shown in Fig. 3) – Pia. Vincenzo, aged 26 (Table I).
No history of eye diseases and of consanguinity in the family. Normal ocular

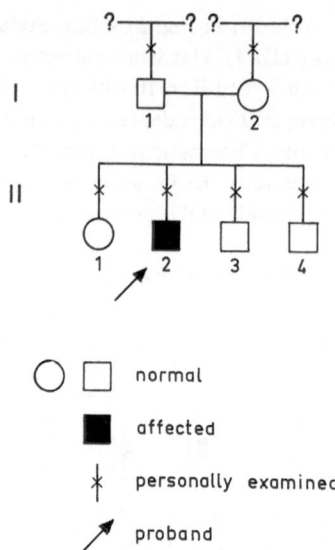

I

II

○ □ normal

■ affected

⚹ personally examined

↗ proband

Fig. 3. Pedigree of family Pia. (Congenital night-blindness with autosomal recessive inheritance).

findings observed in the subject's parent, brothers and sisters. Both eyes: visual acuity, 10/10; media, clear; fundus oculi, normal; visual field, slightly constricted and without pathological scotomas; dark adaptation, monophasic curve with final threshold of 10^5 Log units; chromatic discrimination, normal by the Ishihara and Panel D 15 tests; ERG, scotopic response, absent; photopic response, present and normal. EOG, sub-normal LP/DT ratio in both eyes (RE = 115; LE = 120). The vitamin A blood level examined by CARRIER and PRICE test was found normal.

Diagnosis = recessive autosomal night-blindness with sub-normal EOG.

RESULTS AND DISCUSSION

Electro-oculographic findings in our patients affected by congenital stationary night-blindness show that changes of EOG are not necessarily linked to the hereditary type of transmission.

In the first family of our series, in which the inheritance was of dominant autosomal type, patient 1 (IV/1 in Fig. 1) had subnormal EOG and the father (patient 2, III/1 in fig. 1) had normal EOG. In the second family, in which the inheritance was of X-linked recessive type, only one out of three affected patients had subnormal EOG (case 3, III/1 in Fig. 2). A cousin (case 4, III/10) and an uncle (case 5, II/3) had normal EOG. In all the affected members of this family myopia was also present and in two of them (cases 3 and 5) a red-green defect was associated. It is interesting to note that EOG behaviour seems to be unrelated with the association of red-green defect since LP/DT ratio was normal in patient 5 and subnormal in patient 3.

166

In case 6, who had an abnormal EOG, a recessive heredity is probable. As is shown in pedigree of Fig. 3 the examined parents and siblings of the proband were not affected by night-blindness but the lack of family history does not rule out autosomal recessive inheritance. Furthermore, the vitamin A blood level was normal in this case.

Therefore, both a normal or an abnormal EOG may be found in all three genetic types of congenital stationary night-blindness, as has been noted also in previous report (see KRILL & MARTIN, 1971).

The EOG may be used to investigate retinal function and it may help to localize the level of involvement. Since the EOG is a response mediated mainly by the pigment epithelium of the retina and by the receptors (ARDEN et al., 1962), one may deduce that the EOG changes, when they are present, indicate an extension of the retinal damage to these layers and mainly to the pigment epithelium.

In congenital night-blindness, scotopic ERG, which arises from the visual and bipolar cells, is always definitely altered according to the severe functional disturbance of the rod-system. Since the EOG tracing remains normal in some cases it follows that where EOG changes are present there is a dysfunction of the pigment epithelium, in addition to the lesion of the rod-system.

It would seem therefore, that two types of stationary night-blindness can be recognized: one with normal EOG in which the lesion is limited to the visual cells and another one, in which the abnormal EOG suggests that also the pigment epithelium cells are functionally altered. Therefore, definite abnormalities of EOG, in addition to the ERG scotopic changes, prove that the lesions are, in these cases, less circumscribed and that they involve a large retinal zone.

REFERENCES

ARDEN, G. B., BARRADA, A. & KELSEY, G. H. New clinical test of retinal function based upon the standing potential of the eye. *Brit. J. Ophthal.* 46: *449-467* (1962).

FRANÇOIS, J., DE ROUCK, A. & VERRIEST, G. L'éléctro-oculogramme dans l'héméralopie essentielle. *Ann. Ocul. Paris* 204: *1035-1046* (1971).

KRILL, A. E. & MARTIN, D. Photopic abnormalities in congenital stationary night blindness. *Invest. Ophthal.* 10: *625-636* (1971).

PONTE, F. & LAURICELLA, M. L'elettro-oculografia nella pratica clinica. Casistica e considerazioni. Proceedings of the 53rd Congress S.O.I., Malta (1971).

Authors' address:

University Eye Clinic
Palermo
Italy

ELECTRO-OPHTHALMOLOGY OF A FAMILY WITH X-CHROMOSOMAL RECESSIVE NYCTALOPIA AND MYOPIA

H. J. VÖLKER-DIEBEN, G. H. M. VAN LITH, L. N. WENT & E. C. DE VRIES-DE MOL

(Leyden and Rotterdam)

ABSTRACT

Sixteen patients of a family suffering from nyctalopia with myopia, X-chromosomal recessively inherited, were examined ophthalmoscopically and psychophysically. Of two other families with X-chromosomal recessive nyctalopia and myopia we examined four affected members. In all these patients we found an almost normal EOG, a lowered scotopic ERG and no oscillatory potentials. The photopic ERG appeared to be very specific, viz. the a-wave was deep and broad, the b-wave very small, often consisting of several peaks. On account of these data the disturbance has to be post-receptoral.

Night blindness or nyctalopia is known as a symptom of some types of retino-pathy, as a symptom of severe vitamin A deficiency and as an inherited static defect. Congenital nyctalopia can be a dominant, recessive or recessive X-chromosomal inherited disease.

This paper reports on a study, started in 1972, on a large family affected by X-linked recessive nyctalopia and myopia.

Two brothers, 7 and 9 years old, were seen at the Department of Ophthalmology of the University of Leiden because of a convergent squint and amblyopia, alternating sursumduction, abnormal head posture and nystagmus.

The ophthalmological examination revealed the following:
– diminished visual acuity with correction of the nonamblyopic eye;
– dystrophy of the pigment epithelium in the posterior pole;
– nyctalopia.

The mother told us that her eldest son had identical problems, as well as her father and his grandfather. This information triggered us to investigate this family.

The pedigree (Fig. 1) clearly shows an X-chromosomal recessive inheritance; the female carriers had a normal visual acuity without myopia or nyctalopia. Of the 207 living members of this family, 18 appeared to be affected, while 5 deceased members were affected according to the case history. Of the 18 living members, 16 were extensively examined. Two were too young, being only 2 and 4 years old. The ages of the members examined varied between 6 and 77 years.

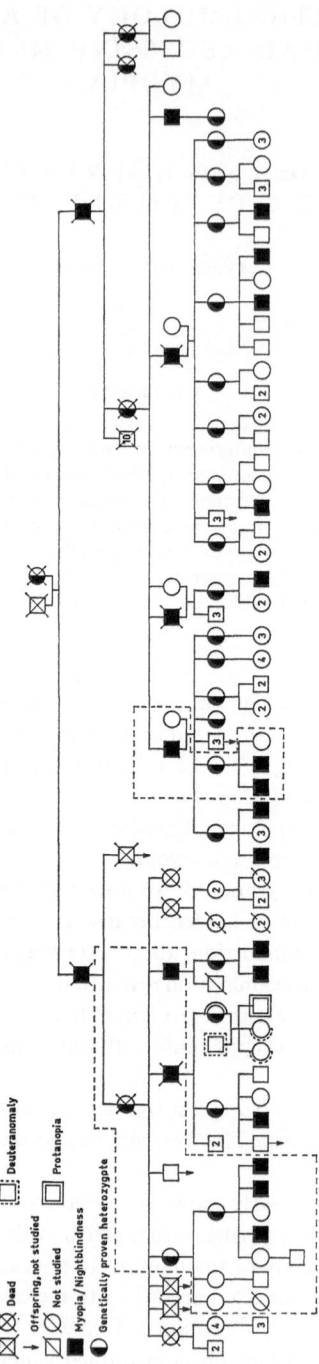

Fig. 1. Pedigree B; X linked chromosomal recessive nyctalopia and myopia

Visual acuity

Table I shows that the visual acuity ranged between 4/60 and 0.6 and the myopia between 3.5 and 19 D. In 13 cases there was also an astigmatism. The degree of anisometropia amounted to max. 1.75 D. No relation appeared to exist between patient age and the visual acuity or degree of myopia.

TABLE I

Clinical findings in 16 patients of pedigree B.

Age yrs	Myopia		Astigmatism		Visual acuity		Squint			alt. sursumduction	Nystagmus
	RE	LE	RE	LE	RE	LE	RE	Alt.	LE		
6	− 3.5	− 3.5	−0.5	−1.5	0.2	0.5	eso			−	+
8	− 9.0	− 9.0	−	−2.0	0.2	4/60			eso	+	+
9	− 6.0	− 6.0	−0.5	−0.5	0.4	0.4		exo		+	+
9	− 9.0	− 9.0	−1.0	−1.0	0.4	0.5		−		+	+
10	− 7.25	− 7.25	−	−	0.5	0.16			eso	+	+
13	− 8.5	− 7.5	−	−	0.5	0.1			eso	+	+
13	− 1.0	− 2.75	−3.5	−2.5	0.5	0.5	eso			−	+
14	− 9.5	− 9.0	−0.5	−1.0	0.6	0.5			exo	+	+
17	− 6.5	− 6.75	−6.0	−5.5	0.3	0.2	eso			−	+
18	− 5.0	− 5.0	−1.5	−2.0	0.6	0.6	−			−	+
20	− 7.75	− 7.0	−1.5	−1.0	0.6	0.4			exo	+	+
20	−17.0	−18.0	−2.0	−2.0	0.5	0.5	exo			−	+
22	− 3.5	− 4.5	−2.0	−1.0	0.5	0.3			eso	+	+
24	−19.0	−19.0	−	−1.0	0.4	0.2	eso			−	+
76	− 8.0	− 8.0	−	−	0.3	0.3	−			+	+
77	− 4.5	− 3.0	−	−2.0	0.5	0.3		exo		+	−

Visual fields

Visual fields analysed with the Goldmann perimeter were normal and not constricted, as described in literature. (NETTLESHIP, 1912).

Squint

Eight patients had an esotropia, five patients an exotropia. In three patients no squint was found. Apart from the eso- and exotropia, ten patients had an alternating sursumduction.

Nystagmus

Fifteen out of 16 patients showed a fine or coarse nystagmus which was mostly horizontal. In 7 patients the horizontal nystagmus had also a fine rotatory component.

Dark adaptation curves

Testing was performed on a Goldmann-Weekers Adaptometer (Figure 2). The subject was light adapted for 10 min to a luminance of 500 Lux. Thresholds during dark adaptation were measured for a white circular test field of 11 degrees. Dark adaptation curves were always monophasic; no measurable scotopic function could be obtained.

Colour vision

With the colour vision tests of Ishihara, H.R.R, Farnsworth panel D15 and Farnsworth-Munsell 100 Hue test we could not detect specific colour vision defects in these patients.

Fundus

All patients showed a strikingly similar fundus picture. Apart from the myopic changes in the posterior pole, the atrophy of the choriocapillaris and the dystrophy of the pigment epithelium were more diffuse than may be expected in degenerative myopia only. This was seen in both the older and the younger patients. In the macular region irregular pigmentations were seen in all patients. Dystrophy of the pigment epithelium was proved by means of fluorescein angiography (Fig. 3). The choroidal vessels in the macular region were far too obvious as compared with the normal fluorogram.

We do not know whether the alterations in the pigment epithelium developed later or were present at birth, i.e. it may be a dystrophy or a dysgenesis. Since these alterations were the same in the old as well as the young patients, even in the patient aged 2 years, we suppose that it is a dysgenesis rather than a dystrophy.

Electro-ophthalmological examination

The following electro-ophthalmological examinations were carried out: the EOG and the ERG with its components, the scotopic b-wave, the photopic a-wave and the oscillatory potentials.

The EOG was registered with the semi-automatic system described by HENKES et al. (1968). Stimulation for the ERG has been carried out with a xenon light flash stroboscope, built into a ball stimulator (VAN LITH et al., 1973). After amplification, the recordings were averaged with a C.A.T. (computer of average transients). The OPs were evoked with a light flash of 40 J after 10

172

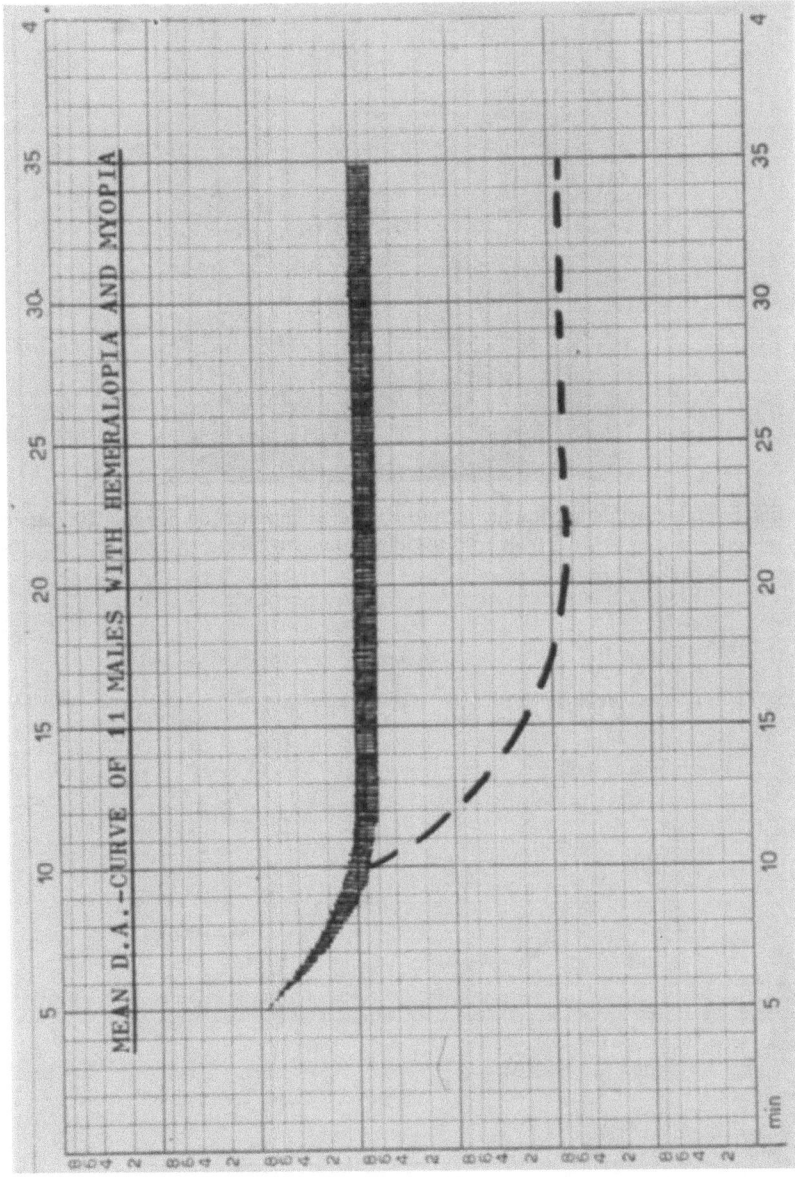

Fig. 2. Mean D. A. curve of 11 males with nyctalopia and myopia. The dotted line
is the normal value.

minutes dark adaptation. They were recorded photographically from the screen
of an oscilloscope. Fig. 4 represents the recordings of a normal subject.

In Fig. 5 the recordings of one of the young patients are shown. The alterations are typical for all other patients. The EOG has a light rise of about 2.03.

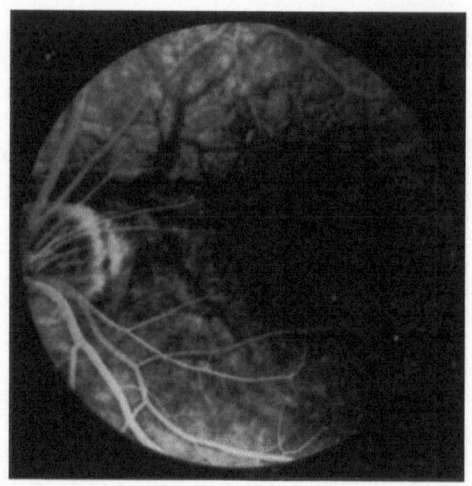

Fig. 3. Fluorescein angiographic picture 1'51" after injection of due in a 20 years old male with nyctalopia and myopia.

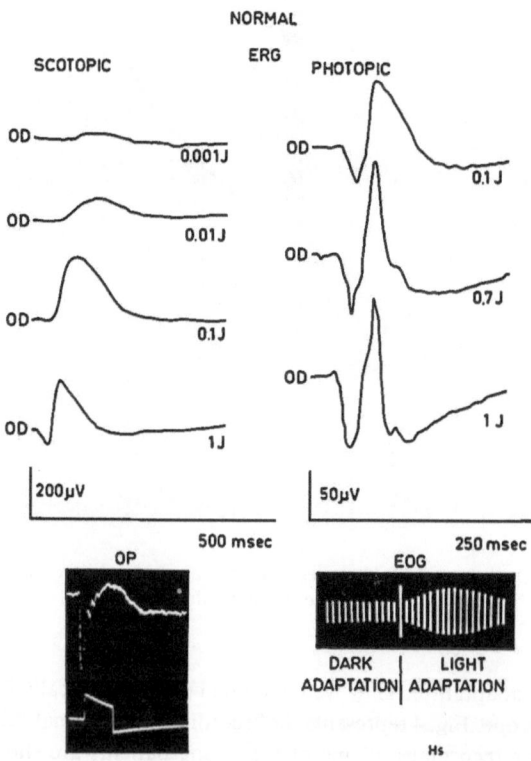

Fig. 4. Represents the recordings of a normal subject.

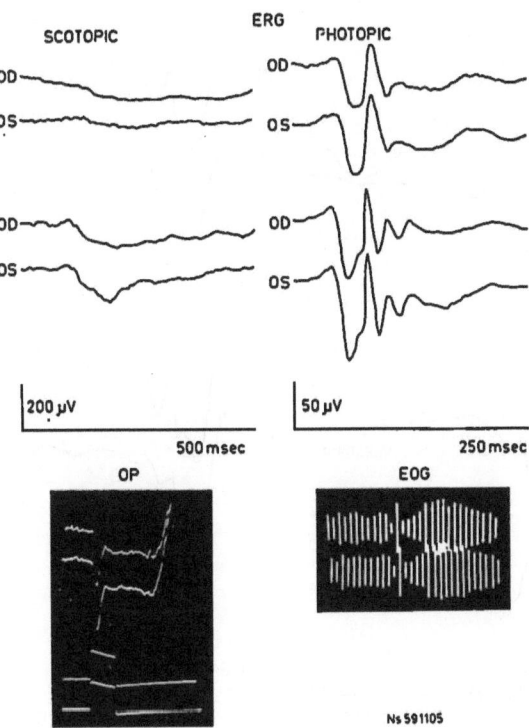

Fig. 5. Electro ophthalmologic recordings of a 13 years old male with nyctalopia and myopia.

An exact measurement was not possible as the patient did not watch the fixation lights regularly.

The scotopic b-wave of the ERG was extremely low and amounted to about 25 muV, i.e. 10% of the normal value. The peak time was normal (80 msec).

Although the a-wave in the photopic ERG is of normal height (80 muV) and has generally a normal latency time (10 msec), this wave is much broader than normal. This is only partly reflected in a lengthened implicit time of the a-wave (60 msec, normally less than 50 msec); it is more remarkable if the implicit time of the photopic b-wave is measured.

The photopic b-wave is not only reduced, but its form is also altered. Instead of one clear positive peak, which should be twice as high as the a-wave in our set up, we observed some small potentials of short duration. They have the appearance of the well known oscillatory potentials. The latter, however, have a much shorter implicit time and are superimposed on the ascending limb of the b-wave. The normal OPs are absent as can be seen in the figure.

In figure 6 the recordings of the photopic ERG of the other members of the family are shown. All the recordings show the same peculiar and specific deep and broad a-wave and the small positive peaks; sometimes one peak is seen.

In order to check whether the alterations found are typical for this family

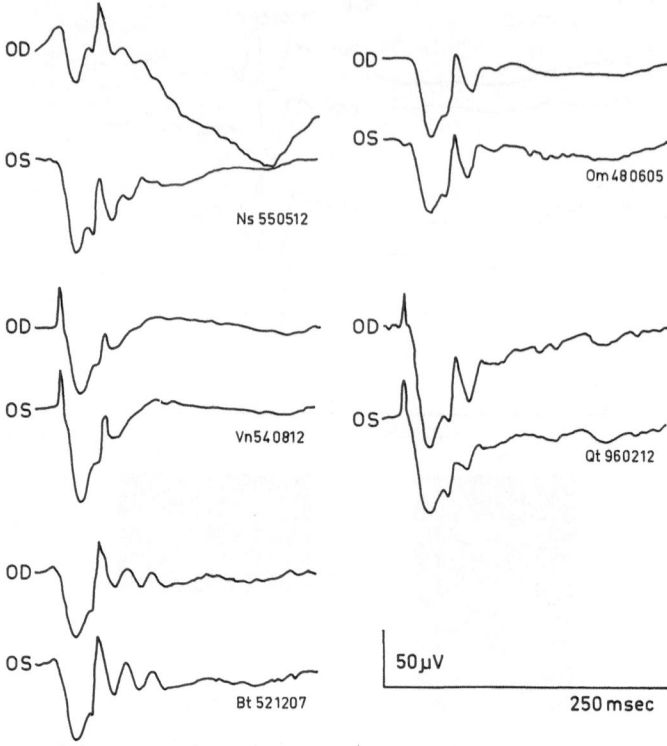

Fig. 6. Recordings of the photopic ERG of 5 males with myopia and nyctalopia.

only or are typical for the X-chromosomal recessive nyctalopia with myopia in general, some members of two other families with the same disorder have been examined. The results were identical.

CONCLUSION

We found an almost normal EOG in patients with X-chromosomal recessive form of nyctalopia with myopia. Together with the normal a-wave in the ERG it means that the receptor system is functioning normally. The scotopic and photopic b-waves are lowered, indicating that the disturbance has a post-receptoral localization. The absent OPs are in accordance with this assumption.

DISCUSSION

CARR et al. (1966) also found a post-receptoral disturbance in the recessive form of nyctalopia. They not only found a normal EOG and receptor potential in the ERG, but also a normal concentration and regeneration of rhodopsin. In the dominant form they localized the disturbance in the receptor inner segments, as a normal concentration and regeneration of rhodopsin was combined with a lowered EOG and a-wave in the ERG.

176

Comparing their electrophysiological data with ours, one can conclude that the X-chromosomal recessive nyctalopia may be the same as that of the recessive form. It is not known yet whether in the latter the broad a-wave and peculiar wave form of the b-wave also exist.

Concerning the broad photopic a-wave our results confirm those of KRILL & MARTIN (1971). They were the first to stress, that in congenital night blindness photopic disturbances can also be found. They describe identical peak times of the scotopic and photopic b-waves as a characteristic abnormality for all forms of congenital night blindness. The typical alterations we found in the photopic ERG are not obvious in their recordings. AUERBACH et al. (1969) and MERIN et al. (1970) investigated the X-chromosomal and the recessive form of nyctalopia. Usually they found an ERG of the Schubert-Bornschein (1952) type, i.e. a deep normal a-wave of normal implicit time and a small b-wave. They do not describe differences between both types of nyctalopia. Therefore, we can not say at this moment whether the alterations we found are exclusive for the X-chromosomal recessive form of nyctalopia. Other families have to be examined.

REFERENCES

AUERBACH, E., GODEL, V. & ROWE, H. An electrophysiological and psychophysical study of two forms of congenital night blindness. *Invest. Ophthal.* 8: *332* (1969).

CARR, R. E., RIPPS, H., SIEGEL, I. M. & WEALE, R. A. Rhodopsin and electrical activity of the retina in congenital night blindness. *Invest. Ophthal.* 5: *497* (1966).

CARR, R. E., RIPPS, H., SIEGEL, I. M. & WEALE, R. A. Visual functions in congenital night blindness. *Invest. Ophthal.* 5: *508* (1966).

HENKES, H. E., DENIER VAN DER GON, J. J., VAN MARLE, G. W. & SCHREINEMACHERS, H. P. Electro-oculography, a semi-automatic recording procedure. *Brit. J. Ophthal.* 52: *122-126* (1968).

KRILL, A. E. & MARTIN, D. Photopic abnormalities in congenital stationary night blindness. *Invest. Ophthal.* 10: *625* (1971).

VAN LITH, G. H. M., MEININGER, J. & VAN MARLE, G. W. Electro-physiological equipment for total and local retinal stimulation. Xth I.S.C.E.R.G. Symposium, Los Angeles, 1972. Junk, The Hague (1973).

MERIN, S., ROWE, H., AUERBACH, E. & LANDAU, J. Syndrome of congenital high myopia with nyctalopia. *Amer. J. Ophthal.* 70: *541* (1970).

NETTELSHIP, E. A pedigree of congenital night blindness with myopia. *Trans. Ophthal. Soc. U.K.* 32: *21* (1912).

SCHUBERT, G. & BORNSCHEIN, H. Beitrag zur Analyse des Menschlichen Elektroretinogramms. *Ophthalmologica (Basel)* 123: *396* (1952).

Authors' addresses:

H. J. VÖLKER-DIEBEN
L. N. WENT
E. C. DE VRIES-DE MOL
Depts. of Ophthalmology and
Human Genetics
University of Leiden
The Netherlands

G. H. M. VAN LITH
Eye Hospital
Erasmus University
Rotterdam
The Netherlands

PSYCHOPHYSICAL AND VECP EXAMINATION OF A ROD MONOCHROMAT AND A CONE MONOCHROMAT

E. ADACHI-USAMI, V. GAVRIYSKY, J. HECK, E. SCHENKEL & H. SCHEIBNER.

ABSTRACT

The spectral sensitivity was studied by measurement of the sensory threshold and by recording the visually evoked cortical potential (VECP) in a rod monochromat and a cone monochromat.

In the rod monochromat, the loss of sensitivity with increasing background illumination was higher as compared to a normal observer. The relative spectral sensitivity in the dark adapted state and during light adaptation was the same and corresponded closely to the CIE scotopic luminosity curve. In the cone monochromat, the photopic sensitivity curve was greatly reduced at longer wavelengths as compared to a normal observer. He may be classified as a protan type cone monochromat.

The aim of this study was to determine the spectral sensitivity function of a rod monochromat and of a cone monochromat by measuring the sensory threshold as well as recording the visually evoked cortical potential (VECP).

APPARATUS AND METHODS

Fig. 1. shows the experimental set up. The optical stimulator consists of two beams, both originating from the same xenon 150 Watt lamp. The subject lies supine on a couch, his head fixed. In Maxwellian view he fixes the center of a circular adaptation field, 15 degrees in diameter, on which the test light, 10 degrees in diameter, is concentrically superimposed. For measurements under scotopic conditions, the adaptation beam provides a dim red light of a half degree for the purpose of fixation.

The so-called retinal illumination, I, which in reality is a luminous intensity (DIN 5031, 1967; SCHEIBNER, 1973), was measured by applying the inverse square law $I = E \cdot d^2$, where E is the illuminance in a distance d behind the plane, where the subject's pupil would be.

The pupil of the eye was dilated, the other eye being occluded with an eye patch. Light pulses of 20 ms duration were presented for photopic measurements and 100 ms duration for scotopic measurements. The repetition rate of the stimulus was 2.3 per second. The potentials were led off with a gold disk electrode placed 3 cm above the inion; they were amplified, led through a band-pass filter of a 0.8-250 Hz and fed into an oscilloscope, which in turn was connected to a BIOMAC computer.

179

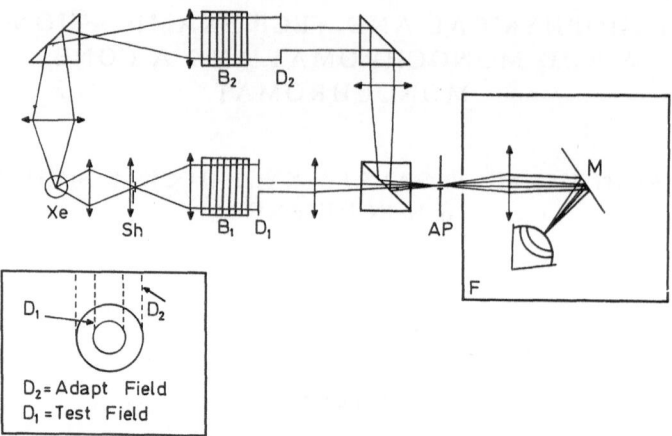

Fig. 1. Optical system. XE = Xenon arc lamp 150W; Sh = electromagnetic shutter; B_1 and B_2 = filter boxes; D_1 and D_2 = diaphragms in the test and adapting beams; Ap = artificial pupil; M = mirror; F = Faraday cage.

Measurements were made a) by determining the sensory threshold and b) by determining the amplitude from the first negative trough (N_1) to the first positive peak (P_1) of the VECP, both in dependence of the radiant power of the test light.

RESULTS

A. *Rod monochromat.*

S. P., male, 11 years old, exhibiting photophobia and nystagmus. The visual acuity of his both eyes was about 0.1. A central scotoma could not be clearly established. Colour discrimination was typical for achromatopsia. In Fig. 2, the rod monochromat's anomaloscope matches lie on a steep curve (dots).

Fig. 3 shows, on the left side for comparison, the VECPs obtained from an 11 year old *normal* observer, and on the right side those of the rod monochromat. At the top, the responses to red light of wavelength 650 nm, without any background illumination, are plotted; in the middle and at the bottom, the responses to 650 nm with a blue background of 462 nm amounting to 100 troland and 1000 troland are shown. To produce the two comparable responses without background shown at the top of this figure, the rod monochromat needed a test light almost 4 logarithmic units higher than the normal observer. With a background of 100 troland, the VECPs of the rod monochromat are seen to be smaller than that of the normal. With a background of 1000 troland, sufficient to suppress the activity of the rods, no response could be recorded from the rod monochromat, while a clear response was obtained from the normal observer (bottom of Fig. 3).

After dark adaptation, the VECPs were much smaller than the VECPs of a normal subject. Under photopic conditions of 10 troland suited for the rod

180

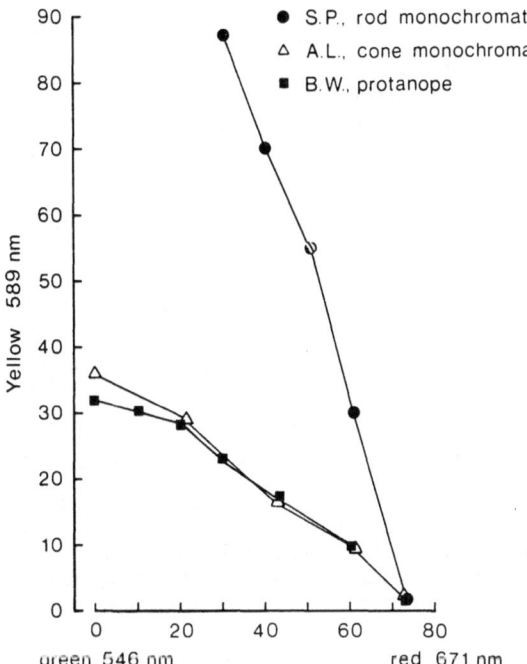

Nagel anomaloscope

- ● S.P., rod monochromat
- △ A.L., cone monochromat
- ■ B.W., protanope

Fig. 2. Colour matches made on a Nagel anomaloscope by a rod monochromat (dots), cone monochromat (triangles), and a protanope (filled squares). Abscissa: red-green mixture. Ordinate: brightness of the yellow comparison light. The mean value of normal trichromats is 43 (red-green mixture) and 16 (yellow).

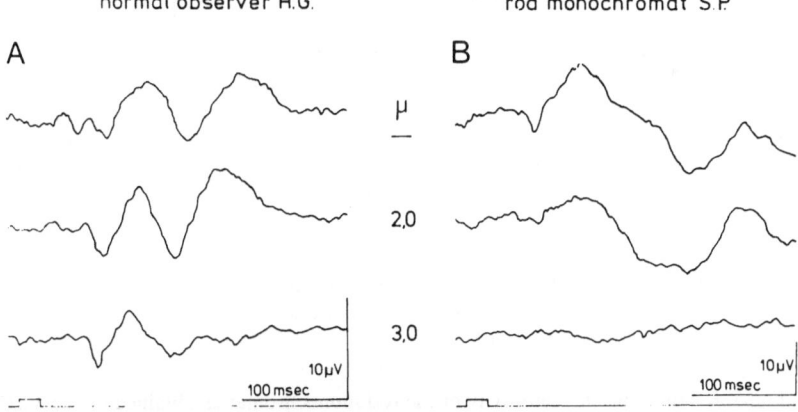

normal observer H.G.   rod monochromat S.P.

A   B

μ —

2,0

3,0

10μV
100 msec

10μV
100 msec

Fig. 3. VECPs of a normal (A) and the rod monochromat (B) in response to red stimuli (λ = 630 nm) of 10° diameter in darkness (top) and with background of blue light (467 nm) of 10^2 td and 10^3 td (μ) (middle and lower records). The strength of the test light in the dark adapted recordings is 100 td for the normal observer and 700000 td for the rod monochromat. In the light adapted recordings, it is 7000 td for the normal observer and 700000 td for the rod monochromat. The light pulse is indicated by upward deflection of the line drawn at the bottom.

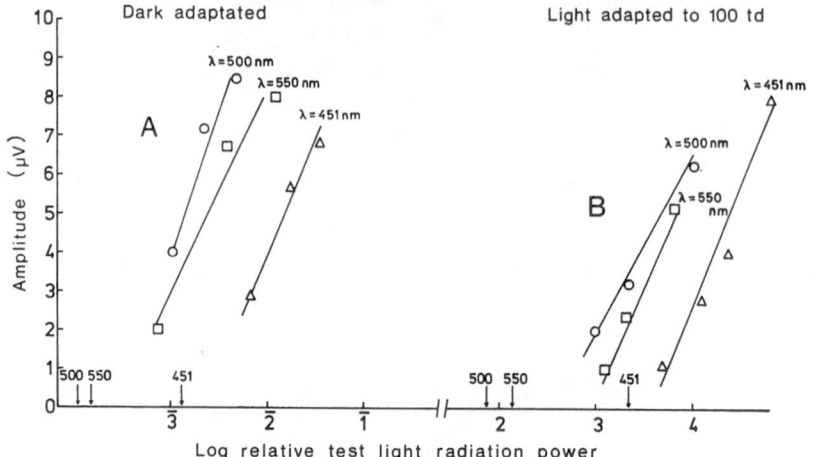

Fig. 4. Rod monochromat. Amplitudes of electropositive VECPs in μV as a function of the logarithm of the test light power determined for the test wavelengths λ = 451, 500 and 550 nm. Scotopic data as obtained after 30 minutes of dark adaptation (A), photopic data as obtained during exposure to a *white* background of 100 troland (B). Results of sensory determination as indicated by arrows on the abscissa.

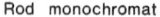

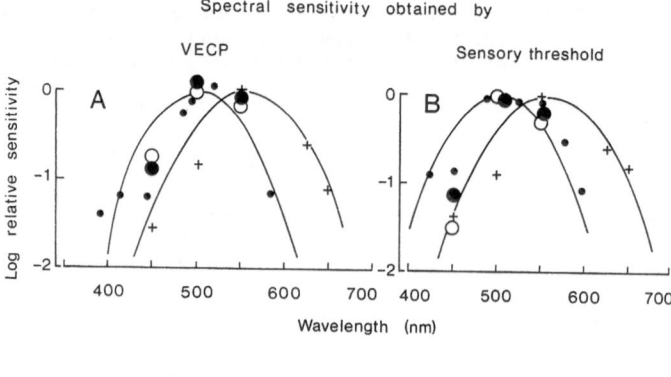

Fig. 5. Relative spectral sensitivity of the rod monochromat as obtained by the VECP (A) and by the sensory threshold (B) in the dark adapted eye (large filled circles) and during exposure to 100 troland white light (open circles). In the VECP determination, 4.5 μV was the criterion amplitude. For comparison, the data of two normal observers are included, measurements in dark adapted state of one (HUBER & ADACHI-USAMI, 1972) are marked by small dots, those in light adapted state of another, S. G., by crosses. The continuous lines are the CIE scotopic and photopic spectral luminosity curves.

182

monochromat, he needed 400 times more light for a minimum VECP than a normal subject adapted to 100 troland.

In order to determine the spectral sensitivity function of the rod monochromat under scotopic and photopic conditions, the amplitudes of the first negative (N_1) to the first positive (P_1) deflection of the VECP were plotted as a function of the test light power in logarithmic units for the wavelengths 451, 500 and 550 nm, (Fig. 4).

In the same figure, the results for the sensory thresholds are indicated by arrows on the abscissa. From the VECP curves the test light power necessary for a criterion amplitude of 4.5 μV was read and, Fig. 5, its reciprocal was plotted against stimulus wavelength. Both in the VECP curve and in the sensory curve, the peak of the spectral sensitivity function of the rod monochromat is at about 500 nm. This is true in the dark adapted as well as in the light adapted state. Fair agreement with the CIE scotopic spectral luminosity curve is existent in particular with the VECP data. Thus, no Purkinje shift can be observed in the rod monochromat during light adaptation, where the measurement is based on photopic VECPs of short latent period, a feature which normally makes the spectral luminosity curve shift to a peak of 560 nm. Nevertheless, the significant increase of the test light that was necessary to reach the VECP threshold as well as the sensory threshold indicates that the rod monochromat's photopic mechanism is greatly deteriorated. Similar results in another rod monochromat have been obtained by means of the electroretinogram (DODT et al., 1967) and the pupillary light reflex (ALEXANDRIDIS & DODT, 1967).

B. *Cone monochromat.*

A. L., male, 25 years old. The visual acuity was 0.8 in both eyes. The subject was unable to discriminate any colours since childhood. No photophobia or nystagmus could be noticed. Colour discrimination was tested with various methods. The Nagel anomaloscope indicated him as a protanope, as is shown in Figure 2 (triangles). He can be classified as a protan type cone monochromat (JAEGER, 1972). In a short test on a visual colorimeter, he turned out to accept colour matches, in particular with respect to brightness, of a protanomalous for wavelengths greater than 500 nm, but *not* of a normal trichromat of the same wavelength range.

The spectral sensitivity of the cone monochromat between 421 nm and 650 nm was determined by means of the positive amplitude of the VECP and the sensory threshold during a *white* background of 1000 troland. The final results are shown in Fig. 6. While the shape of his VECP in its temporal course was about the same as in normal observers, his positive amplitude in the VECP was distinctly smaller than in the normal observer, as can be seen in the upper part of this figure. Therefore, a criterion amplitude of 3.0 μV instead of 4.5 μV was chosen for the measurement of the relative spectral VECP sensitivities. As shown in this figure, his relative spectral sensitivity was higher in the blue and much smaller at longer wavelengths as compared to the CIE photopic luminosity curve. This can be seen both for the VECP and for the sensory data. This phenomenon seems to be in accord with the results on the visual colorimeter. Moreover, the spectral sensitivity functions of the cone monochromat investigated here are compatible with the data of another cone monochromat reported by WEALE (1953) and indicated by broken lines in the lower parts of Fig. 6.

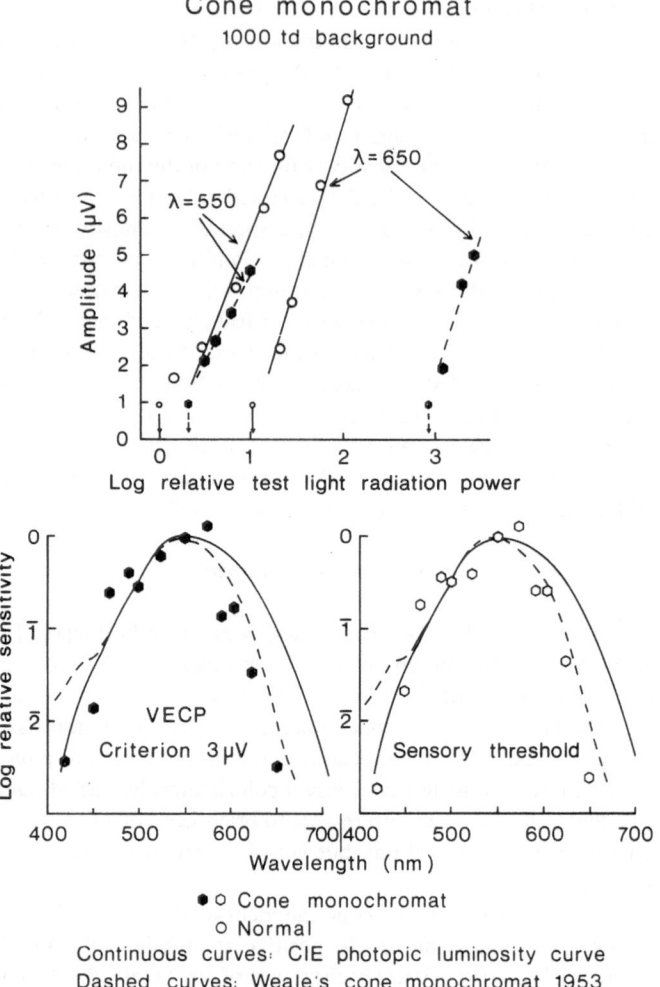

Fig. 6. Data derived from the VECPs of a normal observer (circles), and a cone monochromat, A. L. (hexagons). The upper part shows the amplitude N_1-P_1 in μV as a function of the radiant power of test flashes, $\lambda = 550$ nm and 650 nm, the abscissa being scaled in logarithmic units. The sensory thresholds are denoted by arrows pointing to the abscissa. Left in the lower part is shown the spectral sensitivity of the cone monochromat, A. L., obtained through the VECP (3.0 μV as a criterion), right through the sensory threshold. The continuous line indicates the CIE photopic spectral luminosity curve, the broken line indicates the curve for a cone monochromat, A. B. (WEALE, 1953).

In measuring the VECP, the effect of stray light can be neglected, because there is no contact lens and the light energy for a threshold response is close to the sensory threshold. Sensitivity measurements based on the photopic VECP are in good agreement with psychophysical data except for a somewhat higher sensitivity in the region of longer wavelengths (RIGGS & WOOTEN, 1972). Correspondence is found also for the scotopic VECP data with the psychophysical ones all over the spectrum (HUBER & ADACHI-USAMI, 1972).

While *electroretinographic* determinations of the spectral sensitivity function in man under photopic conditions can be made only with the help of special auxiliary actions not to be discussed here, similar procedures are not necessary for obtaining photopic sensitivity data based on the VECP. Moderate light adaptation prior to measurement is ever sufficient. Only ARMINGTON (1966) reported that the photopic VECP sensitivity between 425 to 475 nm is about 0.5 log units higher than the sensory one, while CAVONIUS (1965), SIEGFRIED (1970), DE VOE et al., (1968) and HUBER & ADACHI-USAMI (1972) found a good correspondence between the two sets of data.

As the spectral sensitivity function obtained by the VECP under both scotopic and photopic conditions shows a better relation with the psychophysical data than the ERG, the study of colour defective subjects by means of the VECP may be considered as useful.

In our experience, the curve describing the VECP amplitude versus the logarithm of the test light power does exhibit linearity only within a radiant power range between 0.15 and 1.5 logarithmic units above the sensory threshold. Within this range of radiant power we missed the doubled positive waveform reported by SHIPLEY et al. (1968).

We consider the VECP method a feasible objective diagnostic tool in cases of colour blindness. However, cooperation of the subject is required throughout a relatively long period of testing, about 20 minutes for *one* stimulus wavelength. Further developments may hopefully shorten the procedure.

REFERENCES

ALEXANDRIDIS, E. & DODT, E. Pupillenlichtreflexe und Pupillenweite einer Stäbchenmonochromatin. *Albrecht v. Graefes Arch. klin. exp. Ophthal.* 173: *153-161* (1967).

ARMINGTON, J. C. Spectral sensitivity of simultaneous electroretinogram and occipital response. In: Clinical Electroretinography, 3rd ISCERG Symp. 1964, ed. by H. M. BURIAN & J. H. JACOBSON, Pergamon Press, London 1966 (Supplement to *Vision Research* 6, 1966).

CAVONIUS, C. R. Evoked response of the human visual cortex, spectral sensitivity. *Psych. Sci.* 2: *185-186* (1965).

Deutsche Normen, Din 5031: Strahlungsphysik im optischen Bereich und Lichttechnik, Größen, Bezeichnungen, Einheiten. Blatt 6: Pupillen-Lichtstärke als Maß für die Netzhautbeleuchtung. Beuth-Vertrieb, Berlin (1967).

DE VOE, R. G., RIPPS, H. & VAUGHAN, H. G. Cortical responses to stimulation of the fovea. *Vision Res.* 8: *135-147* (1968).

DODT, E., VAN LITH, G. H. M. & SCHMIDT, B. Electroretinographic evaluation of the photopic malfunction in a totally colour blind. *Vision Res.* 7: *231-241* (1967).

HUBER, C. & ADACHI-USAMI, E. Scotopic visibility curve in man obtained by the VER. In: The visual system: Neurophysiology, Biophysics and their Clinical Applications. Proc. 9th ISCERG Symp., 1971, edited by G. B. ARDEN, New York, London 1972. (*Ady. Exp. Med. and Biol.* 24: *189-198*).

JAEGER, W. Genetics of congenital colour deficiencies. In: Handbook of sensory physiology, VII/4, Visual Psychophysics, edited by D. JAMESON & L. M. HURVICH, Springer-Verlag, Berlin, Heidelberg, New York (1972).

RIGGS, L. A. & WOOTEN, B. R. Electrical measures and psychophysical data on human vision. In: Handbook of Sensory Physiology Vol. VII/4, edited by D. JAMESON & L. M. HURVICH, Springer-Verlag, Berlin, Heidelberg, New York (1972).

SCHEIBNER, H. Allgemeine Diskussion. Zur Spezifikation von Lichtreiz-Größen. In: Die normale und die gestörte Pupillenbewegung, Normal and Disturbed Pupillary Movements. Herausgeg. von E. DODT & K. E. SCHRADER, p. 286-287, Verlag J. F. Bergmann, München (1973).

SHIPLEY, T., WAYNE, J. & FRY, A. Spectral analysis of the visually evoked occipitogram in man. *Vision Res.* 8: *409-431* (1968).

SIEGFRIED, J. B. The relationship between stimulus wavelength and the waveform of averaged visual evoked cortical potentials. *Amer. J. Optom.* 47: *282-286* (1970).

WEALE, R. A. Cone-monochromatism. *J. Physiol. (Lond.)* 121: *548-569* (1953).

Authors' address:

Dr. H. Scheibner
Max-Planck-Institut für physiologische und klinische Forschung, W. G. Kerckhoff-Institut.
D-6350 Bad Nauheim
West-Germany

ACHROMATOPSIA WITH MYOPIA IN A GENETIC ISOLATE*

RONALD E. CARR & IRWIN M. SIEGEL

(New York)

ABSTRACT

A high percentage of a genetically isolated population from the island of Pingelap was found to have symptoms of poor visual acuity, loss of color vision, nystagmus, and photophobia. History indicated a high degree of ancestral consanguinity, and study of family groups showed the disorder to be transmitted as an autosomal recessive trait. Ocular examination, including subjective psychophysical testing as well as electroretinography, was performed on affected patients and known carriers and revealed the disease to be congenital achromatopsia. This condition, relatively rare in the general population, was present in 6% of these islanders. In addition, about 80% of the affected individuals had associated myopia, the majority in the pathologic range.

Patients with congenital achromatopsia (total color blindness, rod monochromatism) typically complain of poor visual acuity and aversion to bright lights, since these symptoms are produced by widespread loss of functioning retinal cones. (HARRISON et al., 1960). The incidence of this unusual vision disturbance is much lower than the commonly occurring forms of sex-linked color deficiencies, and affects males and females in equal numbers. The high rate of ancestral consanguinity (31% in Europe and 75% in Japan) in pedigrees with affected members indicates that the mode of inheritance is autosomal recessive. (FRANçOIS, 1961). HOLM & LODBERG (1940), in their study of seven generations, including about 300 people, all from a small island off the coast of Denmark, found 20 persons with achromatopsia.

In 1970 and again in 1972 we studied a group of South Pacific Islanders, the Pingelapese, a large number of whom were reported to have poor acuity and loss of color vision. The initial study was designed to determine the nature of the condition, which was found to be achromatopsia, while the more recent study concentrated on the observed high incidence of achromatopsia combined with high myopia.

* This study was supported in part by Research to Prevent Blindness Inc., grant EY 00213 from the Public Health Service, National Eye Institute, National Institutes of Health, and the National Science Foundation under grants NSF GA 34948 and NSF GD 34462 to the Scripps Institution of Oceanography for operation of the Alpha Helix Research Program.

Pingelap atoll is located in the Eastern Caroline Islands, part of the huge archipelago known as Micronesia. This three-million square mile area of the Pacific Ocean includes the Caroline, Marshall, and Mariana islands groups, and since the end of World War II is known collectively as the Pacific Trust Territory of the United States, Over a period of 250 years, many nations, including Spain, England, Germany, Japan, and America have instituted cultural and social changes on these islands, but it was a natural catastrophe two centuries ago which brought about the high incidence of achromatopsia in the Pingelapese. In the late 18th century a typhoon of great intensity struck the tiny atoll. Deaths from injuries, disease, and starvation reduced the population markedly, but the survivors lost little time in rebuilding and repopulating their community, and by the early 1900s they numbered several hundred. At this time, the (German) administrators of the district, to alleviate overcrowding on Pingelap, assigned more than 100 natives to the large island of Ponape. Subsequently, many other Pingelapese followed these early migrants, and it is now estimated that there are about 900 on Ponape and 600 remaining on Pingelap. Although Ponape contains several enclaves of immigrant populations from neighboring atolls each engages in endogamous marriage practices, so that even in contemporary times the Pingelapese maintain in their population a high frequency of the gene for achromatopsia. Our original survey (CARR et al., 1971) showed that the incidence of affected persons in the Pingelap Island population was 6%. Using the Hardy-Weinberg formula, (STERN 1960) the calculated incidence of the carrier state in this group is 37%. In a general population, on the other hand, one out of 30,000 persons was reported to be affected with achromatopsia, (GÖTHLIN, 1924) and only about 1% are carriers for the disorder.

MATERIALS AND METHODS

A total of 65 patients with achromatopsia, 174 unaffected family members, and a control series of 156 unselected patients were examined on both the island of Ponape, in two separate Pingelapese settlements, and on the island of Pingelap itself. This latter, remote area was reached through the services of the R/V Alpha Helix, a laboratory vessel of the Scripps Institute of Oceanography and the National Science Foundation.

Routine testing

With the help of Peace Corps volunteers who were fluent in Pingelapese and local dialects, we were able to obtain histories and perform subjective testing. Every patient was tested on the standard Snellen eye chart or illiterate E test at a distance of 20 feet. For children and those adults with severely reduced vision, the flash-card vision test of the New York Association for the Blind was used at a distance of five feet. During the initial study refractions were performed only on patients with a visual acuity of less than 20/30, but in the second, more intensive phase of the study, retinoscopy was done on all individuals seen. Direct and indirect ophthalmoscopy was routinely done on all patients after dilatation, and photographs were taken with a portable (Model PRV Olympus Corp) fundus camera.

Color vision

The Ishihara and the Hardy-Rand Rittler pseudoisochromatic tests were administered under standard illumination by placing a Macbeth Illuminant 'C' filter in front of a 100 watt frosted tungsten bulb. Patients with color defects were further tested with the Farnsworth D-15 panel, and Sloan achromatopsia strips.

Special testing

Determination of final dark adapted thresholds and electroretinography (ERG) were performed on patients with unusual visual problems, those suspected of being achromatic, and those known to be achromatopsia carriers. The ERG was recorded using a slightly modified Cambridge Model VS III portable electrocardiograph machine. A small solid state amplifier allowed the 'sync-out' pulse from the Grass PS-2 photostimulator to activate the marker pen whenever the flash tube was pulsed, thus obtaining a stimulus mark on the record. In addition, the response to very low frequencies was reduced to eliminate pen drift by inserting an appropriate R-C network into the accessory jack receptacle. Electrical shielding of the patient was not necessary because the amplification system receives the ERG signal plus background, and returns the inverted common mode signal to the subject through the ground lead. This inverted 'driven ground' signal, while allowing amplification of the differential signal, tends to eliminate in-phase activity such as AC hum. After mydriasis and anesthetization of the cornea, a Burian-Allen type contact lens electrode containing a drop of Isopto Alkaline, was placed on the patient's eye. Metal disk reference and ground electrodes were fixed to the forehead and wrist with saline paste. For optimum recording, it was important to thoroughly cleanse and slightly abrade the skin area to which electrodes were attached with alcohol-soaked gauze sponges.

Final dark-adapted thresholds were obtained with a small box containing a light source powered by the ophthalmoscope transformer, a camera shutter set at 1/25 second, removable neutral density filters, and a pair of polaroid plates which could be varied to obtain small changes in stimulus intensity. A small red fixation light ensured that the stimulus, which subtended an angle of about 4.5°, fell 15° temporal to the fovea. Typically, the patient would have his right eye dilated and securely patched for at least one-half hour before the test. During this period of dark adaptation the examiner would explain the nature of the test and demonstrate what would be required. There was little difficulty obtaining reliable data once the patient understood the task.

During the initial study performed in 1970 efforts were primarily directed towards establishing a diagnosis. A total of 26 affecteds were examined at that time and found to have absent color vision, reduced visual acuity, nystagmus, and an extinguished ERG flicker response; all findings in accord with a severe, generalized dysfunction of the cone system. In those patients who did not have any significant degree of myopsia the scotopic system was found to be normal on the basis of dark adapted final thresholds and the scotopic ERG. However, the results of both these latter tests were abnormal in the majority of affecteds tested during this initial survery. It was in these individuals, with abnormalities related to both photoreceptor systems, that significant degrees of myopia were noted. The effect of myopia on retinal function has been reported previously (BLACH et al., 1966; FRANCESCHETTI et al., 1959) and thus seemingly accounts for this more generalized abnormality. These changes are, however, easily distinguished from the cone-rod form of generalized retinal degeneration. (GOODMAN et al., 1963). The association of myopia and achromatopsia in this population was made clear in the second survey in which a total of 50 affecteds were studied of whom 40 had myopia, an incidence of 80%. Refractive errors (spherical equivalents) ranged from $+2.00$ to -16.00 with a median of -5.4 diopters. Of this group of myopes, 24 had refractive errors greater than -5.00 diopters.

Most of the achromatic subjects showed macular granularity or a lack of the foveal reflex. Several showed true macular degenerative changes and those having high myopia also showed fundus pathology associated with that disorder. Several affected patients had retinal changes that were independent of the achromatopsia and/or myopia. Among these latter was one patient with peripapillary choroidal sclerosis with generalized retinal pigmentation and two with lesions typical of congenital toxoplasmosis.

Examinations were performed on 174 unaffected family members of whom 70 were known carriers (i.e. persons who had one affected parent or women who had affected children). Of these, all but 3 older individuals had corrected acuities of 20/30 or better and most read the 20/15 line with ease. In those carriers who were fully tested, all but one had normal color vision tests, dark adaptometry, and ERG studies. The single exception, a woman who was a known carrier, had severe vascular retinopathy and findings indicative of an acquired form of the cone-dysfunction syndrome.

Ophthalmoscopic examination of the unaffected population revealed a variety of retinal changes, most of which are found in the general population as a result of aging. Of particular note was the finding of angoid streaks in three of the older carriers. In two patients this was associated with reduced vision and macular degeneration. These latter changes were, however, more typical of the senile form of macular dystrophy. About a third of the carriers showed Gunn's dots (GUNN, 1883) (hyaline verrucosities of the internal limiting membrane), which gave a pinpoint refractile appearance in the peripapillary area. Due to the superficial nature of these tiny nodules and their commun occurrence in otherwise normal eyes, no significance can be attributed to them.

A second control series of 156 unaffected subjects had ocular examinations including retinoscopy and ophthalmoscopy. None of the individuals had any relationship to those patients with achromatopsia. They ranged in age from 6 to 14 and were students of the school on Pingelap. Surprisingly only one myope was found, all other individuals being either emmetropic or hyperopic. All those tested, including the corrected myope, had visual acuities of better than 20/25 with 96% having acuities of 20/15 O.U.

DISCUSSION

Pedigree analysis of the Pingelap population with regard to achromatopsia indicates that the mode of transmission is autosomal recessive. Typically, affected offspring had unaffected parents, who themselves had a parent with achromatopsia or who had affected siblings. Usually, consanguinity of some degree between parents of affected children could be proven.

One of the outstanding features of our achromatic population is the large percentage of associated high myopia. This was not noted by HOLM & LODBERG (1940), in the literature review by FRANÇOIS and associates (1961), or in the 50 patients representing complete and incomplete forms of the syndrome studied by GOODMAN and his colleagues (1963). We are therefore reluctant to assume that high myopia is an effect of the gene for achromatopsia, although this possibility cannot be excluded. There seems little doubt that high degrees of myopia itself are transmitted as an autosomal recessive (FRANÇOIS, 1961), and if these genes are present in a highly inbred population such as the Pingelapese, the incidence should be much greater than in the general population.

While it is of interest to pursue this relationship between achromatopsia and myopia in this group, any discussion of the genetic probabilities must be theoretical, however, since matings between affected individuals have not been observed in this population.

There is good evidence against the gene loci for achromatopsia and myopia being on different pairs of chromosomes since no high myopes without achromatopsia were found. A much more probable explanation would be that the two traits exist as linked pairs on one chromosome. This hypothesis, however, does not fully explain the absence of high myopia alone nor the presence of emmetropic achromats.

The absence of any significant degree of myopia in the Pingelapese is of interest in light of the recent studies of both SAFIR, who demonstrated in the Negro population of New York City an almost total absence of myopia, and HOLM (1937), who likewise showed a very low incidence of myopia in Palaeonegrids of Africa. This is in distinct opposition to the higher incidence found in both the White and Puerto Rican races (SAFIR).

The Pingelap Islanders are not an exceptional genetic isolate; many similar isolates have been reported from other remote areas and no doubt several more with different ocular problems will be discovered. The combination of swift transportation and portable diagnostic equipment afford the ophthalmologist a unique opportunity to study in detail and possibly treat great numbers of patients afflicted with some of these disorders. For example, in addition to the diagnostic and hereditary studies we were also able to dispense prescription sunglasses to all affected patients. The lenses (courtesy of the American Optical Co.) were a neutral brown (Cosmolite) and had a nominal density of 1.0. Although we could have provided tinted plastic lenses in any density we chose, only a moderately dense value which the myopic-achromats could wear comfortably indoors and still derive some comfort in the bright sun. A recent follow-up report on those patients who received the spectacles indicates that they are able to function more efficiently over a larger range of luminances than had previously been possible.

REFERENCES

BLACH, R. K., JAY, B. & KOLB, H. Electrical activity of the eye and high myopia. *Brit. J. Ophthal.* 50: *629* (1966).

CARR, R. E., MORTON, N. E. & SIEGEL, I. M. Achromatopsia in Pingelap Islanders: Study of a genetic isolate. *Am. J. Ophth.* 72: *746* (1971).

FRANCESCHETTI, A., DIETERLE, P. & SCHWARZ, A. Skotopisches Elektroretinogramm (ERG) bei Myopie mit und ohne Congenitaler Hemeralopie. Acta Fac. Med. Univ. Brun. ERG Symposium Luhacovice 4: *247* (1959).

FRANÇOIS, J. Heredity in Ophthalmology. St. Louis, Mosby (1961).

GOODMAN, G., RIPPS, H. & SIEGEL, I. M. Cone dysfunction syndromes. *Arch. Ophthal.* 70: *214* (1963).

GÖTHLIN, G. Congenital red-green abnormality in color vision and congenital total color blindness from the point of view of heredity. *Acta Ophthal.* 2: *15* (1924).

GUNN, R. M. Peculiar appearance in the retina in the vicinity of the optic disc occurring in several members of the same family. *Tr. Ophth. Soc. U.K.* 3: *110* (1883).

HARRISON, R., HOEFNAGEL, D. & HAYWARD, J. N. Congenital total color blindness, a clinicopathological report. *Arch. Ophthal.* 64: *685* (1960).

HOLM, S. Les états de la réfraction oculaire chez les palénégrides au Gabon, Afrique équatoriale française. *Acta. Ophthal. (Suppl.)* 13: *1-299* (1937).

HOLM, E. & LODBERG, C. A family with total color blindness. *Acta Ophthal.* 18: *224* (1940).

SAFIR, A. Personal communication.

STERN, C. Principles of Human Genetics, chap. 10. 2nd ed. San Francisco, Freeman (1960).

Authors' address:

Dept. of Ophthalmology
New York University School of Medicine
Medical Centre
550 First Ave.
N.Y. N.Y. 10016
USA

VISUAL PIGMENT KINETICS AND ADAPTATION
IN FUNDUS ALBIPUNCTATUS*

RONALD E. CARR, HARRIS RIPPS & IRWIN M. SIEGEL

(New York)

ABSTRACT

Most nightblinding disorders are characterized by elevated scotopic thresholds, irrespective of the time in darkness. In some instances, however, rod sensitivity returns after a prolonged period of dark adaptation. One such variant is fundus albipunctatus in which both the cone and rod branches of the dark adaptation curve are grossly abnormal but final thresholds are normal.

The results of fundus reflectometry indicated that both rhodopsin and the foveal cone pigments regenerate very slowly; the half times of recovery for the rod and cone pigments were 48 and 17 minutes, respectively. The changes in pigment levels paralleled the prolonged scotopic and photopic branches of the dark adaptation curve. Since the most distal stage of the visual system – the visual pigment cycle – is affected in this anomaly, the b-wave of the electroretinogram was attenuated throughout most of the course of dark adaptation, but reached normal amplitudes when maximal sensitivity was attained, i.e. after three hours of dark adaptation.

These findings are in striking contrast to those obtained in other forms of congenital stationary nyctalopia in which we have found normal concentrations of photopigment and normal pigment kinetics. In those patients, the abnormal electrical responses and losses in visual sensitivity appeared to stem primarily from a defect in neural function.

INTRODUCTION

Fundus albipunctatus cum hemeralopia is the descriptive name suggested by LAUBER (1910) to identify a stationary form of congenital night blindness characterized by the punctate whitish lesions that dot the fundus. Although similar ophthalmoscopically to retinitis punctata albescens (NETTLESHIP, 1908), it lacks the usual concomitants of a degenerative retinal disease; namely, visual field loss, pigmentation, and vascular constriction. In addition, later studies have shown that the loss of scotopic (rod) function is often transitory; i.e., rod adaptation may be greatly retarded and the normal threshold reached only after a prolonged stay in darkness (McDONALD & ADLER, 1940; FRANCESCHETTI & CHONE-BERCIOUX, 1951; SMITH, RIPPS & GOODMAN, 1959). It will be recalled that this peculiar feature is seen also in Oguchi's disease (OGUCHI, 1912; CARR & GOURAS, 1965; CARR & RIPPS, 1967), and at least one author (GIANNINI,

* This study was supported by grants EY 00213, EY 00285, and EY 18766 from the National Eye Institute, U.S. Public Health Service, National Institutes of Health.

1934) has attempted to draw a parallel between the two conditions.

It is now possible to test selectively (and objectively) the functional integrity of the different retinal layers, and thereby obtain information as to the sites affected by various pathological processes (CARR, RIPPS, SIEGEL & WEALE, 1966 a). In the case of Oguchi's disease, for example, we discovered (CARR & RIPPS, 1967) an upset in the orthodox relation between visual pigment regeneration and subjective adaptation (DOWLING, 1960; RUSHTON, 1961). In fact, the results of electrophysiological and fundus reflectometric examination have shown that the slow rate of dark adaptation is due not to abnormalities in the rhodopsin cycle, but to a defect in neural activity within the retina.

We have since employed similar test procedures to analyze retinal function in fundus albipunctatus. The results reported here illustrate the striking differences between this condition and other congenital, stationary night-blinding disorders.

METHODS

History and Preliminary Examination

Our two subjects were brothers, ages 42 and 44, born on the Dutch island of Saba. Although there is no history of parental consanguinity, there is the likelihood that some inbreeding had occurred in former generations. Both subjects were aware of difficulty seeing at night, but felt that this problem was minor since visual performance tended to improve if they remained in darkness for an hour or two. Their parents and two sisters were said to have normal night vision.

On routine ophthalmological examination, both subjects gave similar findings. Visual acuity was 20/20 after correction of a small refractive error, and with the exception of the fundus appearance, all other preliminary test results (e.g. color vision, central and peripheral fields, etc.) were within normal limits. Ophthalmoscopically, their fundi showed a diffuse array of whitish punctate opacities encircling the posterior pole and situated deep to the retinal vessels; there were fewer lesions in the far periphery, and the area of the macula was entirely spared (Fig. 1).

With regard to the investigative procedures described below, only the younger brother could be prevailed upon to return for periodic testing, and consequently, most of the data refer to the results obtained on one subject (L.D.).

The New York Reflectometer

The apparatus used for studying the bleaching and regeneration kinetics of human visual pigments was a modified version of the London reflectometer designed by WEALE (1959). Detailed descriptions have appeared in earlier publications (CARR, RIPPS, SIEGEL & WEALE, 1966; CARR & RIPPS, 1967); only a brief account of the principles and method is given here.

When the fundus is viewed ophthalmoscopically, the light emerging through

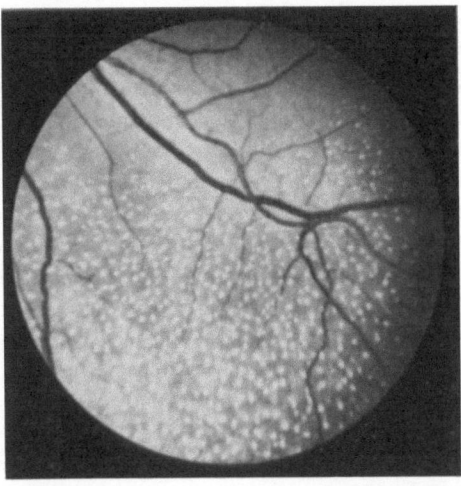

Fig. 1. Fundus photograph of the retina of subject L.D. showing the large band of discrete white spots surrounding the macula.

the pupil has twice traversed the eye. Much of the energy in the incident beam has been lost due to absorption, diffuse reflection and scatter by the semi-transparent ocular tissues and the heavily pigmented layers of the retina and choroid. However, a fraction of this loss is attributable to the visual pigments, since after these have been bleached to relatively colorless photoproducts, more light emerges than from a dark-adapted eye. This small difference in transmissivity between the dark- and light-adapted retina can be detected with a photomultiplier, and analyzed spectrally by using test lights of various wavelengths. In the present system, the test wavelengths are derived from a beam of white light that is passed sequentially through 29 interference filters mounted in spectral order (from 400-680 nm) on a rotating wheel. Consequently, the photomultiplier output is a series of deflections, each of which corresponds to a particular test wavelength; these signals are then digitized and fed to a computer for processing (RIPPS & SNAPPER, in press). The method is entirely objective, demanding neither wedge settings nor null readings on the part of the experimenter (CAMPBELL & RUSHTON, 1955; HOOD & RUSHTON, 1971).

The procedure was such as to obtain spectral scans of the test region (either foveal or peripheral), first with the eye fully dark adapted, and again after it had been exposed to an intense bleaching light for 30 seconds. From these measurements it was possible to construct a difference spectrum i.e., the difference between the density spectrum of the visual pigments and that of the products into which they are transformed by bleaching. The rate at which the bleached photopigments regenerate was obtained from reflectivity measurements taken at various times after the bleaching light was extinguished. In all instances, the test area was smaller than, but concentric with, that used for the measurement of dark adaptation.

Dark Adaptometry

The course of dark adaptation was determined monocularly on a modified Goldmann-Weekers Adaptometer; all experimental runs were made after the subject's pupil had been dilated with 2 per cent cyclopentolate hydrochloride (Cyclogyl). Peripheral thresholds were measured with a white, circular test field subtending 4 degrees at the eye and stimulating an area of the temporal retina located 16° from the fovea. Foveal thresholds were tested with a 1 degree field, centered within a circular array of dimly illuminated red spots. Test flashes were 0.7 sec in duration. Since the light-adapting exposures varied in accordance with the objectives of the experiment, they are given in the description of the results, but in all cases the dimensions of the adapting field exceeded that of the test area.

Electro-oculography

The method is essentially that of ARDEN & KELSEY (1962). With electrodes taped to the skin near the canthi of each eye, the subject fixated alternately two small neon lamps which were located in the horizontal plane and subtended a visual angle of 20 degrees; the lamps flashed sequentially every 0.8 sec. The potentials generated by these saccades were recorded on an ink-writing oscillograph during periods of light- and dark-adaptation. A measure of the light-induced change in the eye's standing potential was obtained by determining the ratio of the maximum potential elicited during exposure to a luminance of 2800 mL (the light peak), to the minimum of the dark-adapted eye (dark trough). In the normal eye this ratio exceeds 180 per cent.

Electroretinography

Electro-retinal reponses to a brief flash of light were recorded on an ink-writing polygraph. The stimulus lamp (Grass Model PS-2) delivered, at the setting for maximum intensity, a luminance of 6.8×10^7 cd/m^2. Electrical activity was recorded as the change in potential between a Burian-Allen corneal electrode and a silver disc reference electrode taped to the forehead. In addition to our usual routine of recording responses to single and intermittent flashes in the light-adapted state and after a short period of dark adaptation, electroretinograms to dim blue flashes were also obtained at various intervals during a prolonged (3 hour) course of dark adaptation.

RESULTS

Subjective Adaptometry

Figure 2 shows the results of adaptometry for L.D. (data points) as compared with the normal (dashed line); clearly, both branches of L.D.'s dark-adaptation curve are grossly abnormal. Although there is a rapid fall in threshold for

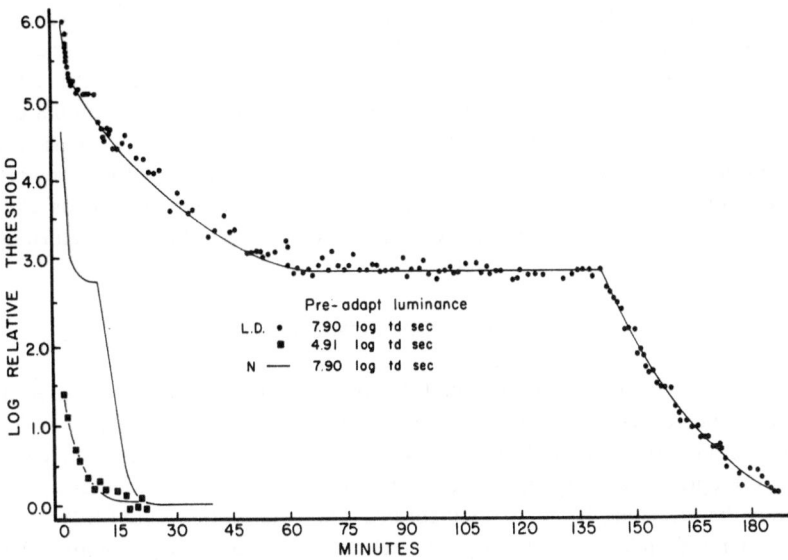

Fig. 2. Course of dark adaptation of subject L.D. following exposure to the luminances indicated. A normal curve (N) obtained after pre-adaptation to the higher luminance is shown for comparison. Free hand curves were drawn through the experimental data.

a brief period after the light-adapting field is extinguished, the rate of descent slows considerably thereafter, and the cone plateau is reached after an hour of dark adaptation. Thresholds then remain constant for an additional 80 min, at which time there is an abrupt transition to the second (rod) branch of the curve. Once again the decline in threshold is much slower than in the normal, and more than three hours in darkness are required before thresholds attain the final, dark-adapted level. But, in spite of the extremely slow rate at which the rod and cone mechanisms recover sensitivity, the final thresholds of both correspond almost exactly with those of the normal.

Another interesting feature of L.D.'s adaptation curve concerns the time at which the cone-rod transition occurs. Since rod thresholds are masked by the greater sensitivity of the cone mechanism during the first 140 min of dark adaptation, it is not possible to establish the form of the rod curve during this entire period. Nevertheless, if it is assumed that the curve describing the rod segment decays exponentially, then extrapolating back to earlier times indicates that rod threshold is indeterminate (e.g. > 20 log units above the absolute level) for almost two hours into dark adaptation. Thus, the delayed appearance of the scotopic segment of the dark adaptation curve suggests the possibility that there is a prolonged 'silent period', during which time rods are completely suppressed (DOWLING & RIPPS, 1970, 1972), or their neural pathways pre-empted by cone signals (GOURAS & LINK, 1966). Electrophysiological data, i.e., the long-lasting depression of a- and b-wave amplitudes (see below), tend to support the former alternative.

197

Adaptometry was performed also after exposure to a much weaker pre-adapting field (triangles). The retinal illuminance (4.9 log td-sec) was selected so as to match the value used previously in testing a subject with Oguchi's disease (CARR & RIPPS, 1967). Although this intensity bleaches less than 0.8 per cent of the available rhodopsin, it will be recalled that in Oguchi's disease the exposure elevated rod threshold above the cone level and caused it to remain there for more than 30 min of subsequent dark adaptation. In fundus albipunctatus, on the other hand, there is far less of an effect; thresholds returning rapidly to the dark-adapted level.

The Visual Pigments

Fig. 3 shows difference spectra for L.D. and a normal subject as measured in the peripheral retina (16° temporal to the fovea) at various times after exposing the test area to a retinal illuminance of 7.5 log td-sec. The density differences ($\triangle D$) represent changes measured from an initial recording taken immediately after the bleaching light was extinguished; they are plotted $\triangle D$ ($\times 2$) to account for double transit through the retina. It is immediately apparent that rhodopsin regeneration is extraordinarily slow in L.D. After 20 min in darkness, when regeneration is nearly complete in the normal, it has only just begun to make an appearance in L.D. In fact, the difference spectra continue to increase in magnitude for almost 2 hours, at which time all that was bleached has reformed. At its maximum, the density change is somewhat less than in the normal subject, but still within normal limits.

Fig. 4 illustrates graphically the time course of regeneration for rhodopsin (circles) as well as for the foveal cone pigments (squares). The data points were obtained from curves like those of Fig. 3, but here refer to density changes at a single wavelength relative to the maximum $\triangle D$ for that wavelength. Hence we obtain per cent regeneration as a function of time after the bleach. To minimize the influence of absorbing photoproducts, 540 nm and 590 nm were selected as measuring wavelengths for the rod- and cone-pigment data, respec-

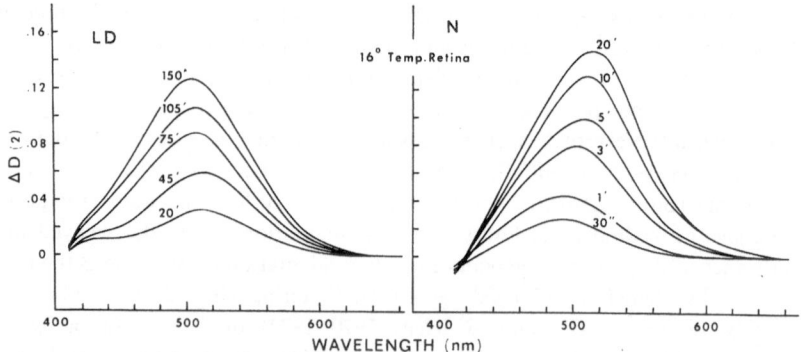

Fig. 3. Density difference spectra measured in the peripheral retina during the course of dark adaptation. Density differences refer to spectral recordings taken before and at the times indicated after exposure to a retinal illuminance of 7.5 log td sec.

198

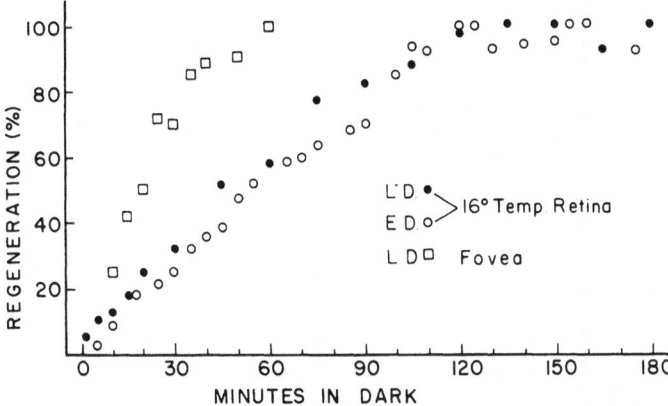

Fig. 4. The regeneration of visual pigments in fundus albi punctatus. See text for details.

tively. The time required for each function to attain the 50 per cent mark provides a reasonable estimate of the regeneration rates, and illustrates how surprisingly slow these processes are in fundus albipunctatus. For rhodopsin the half-time is about 60 min, for the cone pigments about 20 minutes; values approximately 20 times and 16 times greater than those found in normal subjects (RIPPS & WEALE, 1969; HOLLINS & ALPERN, 1973).

Another important difference between the results for L.D. and those of the normal is in the peak wavelengths (λ_{max}) of the regeneration-difference spectra (Fig. 3). Note that in the normal there is a progressive shift in λ_{max} from about 490 nm after 30 sec, to a λ_{max} of 510 nm after 20 min in darkness. Displacement of the maximum from that of the regenerating rhodopsin has been attributed to the early formation and subsequent decay of an intermediate product of bleaching, presumably metarhodopsin III (Ripps & Weale, 1969). For subject L.D. there is also a spectral shift – but in the opposite direction, i.e. from ∼510 nm at 20 min to approximately 500 nm after 150 min. Our analysis of this phenomenon is still incomplete, although there is the obvious possibility that a blue-absorbing photoproduct forms slowly and stays about long after the bleaching light is extinguished.

Electrical Responses

Having shown that the slow rate of dark adaptation occurs at the most distal and central ends of the visual pathway, it was no surprise to find that the phenomenon could be observed also at any intermediate stage. In both the ERG and EOG, the functional disturbance was manifest as an increase in the time required to evoke normal light-induced potentials. With the EOG, for example, it is standard procedure to derive a light:dark ratio by determining the maximum voltage elicited in bright ambient conditions relative to the minimum value obtained during a preceding 15 min dark adaptation (Fig. 5). For L.D., this yielded a ratio of 135 per cent; i.e., not significantly greater than would

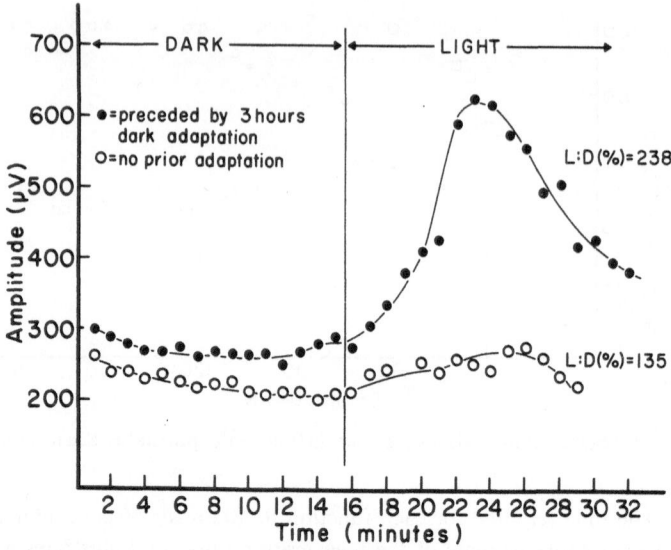

Fig. 5. Light-induced changes in the EOG of subject L.D. after a 15 min period in the dark (open circles) and following three hours of adaptation to darkness (dots). The light: dark ratio (in percent) reaches normal values, i.e. >180% only after the prolonged stay in the dark.

result from baseline oscillations. However, very different results were obtained when our subject was dark-adapted for 3 hours prior to the experimental session (filled symbols); the light peak to dark trough ratio of 238 per cent is well above the lower limit of the normal range.

The amplitude of the ERG b-wave provides another parameter by which to demonstrate the slow recovery of function after photic exposure. As shown in Fig. 6, electrical responses to a dim (S_1) blue flash are greatly depressed by light adaptation, but return to normal amplitudes after 140 min of dark adaptation. Following the same light exposure, the ERG of a normal subject requires only 20 min to recover fully its maximum amplitude. The attenuated amplitude for L.D. at the 20 minute mark cannot be increased appreciably by increasing the flash intensity. The response to a maximum intensity (S_{16}) flash of white light shows that it elicits only a small photopic ERG in L.D., whereas it effects a huge increase in the normal response.

DISCUSSION

The night-blinding disorders constitute a remarkably heterogenous group with regard to mode of inheritance, extent of visual loss, fundus appearance, and prognosis. Even the term 'nyctalopia' may be inappropriate, referring in some instances to any abnormality in the scotopic portion of the dark-adaptation curve, e.g. a moderately elevated final threshold, a retarded rate of dark adaptation, or a delayed onset for the rod segment of the curve. Moreover, many

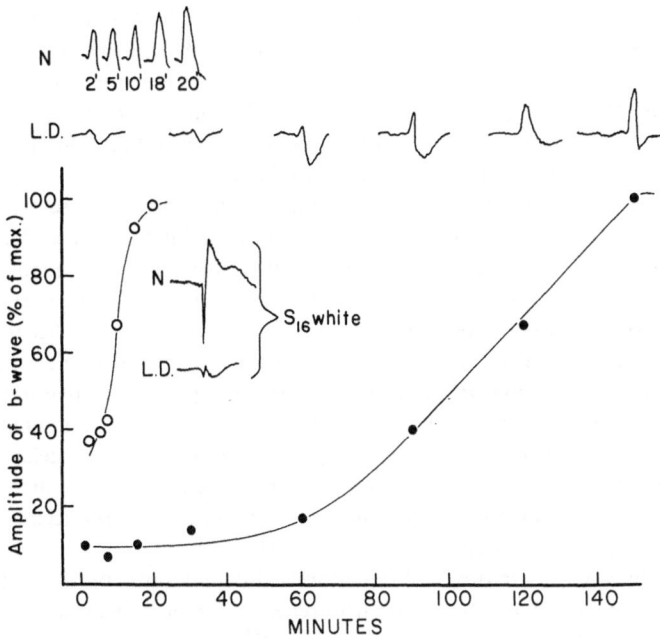

Fig. 6. Growth of b-wave amplitude to a dim blue flash following preadaptation to a luminance of 8.02 log td sec for subject L.D. (dots) and a normal (open circles). Some of the actual ERG tracings obtained at selected time intervals are shown above the graphs. Inset: after 20 min in the dark, a normal subject shows a full amplitude ERG to a bright (S_{16}) flash while L.D.'s response to the same stimulus is very reduced.

'night-blind' patients suffer also from defects in photopic function (cf. AUERBACH, GODEL & ROWE, 1969).

Fundus albipunctatus provides a case in point. The curve of Fig. 2 shows that the functional integrity of both the rod and cone systems is impaired. In both, however, the visual loss is transitory; i.e., the cone plateau as well as the final dark threshold are within normal limits – but the rates at which they are reached are grossly abnormal. Particularly noteworthy in this connection are the slow regeneration rates of the rod and cone pigments (Fig. 4), pointing clearly to a defect involving the initial stage of the visual process. It is not surprising, therefore, that the consequences of the disturbance are manifest at subsequent stages in the visual pathway. As shown in Figs. 5 and 6, the period of dark adaptation required for the EOG to exhibit a normal light-induced voltage increment, and the time for full recovery of ERG amplitude following light adaptation, are greatly prolonged as compared to the normal functions.

These results are in marked contrast to our earlier observations in subjects with congenital, stationary night blindness (CARR et al., 1966a,b). In those cases, rhodopsin kinetics were entirely normal, a finding confirmed recently by ALPERN, HOLLAND & OHBA (1972). While it was apparent from the nature of the electrophysiological responses that the defect was of retinal origin, neither the electrical nor the psychophysical data gave any indication that the adaptive mechanism was merely slow in adjusting to different ambient levels; the subjects were indeed night blind. Furthermore, the fact that the rhodopsin cycle was not affected, suggests that the functional properties of the pigment epithelium and its purported role in visual pigment regeneration (DOWLING, 1960) are not significantly affected by the pathological process.

Fundus albipunctatus differs also from Oguchi's disease in several important respects, although both conditions typically exhibit extended dark-adaptation curves. First of all, our previous results in Oguchi's disease indicate that the rod mechanism is selectively affected; the cone branch of the dark-adaptation curve proceeds at the normal rate (CARR & RIPPS, 1967). Secondly, the rate at which rhodopsin regenerates is very nearly normal, the defect presumably occurring proximal to the receptors. And lastly, the adaptive mechanism of the rods performs in an aberrant fashion even when trivial amounts of rhodopsin are bleached, i.e. relatively weak illumination suffices to delay the appearance of the rod branch of the dark adaptation curve by more than 30 min. Exposure to a similar luminance in fundus albipunctatus produced far less of an effect on the time course of adaptation (Fig. 2).

We are faced, therefore, with an entirely different situation in fundus albipunctatus, where the findings appear to reflect an upset in the intimate relation between the photoreceptors and pigment epithelium. It is well known that the latter is essential for regeneration of visual pigments (KUHNE, 1878), and serves as a site for the storage and metabolism of vitamin A (WALD, 1935-36). An abnormality in this tissue might well account for the unusually slow rate at which bleached rod- and cone-pigments regenerate. Alternatively, the receptors may be unable to efficiently transport their photoproducts or utilize the the vitamin A stores of normally-functioning epithelial cells. The key to the locus of the defect may lie in the punctate lesions that dot the fundus, but we are uncertain as to their composition or their level within the retina. However, they do not appear to be depigmented foci in the pigment epithelium, since choroidal fluorescence is not seen at these sites during angiography.

In the normal retina, the rate-limiting step in the dark-adaptation process seems to be the regeneration of bleached visual pigments; both DOWLING (1960) and RUSHTON (1961, 1965) have reported a log-linear relation between visual sensitivity and photopigment concentration. On this view, the biphasic curve of subjective adaptation is governed by the recovery rates of the cone and rod photopigments. We are not in a position to judge whether this relationship applies in our subjects. Although the curves of dark adaptation and pigment regeneration are superficially similar (Figs, 2 and 4), a cursory glance at the scotopic functions shows that subjective thresholds remain elevated long after rhodopsin has completely regenerated. It should be noted, however, that the two sets of data were obtained following very different light-adapting conditions (particularly in regard to exposure duration); previous light history is known to influence the temporal course of adaptation in normal observers (THOMSON, 1949; HECHT et al. 1948).

It is necessary also to consider the possibility that the prolonged period over

202

which rod and cone thresholds remain elevated is due to the presence of products of bleaching, which may decay slowly in fundus albipunctatus. According to ERNST & KEMP (1972), photoproducts in the rat retina exert a profound effect on the responses of its photoreceptors. Because our subjects were available for only a limited period, we were unable to examine in greater detail the influence of photochemical changes on the visual responses. Nevertheless, it is clear that conditions such as fundus albipunctatus provide unique opportunities for studying the relation between photochemical events, electrical responses and visual sensitivity.

REFERENCES

ALPERN, M., HOLLAND, M. G. & OHBA, N. Rhodopsin bleaching signals in essential nightblindness. *J. Physiol.* 225: *457-476* (1972).

ARDEN, G. B. & KELSEY, J. H. Changes produced by light in the standing potential of the human eye. *J. Physiol.* 161: *189-204* (1962).

AUERBACH, E., GODEL, V. & ROWE, H. An electrophysiological and psychophysical study of two forms of congenital night blindness. *Invest. Ophthal.* 8: *332-345* (1969).

CAMPBELL, F. W. & RUSHTON, W. A. H. Measurement of the scotopic pigment in the living human eye. *J. Physiol.* 130: *131-147* (1955).

CARR, R. E. & GOURAS, P. Oguchi's disease. *Arch. Ophthal.* 73: *646-656* (1965).

CARR, R. E. & RIPPS, H. Rhodopsin kinetics and rod adaptation in Oguchi's disease. *Invest. Ophthal.* 6: *426-436* (1967).

CARR, R. E., RIPPS, H., SIEGEL, I. M. & WEALE, R. A. Rhodopsin and the electrical activity of the retina in congenital night blindness. *Invest. Ophthal.* 5: *497-508* (1966a).

CARR, R. E., RIPPS, H., SIEGEL, I. M. & WEALE, R. A. Visual functions in congenital night blindness. *Invest. Ophthal.* 5: *508-514* (1966b).

DOWLING, J. E. The chemistry of visual adaptation in the rat. *Nature (Lond.)*, 188: *114-116* (1960).

DOWLING. J. E. & RIPPS, H. Visual adaptation in the retina of the skate. *J. Gen. Physiol.* 56: *491-520* (1970).

DOWLING, J. E. & RIPPS, H. Adaptation in skate photoreceptors. *J. Gen. Physiol.* 60: *698-719* (1972).

ERNST, W. & KEMP, C. M. The effects of rhodopsin decomposition on P_{III} responses isolated rat retinae. *Vision Res.* 12: *1937-1946* (1972).

FRANCESCHETTI, A. & CHOME-BERCIOUX, N. Fundus albipunctatus cum hemeralopia. *Ophthalmologica* 121: *185-193* (1951).

GIANNINI, D. Ccntributo clinico allo studio del 'fundo albino puntato' e considerazioni sui rapporti colla 'malattia di Oguchi'. *Ann. Ottal.* 62: *752-762* (1934).

GOURAS, P. & LINK, K. Rod and cone interaction in dark-adapted monkey ganglion cells. *J. Physiol.* 184: *499-510* (1966).

HECHT, S., HENDLEY, C. D., ROSS, S. & RICHMOND, P. N. The effect of exposure to sunlight on night vision. *Amer. J. Ophthal.* 31: *1573-1580* (1948).

HOLLINS, M. & ALPERN, M. Dark adaptation and visual pigment regeneration in human cones. *J. Gen. Physiol.* 62: *430-447* (1973).

HOOD, C. & RUSHTON W. A. H. The Florida retinal densitometer. *J. Physiol.* 217: *213-229* (1971).

KÜHNE, W. Zur Photochemie der Netzhaut. *Untersuchungen. physiol. Inst. Univ. Heidelberg.* 1: *1-14* (1878).

LAUBER, H. Die sogenannte Retinitis punctata albescens. *Klin. Mbl. Augenh.* 48: *113-148* (1910).

MCDONALD, R. & ADLER, F. H. Clinical evaluation of tests of dark adaptation. *Arch. Ophthal.* 24: *447-461* (1940).

NETTLESHIP, E. Retinitis punctata albescens. *Roy. London Ophthal. Hosp. Rep.* 17: *377-393* (1908).

OGUCHI, C. Über die eigenartige Hemeralopie mit diffuser weissgraulicher Verfarbung des Augen hintergrundes. *v. Graefe Arch. F. Ophth.* 81: *109-117* (1912).

RIPPS, H. & SNAPPER, A. G. Computer analysis of photochemical changes in the human retina. Computers in Biol. and Med. in press. (1974).

RIPPS, H. & WEALE, R. A. Rhodopsin regeneration in man. *Nature (Lond.)* 222: *775-777* (1969).

RUSHTON, W. A. H. Rhodopsin measurement and dark adaptation in a subject deficient in cone vision. *J. Physiol.* 156: *193-205* (1961).

RUSHTON, W. A. H. Visual adaptation. *Proc. Roy. Soc.* B162: *20-46* (1965).

SMITH, B. F., RIPPS, H. & GOODMAN, G. Retinitis punctata albescens. *Arch. Ophthal.* 61: *93-101* (1959).

THOMSON, L. C. The influence of variations in the light history of the eye upon the course of its dark adaptation. *J. Physiol. (Lond.)* 109: *430-438* (1949).

WALD, G. Carotenoids and the visual cycle. *J. Gen. Physiol.* 19: *351-371* (1935-36).

WEALE, R. A. Photo-sensititive reactions in foveae of normal and cone monochromatic observers. *Optica Acta* 6: *158-173* (1959).

Authors' address:

Dept. of Ophthalmology
New York University School of Medicine
Medical Centre
550 First Ave.
N.Y. N.Y. 10016
USA

EFFECTS OF DURATION AND INTENSITY OF ILLUMINATION ON THE LIGHT-INDUCED CHANGE IN THE AMPLITUDE OF THE HUMAN ELECTRO-OCULOGRAM*

VALTER ELENIUS & EERO AANTAA

(Turku, Finland)

The slow light-induced change in the amplitude of the human electro-oculo-gram (EOG) (KRIS, 1958; KOLDER, 1959; ARDEN & KELSEY, 1962) has been measured in the present study by using stimulation lights varying both in duration and intensity.

The averaged results have been used to study the relationship between the peak time and the amplitude of the first maximum as well as between the amplitude of the first maximum and first minimum of the potential.

METHODS

The EOG was recorded bilaterally with the use of chlorided silver electrodes (6 mm in diameter) placed on the skin near the temporal canthi of the lids of both eyes. The skin was cleaned with ether, electrode jelly was applied, and the electrodes were fastened with adhesive tape. An earthed electrode was placed on the skin of the forehead. For all recordings, a condenser coupled differential amplifier with a one-second time constant was used. The subject to be examined was in a sitting position. Two small fixation lights were used to control the magnitude (30°) of the rapid horizontal eye movements made on command. A check was made to ensure that the subject could not make compensatory head movements. A projector was used to illuminate a square area of 80 × 80 cm on a white screen placed 120 cm in front of the subject's eyes. The pupils were not dilated. The maximal intensity of light (2800 K°) used for stimulation was 10000 photopic troland.

The series of normal subjects comprised of 89 individuals of both sexes aged 19 to 40 years. In no case there was a history of previous eye disease. A check was made to ensure that in all subjects the visual acuity was at least 0.9 without correction with glasses. Cases of squint or apparent heterophoria were excluded.

Before examination the subjects waited for half an hour in a moderately illuminated room. Each subject was tested only with one test light. Before illumination there was a period of dark adaptation of 15 min duration. The measurements of the amplitude were made directly from the afterglow on the oscilloscope screen, each measurement being the average of the response to a

* This work has been supported by a grant from the Finnish-Norwegian Medical Research Foundation.

series of ten rapid horizontal eye movements. The final averaged results are based on measurements made on at least ten subjects. The results obtained with test lights of 9 min duration (10000 and 1000 troland intensity) and with the test light of 1 min duration (10000 troland intensity) are based on measurements made on 16, 19 and 14 subjects respectively.

RESULTS

Average results are illustrated in Fig. 1. Evidently, a large increase in the amplitude of the EOG can be evoked only with light of relatively long (at least 7 min) duration. With shorter duration of illumination (3 min or less) there is much less increase in the amplitude and its decline starts earlier. It is also evident that light of 10000 troland intensity (circles) as compared with light of 1000 troland intensity (dots) of the same 9 min duration caused a much larger increase in the amplitude.

The maximum and minimum of the curves of Fig. 1 are in Fig. 2 presented in per cent of the average amplitude previously measured after 15 min of dark adaptation and plotted against time after beginning of illumination. It appears (Fig. 2, A) that the average maximum of the positive light-induced response evoked with light of 9 min and 1 min duration (constant 10000 troland intensity) is 69% (SD 43) and 34% (SD 20) respectively, the average peak times being 8 min (SD 0.8) and 6 min (SD 0.85). In comparison the average maximum of the positive response evoked with light of 1000 troland intensity and of 9 min duration is 36% (SD 32) the peak time being 7 min (SD 0.67).

Variation in the intensity of illumination (duration constant) does not seem to be related to a measurable alteration in the magnitude of the average negative response (Fig. 2, B; circle and dot) while after an equally large average positive response caused by short (1 min) illumination of 10000 troland intensity and long (9 min) illumination of 1000 troland intensity the average negative response is much smaller after illumination of short duration.

COMMENT

KOLDER (1959) and ARDEN & KELSEY (1962) have shown that re-illumination of the previously dark adapted human eye causes a large rise of the EOG potential the magnitude of which varies with the logarithm of the intensity of illumination and with the duration of dark adaptation. They also showed that during the succeeding falling phase of the potential the amplitude is independent of the intensity of illumination, a fact which is in agreement with the results of the present study. The idea of the positive and negative components of the light-induced alteration in the standing potential being two separate processes is further supported by the fact that in the monkey eye the positive component of the slow light-induced DC response is abolished by interruption of central retinal artery circulation leaving a negative DC component which is maintained during illumination (GOURAS & CARR, 1965). An interesting result of the present study is that the relationship between the relative magnitude of the

206

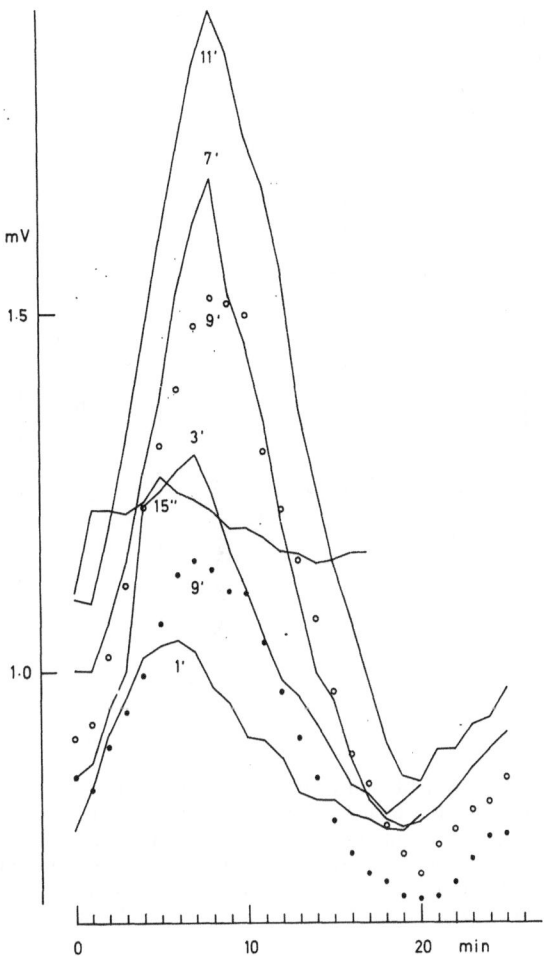

Fig. 1. Curves illustrating light-induced alteration in the amplitude of the EOG. First measurement after 15 minutes of previous dark adaptation. Intensity of illumination 10,000 photopic troland (solid lines and circles) and 1000 troland (dots). Duration of illumination marked near the maximum of each curve. The curves marked with circles and dots (9 min illumination) and the curve obtained with illumination of 1 min duration show averages of 16, 19 and 14 subjects respectively. All other curves show averages of 10 subjects.

positive and negative light-induced response of the indirectly recorded human standing potential depends on the duration of illumination, shorter illumination altering the balance in favor of the positive response.

In the present series there is large variation (Fig. 2, A) in the maximum amplitude of the positive light-induced response but much less variation in the peak time. With shorter duration of illumination there is a shift to earlier occurrence of the maximum, i.e. the potential declines earlier. Apparently also

207

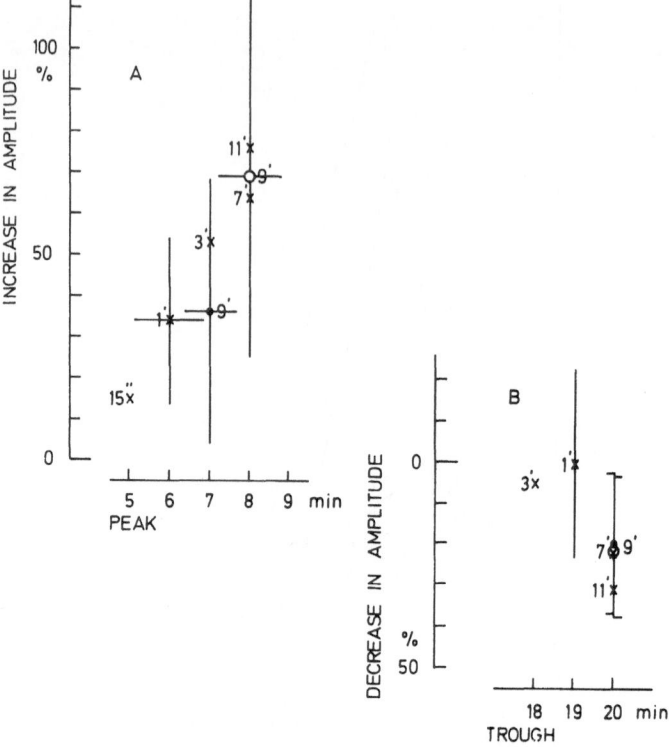

Fig. 2. Maximum of the light-induced increase (A) and of the subsequent decrease (B) in the amplitude of the EOG shown in percent of the amplitude previously measured after 15 minutes of dark adaptation and plotted against time after beginning of illumination. Crosses, circles and dots (marked with respective duration of illumination) refer to corresponding maximum and minimum amplitudes of the average curves of Fig. 1. Vertical and horizontal bars indicate twice the standard deviation.

reduced intensity of illumination may be related to earlier decline of the potential, however in the present study, only a very limited range of intensities (1 log unit) were tested.

In a small series of experiments published earlier (ELENIUS & AANTAA, 1973) it was shown that when coloured lights of the strength comparable to those used in the present study were used for stimulation, there was no difference in the peak time of responses of equal amplitude evoked with blue and red lights. Spectral sensitivity studies performed on normal and totally colour-blind human eyes showed, that these coloured lights activated both the rod and cone mechanisms.

REFERENCES

KRIS, C. Corneo-fundal potential variations during light and dark adaptation. *Nature* 182: *1027* (1958).

KOLDER, H. Spontane und experimentelle Änderungen des Bestandpotentials des menschlichen Auges. *Pflügers Archiv*. 268: *258-272* (1959).

ARDEN, G. B. & KELSEY, J. H. Some observations on the relationship between the standing potential of the human eye and the bleaching and regeneration of visual purple. *J. Physiol*. 161: *205-226* (1962).

GOURAS P. & CARR, R. E. Light-induced DC response of monkey retina before and after central retinal artery interruption. *Invest. Ophthal*. 4: *310-317* (1965).

ELENIUS, V. & AANTAA E. Light-Induced Increase in Amplitude of Electro-oculogram Evoked With Blue and Red Lights in Totally Color-Blind and Normal Humans. *Arch. Ophthal*. 90: *60-63* (1973).

Authors' address:

Dept. of Ophthalmology
and Oto-rhino-laryngology
University of Turku
Finland

THE STEADY STATE IN EOG

A. THALER & P. HEILIG

(Vienna)

ABSTRACT

The influence of steady state and preadaptation on the EOG was examined. With low light-intensity (20 asb) a steady state can be attained after about 35 minutes. This preadaptation appears to be the most reliable basis for electrooculography.

Since electro-oculography was introduced to clinical ophthalmology by FRANÇOIS and coworkers the main problem of this method is the wide range of variability (DAVIS & SHACKEL, 1960; SHACKEL & DAVIS, 1960; KELSEY, 1967; VAN LITH & BALIK, 1970; MÜLLER & HAASE, 1970; KOLDER & HOCHGESAND, 1973; HOCHGESAND & SCHICKETANZ). A couple of factors responsible for the variations, e.g., age of patient (SCHMID), interindividual differences of standing potential, cannot or can hardly be influenced. Some of the factors, e.g., position of electrodes, can be eliminated by the use of dark-light ratio (ARDEN and coworkers, 1962). Errors can be avoided by an exact method of examination, e.g., DC-amplification. It is the purpose of this study to investigate the influence of preadaptation on the course of EOG, in order to reduce its variability and to make this valuable tool for diagnosis in tapetoretinal degenerations more reliable.

METHODS

In three normal male subjects of 28 to 33 years 11 tests were carried out, lasting from 2 1/2 to 5 hours. The examinations were performed in front of an Ulbricht ball (r = 35 cm), which could be illuminated evenly by 4 low intensity bulbs as well as by 3 fluorescent tubes. Four different intensities were used: 0 asb, 20 asb, 700 asb and 2100 asb. Every minute the subject had to perform eye movements of 30 degrees for about 20 seconds. Each fixation light was illuminated for 2 seconds. At the culmination of the light peak continuous registration was carried out. On the inner and outer canthi silver-silver-chloride electrodes (Beckman 16 mm, Beckman electrode paste) were fixed with collodium. The potential was led off to an oscilloscope (Tectronix RM 565) using DC-amplification (Tectronix 3A9) and filmed from the screen (Nihon-Kohden PC-2A). All tests were carried out in the afternoon. No mydriatics were used. The examination was started after 35 minutes of preadaptation, when the potential

211

could be expected to be stable and the impedance was lower than 0,5 k-Ohm. Recordings were projected onto a screen. The amplitudes of 10 eye movements/ min were measured and averaged. For the statistical analysis two nonparametric tests were used: 1) Wilcoxon's matched-pairs-signed-value test, 2) a nonparametric test similar to the ordinary t-test (PFANZAGL, 1966).

RESULTS

1. steady state

In 11 tests a steady state was obtained 35 times. In each experiment at least two, but mostly three or four steady states could be compared. Statistical analysis showed that steady states in 2100 asb were significantly higher than those in darkness (t = 2,49, d.f. 11) and those in 20 asb (t = 3,16, d. f. 7). No difference could be proved between steady states in darkness and in 20 asb (t = 0,13, d.f. 7). The amplitudes of steady states in 700 asb were as high as in 2100 asb (fig. 1). These results are in good accordance with KRIS' findings. Tab. 1 shows mean and standard deviation of steady states in different light intensities.

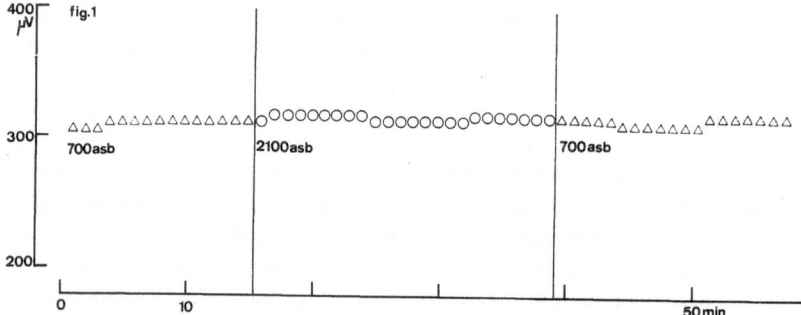

Fig. 1. No discernible alteration of steady state when illumination was increased from 700 (△) to 2100 (○) asb and decreased from 2100 (○) to 700 (△) asb.

TABLE 1

Mean values and standard deviations of steady states in different light intensities.

	0 (n = 13)	20 asb (n = 8)	2100 asb (n = 10)
M	305 μV	302 μV	339 μV
S	50	72	42

2. dark trough

The lowest point in dark trough was found to be independent of the previous steady states' light intensity (KOLDER). This fact could only be observed when light-steady states were succeeded by darkness. When the light-intensity was reduced to a lower level, there was no (2100 to 700 asb (fig. 1)) or a small (2100 to 20 asb, 20 asb to darkness (fig. 2)) decrease of the standing potential. A second trough could be observed when illumination was reduced in two steps. This observation shows that the dark trough is no all-or-nothing phenomenon. When darkness was started in the decreasing slope of light peak, the level of the dark trough was significantly lower than when darkness was started from a steady state (t = 4,4, d.f. 9) (fig. 3). This was found to be true in 9 of 10 tests, in one experiment the potential reached the same level.

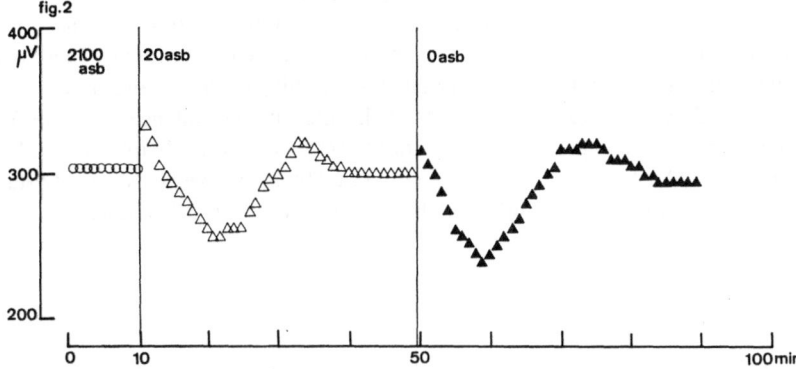

Fig. 2. Decrease of light intensity in two steps from 2100 (○) to 20 (△) to 0 (▲) asb.

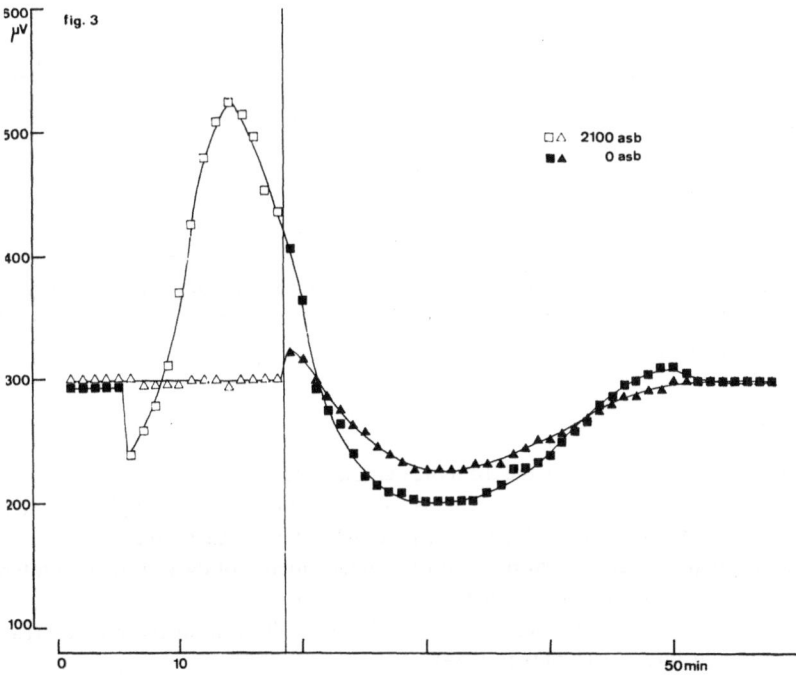

Fig. 3. Dark through (▲) following steady state in 2100 asb (△) and dark trough (■) following light peak in 2100 asb (□).

213

The dark trough stopped slow oscillations of the standing potential, but it was influenced by these oscillations (ARDEN & KELSEY).

3. light peak

The light peak was found to be dependent on light intensity (fig. 3, fig. 4) as reported by KRIS and KOLDER and others. There was no consistent difference of light peak starting from steady state in darkness or starting from a dark trough in the 13th minute after onset of darkness.

When light-intensity was increased in steps no (700 to 2100 asb (Fig. 1)) or lower (0 to 20 asb, 20 to 2100 asb (Fig. 4)) light peaks could be found. Therefore, the light peak does not appear to be an all-or-nothing phenomenon, either.

We did not evaluate statistically the light-intensity dependance of 2nd or 3rd light peak as it was performed by GLIEM (1971). But it was obvious that in low intensity (20 asb), no 3rd light peak could be obtained. The 20 asb-steady state was reached after the 2nd light peak between the 30th and 35th minute.

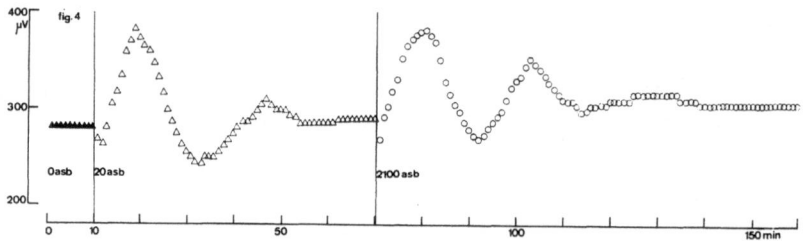

Fig. 4. Augmentation of light intensity in two steps from 0 (▲) to 20 (△) to 2100 (○) asb.

4. light trough

No statistical difference could be proved between light trough and comparable dark trough. These results are in good accordance with ARDEN & KELSEY's findings (1962).

DISCUSSION

Two statements can be made from the demonstrated results:
1. There are two different mechanisms which are generating light peak and dark trough (KOLDER, 1959). This is confirmed by at least three facts:
a. the dependence of light peak and the independence of dark trough on intensity of illumination (KRIS, KOLDER and others).
b. the different frequencies of slow oscillations following increase or decrease of light-intensity (KOLDER, 1959).
c. the resulting deeper deflection when light trough and dark trough are superimposed (fig. 3).

214

2. A steady state appears to be the most reliable basis for comparable electro-oculography. An ill-defined preadaptation can cause an irregular oscillation of standing potential which can hardly be used as a basis for comparable results, as it is shown by the example demonstrated in Fig. 5. It can be assumed that any preadaptation which is too short to reach a steady state is causing an irregular condition. (When electrodes are fixed in a dimly illuminated room – as it is usually done in most EOG laboratories – the state of adaptation can approach the postulated conditions.) When the steady state is followed by a period of darkness, the light intensity of preadaptation is of no significance because of the independence of dark trough of preceding light intensity. The possibility to reach the steady state in a shorter time is an argument for preadaptation to low light-intensity. As it could be shown, superposition of light- and dark trough results in a deeper deflection and in a higher dark-light ratio. Under these conditions the influence of the two generators of EOG cannot be studied separately. Therefore, ARDEN and coworkers' (1962) course of examination appears to be preferable, yielding a true dark trough. The later light peak was not found to be influenced by the preceding dark trough.

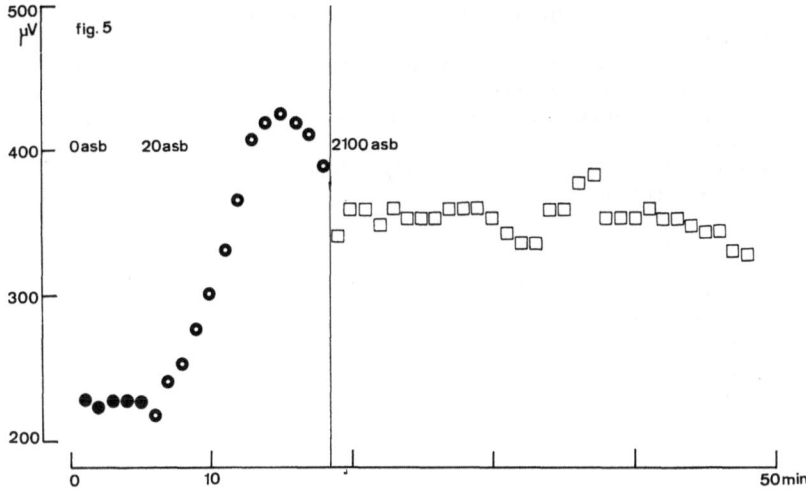

Fig. 5. Irregular oscillations of standing potential caused by high light intensity (2100 asb [□]) following a short time (13 min) of low intensity preadaptation (20 asb [○]).

ACKNOWLEDGMENT

We thank Dr. J. GORDESCH, Computer Centre of the University of Vienna (Director: Prof. Dr. L. SCHMETTERER) for his help in the statistical analysis.

215

REFERENCES

ARDEN, G. B., BARRADA, A. & KELSEY, J. H. New clinical test of retinal function based upon the standing potential of the eye. *Brit. J. Ophthal.* 46: *449-467* (1962).

ARDEN, G. B. & KELSEY, J. H. Changes produced by light in the standing potential of the human eye. *J. Physiol. Lond.* 161: *189-204* (1962).

ARDEN, G. B. & KELSEY, J. H. Some observations on the relationship between the standing potential of the human eye and the bleaching and regeneration of the visual purple. *J. Physiol. Lond.* 161: *205-226* (1962).

DAVIS, J. R. & SHACKEL, B. Changes in the electrooculogram potential level. *Brit. J. Ophthal.* 44: *606-618* (1960).

FRANÇOIS, J., VERRIEST, G. & DE ROUCK, A. L'électrooculographie en tant qu'examen fonctionnel de la rétine. *Progr. Ophthal. S. Karger* 7: *1-67* (1957).

GLIEM, H. Das Elektrookulogramm. VEB Georg Thieme, Leipzig (1971).

HOCHGESAND, P. & SCHICKETANZ, K. H. Aspekte bei der Normwertgewinnung von Parametern des EOG's. *Klin. Mbl. Augenheilk.* in Druck.

KELSEY, J. H. Variations in the normal electro-oculogram. *Brit. J. Ophthal.* 51: *44-49* (1967).

KOLDER, H. Spontane und experimentelle Änderungen des Bestandpotentials des menschlichen Auges. *Pflügers Arch. ges. Physiol.* 268: *258-272* (1959).

KOLDER, H. E. & HOCHGESAND, P. Empirical model of electrooculogram. *Doc. Ophthal.* 34: *229-241* (1973).

KRIS, CH. Corneo-fundal potential variations during light and dark adaptation. *Nature* 182 (II): *1027-1028* (1958).

LITH VAN, G. H. M. & BALIK, J. Variability of the electrooculogram. *Acta Ophthal.* 48: *1091-1096* (1970).

MÜLLER, W. & HAASE, E. Inter- und intraindividuelle Streuung im EOG. *Graefes Arch. Ophthal.* 181: *71-78* (1970).

PFANZAGL, J. Allgemeine Methodenlehre der Statistik II. W. de Gruyter, Berlin, 142, (1966).

SHACKEL, B. & DAVIS, J. R. A second survey with electrooculography. *Brit. J. Ophthal.* 44: *337-346* (1960).

Authors' address:

IInd Eye Department
School of Medicine
University of Vienna
Alserstr. 4
A–1090 Vienna
Austria

THE FOVEAL ELECTRO-OCULOGRAM*

P. HOCHGESAND & K. HACKENBERG

(Mainz)

The Electro-Oculogram (EOG) represents the indirectly measured resting potential of the retina and is considered as a mass response of the entire retina, mainly the pigment epithelium, the neuroepithelium and the choriocapillaris of the chorioid. The application of the EOG as a clinical test (FRANÇOIS et al., 1956; ARDEN et al., 1962; ARDEN & KELSEY, 1962) is restricted by different factors: the amplitude of the EOG potential is not only dependent on the corneo-retinal potential, but also on the extent of eye movements, the position of electrodes, the indirect recording and the retinal illumination. FINKELSTEIN & GOURAS (1969), KRIS (1958) and KOLDER (1959) first described the oscillations of the resting potential. The EOG shows considerable variability. In particular, there is a large interindividual variability, while day and daytime variations are of less importance. (KELSEY, 1967; VAN LITH & BALIK 1970 and 1971; MUELLER & HAASE, 1970; GLIEM, 1971; HOCHGESAND & SCHICKETANZ, 1973). Repeatedly, workers have tried to describe the puzzling oscillations by mathematical or empirical models (HOMER & KOLDER, 1966; KOLDER & HOCHGESAND, 1973).

Since the EOG demonstrates a mass response of the entire retina, local diseased areas of the retina are not detectable. The EOG gives little information in most cases of macular disorders. It is not yet known, for sure, how much the macular structures contribute to the characteristic oscillations. Since macular diseases appear frequently and since there is a basic difference in the structure of the macula as compared with the periphery of the retina, it would be of great value to have an objective functional test based on the electrical activities of the retina. The studies deal with the possibility of a 'foveal EOG' test, and whether such a test could eventually be introduced into clinical applications.

MATERIAL AND METHODS

When stimulating the macula by light, some primary methodical problems have to be considered. Foveal stimulation excites the surrounding rods and cones by stray light, and for that reason no pure foveal response results. To record a foveal EOG, the disturbing stray light must be eliminated as with the

---

* Supported by the Deutsche Forschungsgemeinschaft.

foveal ERG (ARDEN & BANKES, 1966). A preliminary test was performed as follows: a white stimulus of 2° visual angle and 9×10^5 asb was projected in the dark adapted eye on the blind spot for a duration of 0,1 second. Due to the stimulation of the sensory receptors arranged around the papilla, it was possible to record an ERG by means of corneal electrodes (type BURIAN-ALLEN). By a smooth increase of a blue-green background illumination this 'diffuse ERG' is eliminated, and consequently also the disturbing stray light. The threshold determination of the background illumination was performed with the help of an averager.

However, the background illumination had a considerable influence on the light response of the EOG. First of all, this influence had to be evaluated using various intensities and wavelengths. Examination of the spectral sensitivity of the EOG has been done by ELENIUS & LEHTONEN (1962), and ARDEN & KELSEY (1962).

The foveal EOG was recorded on healthy subjects between 18 and 32 years, with refraction between $+ 1,0$ s and $-1,0$ s. Thereafter, a standard EOG was recorded on the same persons at an interval of ten minutes as a control. Recording technique: placement of the skin electrodes (BECKMANN) at the inner and outer canthus of the eye, pupils were not dilated and the test was done under normal room light conditions. During the initial dark period of 12 minutes, eye movements were initiated at an angle of 35° by two alternating flashing fixation lights with a repetition cycle of ten seconds. This was followed by a 12 minute light period while focussing on the left light and after one second changing over to the right light. After another second a 1° visual angle stimulus was shined through a half-silvered mirror for 8 seconds; the stimulus and the right fixation light were switched off, and a new cycle started. The right fixation light was pre-switched to prevent a retinal illumination tail produced by eye movements. The light adaptation was interrupted less than two seconds during the light period. The test was performed using two stimulus intensities:
a. same intensity of illumination as used for the standard EOG (1800 asb),
b. 9×10^5 asb.

No background illumination was used. D.C.-amplification was used, and the potential was observed on an oscilloscope and recorded on paper moving at a rate of 1 cm/min. Calibration was done before and after testing.

A foveal EOG was done on 13 patients with different stages of macular degeneration. Foveal EOG's and standard EOG's were compared.

RESULTS

Stray light problem: the stray light potential – generated by a stimulus of 9×10^5 asb – amounts to 250 microvolts after averaging without any background illumination (Fig. 1). It can be reduced to 50 microvolts by slowly increasing the intensity of a blue-green background illumination. Four persons were tested first by means of a standard EOG and foveal EOG with the prescribed background illumination (Fig. 2): comparing the dark trough, the light peak, the ratio of the two and the absolute potential values, no significant difference

218

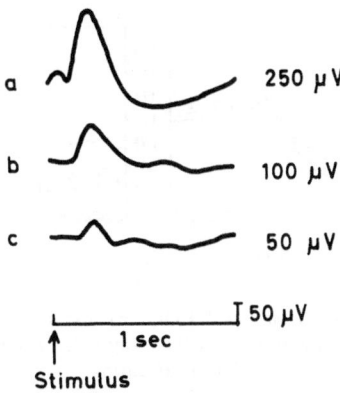

Fig. 1. ERG recorded using the blind-spot technique. Stimulus 2° visual angle; 9×10^5 asb. Blue-green background illumination a. 70% less than b. b. 1800 asb, covered with a blue-green filter. c. 15% asb more than b. Potential averaged from 16 responses.

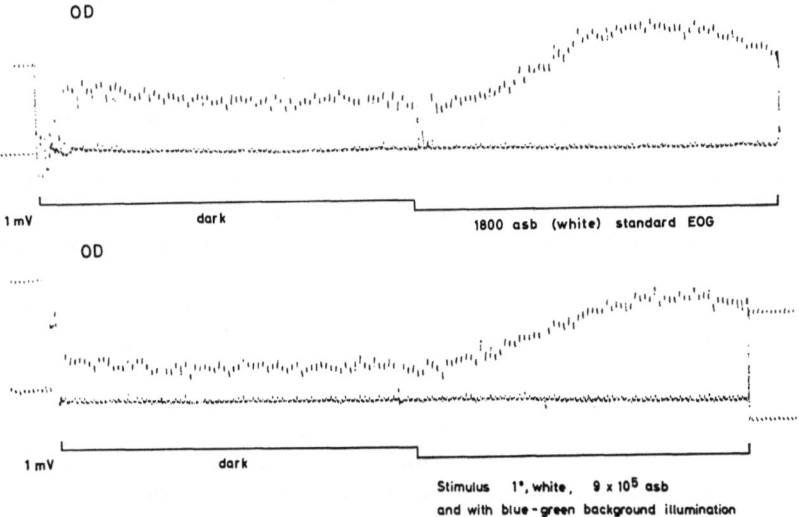

Fig. 2. Original EOG tracings from the third person. Both recordings from the right eye. No difference between standard EOG and foveal EOG with background illumination.

appears except an amplitude decrease at the beginning of the dark trough of the foveal EOG. However, this effect may be caused by the previous recording of the standard EOG. The graphical comparison of both EOG groups is shown in Fig. 3. The influence of a background illumination on the light response of the resting potential is shown in Figures 4a – d and 5a – b: when removing the blue-green filter (Cinemoid Sheet) after 12 minutes, no potential rise in white light can be observed (Fig. 4b). The two EOG's in Fig. 4c and 4d represent the dependence of light response upon retinal illumination: i.e. not only for white

219

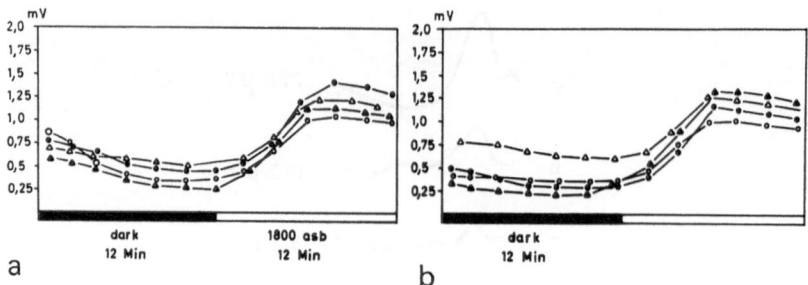

Fig. 3. Comparison between standard EOG (a) and foveal EOG with background illumination (b), eliminating almost all the stray light. Four persons: dark-trough to light-peak ratios:

	a	b
△	240	235
○	220	230
●	235	255
▲	265	295

Foveal stimulation 1°, 9×10^5 asb with background illumination.

but also for blue-green light, the light response is directly dependent on the retinal illumination. However, the light response to white light is higher at equal illumination. There is a spectral sensitivity factor in the light response of the EOG: a blue light produces a larger light response than a red one at the same illumination level (Fig. 5a and 5b). This leads to the conclusion: the peripheral retina is of more importance to the light response than the central part of the retina.

As an 85% reduced light intensity, which is necessary to avoid stray light, still causes considerable light response, a foveal EOG can only be recorded without background illumination. Therefore, a certain stray light effect must be taken into consideration.

Ten subjects had a foveal EOG's performed with macular stimulation reduced to the same level of illumination as used in the standard EOG (Table 1). Averaging 20 responses recorded during a pre-test, the blind spot ERG at 1800 asb indicated a stray light response under 10 microvolts.

The mean value of the ten ratios is 144 at a confidence limit of 130 to 158; the ratio from the standard EOG of the ten persons recorded on the same day is 232 at a confidence limit o 213 to 251.

Since, physiologically, a slow potential increase begins after ten minutes dark adaptation, a good separation of the foveal EOG at 1800 asb and the physiological oscillation is only partially possible. For that reason, a foveal EOG stimulus was selected with 2.7 log units more illumination than that used in the standard EOG. For five subjects an average ratio value of 170 was reached with a range of 152 to 188. Tests were performed without background illumination. The 2.7 log unit stronger stimulus never resulted in a ratio over 190. There is a good separation from the standard EOG ratio and a sufficiently limited stimulation of the macular area. A highly significant (a = 1%0) mean value differ-

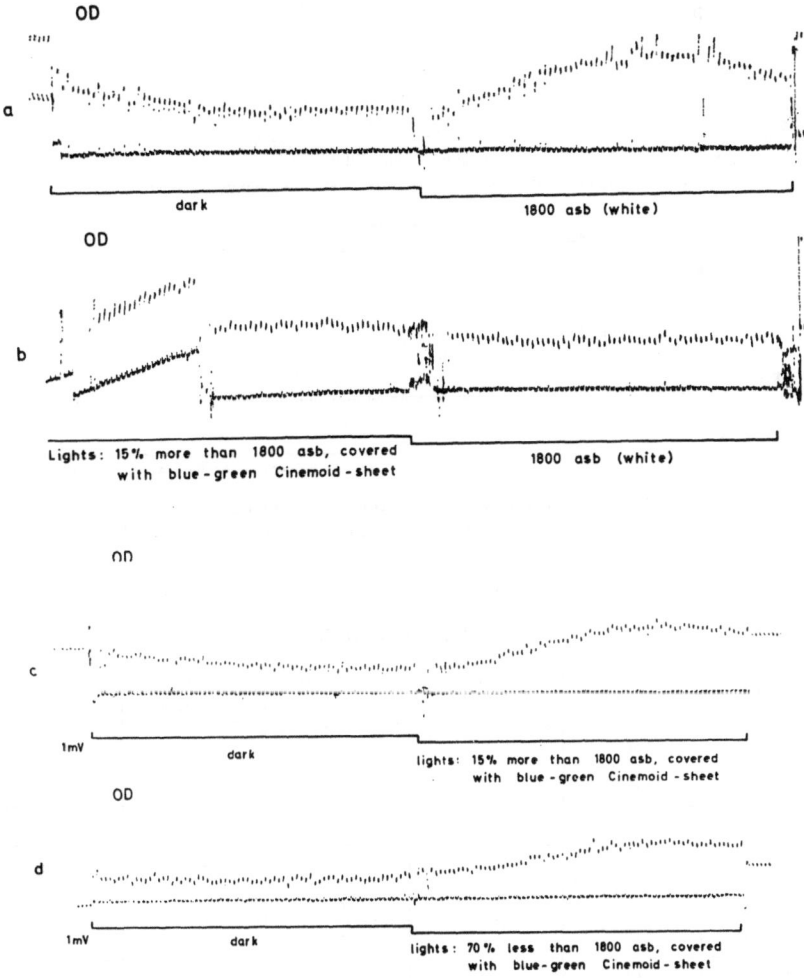

Fig. 4a–c: Dependance of the light response upon the background illumination. b: shows, that there is no further light response upon removing the blue-green filter after 12 minutes. c and d: not only for white but also for blue-green light the light response is directly dependent upon the retinal illumination.

ence can be observed in the t-test for combined trial against the ratio of the standard EOG. Additionally, the stray light effect will be only around 250 microvolts, whereas the EOG potential is within a range of one and two millivolts.

Fig. 6a–c shows the original EOG tracings from the same person:

a. standard EOG,

b. foveal EOG with a foveal stimulation of 9×10^5 asb and

c. with a foveal stimulation of 1800 asb.

As a control, to determine whether the EOG response was really macular,

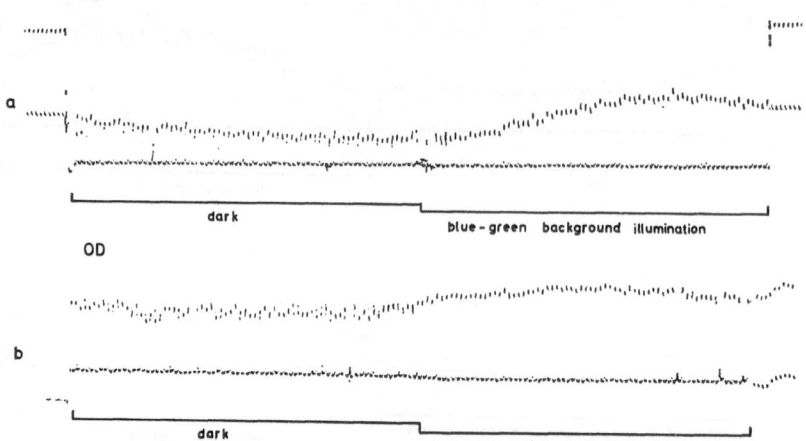

Fig. 5a and b: The light response depends on the wavelength used: blue generates a larger peak than red light. Fig. 4 and 5 from the same person.

TABLE 1: EOG ratios of the various tests on the ten subjects.

EOG - Ratios

Testperson	Stimulation 1°, 1800 asb	Stimulation 1°, 9 x 10⁵ asb	Standard - EOG (1800 asb)	Stimulation 20° parafoveal	24 Min dark, no stimulation
1	200	—	300	—	140
2	135	165	215	130	—
3	130	155	215	—	—
4	140	—	230	—	115
5	140	180	220	—	—
6	135	—	225	—	—
7	140	190	230	—	—
8	135	—	210	—	—
9	135	160	220	130	—
10	140	—	250	—	—

the stimulus was shifted 20° paramacularly (Fig. 7a–c): in paramacular simulation the light response is considerably lower for the same light intensity and subject, and the response peak is reached much later than 8 minutes as compared to the foveal EOG or even the standard EOG: i.e. the macula is involved in the light response to a lesser degree than the periphery, but to a greater degree than a comparable spot of the retina. The cones, concentrated in the macula, the central part of the choriocapillaris and the central pigment epithelium do not play a significant role in the EOG while the more light-sensitive peripheral rods do.

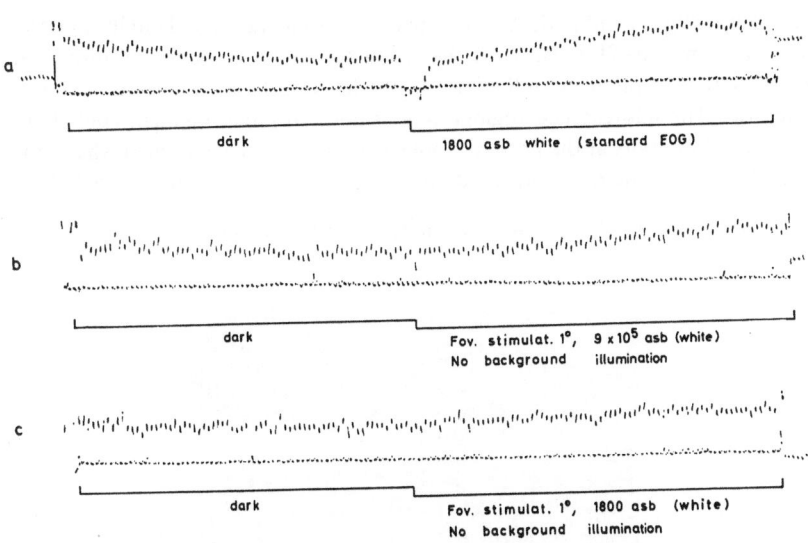

a   dark   1800 asb white (standard EOG)

b   dark   Fov. stimulat. 1°,   9 x 10⁵ asb (white)
     No background   illumination

c   dark   Fov. stimulat. 1°,   1800 asb (white)
     No background   illumination

a - c recorded from the same person. Ratios: a: 210,   b: 160,   c: 135

Fig. 6a–c: EOG's recorded from the same person: a: standard EOG, ratio 210. b: foveal EOG with 9×10^5 asb, ratio 160. c: foveal EOG with 1800 asb, ratio 135

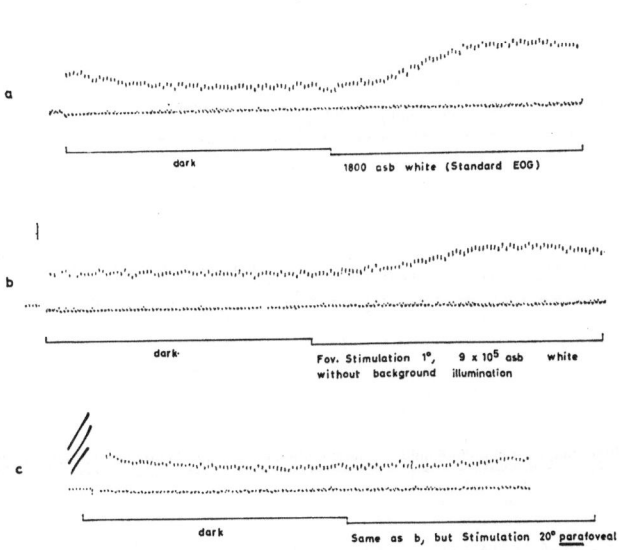

a   dark   1800 asb white (Standard EOG)

b   dark   Fov. Stimulation 1°,   9 x 10⁵ asb   white
     without background   illumination

c   dark   Same as b, but Stimulation 20° parafoveal

Fig. 7a–c: EOG's recorded from the same person on the same day. a. standard EOG, ratio 225, b. foveal EOG, ratio 160, c. parafoveal EOG, ratio 130.

Case 1 is a 49-year-old patient with a macular degeneration of Hutchinson Tay type in the macula (Fig. 8a + b). The right eye shows a rough and disciform accumulation of pigment epithelium. In the left eye these alterations were less extensive. The fluorescence angiography* shows an intact pigment epithelium over the white spots at the posterior pole, except in the macular area where it is fully destroyed. The recorded standard EOG of the right eye shows a definitely

* We thank PROF. DR. STEINBACH for the fluorescence fundus angiography.

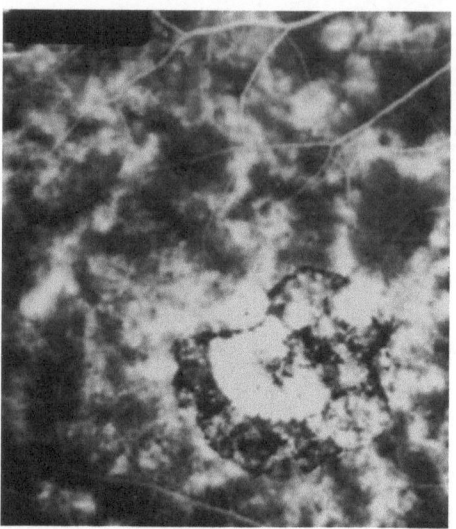

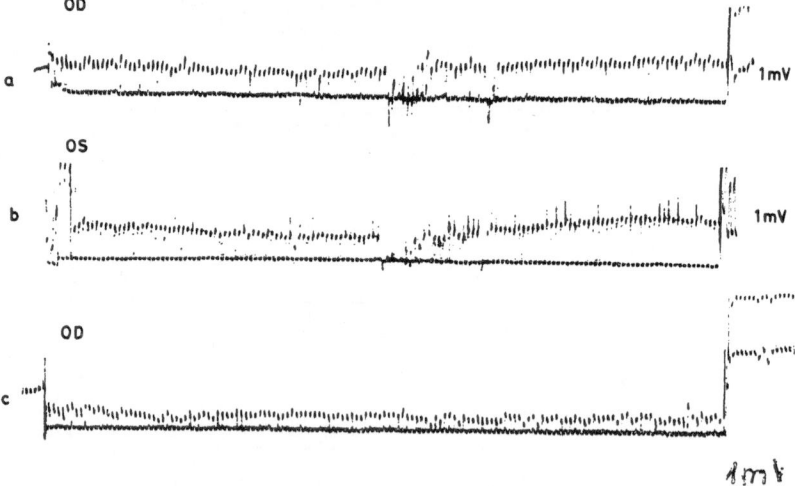

Fig. 8a + b: 49-year-old patient with macular degeneration. Visual acuity OD: 0,07 OS: 0,4. a. fluorescence angiogram. b. *a.*standard EOG OD, ratio 150. *b.* standard EOG OS, ratio 190. *c.* foveal EOG.

pathological EOG value; on the left eye it is at the lower limit of normality. In the foveal EOG there is no light response at all.

Case 2 is a 60-year-old female, as shown in Fig. 9a–c, with a disciform macular degeneration in the left eye. The macula shows a bubbly edema with whitish precipitates. Below there are hard exudates, nasal fine pale yellow scars. The subretinal exudate fluoresces in the macular area. The ratio of the standard EOG is 174, of the foveal EOG 115.

Case 3 Fig. 10a and b show the case of a 30-year-old male with a dry macular degeneration in the left eye. The ratio of the standard EOG is 200, of the foveal EOG 125.

Case 4 Fig. 11a and b is a 65-year-old female with a dry macular degeneration in the left eye. An aggregate of rough granules is seen in the macular area. With

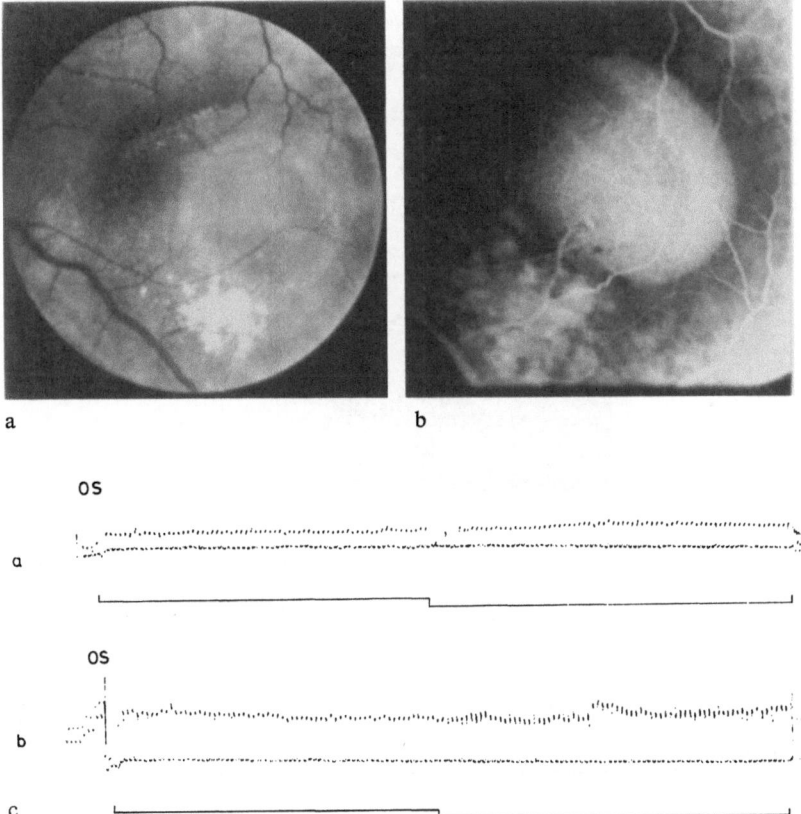

a   b

Fig. 9a–c: 60-year-old female with disciform macular degeneration of the left eye. Visual acuity OD: 1,0. OS: 0,6. a. fundus photo. b. fluorescence angiogram. c. *a*. standard EOG, ratio 174. *b*. foveal EOG, ratio 115.

225

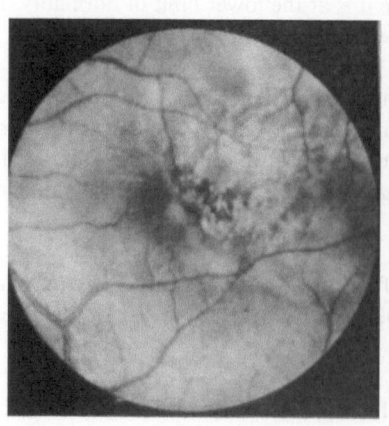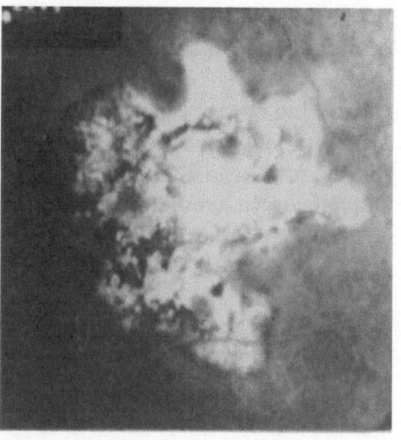

Fig. 10a and b: 30-year-old male with a dry macular degeneration. a. fundus photo. b. fluorescence angiogram. Ratio of the standard EOG 200, of the foveal EOG 125.

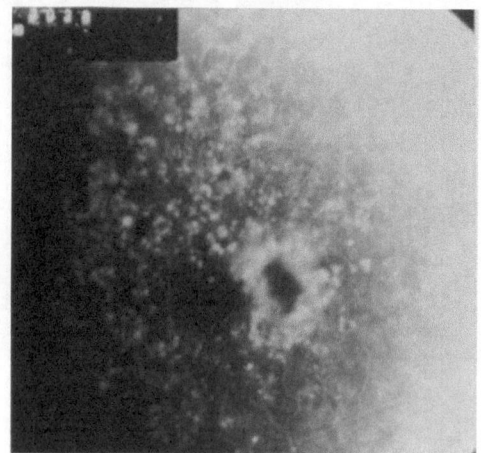

OS

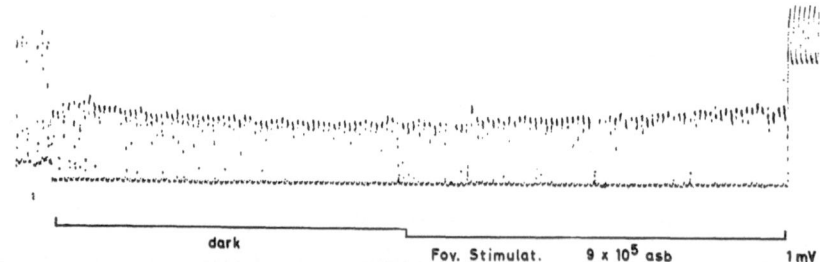

dark   Fov. Stimulat.   9 x 10⁵ asb   1 mV

Fig. 11a and b: 65-year-old female with macular degeneration OS. Visual acuity 0,3.
a. fluorescence angiogram. b. foveal EOG, ratio 120.

the beginning of the chorioidal fluorescence, there appears a patchy fluorescence, which is ringshaped at the posterior pole. In the central area, fluorescence is absent, possibly due to bleeding. The ratio of the foveal EOG is 120.

DISCUSSION

Recording of the testing potential of an isolated macular area seems to be possible. Also, using much higher retinal illumination as compared to the standard EOG smaller ratios are generated. The recording must take place without any background illumination, because of its considerable influence on the light response. The macula participates in the oscillations, but only to a small degree. Totally, the influence is not as great as the peripheral parts of the retina. This is in agreement with ELENIUS & KARO (1966), and GOURAS & CARR (1965), who already pointed out that the cones play a role in the light response, and not just the rods, as presumed previously.

In a number of cases of extensive macular degeneration which remarkably decreased visual acuity and distinctly altered pigment epithelium, flat foveal EOG's were found. In cases of slightly altered maculas the foveal EOG did not differ significantly as compared with the foveal EOG of normal persons. It seems that only extensive alterations in the central retina can be detected by the foveal EOG. The clinical application of the foveal EOG is influenced by a number of factors: the usually elderly patient should be cooperative during recording, should be able to endure the recording procedure of approximately 30 minutes, and the visual acuity should be good enough to permit recognition of the fixation light.

ACKNOWLEDGMENT

Thanks are given for the technical assistance of Mr. H. LEITNER, 'Klinik für Kommunikationsstörungen'.

REFERENCES

ARDEN, G. B., ADEL BARRADA & KELSEY, J. H. New clinical test of retinal function based upon the standing potential of the eye. *Brit. J. Ophthal.* 46: *449-467* (1962).

ARDEN, G. B. & BANKES, J. L. K. Foveal electroretinogram as a clinical test. *Brit. J. Ophthal.* 50: *740* (1966).

ARDEN, G. B. & KELSEY, J. H. Some observations on the relationship between the standing potential of the human eye and the bleaching and regeneration of visual purple. *J. Physiol.* 161: *205-226* (1962).

ARDEN, G. B. & KELSEY, J. H. Changes produced by light in the standing potential of the human eye. *J. Physiol.* 161: *189* (1962).

ELENIUS, V. & KARO, T. Cone activity in the light-induced response of the human electrooculogram *Pflueger Arch. Ges. Physiol.* 291: *241* (1966).

ELENIUS, V. & LEHTONEN, J. Spectral sensitivity of the standing potential of the human eye. *Acta Ophthal.* 40: *559* (1962).

FINKELSTEIN, D. & GOURAS, P. Visual electrophysiology. An introduction to the ERG, EOG, ERP and VER. *International Ophthalmology Clinics* Vo. 9 No. 4 (1969).

FRANCOIS, J., VERRIEST, G. & DE ROUCK, A. Electro-oculography as a functional test in pathological conditions of the fundus. I. First results. *Brit. J. Ophthal.* 40: *108-112* (1956).

GLIEM, H. Das Elektrookulogramm. *VEB Georg Thieme, Leipzig* (1971).

GOURAS, P. & CARR, R. Cone activity in the light induced D-C response of monkey retina. *Invest. Ophthal.* 4: *318* (1865).

HOCHGESAND, P. & SCHICKETANZ, K. H. Wie weit läßt sich durch die Faktoren Person, Tag und Tageszeit die Variabilität des EOG erklären? Aspekte bei der Normwertgewinnung von Parametern des EOG's. Vortrag: 16. Tagung der Österreichischen Ophthalmologischen Gesellschaft und Tagung der Vereinigung Bay. Augenärzte in Würzburg vom 31.5.–2.6. 1973.

HOMMER, L. D. & KOLDER, H. Mathematical model of oscillations in the human corneo-retinal potential. *Pflügers Archiv.* 287: *197-202* (1966).

KELSEY, J. Variations in the normal electrooculogram. *Brit. J. Ophthal.* 51: *44* (1967).

KOLDER, H. Spontane und experimentelle Änderungen des Bestandpotentials des menschlichen Auges. *Pflueger Arch.* 261: *258* (1959).

KOLDER, H. E. & HOCHGESAND, P. Empirical model of electro-oculogram. *Documenta Ophthalmologica* 34: *229-241* (1973).

KRIS, C. Corneo-fundal potential variations during light and dark adaptation. *Nature* 182: *1027* (1958).

VAN LITH, G. H. M. & BALIK, J. Variability of the electrooculogram (EOG). *Acta Ophthal.* 48: *1091* (1970).

VAN LITH, G. H. M. & BALIK, J. The variability of the EOG in the same person. *Ophthalmologica* 163: *63* (1971).

MÜLLER, W. & HAASE, E. Inter- und intraindividuelle Streuung im EOG. *v. Graefes Arch. Klin. exp. Ophthal.* 181: *71-78* (1970).

Author's address:

Univ.-Eye-Clinic Mainz
Langenbeckstr. 1
65 Mainz 1
West-Germany

A NEW METHOD FOR D.C. REGISTRATION OF THE HUMAN ERG AT LOW AND CONVENTIONAL STIMULUS INTENSITIES*

SVEN ERIK G. NILSSON & BENGT KNAVE

(Linköping)

ABSTRACT

A new method developed for d.c. registration of the human ERG made it possible to study retinal functions that have not previously been studied clinically, e.g. the retinal responses below the b-wave threshold and the c-wave. It is hoped that this new method may make it possible to diagnose earlier certain pigment epithelial and retinal disorders induced by drugs or caused by other factors.

On the basis of d.c. recordings on the dark adapted sheep eye of the ERG responses below the conventional b-wave threshold KNAVE, MØLLER & PERSSON (1972) recently proposed a reinterpretation of the major components of the ERG. Indications of positive and negative d.c. responses from the inner nuclear layer were found, in addition to the rod receptor potential. The c-wave could be recorded at stimulus intensities above the b-wave threshold. This method for d.c. registration of the sheep ERG also proved to be useful when studying the effects on retinal function of neuro-pharmacologically active substances and drugs, such as alcohol (BERNHARD et al., 1973) and barbiturate (KNAVE, NILSSON & PERSSON, 1973). Selective effects on the c-wave, representing the pigment epithelial cells, could be induced by single i.v. injections to the sheep of the new antituberculous drug rifampicin (KNAVE, PERSSON, CALISSENDORFF & NILSSON, 1973), the melanin affinity of which has recently been shown auto-radiographically (BOMAN, 1973). The fact that rifampicin, as well as other drugs with known melanin affinity, e.g. chlorpromazine and chloroquine, are given therapeutically for years, calls for studies of the long-term effects on the pigment epithelium and the retina of these drugs experimentally and clinically. Thus, a method for d.c. recordings of the human ERG must be developed. The routine method for clinical ERG (KARPE, 1945, 1948, 1962; RIGGS, 1941) is based on a.c. registration of the a- and b-waves, and the silver – silver chloride electrode system used does not fulfil the stability requirements for d.c. recordings. The present paper describes a new method for d.c. registration of the human ERG. A more detailed report is being published elsewhere (KNAVE, NILSSON & LUNT, 1973).

* This investigation was supported by grants from the Swedish Medical Research Council (Projects No. 12x-734 and 04x-3119) and the Magn. Bergwall Foundation.

Healthy volunteers with previously dilated pupils were kept in darkness for one hour. Thereafter, in an illumination not exceeding 5 Lux, a slightly opaque scleral contact lens (Fig. 2), modified from KNAVE (1970), was applied to the eye, and a plastic chamber (Fig. 2) for the tip of the reference electrode was placed on the forehead (Fig. 3). The contact lens and the chamber were both filled with Methocel ^{R} (Baeschlin). One of the forearms was grounded.

The matched calomel half-cells used as recording and reference electrodes were connected to the contact lens and the chamber on the forehead by means of saline bridges in 60-cm-long agar-filled polyethylene tubes (Figs. 1 and 2), changed for every volunteer, so that calomel could never reach the eye. To ensure a good contact with the Methocel, pieces of surgical swab (Sponcal) were put in the tips of the recording tubes (Fig. 1). The swab was not allowed to touch the cornea. The electrodes were connected to the differential inputs of a

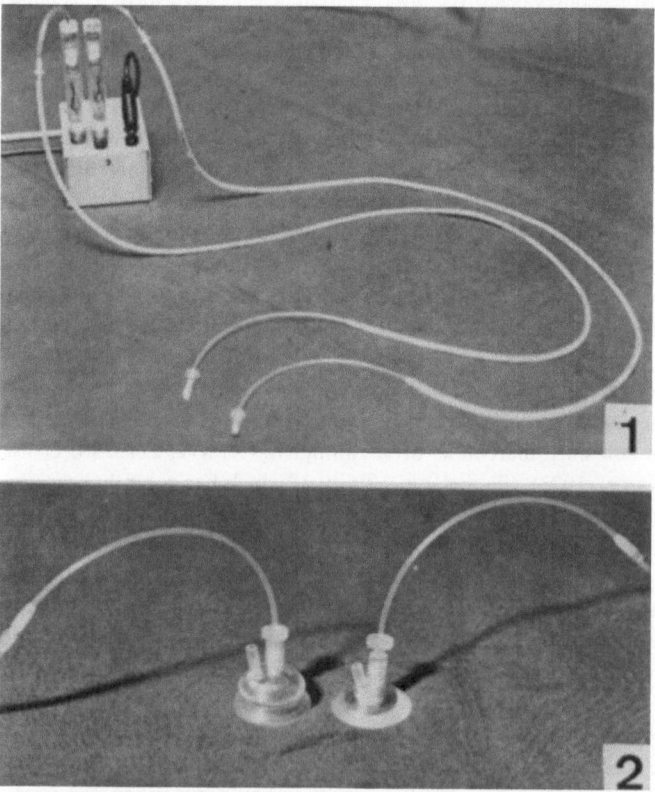

Fig. 1. The matched calomel half-cells used as recording and reference electrodes. Between the half-cell and the electrode tip is a saline bridge in an agar-filled polythylene tube.

Fig. 2. The scleral contact lens to the left and the plastic chamber for the forehead to the right. The electrode tips are inserted in their holders.

low drift d.c. amplifier (Fig. 5). The potentials were lowpass-filtered (220 Hz cut off, 18dB/octave) and fed into a Hewlett-Packard signal analyzer 5480 S. The noise level of the electrode system was 5–10 μV and the d.c. drift 10–15 μV/hr. Before taking a photograph four to 50 responses were usually averaged by the signal analyzer.

The stimulus light source was a 150 Watt ozone-free Osram XBO xenon lamp with an approximately flat spectral emission curve within the visible part of the spectrum. The heat was controlled by a heat reflection and a heat ab-

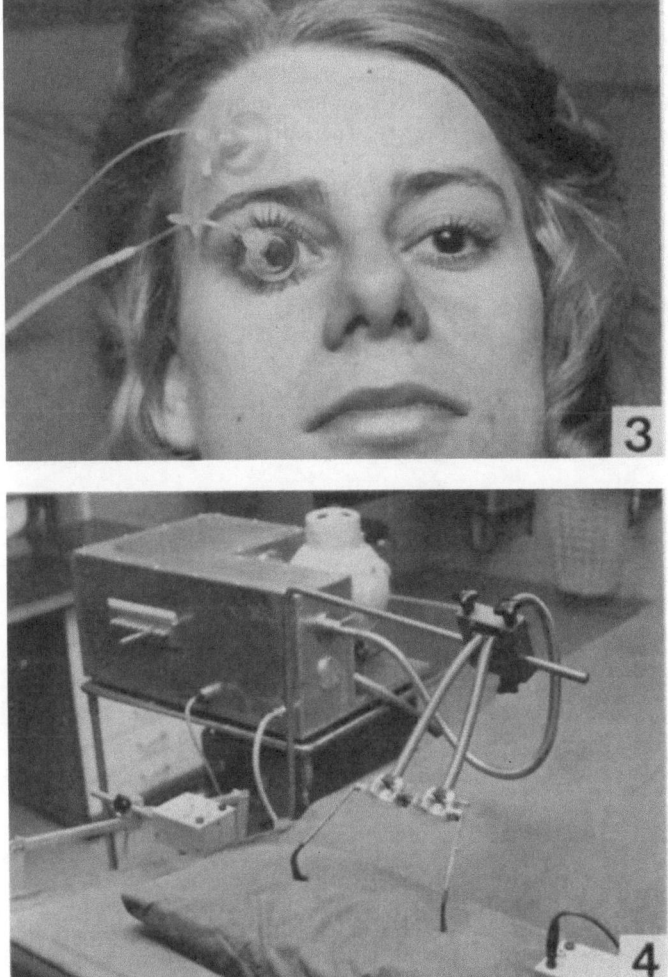

Fig. 3. The contact lens on the eye. The chamber into which is led the tip of the reference electrode is attached to the forehead by means of a ring-shaped two sided adhesive tape.

Fig. 4. The stimulus light unit including a xenon lamp, filters, an electronic shutter and a Y-shaped fiber optics attached to an adjustable spectacle frame.

231

sorbing filter (Zeiss) and the light intensity was changed by means of neutral density filters (Balzer). The intensity eliciting a single flash b-wave (threshold at 30–40 μV) is referred to as log relative intensity O. Stimulus duration was varied with the aid of a Zeiss electromagnetic shutter, placed in a focal plane of the beam. The interval between the test flashes was 10 sec for log relative intensity −0.5, 30 sec for log relative intensity 0.5 and 2 min for log relative intensity 4.5. In order to control more accurately the light reaching the pupil the stimulus light was led to the patient's eyes through a Y-shaped quartz fiber optics (Schott) (Fig. 4). By means of a special spectacle frame the tips of the fiber bundles could be adjusted in two planes so as to fit precisely the position of the pupils.

Finally a shielding wire-net cage was lowered over the upper part of the volunteer and over the electrode system in order to exclude artefacts from alternating current, etc. (Fig. 5). Thereafter, the eyes were allowed to dark adapt for about 30 min.

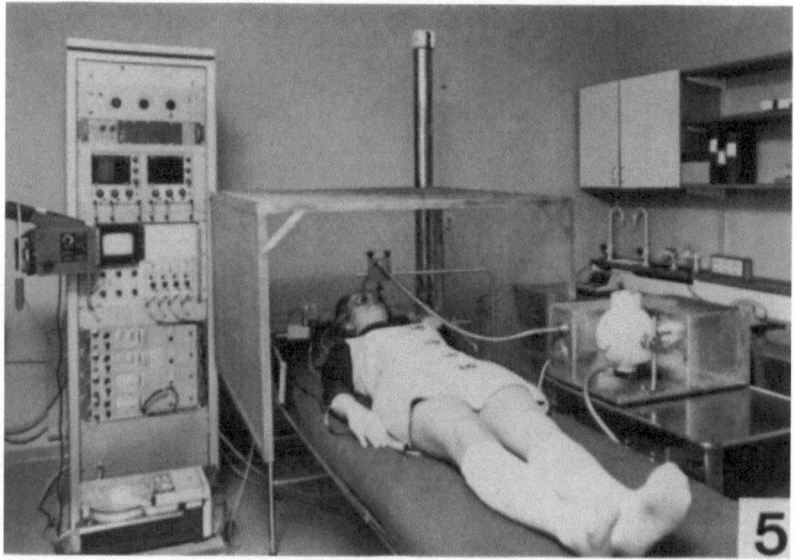

Fig. 5. A volunteer prepared for d.c. recording of the ERG. The fiber optics in place. A shielding wire-net cage is lowered over the volunteer and the electrode system to exclude artefacts form alternating current etc. The calomel half-cells are connected to one of the four low-drift d.c. amplifiers in the rack, which in addition contains a Hewlett-Packard signal analyzer, two more oscilloscopes and electronics for the trigger system and for the stimulus light shutter. A tape punch (seen at the bottom of the rack) was used to collect the data for possible future need of a more detailed computer analysis.

Some typical responses will be shown in the present paper only as a demonstration of the main features and possibilities of the new method for d.c.
registration of the human ERG. A more systematic analysis of the results will
be presented in following papers.

Fig. 6 shows the d.c. recorded human ERG in response to a relative stimulus
intensity of 4.5 log units. With a stimulus duration of 0.1 sec and a sweep time
of 0.45 sec a small a-wave and a predominant b-wave are found (6A). In response to a stimulus of longer duration (1 sec) and with a longer sweep duration
(4.5 sec) a c-wave, representing the activity of the pigment epithelial cells
(Noell (1953) and others), is also seen (6B).

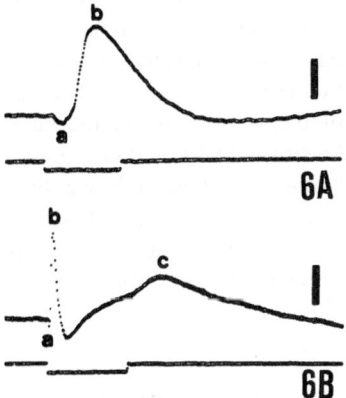

Fig. 6. The d.c. recorded human ERG in response to a relative stimulus intensity of
about 4.5 log units above b-wave threshold. Stimulus duration (indicated on lower line)
0.1 sec (A) and 1.0 sec (B). Amplitude calibration 250 μV.

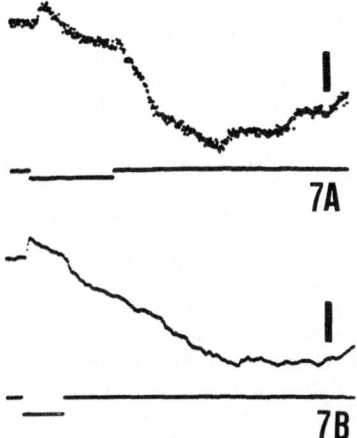

Fig. 7. The d.c. recorded human ERG in response to a relative stimulus intensity of
about 0.5 log unit be ow (A) and above (B) b-wave threshold. Stimulus duration 1.0
sec. Amplitude calibration 25 μV (A) and 250 μV (B).

Fig. 7A demonstrates the ERG in response to a stimulus with an intensity of −0.5 relative log unit. A positive d.c. shift of about the same duration as the light stimulus and with an amplitude of about 10 μV is seen superimposed on a slow, cornea-negative potential with an amplitude maximum about 1.5 sec after cessation of light. The positive d.c. shift of this ERG response below the conventional b-wave threshold (30–40 μV) well corresponds to the so-called positive d.c. response of the low-intensity ERG of the sheep shown by KNAVE, MØLLER & PERSSON (1972). It seems that the cornea-negative potential represents the rod receptor potential.

A recording just above the b-wave threshold (0.5 relative log unit) is shown in Fig. 7B. Although the configuration of this ERG response is similar to the 'low-intensity' ERG demonstrated in Fig. 7A, the positive d.c. shift now exceeds the conventional threshold (30–40 μV) in electroretinography. The initial part of the positive d.c. shift thus represents the b-wave of the ERG. The slow, negative shift following the positive d.c. potential corresponds to the remnant negativity first described by GRANIT & RIDDELL (1934).

The new method for d.c. registration of the human ERG thus makes it possible to study the neuro-retinal functions below the b-wave threshold as well as the c-wave and other slow potentials, e.g. the so-called remnant negativity, which have not earlier been investigated clinically. There are reasons to hope that the method in the future might lead to an earlier diagnosis than before of pigment epithelial and retinal disorders induced by drugs or based on other pathological conditions.

REFERENCES

BERNHARD, C. G., KNAVE, B. & PERSSON, H. E. Differential effects of ethyl alcohol on retinal functions. *Acta Physiol. Scand.* 88: *373-381* (1973).

BOMAN, G. Melanin affinity of a new antituberculous drug, rifampicin, investigated by whole body autoradiography. *Acta Ophthal. (Kbh.),* 51: *367-370* (1973).

GRANIT, R. & RIDDELL, L. A. The electrical responses of light – and dark-adapted frogs eyes to rhythmic and continuous stimuli. *J. Physiol. (Lond.)* 81: *1-28* (1934).

KARPE, G. The basis of clinical electroretinography. *Acta Ophthal. (Kbh.),* Suppl. 24 (1945).

KARPE, G. Apparatus and method for clinical recording of the electroretinogram. *Doc. Ophthal.* 2: *268-276* (1948).

KARPE, G. A routine method of clinical electroretinography. *Acta Ophthal. (Kbh.),* Suppl. 70: *15-31* (1962).

KNAVE, B. Long-term effects of high intensity flashes on the ERG of the rabbit. *Acta Physiol. Scand.* 78: *478-490* (1970).

KNAVE, B., MØLLER, A. & PERSSON, H. E. A component analysis of the electroretinogram. *Vision Res.* 12: *1669-1684* (1972).

KNAVE, B., NILSSON, S. E. G. & LUNT, T. The human electroretinogram: DC recordings at low and conventional stimulus intensities. Description of a new method for clinical use. *Acta Ophthal. (Kbh.)* 51: *716-726* (1973).

KNAVE, B., NILSSON, S. E. G. & PERSSON, H. E. in preparation for publication (1973).

KNAVE, B., PERSSON, H. E., CALISSENDORFF, B. & NILSSON, S. E. G. Selective effects of a new antituberculous drug, rifampicin, on the c-wave of the sheep electroretinogram. *Acta Ophthal. (Kbh.)* 51: *371-374* (1973).

NOELL, W. K. Experimentally induced toxic effects on structure and function of visual cells and pigment epithelium. *Am. J. Ophthal.* 36: *103-116* (1953).

RIGGS, L. Continuous and reproducible records of the electrical activity of the human retina. *Proc. Soc. Exp. Biol. & Med.* 48: *204-207* (1941).

Authors' address:

Dept. of Ophthalmology
University of Linköping
University Hospital
S-581 85 Linköping
Sweden

THE ELECTRORETINOGRAM
A REINTERPRETATION OF ITS BASIC
COMPONENTS.

B. KNAVE, A. MØLLER & H. E. PERSSON

(Stockholm)

At quite an early date the gross ERG was considered to be composed of several component potentials of different sign and amplitude. In a large number of investigations the ERG components have been analysed and fixed (see e.g. GRANIT, 1933; BROWN, 1968; TOMITA, 1970, 1972). Recent studies on the intracellular responses from the receptors and neurones in the vertebrate retina have revealed the response characteristics of different retinal cells (see e.g. KANEKO & HASHIMOTO, 1969; KANEKO, 1970 and review TOMITA, 1970; 1972). In the present study the ERG and its components were studied with a new technique (low-intensity ERG) and analysed taking into special consideration the relations and functional similarities of the ERG and the intracellular retinal potentials. The corneal low-intensity ERG to repetitive sub-liminal light stimuli was d.c.-recorded with matched calomel half-cells and averaged (summated) on a computer (Didac Intertechnique 800). The experimental technique and recording procedure has been described in detail (KNAVE, MØLLER & PERSSON, 1972). With this technique, it is possible to study the details of the ERG at intensities below the b-wave thresholds in long-term sessions during constant experimental conditions.

It was found that the averaging technique enabled recordings of ERG responses within an intensity range about 2.5 log units below the single flash b-wave threshold of the dark-adapted eye. Fig. 1 shows averaged responses to 1-sec flashes at an intensity of the lower limit of this range. The first response to appear consisted of a slow, cornea-negative transient potential outlasting the stimulus by several seconds. The configuration of this slow negativity is similar to the isolated rod receptor potential (rod RP) intraretinally recorded in the night monkey (BROWN & WATANABE, 1962b) and to the intracellular rod RP in response to low stimulus intensities in the isolated frog retina (TOYODA et al., 1970). Furthermore, the intensity-amplitude curve of the slow negativity (the amplitude increased almost linearly with logarithm of intensity, see dashed line in Fig. 4) was found to be similar to rod receptor intensity-amplitude curves obtained with other techniques. Thus, there is evidence to suggest that the slow negative response of the dark-adapted eye obtained at lowest stimulus intensities below b-wave threshold represents the isolated rod RP.

When successively increasing the stimulus intensity, the responses underwent a series of characteristic alterations (Fig. 2). At somewhat higher intensities

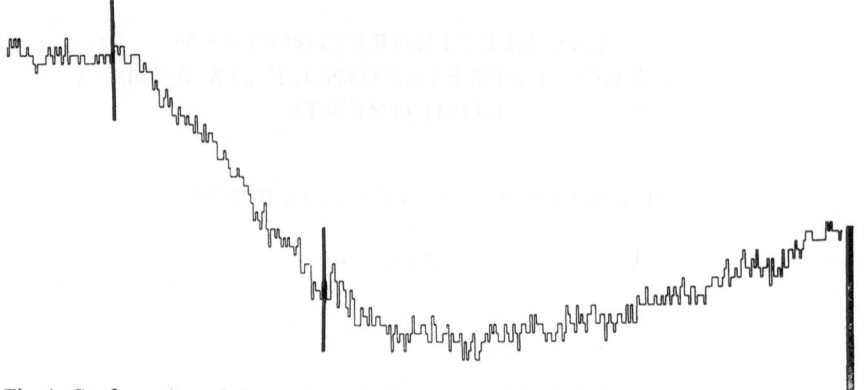

Fig. 1. Configuration of the summated ERG in response to a light stimulus with an intensity of 2.4 log units below the *b*-wave threshold of the dark-adapted eye. Onset and cessation of light stimulus (1 sec.) is marked by vertical bars in the record. Amplitude calibration: 5 μV. 200 responses were summated. Interval between stimuli: 10 sec.

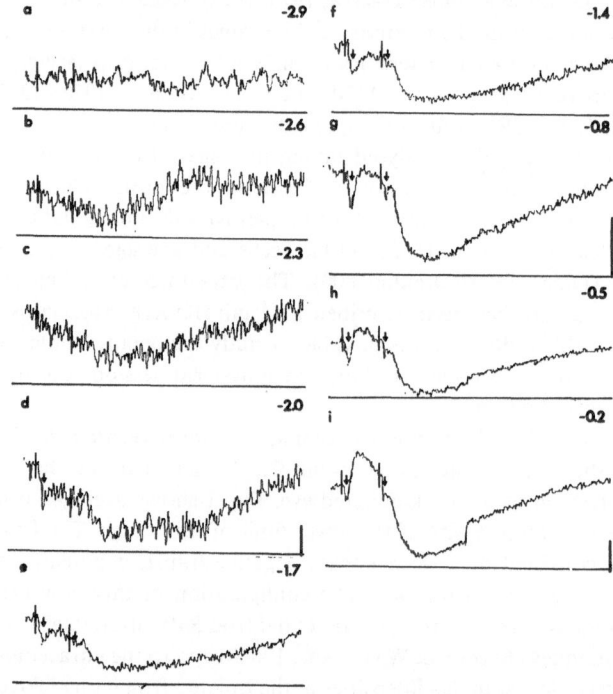

Fig. 2. Effects of stimulus intensities on ERG responses below *b*-wave threshold of the dark adapted eye. Onset and cessation of light stimulus (1 sec.) is marked by vertical bars in the records. Logarithm of stimulus intensities at the right of each record. The intensity eliciting a single flash *b*-wave threshold of 30-40 μV is referred to as log relative intensity 0. Amplitude calibration: 2 μV (a-d), 10 μV (e-g) and 10 μV (h-i). Arrows (d-i) indicate two negative deflections on both sides of a positive shift, which developed successively superimposed on the falling phase of the initial transient slow negativity. Fifty to 200 responses were summated. Interval between stimuli: 10 sec. (the positive shift appearing in h and i about 3 sec. after the cessation of the light stimulus was not a constant finding and, as a consequence, was not further investigated).

238

than those eliciting the slow negativity (Fig. 2b, c) two small negative deflections (marked by arrows, Fig. 2 d–i), surrounding a positive shift, developed successively, superimposed upon the falling phase of this slow negativity. The two small negative deflections coincided in time with the onset and cessation of the light stimulus. For reasons to be presented, the falling phase at 'on' and the rising phase at 'off' of these negative waves are considered to represent the beginning and end of a negative d.c. response, which in the following is referred to as the 'negative d.c. response'. The interposed positive plateau is referred to as the 'positive d.c. response'. A tentative scheme for the diagrammatic representation of the components, suggested above, is shown in Fig. 3. The upper diagram depicts a typical ERG below b-wave threshold (cf. Fig. 2 g), which is assumed to be built up of the slow negative transient response (lower diagram) and the d.c. responses (middle diagrams). In this connection it is relevant to refer to recent findings by KANEKO & HASHIMOTO (1969) on the intracellular responses from single neurones in the inner nuclear layer of the carp retina. Different types of responsive units were found: 1. 'on'-type units, which depolarize during illumination, resulting in extracellular, cornea-positive d.c. responses; 2. 'off'-type units resulting in negative d.c.-responses and 3. 'on-off'-type units which depolarize transiently both at the beginning and cessation of light.

At lower intensities, the amplitudes of the d.c. shifts of the present study

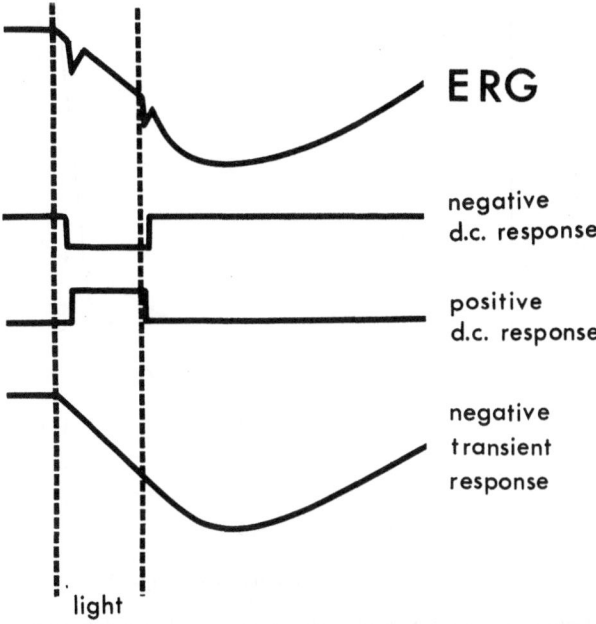

Fig. 3. Schematic representation of ERG components below b-wave threshold of the dark-adapted eye. Upper diagram depicts a typical low-intensity ERG, which is assumed to be built up of the slow negative transient response (lower diagram), and a negative and a positive d.c. response (middle diagrams).

239

were of the same order of magnitude but at higher intensities the amplitude of the positive d.c. response increased more than the negative one (Fig. 2 g–i).

In fact, the intensity-amplitude patterns of these positive and negative d.c. responses agree quite well with those of the 'on' and 'off' units, respectively, reported by KANEKO & HASHIMOTO (1969). The amplitude of the potentials of the 'on' units increased slowly at low intensities. The increase was then greater and almost linear to the logarithmic scale of the light intensity over 2 log units prior to saturation. The intensity-amplitude curve of the 'off' units was usually of a staircase shape, having two saturation levels at considerably lower amplitudes than of the 'on' units. In the present study the positive d.c. response was found to have a wide dynamic range, with no sign of saturation at low stimulus intensities (Fig. 4, solid line). The negative d.c. response (Fig. 4, dotted line) was found to saturate (and be gradually masked by the positive d.c. response) at low intensities, as was the case for the 'off' units in the carp retina. On the basis of the foregoing discussion, it is tempting to suggest that the positive and negative d.c. responses obtained with corneal electrodes from the intact eye, in the present study, might correspond to the 'on' and 'off' d.c. shifts led off intracellularly by KANEKO & HASHIMOTO (1969).

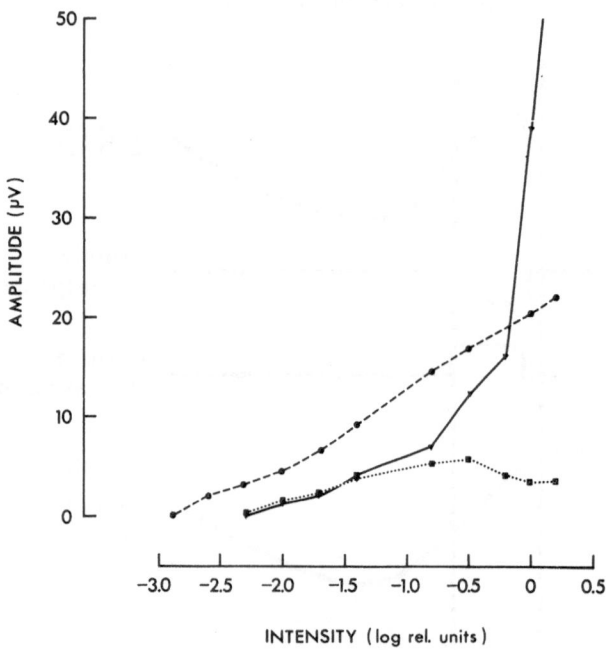

Fig. 4. Intensity-amplitude curves of ERG components below b-wave threshold of the dark-adapted eye. Transient negative response: dashed line. Positive d.c. response: solid line. Negative d.c. response: dotted line. Stimulus intensity in log units; the intensity eliciting a single flash b-wave threshold of 30-40 being referred to as log relative intensity 0. Amplitude in μV.

240

The reinterpretation of the ERG components, as suggested above, is based upon studies of the low-intensity ERG. In order to test whether or not such a reinterpretation may be valid also for the single flash, suprathreshold ERG we studied the conventional ERG of the light-adapted eye before and after raising the intraocular pressure. By light-adapting the eye the interfering c-wave was eliminated (Fig. 5). It was assumed that raising the intraocular pressure would block the retinal as well as the chorioidal circulation and consequently the oxygen supply to the retina. Since the receptor cells are less sensitive to asphyxia than the neurones in the retina, expressions for receptor cell activity in isolation were expected to be obtained using this technique. The intraocular pressure was raised by injecting 0.4 ml Ringer solution into the vitreous and recordings were thereafter taken at different time intervals (Fig. 5 b–g).

Fig. 5a shows the light-adapted ERG before raising the intraocular pressure. The a- and b-waves are seen to be followed by a negativity corresponding to the so-called remnant negativity (GRANIT & RIDELL, 1934). At 0.5 and 1.5 min after the injection (Fig. 5b and c, respectively) only a slow, negative response was obtained, similar to that of the dark-adapted eye at very low stimulus intensities (Figs. 1 and 2c). At 3.5 min after the injection (Fig. 5d), a positive component,

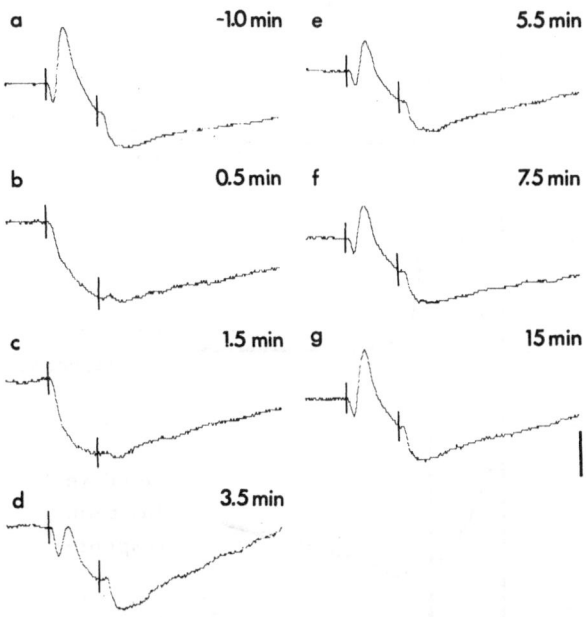

Fig. 5. Effects of raising the intraocular pressure on the light-adapted ERG. The intraocular pressure was raised by injecting 0.4 ml Ringer solution into the vitreous. ERGs were taken before (a) and at different intervals thereafter (b–g). Time intervals at the right of each record. Background light illumination 600 lm/m². Light stimulus (0.1 sec) marked by vertical bars in the records. Stimulus intensity: 5.3 log units above the b-wave threshold of the dark-adapted eye. Amplitude calibration: 50 μV.

lasting as long as the light stimulus, appeared imposed on the slow negativity. The amplitude of this positive component successively increased with time (Fig. 5 e-g), and 15 min. after injection (Fig. 5g) the ERG reverted to its original shape and amplitude, as an expression for an expected normalization of the intraocular pressure.

By clamping the retinal circulation, it was shown that in some species the receptor cell response can be isolated (BROWN & WATANABE, 1962 a,b). Since our recordings are similar to those obtained by these authors, we have good reasons to believe that the isolated negativity in the present experiment represents receptor cell activity, although our technique was different from theirs. By intergrating this isolated negativity with tentative positive and negative d.c. responses, the ERG configuration before raising the intraocular pressure was obtained. This is illustrated in Fig. 6, where the upper diagram depicts the light-

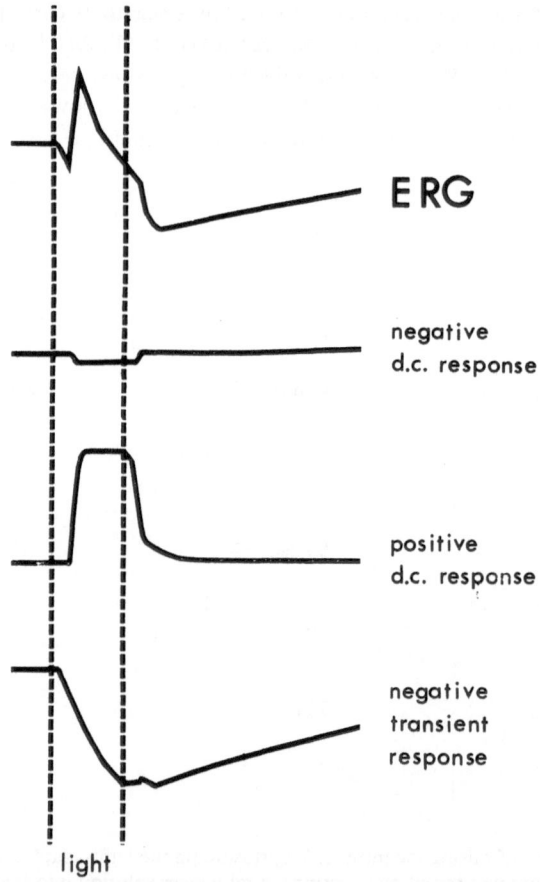

Fig. 6. Schematic representation of ERG components in the light-adapted eye. Upper diagram depicts a typical light-adapted ERG (cf. Fig. 5a), which, it is suggested, is built up of the slow negative transient response (lower diagram; cf. Fig. 5b, c) and a negative and a positive d.c. response (middle diagrams).

242

adapted ERG (Fig. 5a), which, it is suggested, is built up of the slow, negative transient response (Fig. 5b; Fig. 6, lower diagram) and the d.c. responses (middle diagrams). The amplitude chosen for the tentative, negative d.c. response was smaller than for the positive, since the negative d.c. response was found to be much smaller than, and even masked by, the positive d.c. response at higher stimulus intensities in the dark-adapted eye (see e.g. the intensity-amplitude curves in Fig. 4).

Finally, it should be pointed out that the components suggested are not to be considered as new compared to the ones proposed by GRANIT (1933) and MURAKAMI & KANEKO (1966). There are good reasons to believe that the positive d.c. response of the present study is identical with the 'square, positive' P II in response to a reduced stimulus intensity (GRANIT, 1962). We assume that the change in P II configuration into an initial, transient phase followed by a steady phase at high stimulus intensities is due to the fact that the 'square, positive' P II is imposed on the negative receptor responses. Furthermore, there are several findings which support the view that the receptor potential and the negative d.c. response might correspond to the distal and proximal P III, respectively, as recorded in the coldblooded (MURAKAMI & KANEKO 1966; SILLMAN, ITO & TOMITA, 1969) and warmblooded vertebrate retinas (HANITZSCH & TRIFONOW 1968; PAUTLER, MURAKAMI & NOSAKI 1968).

This work was supported by grants from the Swedish Medical Research Council, the Magn. Bergvall Foundation for Scientific Research, the Hierta Foundation for Ophthalmological Research and Karolinska Institutet.

REFERENCES

BROWN, K. T. The electroretinogram: its components and their origins. *Vision Res.* 8: *633-677* (1968).

BROWN, K. T. & WATANABE, K. Isolation and identification of a receptor potential from the pure cone fovea of the monkey retina. *Nature, Lond.* 193: *958-960* (1962a).

BROWN, K. T. & WATANABE, K. Rod receptor potential from the retina of the night monkey. *Nature, Lond.* 196: *547-550* (1962b).

GRANIT, R. The components of the retinal action potential in mammals and their relation to the discharge in the optic nerve. *J. Physiol., Lond.* 77: *207-239* (1933).

GRANIT, R. In: The Eye (edited by H. DAVSON), Vol. 2, p. 607. Academic Press, New York (1962).

GRANIT, R. & RIDDELL, L. A. The electrical responses of light- and dark-adapted frogs eyes to rhythmic and continuous stimuli. *J. Physiol., Lond.* 81: *1-28* (1934).

HANITZSCH, R. & TRIFONOW, J. Intraretinal abgeleitete ERG-komponenten der isolierten Kaninchennetzhaut. *Vision Res.* 8: *1445-1455* (1968).

KANEKO, A. Physiological and morphological identification of horizontal, bipolar and amacrine cells in goldfish. *J. Physiol., Lond.* 207: *623-633* (1970).

KANEKO, A. & HASHIMOTO, H. Electrophysiological study of single neurons in the inner nuclear layer of the carp retina. *Vision Res.* 9: *37-55* (1969).

KNAVE, B., MØLLER, A. & PERSSON, H. E. A component analysis of the electroretinogram. *Vision Res.* 12: *1669-1684* (1972).

MURAKAMI, M. & KANEKO, A. Differentiation of P III subcomponents in cold-blooded vertebrate retinas. *Vision Res.* 6: *627-636* (1966).

PAUTLER, E. G., MURAKAMI, M. & NOSAKI, H. Differentiation of P III subcomponents in isolated mammalian retinas. *Vision Res.* 8: *489-491* (1968).

SILLMAN, A. J., ITO, H. & TOMITA, T. Studies on the mass receptor potential of the isolated frog retina. I. General properties of the response. *Vision Res.* 9: *1435-1442* (1969).

TOMITA, T. Electrical activity of vertebrate photoreceptors. *Q. Rev. Biophys.* 3: *179-222* (1970).

TOMITA, T. In: Handbook of Sensory Physiology (edited by M. G. F. Fuortes), Vol. VII/2, pp. 635-665. The electroretinogram, as analyzed by microelectrode studies. Springer-Verlag, Berlin, Heidelberg, New York (1972).

TOYODA, J., HASHIMOTO, H., ANNO, H. & TOMITA, T. The rod response in the frog as studied by intracellular recording. *Vision Res.* 10: *1093-1100* (1970).

Authors' address:

Dept. of Physiology II
Karolinska Institutet
104 01 Stockholm 60
Sweden

244

AN UNUSUAL CASE OF RECURRENT
HYPOKALEMIA FOLLOWED
ELECTRORETINOGRAPHICALLY

G. CAVALLACCI & A. WIRTH

(Pisa)

The effect of different ions on the electroretinogram (ERG) was studied by
BEUCHELT in 1921, but his method was rather slow to give satisfactory infor-
mations as to the selective effect on the retinal potentials. Later THERMAN
(1938) found that application of 0.5 % potassium chloride in isotonic glucose to
the opened eye of the frog quickly removed the positive responses, leaving an
isolated negative ERG. To quote from GRANIT (1947) the very first effect of
potassium was that of removing the small oscillations superimposed on the
ERG; the next effect was to increase the a – wave and diminish the b – wave.

More recently HAMASAKI (1963, 1964) investigated the effect of various ions
on the isolated retina of the frog and concluded that both the a – and b waves
originate from the photoreceptors. FURUKAWA & HANAWA (1955) using the
retina of the toad treated with aspartate, showed that the a-wave increases with
increasing external sodium concentration. The same was found by SILLMAN,
ITO & TOMITA (1969). These experiments demonstrated that, except at very low
concentrations, the amplitude of the receptor potential (PIII) increased in direct
proportion to the logarithm of the external sodium concentration. With regard
to potassium the relationship was inversely linear (external potassium concentration on a log scale).

We were fortunate in having the opportunity to observe an unusual case of
recurrent hypokalemia, a rare disease in which, as it will be discussed below,
there is an increase of intracellular potassium.

CASE REPORT

The patient A.M., male aged 45, suffered since 5 years from periodic palsies,
lasting on average from 12 to 48 hours. The episodes were characterized by
intense weekness or complete paralysis of limb and trunk muscles. During the
attack the tendon reflexes were absent or greatly reduced, but returned to
normal as strength and tone returned. As in the typical form the attacks were
precipitated by such factors as physical stress or a large high – carbohydrate
meal.

Normal serum potassium of the subject, as measured with flame photometry,
was 4.3 meq/l: during the episodes levels as low as 3.1 meq/l were reached. The

b-wave increased during the attacks, the values ranging from 250 μV (K⁺ =
4.3) to 410 μV (3.1) (see fig. 1).

The *a*-wave was unchanged.

It is interesting to report in this connection that the electrocardiogram was
typical of high potassium level in the heart muscle, the main features of that
being an increase of the P-Q latency and a deepening of the S-T.

E R G (b-wave) μV	K^+ m eq/l	Na^+ m eq/l	Cl^- m eq/l	E C G
......250	4,3	144	101	
μV 294	3,9	143	100	
μV 330	3,5	144	100	
μV 378	3,3	144	101	
......410	3,1	143	102	

DISCUSSION

We have reported a rare case of muscle paralysis caused by a decrease in blood
potassium (hypokalemia) due to an increase of the ion in the muscle cell.

As we have seen, the *b*-wave was increased whereas the *a*-wave remained
unaffected. This poses the following questions:

1. why the *b*-wave is increased
2. why the *a*-wave is unchanged
3. do the results agree with previous experiments on the effect of electrolytes
changes on the ERG.

We suggest the following explanations:

Question 1. The *b*-wave increases because of an elevation of the resting
potential produced by an increase of the intracellular potassium and a corresponding reduction of that of the external medium.

This results is an increase of the electrochemical gradient.

246

That is to say, there should be an increased permeability to potassium of the nerve cells (probably bipolars, according to the current views) and by consequence of the conductance during the dark period with a block under illumination.

Question 2. As to the *a*-wave one cannot be sure that it is unaffected. In fact, it could be increased but masked by the augmented *b*-wave, the recorded ERG being an algebraic sum of the two components.

On the other hand, the *a*-wave could actually be unchanged because the photoreceptors membrane is more resistant to the inward passage of potassium. The lipoproteic structure of the receptor membrane could stress this hypothesis.

Question 3. It is known from the experiments of Tomita et al. that the *b*-wave amplitude is inversely proportional to external potassium concentration (on a log scale).

We have found in experiments on rabbits (Tota & Cavallacci: 1970a, b – 1971) using several diuretics (furosemide, diclorophenamide, thriamterene) that the *b*-wave is sensitive to plasma changes of electrolytes, particularly of potassium.

In these cases there was an hypokalemia due to increase of the urinary excretion and a supernormal b-wave. It is interesting to report that the ethacrinic acid doesn't affect the ERG. Since its diuretic mechanism is similar to the substances mentioned above, the explanation could be in the blocking effect of ethacrinic acid on the membrane ATP asis with consequent block of the sodium-pump, which is necessary to mantain the membrane potential.

REFERENCES

Beuchelt, H. Die Abhängigkeit der photoelektrischen Reaktion des Froschauges von den ableitendem medien. *Z. Biol.* 73: *205-230* (1921).

Furukawa, T. & Hanawa, I. Effects of some common cations on electroretinogram of the toad. *Jap. J. Phys.* 5: *289-300* (1955).

Granit, R. Sensory mechanisms of the retina. Oxford: Oxford University Press (1947).

Hamasaki, D. I. The effect of sodium ion concentration on the electroretinogram of the isolated retina of the frog. *J. Physiol.* 167: *156-168* (1963).

Hamasaki, D. I. The electroretinogram after application of various substances to the isolated retina. *J. Physiol.* 173: *449-458* (1964).

Sillman, A. J., Ito, H. & Tomita, T. Studies on the mass receptor potential of the isolated frog retina. II. On the basis of ionic mechanism. *Vision Res.* 9: *1443-1451* (1969).

Therman, P. O. The neurophysiology of the retina in the light of chemical methods of modifying its excitability. Acta Soc. Sci. Fenn. N.S.B. II, N° 1; Helsingfors (1938).

Tota, G. & Cavallacci, G. Le modificazioni dell'ERG prodotte dal furosemide (Lasix) *Ann. Ottalm.* 96: *93-97* (1970).

Tota, G. & Cavallacci, G. Le modificazioni dell'ERG prodotte dalla diclorofenamide. *Ann. Ottalm.* 96: *303-311* (1970).

Tota, G. & Cavallacci, G. L'elettroretinogramma dopo somministrazione di triamterene. *Ann. Ottalm.* 97: *143-153* (1971).

Authors' address:

Clinica Oculistica Universitaria
56100 Pisa
Italy

CORTICAL EVOKED RESPONSES FROM STIMULATION OF VARIOUS REGIONS OF THE VISUAL FIELD*

WILLIAM R. BIERSDORF

(Columbus)

ABSTRACT

Visual evoked responses have been recorded in normal subjects to half field (15° disc) and quarter field stimulation. The stimulus was a flashed checkerboard pattern in a light adapted surround (100 ft-L). Monopolar recording from multiple electrode positions was used to obtain potential graphs and equi-potential contour maps of the posterior scalp.

Evoked responses included a biphasic primary response component peaking at about 80-85 msec, which was positive for contralateral and lower field stimulation, and negative for upper field and ipsilateral stimulation. The potential distributions over the scalp (represented by equivalent dipoles) were mostly localized in the vicinity of the occipital pole. The orientations of the quadrant dipoles, but not the locations, varied between subjects. For all subjects, the summation of the quadrant distributions produced mainly tangential dipoles for the lateral half fields and radial dipoles for the vertical half fields, with opposite half-fields having opposite polarities. It is suggested that these responses may be generated in primary visual projection areas.

The objectives of this research are to study differences in the human visual evoked response from stimulation of various parts of the visual field and to determine the sites of origin of these VER's. The approach has been made by obtaining potential contour maps of the posterior scalp from multiple electrode placements. Previous reports have shown waveform and localization differences over the two cerebral hemispheres from stimulation of the two lateral half-fields. Both blank flash and patterned flash stimulation have been used (NAKAMURA & BIERSDORF, 1971; BIERSDORF & NAKAMURA, 1973). In the present study, stimulation of quadrant fields has been performed and related to the results of stimulation of the vertical and horizontal half-fields.

METHOD

Two types of visual stimulation have been utilized in the present investigation. In the first, a checkerboard patterned flash was presented in a 50 cm light adapted hemisphere illuminated with white light at 100 ft-L. The stimulus was one-half or one-quarter of a 15° disc containing alternate opaque and clear checks subtending 15 minutes at a fixation distance of 50 cm. The checkerboard

* This research was supported in part by USPHS Research Grant No. EY00454.

was transilluminated through a red filter by a xenon flash lamp. The lamp was enclosed in a sound-shielded box, and masking noise provided by a ventilating fan on the shielded recording enclosure made the clicks produced by the lamp inaudible. The subject maintained fixation at the center of the straight edge or at the right angle corner of the stimulus as required.

The second type of stimulation was a tachistoscopic presentation of an appearing or disappearing checkerboard with the two fields equated for average luminance. White light was used at a luminance of 5 ft-L. A checkerboard pattern of the same element size as above was used covering half of a 7° disc. The other half of the disc (blank white) was maintained continuously at the same luminance. Fixation distance was the same as above. The checkerboard appeared for one-half the cycle and disappeared for one-half the cycle at various stimulus frequencies including 1.05, 1.7, 1.95, and 2.35 Hz. The results obtained for vertical and horizontal half-fields with this pure pattern-type stimulation were not found to be reliably localized on the scalp. In addition, the localization sometimes appeared on the wrong side of the head for the primary visual areas.

The data presented here will be that utilizing the first (flashed pattern) type stimulation. A stimulus frequency of 3.3 Hz was used for a summation of 256 flashes. A constant moderate stimulus intensity was used. Stimulation was monocular, with the other eye covered with an opaque black eye patch.

Standard EEG electrodes of chlorided silver were attached to the scalp with electrode paste following the International 10-20 EEG system (with additions). Monopolar recording was employed, with the tip of the nose as the negative electrode, and a ground on the chin at the midline. Other negative electrode locations inluding chin, forehead, and ears, were also investigated. Ten electrodes were recorded simultaneously with a four channel signal averager (Fabri-Tek 1052) and an FM tape recorder. Responses were recorded on an X-Y plotter. For the potential contour mapping, ten electrode positions clustered around the occipital pole were recorded first. Then a second recording covered ten electrode positions on the periphery of the first, with certain positions repeated for reliability.

RESULTS AND DISCUSSION

Evoked responses from one subject for half-field stimulation are presented in Fig. 1. This subject was a right-handed male of 25 years of age with normal vision. In the upper part of the figure are responses to upper and lower half fields from electrodes along the vertical midline. The C_z position is the vertex and IN the inion. As can be seen, the largest responses appear at the intermediate positions O_z (approximately over the occipital pole) and P_z.

For the lower field, the response consists of a surface positive potential at about 80-85 msec, followed by a surface negative potential at 130-140 msec. The responses to the upper half field have similar deflections of opposite polarity.

In the lower part of the figure are the results for the two lateral half-fields.

250

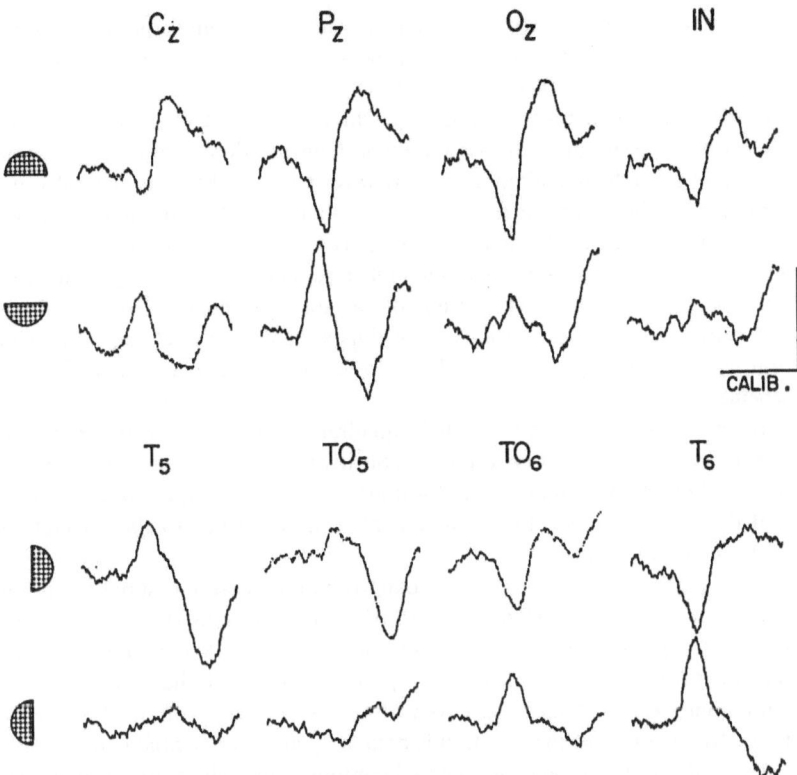

Fig. 1. Visual evoked responses (positive upward) from stimulation of the vertical half fields (upper) and the lateral half fields (lower). IN is the inion, O_z is 10% of distance along the midline toward the nasion, P_z is 30%, and C_z is 50%. TO_5 is 15% of the distance from O_z to the left around the head to the center forehead, and T_5 is 30%. TO_6 and T_6 are the same distances to the right of O_z. Calibration: 5 microvolts, 100 msec. Subject C.

Over the left scalp (T_5, TO_5) the response to the right half field consists of a positive potential also at about 84 msec, followed this time by a negative potential at 150-160 msec. For the same stimulus over the right scalp, the response is surface-negative at 80-85 msec, followed by at least one positive deflection. For left half-field stimulation, the responses are inverted in polarity at electrode positions on both sides of the head.

The positive deflection at 80-85 msec is interpreted as a primary response from stimulation of the contralateral visual field, following the primary visual pathways. Detailed data will be presented here from two subjects, who are representative of other subjects also tested. These subjects have this primary response, which begins with a latency of about 50 msec, reaches a peak near 80 msec, and returns to the baseline near 110 msec. This is usually followed by a negative potential of somewhat more varied time course between subjects. For

251

lateral half visual field stimulation, this primary response appears over the contralateral hemisphere, with often a negative response at the same latency over the ipsilateral hemisphere. As already indicated, responses at the inion are small and larger reponses appear at the parietal area (P_z) which is above the calcarine fissure and the occipital pole. This position is contralateral to the lower half visual field, and appropriately a response of the contralateral waveform appears here in response to the lower half field. The ipsilateral response and the upper half field response in the parietal area are also similar, having a negative potential peaking at about 80-85 msec and then returning to the baseline, followed by positive deflections of variable time course. The lateral half and vertical half evoked responses are thus systematically related. The quadrant field responses were also analyzed to see if they were consistent with this scheme.

In Fig. 2 are presented visual field quadrant responses from the same subject. In general, the primary response is positive (80-85 msec) for lower and contralateral quadrants, and negative for upper and ipsilateral quadrants. In about half the cases, however, these components cancel out due to the orientations of the quadrant sources.

The amplitudes of these visual evoked responses were measured at various latencies which were constant under all stimulus conditions and at all electrode positions. Specifically, amplitudes for the primary peak for subject C were measured from the beginning of the response at 50 msec to the peak at 84 msec. Amplitudes were also measured from 84 msec to 150 msec and for later deflections. One method of presenting this data is by an equipotential contour map.

Fig. 3 illustrates some equi-potential contour maps. These are for half field quarter-field stimulation of subject C. Each map is a view of the back of the head with electrode positions running from the inion at the bottom to the vertex at the top. Electrode positions also range halfway around the head to the right and left of the midline. These maps represent the potential distributions at the 84 msec latency, or the peak of the primary response. Some of the maps have a dotted line representing zero potential, with positive potential lines to one side, and negative potential lines to the other. Each line represents one microvolt. The center four maps represent the voltage distributions from the four visual field quadrants. As the optic pathways place each quadrant in the contralateral cortex, e.g., the lower right quadrant field has been placed here in the upper left position. Analyzing this map, we have a zero line running at an angle through the center, with positive potential lines to the left. This means for electrode positions on the left, positive primary responses were recorded, with negative primary responses recorded on the right. Beside each map there is a symbol which points in the direction connecting the positive and negative potential maxima for that stimulus condition. For both this map and the one below it (upper right quadrant field) the symbols are arrows, which represent voltage distributions which have approximately equal amplitude positive and negative peak potentials. For the lower left quadrant field (upper right map) the voltage distribution is somewhat different. This voltage distribution has a zero line at the lower left with positive potential lines to the right. The symbol

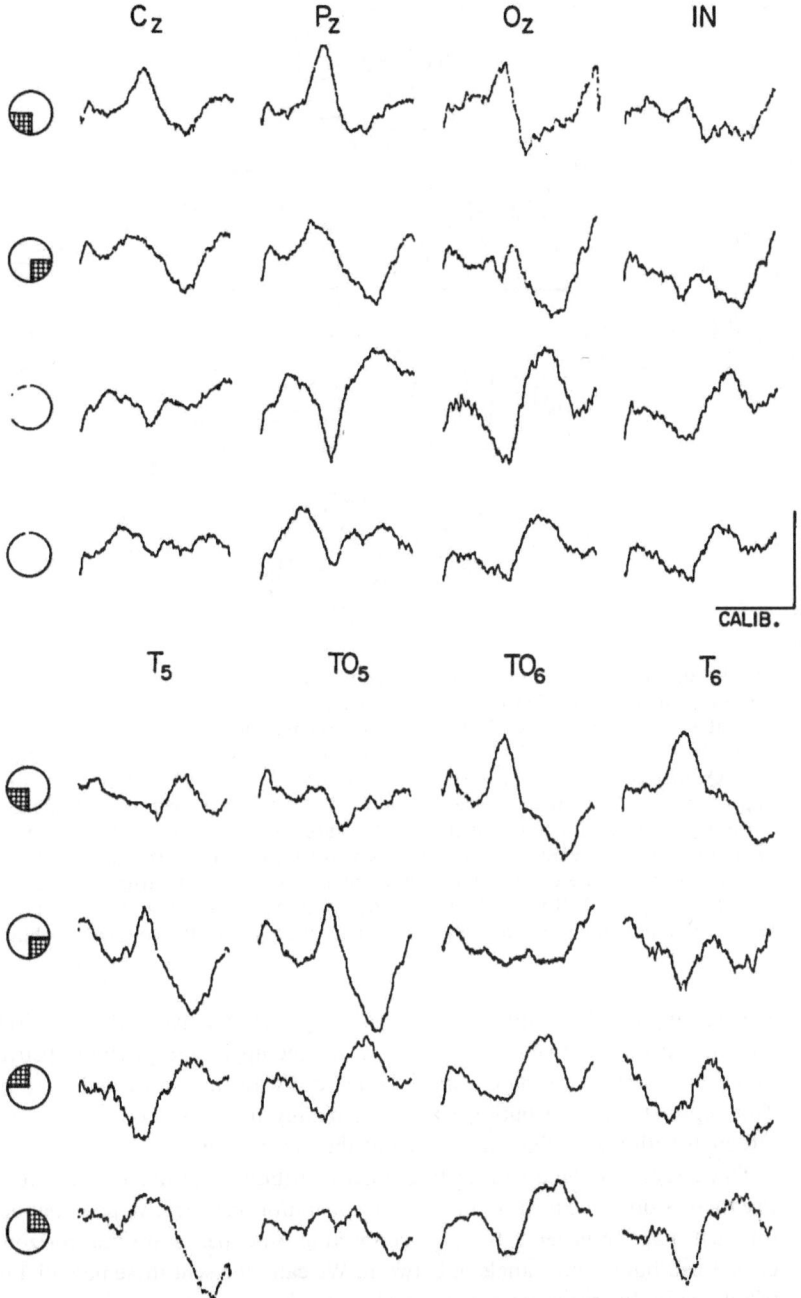

Fig. 2. Visual evoked responses from stimulation of visual field quadrants. Polarity, electrode positions, and calibration same as Fig. 1. Subject C.

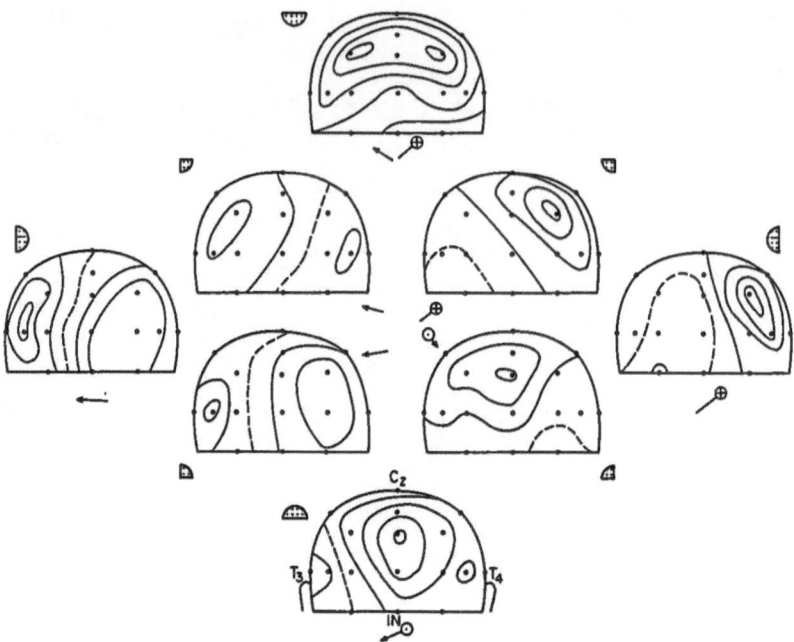

Fig. 3. Equi-potential contour maps for the evoked response amplitudes 50-84 msec, subject C, to half-field and quadrant-field stimulation. Posterior view of scalp with dots at electrode positions. Bottom position on midline is inion. Moving up are electrodes at 10 % distance (O_z), 20 %, 30 % (P_z), and 50 % (C_z). Moving left horizontally from O_z are electrodes at 15 % distance (TO_5), 30 % (T_5), and 50 % (T_3). Shown in the upper left of the map are electrodes P_3 and C_3. Directly below the first electrode to the left of O_z is one on line horizontally with the inion. Similar positions are recorded on the right (even numbered positions). Equi-potential lines every microvolt. Dotted line is zero potential. The center four contour maps are for quadrant-field stimulation, outer four maps for half-field stimulation. Adjacent to each map is an arrow or symbol representing the orientation and type or equivalent dipole for the voltage distribution.

representing this distribution is a line pointing along the axis with an encircled plus sign at the positive end. In contrast, for the upper left quadrant distribution (lower right map) there is an encircled dot with an arrow running from it. This represents a distribution which has mainly negative primary responses, although with a zero line represented at the lower right.

To characterize the quadrant field VER distributions at this latency, we notice there is only one positive potential peak and/or one negative potential peak for each map. In general, the axes connecting these peaks are not horizontal or vertical, but at some angle in between. We can represent these potential distributions by the theoretical concept of an equivalent dipole, which is a small voltage source that can produce the potential distributions shown. Essentially these arrows or arrow-like symbols represent the equivalent dipole source for each voltage distribution. The reason for adopting the dipole concept is to attempt to determine the sites of origin in the head of these visual evoked respon-

254

ses. The dipole is equivalent to a small sheet of dipoles, or voltage sources, which can produce the potential distributions shown on these maps.

These dipoles can be divided into two extreme types. One is the tangential dipole, which produces one positive peak and one negative peak on the head, separated by some distance, and which are of approximately equal amplitudes. This dipole is tangential to the surface of the head, and located somewhere near zero on the axis connecting the two peaks. The right quadrant fields produce VER dipoles of this type. The other extreme type is the radial dipole. This produces only one positive (or negative) peak surrounded by concentric circular lines of equal potential. This equivalent dipole is radial to the surface of the head, and located beneath the peak of the distribution. On this figure, the left quadrant fields are represented by dipoles tipped so much that they are nearly radial dipoles. These are positive radial (lower left quadrant) and negative radial (upper left quadrant).

When a half visual field is stimulated, this is equal to two quadrant fields and we might expect the voltage distribution for the half to equal the sum of the two quarters. To a first approximation, this does hold. On the extreme left of Fig. 3 is the distribution obtained for the right half-field stimulus. It has an approximately horizontal voltage distribution with about equal negative and positive peaks. It is a tangential dipole approximately equal to the sum of the two component quadrant field dipoles. On the extreme right in Fig. 3 is the voltage distribution obtained for the left-half-field stimulus. It is a mainly positive radial distribution, and in this case somewhat different than the sum of the two component quadrant field distributions. A more tangential distribution was expected, and such data was actually obtained in repeat runs.

For the vertical half-field distributions, the sums of the quadrant distributions are fairly well represented. For the lower half field distribution, two positive peaks can still be seen representing the two component quadrant distributions. The upper half field distribution is primarily negative radial, and fairly well represents the sum of the two lower quadrant fields.

In Fig. 4 we have a different way of presenting some of the same evoked response results. These are graphs of the amplitude of the primary response versus horizontal distance through O_z (approximately the occipital pole). Electrode positions are as illustrated in the figure inset (top view of head). These two types of dipoles produce characteristic potential graphs. A radial dipole produces a single potential peak, either positive or negative, that decreases at the same rate on either side of the peak. In this figure, the left quadrants and the left half-field produce distributions which approach a radial dipole form, although the data is not completely symmetrical about the peak. (The dashed line in these graphs is a distribution taken through the peak amplitudes, when they lie off the horizontal). A tangential dipole produces a different type of potential graph. This consists of two potential peaks, one positive, one negative, which are symmetrical about a zero position. In this figure, the right quadrants and the right half-field produce graphs which are more similar to a tangential dipole distribution. A tangential distribution differs from the sum of two opposing radial dipoles in that the potential decreases more gradually

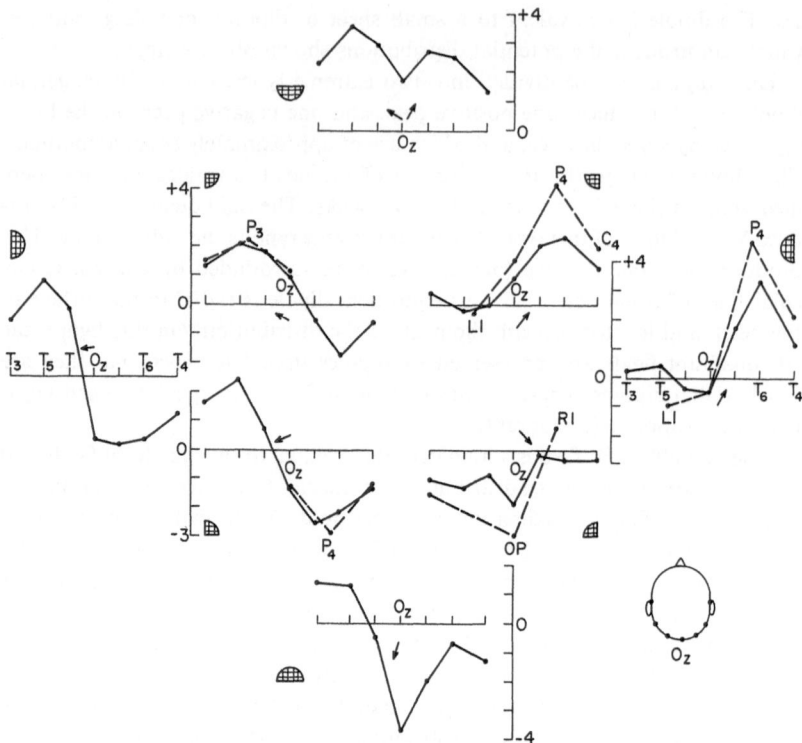

Fig. 4. Graphs of evoked response amplitudes along the horizontal for the various stimulus fields. The solid lines represent data from electrode positions T_3 through O_z to T_4 as described in Fig. 3. Dashed lines represent data from other positions, as labeled when the axis of the potential distribution deviated from horizontal. Center four distributions are for quadrant fields, outer four for half field stimulation. Each graph accompanied by arrow showing approximate orientation of equivalent dipole (surface of head represented by abscissa). Amplitude in microvolts. Subject C.

on the side away from zero than on the zero side. All graphs in this figure are accompanied by arrows showing the approximate orientation and position of the equivalent dipole. The angle of the arrow with the abscissa approximates the angle of the dipole with the surface of the head. (A tangential dipole is parallel to the abscissa, while a radial dipole is perpendicular.)

To characterise the dipoles in this figure, they are all close to the midline position (O_z). The quadrant dipoles may be radial, tangential, or at some angle in between. In general, the lateral half dipoles are more tangential in appearance, while the vertical half dipoles tend to be more of the radial type. (The lower half distribution in this case still reveals its origin with two dipoles from the lower quadrants). Opposite half-field distributions are reversed in polarity. The right half field dipole points to the left, and the other lateral half-field points to the right. The lower half field dipole is surface positive, while the upper half field is mainly surface negative.

256

In Fig. 5 are presented evoked response amplitude graphs for the same subject, but this time along the vertical midline. The electrode positions range from the vertex (C_z) to the inion. The dashed line indicates the distribution when its axis deviates from the vertical. Again the arrows accompanying each graph indicate the approximate position and orientation of the equivalent dipole. To characterize these graphs, most of the dipoles are closer to radial form than to the tangential type. What this means is that a potential dipole that is nearly tangential to the back of the head, can at the same time be more nearly radial to the vertical midline. These potential distributions, or equivalent dipoles, exist in three-dimensional space, and these various graphs provide a

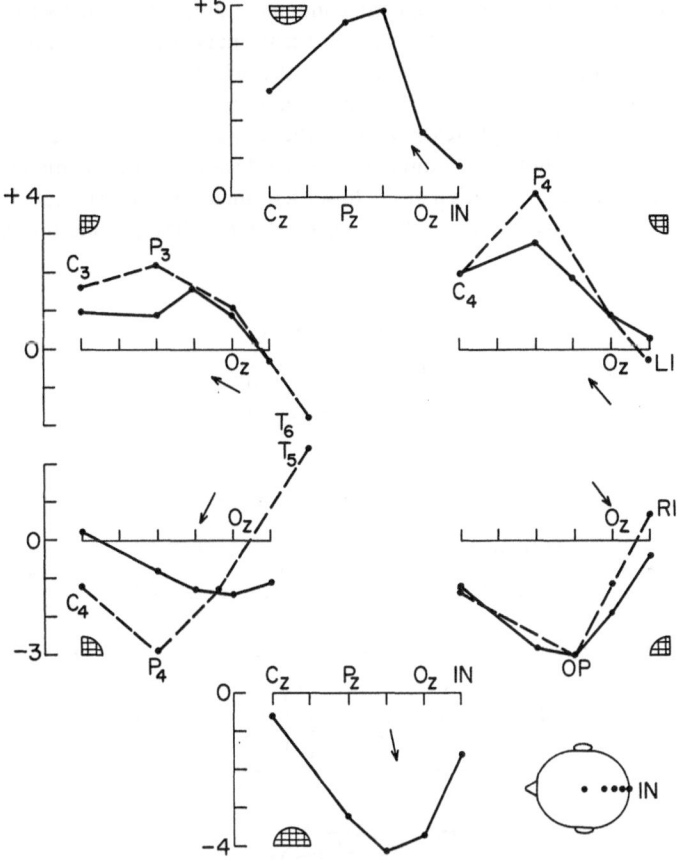

Fig. 5. Graphs of evoked potential amplitudes along the vertical midline for various stimulus fields. Solid lines represent data from electrode positions at the inion through O_z to C_z as described in Fig. 3. Dashed lines represent data from other positions, as labeled, when the axis of the potential distribution deviates from the vertical. Center four distributions are for quadrant fields, upper and lower distributions for vertical half stimulation. Each graph accompanied by arrow showing approximate orientation of equivalent dipole (surface of head represented by abscissa). Amplitude in microvolts. Subject C.

257

means of localizing them in the intracranial cavity. All the dipoles in this figure are located close to the O_z position, but most of them are tilted toward the parietal area (P_z, P_2, P_4). This accounts for the larger amplitude potentials in the parietal area.

Due to shortness of time, only one figure from the second subject will be presented. This subject is a left-handed male of 26 years of age with normal vision. He had a primary response of the same latency and peak latency as the first subject. The same similarity between contralateral and lower half field responses held, being opposite to the upper half field and ipsilateral responses. Like the first subject, the primary response was followed by a potential of opposite polarity, but this subject's latencies for the following components were shorter and he tended to have an extra component during the 200 msec analysis time. The equipotential contour maps for the primary response for this subject are presented in Fig. 6. Some differences in the orientation of the dipoles from the first subject are apparent. This subject had mainly radial potential distributions for the quadrant fields whereas the first subject had some tangential dipoles. Although not shown directly here, the locations of these dipoles were close to O_z, with the exception of the lower left quadrant. This subject's dipoles were mostly directed radially toward O_z or slightly above, while for the first

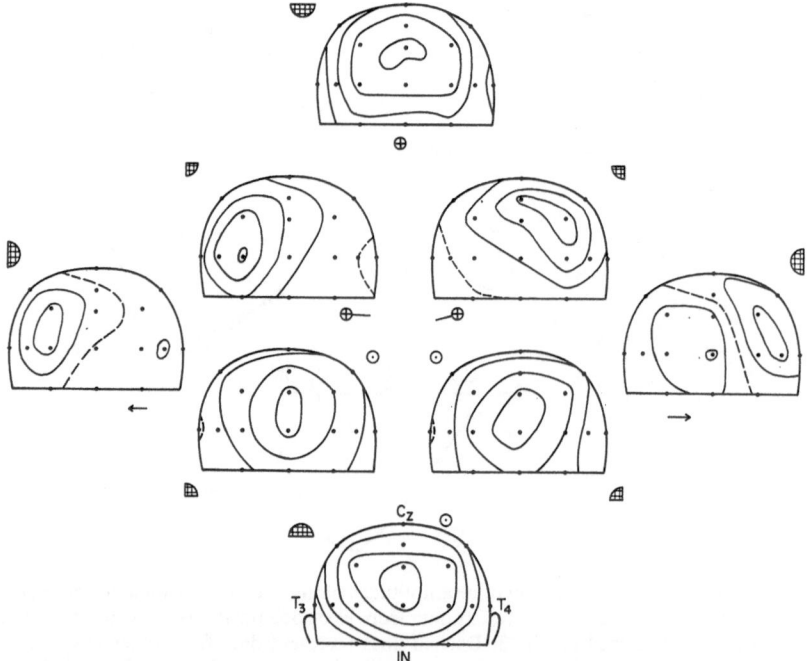

Fig. 6. Equipotential contour maps for the evoked response amplitudes 50-84 msec, subject D, to half field and quadrant-field stimulation. Posterior views of scalp with dots at electrode positions (as in Fig. 3). Adjacent to each map is a symbol representing the orientation and type of the equivalent dipole.

subject they tended to be oriented toward the parietal area.

Despite these minor differences, the summations of the quadrants still produced tangential distributions for the lateral half fields and radial dipoles for the vertical half fields, similar to the results for the first subject. Opposing half field distributions were also reversed in polarity as before. Other negative electrode positions did not significantly change the results.

The results of this investigation suggest that this primary response peaking at 80-85 msec, from stimulation of quadrant and half-fields, is probably localized in the geniculocalcarine pathways or primary visual cortex, although the analysis is not complete as yet. This and other studies have now well established reliable differences in the visual evoked response from stimulation of various areas of the visual field (COBB & MORTON, REGAN & HERON). Differences in obtained waveforms and probable cortical localizations were obtained here than in other similar studies (JEFFREYS & AXFORD, MICHAEL & HALLIDAY).

ACKNOWLEDGMENT

The author wishes to thank JAMES COX, BRUCE DRUM, JAMES ARY, WILLIAM BELL, and DENNIS TONDRYK for their assistance in this research.

REFERENCES

BIERSDORF, W. R. & NAKAMURA, Z. Localization studies of the human visual evoked response. Xth ISCERG Symposium, Doc. Ophth. Proc. Ser. 2: *137-144* (1973).

COBB, W. A. & MORTON, H. B. Evoked potentials from the human scalp to visual half field stimulation. *J. Physiol.* 208: *39-P* (1970).

JEFFREYS, D. A. & AXFORD, J. G. Source locations of pattern-specific components of human visual evoked potentials. *Exp. Brain Res.* 16: *1* (1972).

MICHAEL, W. F. & HALLIDAY, A. M. Differences between the occipital distribution of upper and lower field pattern-evoked responses in man. *Brain Res.* 32: *311* (1971).

NAKAMURA, Z. & BIERSDORF. W. R. Localization of the human visual evoked response. Early components specific to visual stimulation. *Amer. J. Ophth.* 72: *988* (1971).

REGAN, D. & HERON, J. R. Clinical investigation of lesions of the visual pathway: a new objective technique. *J. Neurol. Neurosurg. Psychiat.* 32: *479* (1969).

Author's address:

Ohio State University
Columbus
Ohio
USA

CONTRIBUTION OF THE CENTRAL AND THE PERIPHERAL PART OF THE RETINA TO THE VECP UNDER PHOTOPIC CONDITIONS

Y. OGUCHI & G. H. M. VAN LITH

(Rotterdam)

ABSTRACT

It is a moot point if the retinal periphery contributes substantially to the VECPs. Outside the central retinal area no reasonable cortical potentials can be obtained with localized stimuli. In the experiments described here, the total retina and the whole retinal periphery have been stimulated. Three kinds of responses were observed: a positive foveal potential, a negative para- and perifoveal one and some small peripheral potentials. As to the peaktimes of these various components inter-individual variations occur.

INTRODUCTION

The visually evoked cortical potentials (VECPs) are derived mainly from the cone system, and particularly from the cones of the central part of the retina (VAN HOF et al., 1960; RIETVELD et al., 1965; DE VOE et al., 1968). Inside a 5° eccentricity from the fovea, the height of the VECP made under photopic conditions appears to be dependent on the cone density, whereas outside this 5° eccentricity the height of the VECP suddenly decreases (VAN LITH & HENKES, 1970). This may partly be due to the decrease in the cone density, the convergence of the extrafoveal cones into the ganglion cells, but possibly mainly to the localization of the retinal projection in the area striata (VAN HOF et al., 1966). As the number of cones in the fovea is about 100.000 and the total number of cones is more than 4×10^6 (POLYAK, 1941), the total retina contains 40 times that of the fovea. From this point of view, a recordable VECP may be expected, if at least a large part of the retinal periphery will be stimulated. This idea is supported by the observation that in patients with a central scotoma through an optic neuritis, showing no photopic VECPs with local central stimulation, reasonable VECPs may occur with total stimulation.

The example presented in Figure 1, shows no VECPs with an 8° local stimulation. With total stimulation there are small but reasonable VECPs. That they are small may be understood, as the visual loss includes the center of the visual field and three quadrants. We simulated such a condition by stimulating with a 20° field, and failed to obtain recordable VECPs. Therefore, we have now attempted to stimulate the retina, the center excluded.

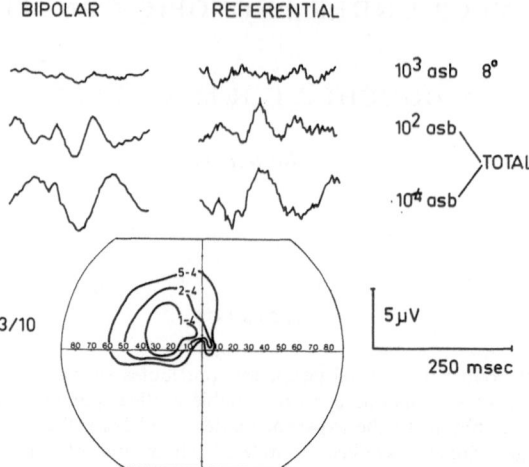

Fig. 1. VECPs of a patient with an optic neuritis Bipolar lead BD, referential lead CE (see Figure 2). 8° foveal and total retinal stimulation under photopic conditions (For stimulus conditions see VAN LITH & HENKES, 1968).

METHOD

The experiments were carried out with a ball stimulator, with which both adaptation light and test light could be presented to the whole visual field (VAN LITH et al., 1973). For the purpose of the present study, a hole was made in the posterior part of the hemisphere of the ball so that the central part of the retina was not illuminated by adaptation light and test light. The hole, subtending a visual angle of 5°, 10° or 20°, could be illuminated by a separate adaptation light, independent of the adaptation light of the hemisphere. With and without hole the inner side of the hemisphere had an adaptive illumination of 2.5 log asb, whereas the adaptive illumination of the hole was 4.9 log asb. A small green patch of 1 mm diameter served as a fixation point. The stimulus was a xenon flash of 1 Joule, the illumination of which could be lowered with neutral density filters in steps of 0.5 log unit. The frequency used was 4 flashes per second. We compared peripheral stimulation using a central hole with total stimulation.

We started our experiments with a dark hole. Subjectively and objectively, however, stray light was conspicuous. The flicker stimulus could be seen in the hole, moreover clear differences in the VECPs between total and peripheral stimulation could not be observed. The size of the hole made practically no difference at all. Therefore, all subsequent experiments were carried out with the strong steady illumination of 4.9 log asb in the hole.

After amplification (time constant 3 sec, no high frequency filter) 1050 responses were averaged on a CAT-computer and recorded with an X-Y plotter

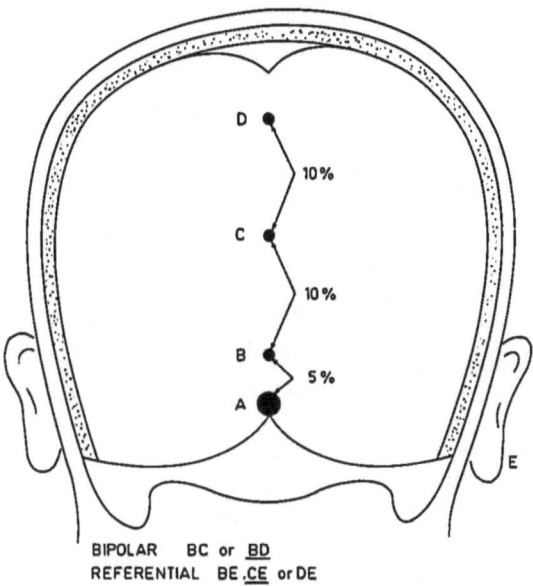

BIPOLAR   BC or BD
REFERENTIAL   BE .CE or DE

Fig. 2. Position of the electrodes.

and a polaroid camera. One bipolar lead over the occipital lobe and three monopolar occipital leads referential to the ear were used. The position of the electrodes and the derivations are shown in Figure 2. The experiments were carried out with 7 normal subjects. Only one eye was stimulated. The pupils of the subjects were always dilated artificially with Mydriaticum.

RESULTS

Three subjects could not properly fix the center of the strong illuminated hole during the averaging time, which was more than 4 minutes. In another subject, the VECPs were too small for further evaluation after total stimulation. The results obtained from these 4 subjects will not be taken into account. The recordings of 2 subjects will be shown in this paper (Figures 3 to 6). Findings in the remaining subject did not essentially differ.

Figures 3 and 4 represent the recordings of subjet YO, obtained with total retinal stimulation and with peripheral stimulation. The peaks in the beginning of each recording are stimulus artifacts. The luminance of the stimulus, represented by the figures between the recordings, was lowered until the responses vanished. In Figure 3 the monopolar derivation BE is shown, in Figure 4 the monopolar derivation DE (compare Figure 2). In both figures, the VECPs regularly decrease, if the stimulus luminance is lowered. With the highest luminance (relative luminance 0), we see a positive peak with a peak time of 102.8

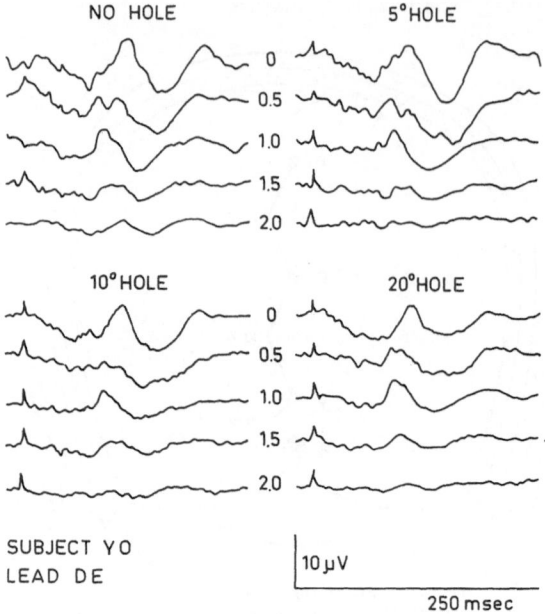

NO HOLE   5°HOLE

0
0.5
1.0
1.5
2.0

10°HOLE   20°HOLE

0
0.5
1.0
1.5
2.0

SUBJECT YO
LEAD DE

10 µV

250 msec

Fig. 3. VECPs (monopolar lead BE) from normal subject YO, obtained with total retinal stimulation and peripheral stimulation using the illuminated holes. The figures between the recordings stand for the relative luminance of the test light.

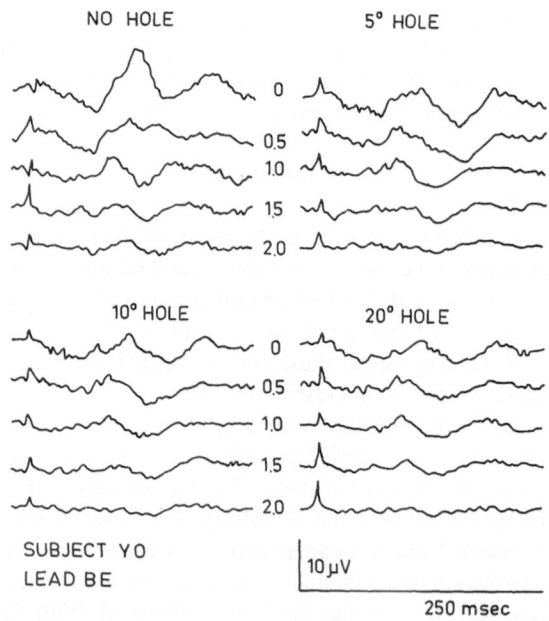

NO HOLE   5° HOLE

0
0.5
1.0
1.5
2.0

10° HOLE   20° HOLE

0
0.5
1.0
1.5
2.0

SUBJECT YO
LEAD BE

10 µV

250 msec

Fig. 4. VECPs (monopolar lead DE) from normal subject YO.

264

msec, a negative wave with a peak time of 133.6 msec and again a small positive wave a peak time of 183.4 msec. It is striking that the first high positive peak is suddenly reduced, going from total stimulation to peripheral stimulation, independent of the size of the hole. This is more marked in Figure 4 than in Figure 3. The negative wave decreases regularly according to the size of the hole. Figure 3 shows this more clearly. As the stimulus luminances decrease, the peak time of the negative wave is reduced.

With the low luminances (0.5, 1.0, 1.5), some small positive and negative waves are obtained. These waves are fairly independent of the size of the hole and also independent of the stimulus luminance.

Apparently, a contradiction exists when the bipolar derivation of Figure 5 is compared to the monopolar derivation of the preceding figures. The positive wave in Figures 5 decreases gradually as the size of the hole increases, while in Figures 3 and 4 the positive wave decreases suddenly. However, we have to consider the bipolar derivation BD as the difference between the monopolar leads BE and DE in Figures 3 and 4. The positive peak in Figure 5 has a peak time of 133.6 msec. Therefore, it is relative to the gradually decreasing negative waves of the monopolar leads of Figures 3 and 4 and not to the positive peaks in the latter figures. As the first positive peaks of the monopolar derivations BE and DE are almost the same, there is only a small wave left in the bipolar derivation BD.

In the other two subjects, comparable results have been obtained. The high

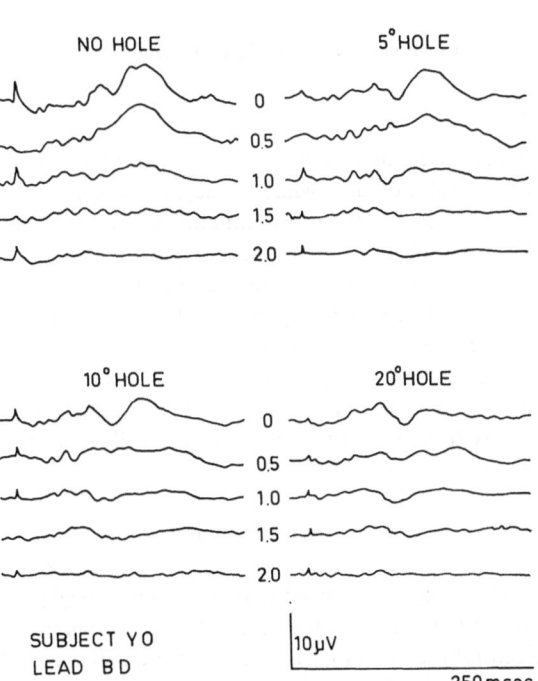

Fig. 5. VECPs (biopolar lead BD) from normal subject YO.

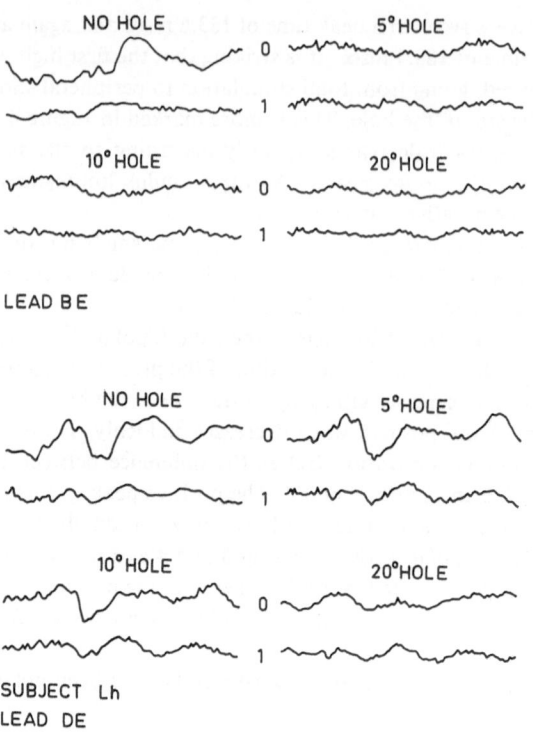

Fig. 6. VECPs (monopolar leads BE and DE) from normal subject Lh.

positive responses after total stimulation with high illumination decreased suddenly in peripheral stimulation, while the negative wave decreased gradually in these subjects. In addition, with low stimulus luminances, total and peripheral retinal stimulation did not show differences (Figure 6).

One marked difference was obtained between the subjects YO and Lh. This becomes apparent if we compare Figures 4 and 6, derivation DE. In subject YO, the gradually decreasing negative waves (a peak time 133.6 msec) are situated behind the suddenly decreasing positive wave (a peak time 102.8 msec). In subject Lh, the negative wave is prior to the positive peak. In the latter subject the negative wave has a peak time of 89.9 msec, while that of the positive wave is 132.7 msec.

DISCUSSION

From the results it may be assumed that stray light is negligible when the high adaptive illumination is used in the holes. If after peripheral stimulation, stray light on the central area takes part in the response, all waves should be higher in experiments with the 5° hole than in those with the 10° or 20° hole. This, however, is only the case with the negative wave. Moreover, the subject did

266

not see any flickering light in the holes, not even with the highest stimulus luminance and smallest hole. In the preliminary experiments without adaptive illumination, i.e. using the dark holes, stray light effects were obvious. The larger the holes, the smaller the response. Perhaps stray light effects were not fully suppressed in the experiments of EASON et al., (1967) and OHBA (1967). They obtained VECPs with a 1° stimulus field even at 40° to 50° from the fovea.

As the high positive peak suddenly decreases, going from total retinal stimulation to peripheral stimulation with the 5° hole, this peak seems to be a reflection of only a 5° central retinal area. The negative wave, decreasing gradually, should then be originating in the para- and perifoveal part of the retina. Since the small waves are almost independent of the size of the hole, they may be assumed to represent a true peripheral response. For several reasons they cannot be stray light responses from the central area. Clear differences in responses between total and peripheral retinal stimulation already occur at the highest stimulus luminance. Moreover, fixation was not more difficult with low test light luminance than with the highest. That poor fixation was not the case may also be deduced from the fact that these low luminance responses are the same with the 20° hole as with the 5° hole. An indication, that the periphery may actually contribute to the VECPs, has also been obtained by JACOBSON et al., (1968) in patients with severely constricted visual fields in two cases of retinitis pigmentosa.

Why in one subject the positive wave is positioned before the negative wave and in the other subject the reverse is seen, cannot yet be explained. It is possible that it is an interindividual variation. To solve this problem more subjects will have to be examined.

The experiments shown here are not in accordance with the findings in patients with a central scotoma. In these patients the VECPs with total retinal stimulation are generally higher than the VECPs found in the normal subjects with peripheral stimulation. An explanation may be, that in patients with a central scotoma some receptors always function within the area of the scotoma. This is not very likely, however, as some function within the scotoma has to be found in those cases psychophysically, too. The observations of FISHMAN & COPENHAVER (1967) do not support this explanation, either. They found normal VECPs with an 11° stimulation in unilateral macular diseases, although with a 3° stimulation the VECPs were lowered.

Another explanation may be, that when a VECP of the central retinal area is present, the peripheral responses are lowered. The question is whether the central part of the retina inhibits a VECP, originating in the para- and perifovea or in the periphery, or if the central VECPs cancel out the peripheral VECPs. The latter may be caused by the configuration of the area striata in the occipital lobe. An inhibition from the central retinal area to the perifoveal area was also suggested by VAN LITH & HENKES (1972), based on their VECP experiments with local stimulation under scotopic conditions.

FINKELSTEIN et al. (1969) pointed out that the contribution of the fovea to the VECP when the entire retina is stimulated, is not clear. Although the cortical representation of the fovea may be one hundred times that of the parafovea, the foveal contribution may represent only a small portion of the total response when the peripheral retina is stimulated in addition to the fovea. This appeared not to be the case in our experiments. The reason may be, that our results are not only based on the photopic condition, as the retinal illumination was aproximately 3000 scotopic trolands. According to AGUILAR & STILES (1954), the rod mechanism is effectively saturated with 2000 to 5000 scotopic trolands. Under scotopic conditions the peripheral contribution to the VECP may be higher. We performed some experiments in this direction, but we were confronted with stray light problems. Further experiments will have to be done.

REFECENCES

AGUILAR, M. & STILES, W. S. Saturation of the rod mechanism of the retina at high levels of stimulation. *Optica acta* 1: *59* (1954).

DE VOE, R. G., RIPPS, H. & VAUGHAN, JR. H. G. Cortical responses to stimulation of the human fovea. *Vision Res.* 8: *135-147* (1968).

EASON, R. G., D. ODEN. B. A. & WHITE, C. T. Visually evoked cortical potentials and reaction time in relation to site of retinal stimulation. *Electroenceph. Clin. Neurophysiol.* 12: *313-324* (1967).

FINKELSTEIN, D. & GOURAS, P. Visual Electrophysiology. An introduction to the ERG, EOG, ERP and VER. In: Electrical responses of the visual system; ed. by S. J. FRICKER, p. *857-881.* Boston, Little & Brown (1969).

FISHMAN, R. S. & COPENHAVER, R. M. Macular disease and amblyopia. *Arch. Ophthal.* 77: *718-725* (1967).

OHBA, N. Visual evoked responses in man by localized retinal stimulation. *Jap. J. Ophthal.* 11: *221-226* (1967).

POLYAK, S. L. The retina. p. 447-448. Chicago, University Press (1941).

RIETVELD, W. J., TORDOIR, W. E. M. & DUYFF, J. W. Contribution of fovea and parafovea to the visual evoked response. *Acta physiol. pharmacol. neerl.* 13: *330-339* (1965).

VAN HOF, M. W. Open-eye and closed-eye occipito-cortical response to photic stimulation of the retina. *Acta physiol. pharmacol. neerl.* 9: *443-451* (1960).

VAN HOF, M. W., VAN HOF-VAN DUIN, J. & RIETVELD, W. J. Enhancement of occipito-cortical responses to light flashes in man during attention. *Vision Res.* 6: *109-111* (1966).

VAN LITH, G. H. M. & HENKES, H. E. The local electric response of the central retinal area. In: Advances in electrophysiology and -pathology of the visual system; Proc. 6th ISCERG Symp., Erfurt 1967; ed. by E. SCHMÖGER, p. 163-170. Leipzig, Thieme (1968).

VAN LITH, G. H. M. & HENKES, H. E. The relationship between ERG and VER. *Ophthal. Res.* 1: *40-47* (1970).

VAN LITH, G. H. M. & HENKES, H. E. Local scotopic responses in ERG and VER. In: The visual system: Neurophysiology, Biophysics, and their clinical applications; Proc. 9th ISCERG Symp., Brighton 1971; ed. by G. B. ARDEN, p. 237-247. New York, Plenum Press (1972).

VAN LITH, G. H. M., MEININGER, J. & VAN MARLE, G. W. Electrophysiological equipment for total and local retinal stimulation; Proc. 10th ISCERG Symp., Los Angeles 1972; ed. by J. T. PEARLMAN, p. 213-218. Den Haag, Junk (1973).

Authors' address:

Eye Hospital
Erasmus University
Rotterdam
The Netherlands

268

STIMULUS AND VISUALLY EVOKED POTENTIAL

H. SPEKREIJSE & L. H. VAN DER TWEEL

(Amsterdam)

INTRODUCTION

The application of evoked potentials (EP's) to the study of the human visual system is based on a number of assumptions which, however, are not always stated explicitly. The first, seemingly trivial, point concerns the assumption of a sensible relation between at least the amplitude of the evoked response and stimulus strength. Since there is fast growing evidence that the visual system treats various stimuli in a different way depending on their characteristic features, one should be quite certain that only *one* feature dominates before even trying to establish a relation between response amplitude and stimulus strength. For example, in the study of contrast EP's firm grounds are needed to exclude contributions due to local luminance changes (SPEKREIJSE, V.D. TWEEL, ZUIDEMA, 1973; PADMOS, HAAIJMAN, SPEKREIJSE, 1973); in the study of EP's to changes in binocularly perceived depth control, experiments are essential to exclude contributions due to displacement of the retinal images across one or both retinae (REGAN & SPEKREIJSE, 1970). Of course, if there were a linear relation between response amplitude and any of the stimulus features, 'cleanness' of stimulus may not be so important, though it will be difficult to untangle which stimulus parameter is relevant for which part of the response. However, as soon as a nonlinear relation exists the stimulus-response plot may even become ambiguous.

This was one of the main reasons for the use of large homogeneous sine wave modulated stimulus fields in our former studies of luminance processing in man (V.D. TWEEL & VERDUYN LUNEL, 1965; SPEKREIJSE & V.D. TWEEL, 1972). With such stimulus fields there is the implicit assumption that lateral interactions are not of first importance. In this paper evidence will be presented that this assumption needs further consideration.

On the other hand, with respect to spatial contrast processing we have stressed the importance of employing stimuli in which the total luminance flux remains constant in time (SPEKREIJSE, 1966; V.D. TWEEL & SPEKREIJSE, 1968). Yet, the luminance modulation per spatial element (check, bar, etc.) may in itself contribute to the response. This problem is not academic, since we could demonstrate, for example, that most if not all of the ERG's to high spatial contrast reversal can be considered as the net result of the addition of responses to luminance increase and decrease, as occurs simultaneously in the two sets of spatial elements (SPEKREIJSE, ESTÉVEZ & V.D. TWEEL, 1973).

It has been hammered – also at ISCERG meetings – that small signal analysis is a safe technique in that it avoids complications due to nonlinear behaviour and especially saturation. Fig. 1 illustrates, however, that the application of small signals is not an absolute guarantee after all. Let us consider the problem of obtaining a constant response or threshold setting for the hypothetical situation of Fig. 1. The compression caused by the saturation element has the result that the amplitude of the stimulus must increase more than proportional to frequency as would be the case for a single RC element. This results in a steeper high frequency fall-off. Hence, static saturation can give an erroneous dynamic characteristic even when a small signal technique is used. Actually, this is because one is fooled by the signal as measured at the output; the input does not fulfil the small signal requirements. On the other hand, large signals can sometimes provide information about dynamic behaviour up to the saturating element. In this paper the usefulness of such a saturation analysis will be illustrated for both luminance and spatial contrast processing in man. The result of this analysis suggests separate colour coded contrast channels, branching off from the luminance channel before colour interaction occurs (REGAN, 1972). The latter seems to account to a large extent for the low frequency attenuation found both in evoked response and psychophysical studies.

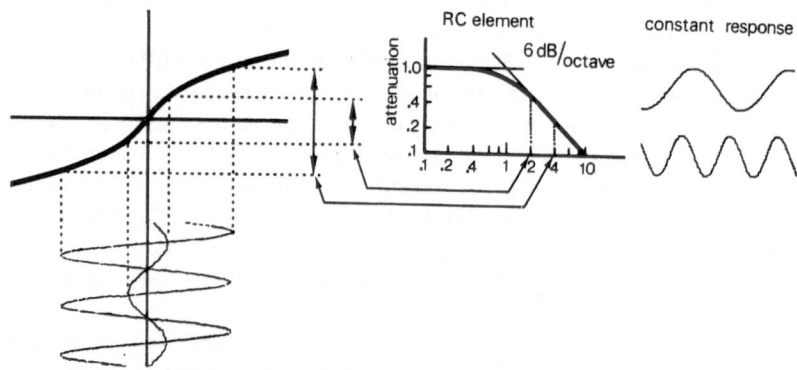

Fig. 1. Example of a nonlinear system for which the constant response method will give erroneously a steeper high frequency fall-off than can be attributed to a single RC-element.

SATURATION IN LUMINANCE EP'S

It is a commonly accepted notion in physiology that a logarithmic relation holds between stimulus strength and neural activity, but our EP data to high frequency luminance modulation show that at first the response grows linearly with modulation depth (Fig. 2) and above a certain modulation starts to flatten (Fig. 3) (SPEKREIJSE, 1966). Since for low modulation depths response ampli-

270

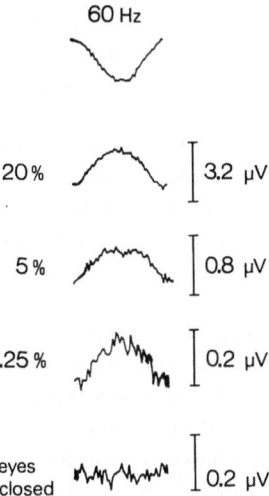

Fig. 2. Visually evoked responses to a white, 60 Hz sine wave modulated 20° field detected by electrodes on the midline (inion-vertex derivation). The number of summations was taken inversely proportional to the modulation depth. Even down to 1.25% modulation the amplitude of the response remains proportional to modulation depth. The luminance of the stimulus field seen in Maxwellian view was 10.000 asb.

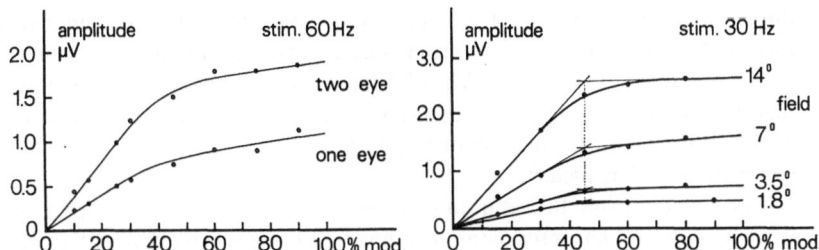

Fig. 3. Amplitude of the VER as a function of modulation depth in case of one and two eye stimulation (left hand graph) and for various sizes of the stimulus field (right hand graph). The left hand data give the amplitude of the fundamental component and the right hand data that of the second harmonic. The mean luminance of the stimulus field was 10.000 asb. The pupils were dilated.

tude grows proportionally with stimulus strength, we prefer to describe the flattening of the response curve by the mathematically noncommittal term saturation.

The left hand data of Fig. 3 give the amplitude of the visual evoked response (VER) as a function of modulation depth of a 60 Hz sine wave modulated 20° field in the case of one and two eye stimulation. Since in both situations saturation becomes evident at the same modulation depth, and since the saturation does not depend on stimulus field size (right hand Fig. 3), the saturation must be assumed to occur early in the visual system and certainly at a site preceding the binocular interaction. From the tacit assumption that early lateral interactions can be neglected in homogeneous field stimulation, it would follow that this saturation will be an individual property of the parallel signal processing channels.

Since there are indications that the saturation is frequency independent (static), the dependence of saturation on stimulus frequency can provide information about distal dynamic processing. If, for example, high frequency attenuation occurs preceding the saturating element, then the saturation point will be reached at higher modulation depth for increasing stimulus frequency. The data of Fig. 4 show that the VER in man saturates at increasingly higher modulation depths for stimulus frequencies below and above 30 Hz, indicating that preceding the saturation per channel, low and high frequency attenuation occurs. It should be noted that this conclusion can be drawn only from the dependence of saturation point on stimulus frequency and *not* from the actual size of the response. In the latter also dynamic processing is reflected which occurs *after* the saturation and which accounts for the fact that the response to 60 Hz stimulation is larger than to, for example, 43 Hz.

If the modulation depths at which saturation occurs are plotted as a function of stimulus frequency, one gets the amplitude characteristic depicted in the left hand of Fig. 5. This amplitude characteristic resembles the psychophysical flicker fusion curves or modulation transfer function (MTF) plots, except for the more shallow high frequency fall-off. Such curves can also be obtained directly from the spike discharge patterns evoked by sinusoidal luminance modulation in single lateral genicule cells of macaque monkey (SPEKREIJSE, v. NORREN & v.D. BERG, 1971). The plotting of the modulation depths required to reach an arbitrary threshold criterion as a function of stimulus frequency resulted in the right hand curve of Fig. 5. The overall similarity between both curves of Fig. 5 is evident.

To conclude: From the saturation of the VER in man to high frequency sine wave modulated light information can be gained about early dynamic charac-

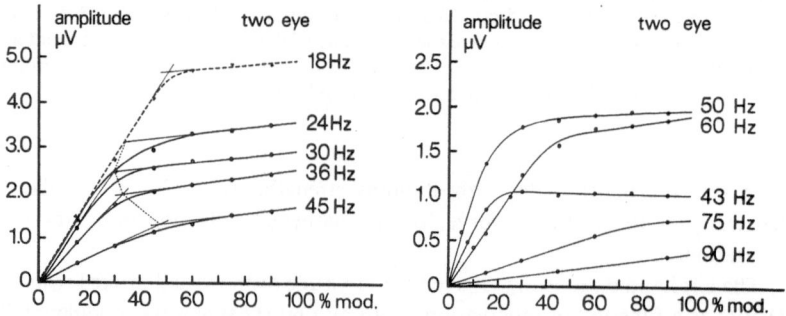

Fig. 4. Saturation of the VER as a function of the frequency of a sine wave modulated 20° Maxwellian field. The mean luminance was 10.000 asb; the pupils were dilated. The left hand data give the amplitude of the second harmonic and the right hand ones that of the fundamental component in the response. For clarity the saturation curve to the 18 Hz stimulus is doubled in amplitude.

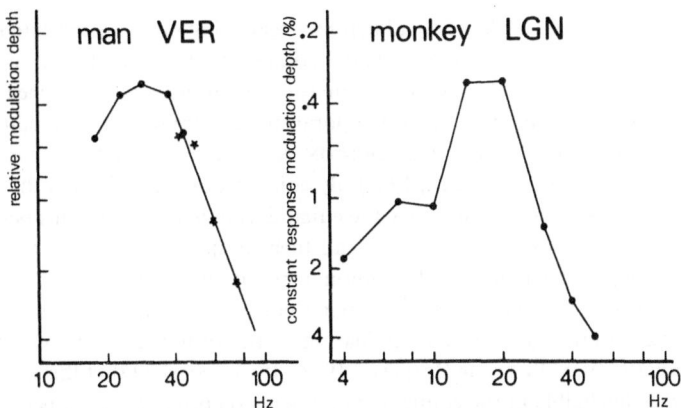

Fig. 5. Amplitude characteristics of distal dynamic processing in man (left side) and monkey (right side). The left hand data are derived from Fig. 4 by plotting the modulation depths at which saturation becomes evident as a function of stimulus frequency. The curve comprises two sets of data: for the frequency range of 18 Hz to 45 Hz the saturation of the second harmonic is used, and for frequencies above 43 Hz the fundamental data are employed. Since the modulation depth at which saturation becomes evident depends on the actual size of the fundamental and second harmonic components at the input of the saturating element, the two sets of data may be shifted along the vertical axis. This is done so that the saturation data of 43 Hz and 45 Hz coincide. The luminance of the binocularly presented 20° stimulus field seen in Maxwellian view was 10.000 asb. The pupils were dilated. The right hand data represent the amplitude characteristics of a yellow$^-$–blue$^+$ LGN cell in macaque monkey determined with blue sinusoidally modulated light at a retinal illumination of 480 troland. This amplitude characteristic is obtained by plotting the modulation depth required for each stimulus frequency to reach a constant response criterion. The Maxwellian field subtended 15°.

teristics. These characteristics exhibit both low and high frequency attenuation and resemble the characteristics that under comparable conditions can be obtained from single cells in the lateral geniculate of monkey, but also from linearizing experiments in man and goldfish (v.D. TWEEL & SPEKREIJSE, 1969; SPEKREIJSE, 1969).

SATURATION IN SPATIAL CONTRAST EP'S

Up till now VER's were presented to stimulus conditions in which lateral interactions were assumed to be of less importance. Now EP's to changes in spatial contrast will be described. These responses are thought to reflect especially lateral interactions. Hence great pains should be taken that they are not contaminated by the responses to a correlated change in average luminance. To overcome this problem we employ a method of spatial contrast stimulation in which the total luminance flux remains constant in time. For a checkerboard pattern – the spatial configuration which we prefer in our experiments – the constant luminance flux criterion can be fulfilled by counterphase modulation of the two sets of checks at equal depths. Depending on the mean intensities of the two sets of checks different spatial stimuli can be generated. In case both sets of checks have the same mean intensity, the bright and dark checks interchange rhythmically at twice the temporal stimulus frequency. This condition is called *pattern reversal* (RIGGS, JOHNSON & SCHICK, 1964; SPEKREIJSE, 1966; COBB, MORTON & ETTLINGER, 1967). By adjusting the intensities of the two sets of checks in such a way that they are equal during half the stimulus period, the checkerboard pattern first appears and then disappears to leave a blank field once during each stimulus cycle. Although also in this *appearance-disappearance* situation the total luminance flux remains constant, yet the luminance modulation per check may cause contamination of the response, as discussed before (SPEKREIJSE, V.D. TWEEL & ZUIDEMA, 1973). It was checked that this contamination was negligible in the contrast experiments reported in this paper.

Fig. 6 shows that in the appearance-disappearance condition an increase in contrast from 6% to 20% and even 60% does not change the response much, indicating directly that also for this stimulus saturation takes place. Moreover, as can clearly be seen from this figure, the appearance response differs from that to disappearance. Considering our starting point that it is preferable to isolate the different signal processing systems by means of a relevant choice of stimulus conditions, and in view of the fact that the disappearance response originates from a different cortical population (ESTÉVEZ & SPEKREIJSE, 1974) we

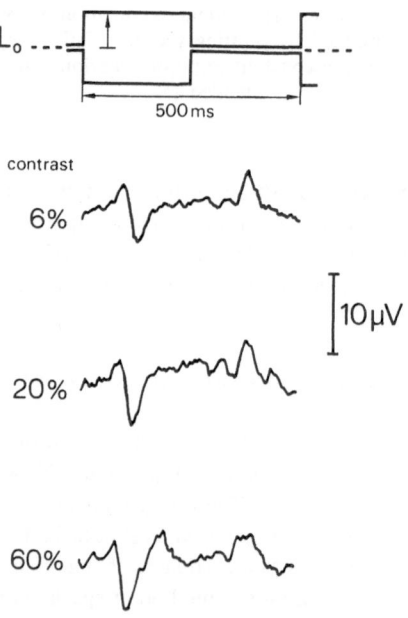

Fig. 6. Occipital responses (inion-ear derivation) to an appearing-disappearing checkerboard with 20' checks as a function of contrast. Mean luminance is 5000 asb; binocular presentation.

prefer abruptly changing patterns at low presentation rates. Since we could show that the pattern reversal response is an unpredictable mixture of both appearance and disappearance components, the appearance-disappearance stimulus was preferred in most of our experiments.

It is well known that under favourable conditions the responses may saturate even at low contrasts. This observation may present an explanation for the following two experimental findings.

Firstly: an initial contrast can reduce considerably the response to a subsequent increase in contrast. Secondly: contrasty steady lines on the edges of an appearing-disappearing checkerboard also suppress the response. These two phenomena are presented in Fig. 7 and 8. Fig. 7 shows that the response to the appearance of a 20% contrast checkerboard is strongly reduced if instead of an initial blank field, at all times a 10% contrast checkerboard is present. Fig. 8 shows that irrespective of the luminance of the lines, steady lines with 20% contrast positioned on the edges of an appearing-disappearing checkerboard are sufficient to halve the responses to a 20% contrast change. In the context of saturation, the size of the response to an increase in contrast can to a first approximation be predicted from the responses to a real appearance of a pattern, if it is assumed that the initial contrast sets the system at a starting point, which is equal to the size of the response to the appearance of a pattern with the same contrast. Hence, as is shown in Fig. 9 a given increase in contrast will elicit a

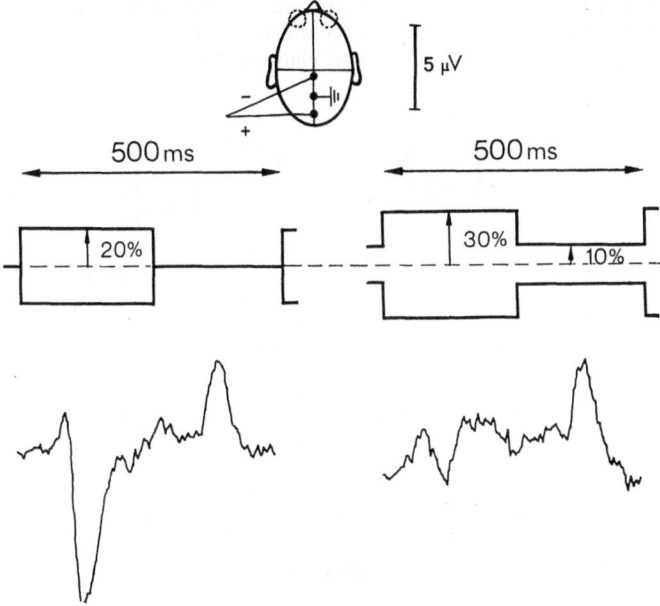

Fig. 7. Occipital response to an appearing-disappearing checkerboard (20' checks) of 20% contrast (left side) and to the same checkerboard but with a contrast varied between 10 and 30%. The response to the increase in contrast is strongly affected by the standing contrast. Mean luminance is 5000 asb; binocular presentation.

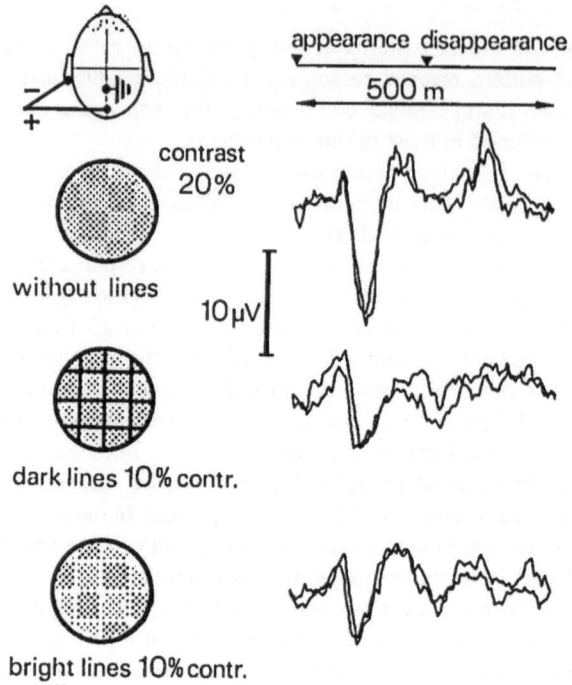

Fig. 8. Steady contrast (20%) lines of 1' on the edges of an appearing-disappearing checkerboard (20' checks) of 20% contrast are sufficient to halve the contrast EPs. Note that this effect is the same irrespective whether the lines are bright or dark. Mean luminance is 5000 asb; binocular presentation.

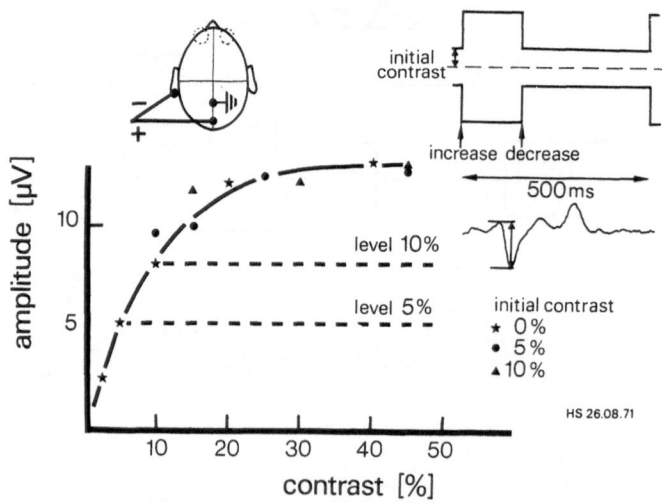

Fig. 9. Amplitude of the appearance response (see insert) as a function of contrast for three levels of initial contrasts of 0%, 5% and 10% respectively. To a first approximation the responses can be described by addition; the initial contrast sets the baseline. Mean luminance in 5000 asb; binocular presentation; the checkerboard with 15' checks subtended 3° of visual angle.

276

smaller response the larger the initial contrast, since the response to the appearance of a pattern saturates. The results obtained with the bright and dark steady lines can be explained by the same mechanism, but apparently the effectiveness of the contrast for reducing the response is the largest if the lines are positioned on the edges. This is also an argument for the true contrast origin of the appearance response. If, however, the steady contrasts are too strong the suppressing effect depends less on the position of the lines.

In Fig. 9 response amplitude is plotted against contrast increase on linear scales. CAMPBELL & MAFFEI (1970), using 8 Hz sine wave gratings, discovered that if the amplitude of the response is plotted against contrast on a logarithmic scale a straight line can be obtained that extrapolates to psychophysical threshold. Our results (Fig. 10) confirm such a relation, but hold over a rather restricted range of contrasts and the correlation with psychophysics is more variable. To our surprise we found that subliminal steady contrasts can enhance the response to the appearance of a pattern. This can be explained as follows. The larger response is obtained (right side Fig. 10) because the initial contrast takes account for the 'dead zone' in the amplitude versus contrast curve. This dead zone occurs because at low luminance levels the to zero extrapolated response curve crosses the horizontal axis at higher contrast. This seeming enhancement of the response by small initial contrasts is in accordance with the psychophysical findings of SHAPLEY & TOLHURST (1973).

Both the reduction of response by high and the enhancement by small initial contrasts imply that a steady contrast is not subject to appreciable adaptation. From this follows the important conclusion that to a first approximation the contrast channels do not exhibit low frequency attenuation.

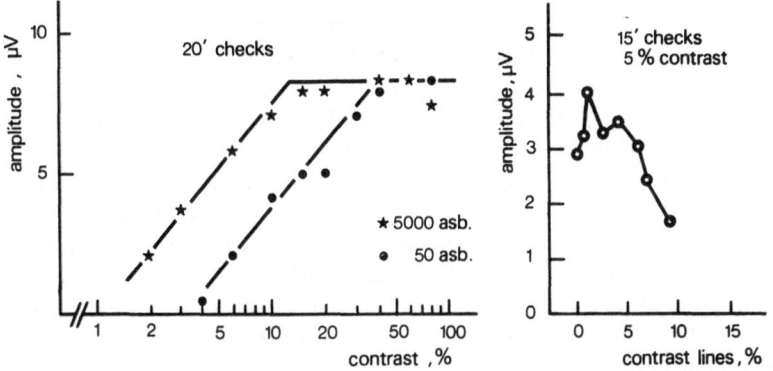

Fig. 10. left side: Amplitude of the appearance response (see insert Fig. 9) as a function of contrast for two levels of retinal illumination. For low contrasts the response to the appearance of a 3° checkerboard with 20' checks seems to increase logarithmically with contrast; saturation becomes evident at lower contrasts the higher the mean luminance. right side: Initial enhancement of the response (inion vertex derivation) to the appearance of a 5% contrast checkerboard with 15' checks by low contrast 'bright' lines (1.2') positioned at the edges of the checks.

Plainly on the basis of the amplitude of the visually evoked potential versus contrast or luminance curves we have reached the conclusion that the luminance channels exhibit low frequency attenuation or adaptation, whereas steady contrasts keep their effectiveness. These results are not surprising considering the functioning of the visual system. The reasoning seems straightforward and the EP data qualitatively in accordance with perception. However, if one wants to make a simple model to account for the two sets of data, we do not feel so confident.

Because of individual functioning of the cones themselves, luminance is the first parameter to be coded and there is no possibility for the contrast system working beforehand. Therefore, there must be a branching somewhere along the visual pathway. Although theoretically other constructions are possible, the most sensible place for this would be at a site preceding the low frequency attenuation exhibited in the luminance channels. In principle such a construction is not unrealistic, since firstly, at receptor and horizontal cell level no low frequency attenuations have been observed (TOMITA, KANEKO, MURAKAMI, PAULTER, 1967; SPEKREIJSE & NORTON, 1970) and secondly, at retinal ganglion cell level low frequency attenuation has been shown to take place after spatial summation (SCHELLART & SPEKREIJSE, 1972).

Spatial interaction does not automatically imply lateral interaction such as the well-known center-surround organization (KUFFLER, 1953; RODIECK & STONE, 1965). There is another type of antagonistic coding namely the colour coding (WAGNER, MACNICHOL & WOLBARSHT, 1960). We have psychophysical evidence that the low frequency attenuation in luminance processing is to a large extent due to interactions between colour coded channels (ESTÉVEZ & SPEKREIJSE, 1974). This finding can best be understood as follows: Suppose that in the human visual system only two cone populations are active, as might be the case for wavelengths longer than 500 nm. Suppose next that these populations with action spectra as depicted in Fig. 11 are stimulated with a patch of light consisting only of wavelengths λ_1 and λ_2 with identical intensities I_1 and I_2. If the wavelengths are so chosen that the sensitivities g_1 and g_2 of the hypothetical green spectral sensitivity curve are equal then alternation of the two monochromatic beams will cause no change in the effective quantum catch per unit of time in this cone population. However, the red cone population will perceive the stimulus as a modulated beam with an effective modulation proportional to the difference of r_1 and r_2. Hence by modulating I_1 and I_2 equally in counterphase, cone population R can be stimulated while keeping the input to cone population G constant.

With this paradigm it is possible to stimulate the human red and green cone populations with different ratios of modulation depths at constant average intensity. Fig. 12 gives the result of such an experiment carried out at two illumination levels (1250 troland for the left and 1.25 troland for the right hand figure). Whereas the shape and position of the high frequency branch of the flicker fusion curve remains constant in accordance with the

278

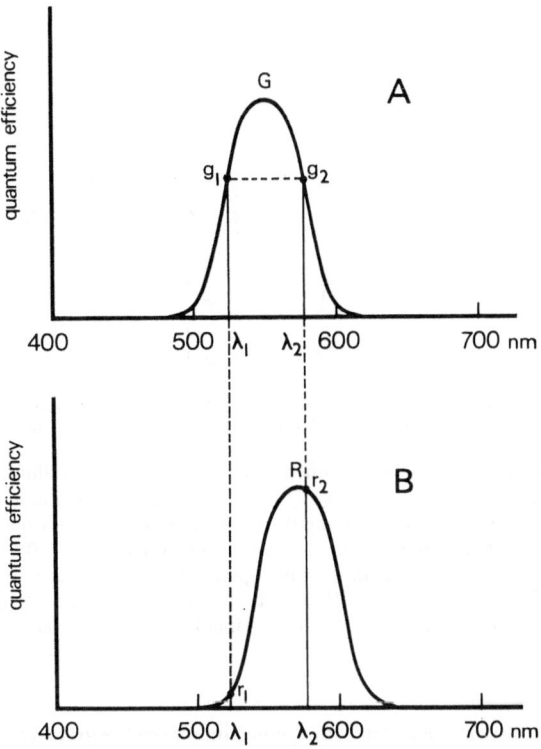

Fig. 11. Schematic presentation of the spectral weights of two monochromatic beams with wavelengths λ_1 and λ_2 respectively. The wavelengths are chosen in such a way that the weights in the hypothetical G(reen) absorption spectrum are equal ($g_1 = g_2$). Necessarily the weights in a different absorption spectrum, such as the hypothetical R(ed) one of Fig. 11B, are not identical ($r_1 \neq r_2$). With the two beams modulated equally in counter phase the quantum catch of system A remains constant, whereas that of system B will be modulated. Both absorption spectra and stimulus intensities are given in quantum efficiency units.

constant intensity used, the low frequency slope increased as the ratio of red to green modulation increased from zero (open triangles) through 0.5 (filled squares) to one (open squares). This means that low frequency attenuation is governed in first instance not by intensity, but by the ratio of red and green cone modulation.

These psychophysical findings have an immediate implication for the organization of the human contrast processing channels. Namely, there should be at least separate red and green coded *contrast* channels. This hypothesis has been verified and tested by a comparative EP study performed on a colour normal and deuteranope subject (REGAN & SPEKREIJSE, 1973). The results are presented in Fig. 13. In the experiment depicted in the upper half of Fig. 13 a given check remained red at all times and its neighbours green. The luminances of the red and green checks were square wave modulated in counterphase, so

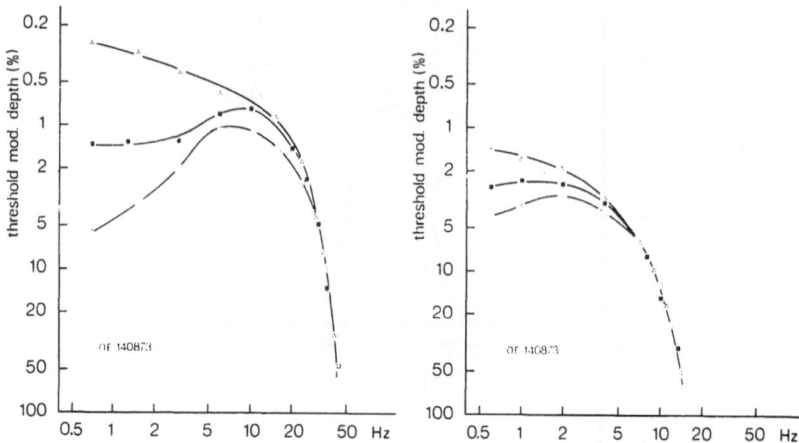

Fig. 12. Corrected MTF plots obtained at two levels of retinal illumination (1250 tld for the left hand and 1.25 tld for the right hand figure) as a function of ratio of effective red to green in phase modulation depth. The data indicated with open triangles were obtained with sole stimulation of the green cone system ($m_R = 0$), those with filled squares with $m_R = \frac{1}{2} m_g$ and those with open squares with $m_R = m_g$. The diameter of the artificial pupil was 3 mm. Wratten filters 25 (transmits wavelengths longer than 590 nm) and 58 (transmits maximally at 530 nm) were used.

that the instant the red check's luminance increased the green check's luminance decreased and vice versa. With photometrically equal luminances of the red and green checks this stimulus elicited in a deuteranopic subject EP's which closely resemble his contrast reversal EP's to black-white pattern-reversal. This, in contrast to the situation for the colour normal subject, where this stimulus gave no response at all. It should be noted that in this experiment pattern reversal is preferred because then an additional criterion, namely symmetry of response, can be used.

These data are in accordance with the concept that in subjects with normal colour vision the physiological signals elicited by the red and green checks remain segregated up to the contrast stage (REGAN, 1972). If, indeed, the red channels compare their outputs independently from the green channels, then the red channels see the 'green' checks as dark and the red checks as bright. Since steady contrasts bring the system into saturation no response and certainly no symmetrical one will be elicited. The same holds for the green contrast channel. Since the deuteranopic subject gives a symmetrical pattern reversal EP to this stimulus, his red and green channels – if present – should be completely fused.

To verify this notion the experiment depicted in the bottom half of Fig. 13. was performed. In this experiment each check was illuminated by the two photometrically equal red and green lights, so that a patternless yellow field was perceived. Next the luminances of the red and green lights were abruptly changed in opposite directions in each set of checks so that the yellow field changed in a

280

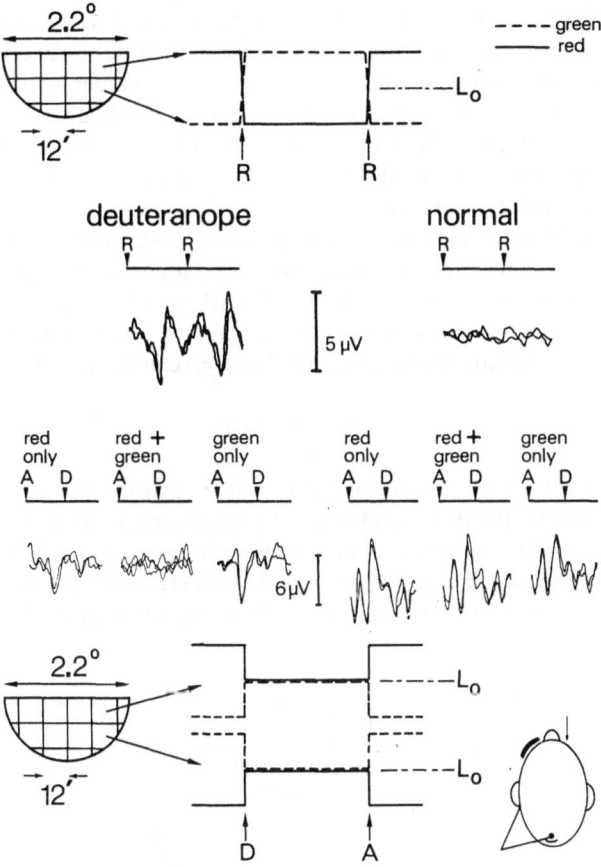

Fig. 13. Transient contrast EP's of a deuteranope (left column) and colour normal subject (right column) to a red-green checkerboard. In the upper half figure the colour of any given check did not change at any time, but its luminance was modulated as illustrated at the top of the figure. When the red and green checks were of equal luminance the deuteranope gave symmetrical pattern-reversal EP's whereas the normal subject gave no discernable EP's. Adjacent checks were modulated in counterphase at 1.85 Hz; mean luminance was 30 asb. The lower half figure shows that the appearance of a pattern of equiluminant red-green checks evoked clear responses for the colour-normal subject but evoked no responses for the deuteranope (compare 'red-green' traces). 'Red only' traces: the stimulus was the abrupt appearance of a pattern of red checks from a previously unpatterned red field. The same for the 'green only' traces. In both situations the total light flux did not change. 'Red-Green' traces: the stimulus was the appearance of a pattern of red and green checks from a previously unpatterned yellow field. There was no change in the net (red + green) luminance at *any* point of the field. The latter stimulus was formed by superposing the 'red only' stimulus upon the 'green only' stimulus as shown at the bottom of the figure. Pattern appearance is marked A and disappearance is marked D. The stimulation rate was 1.85 Hz, maximum contrast was 12% both for the red and green components of the pattern; mean luminance was 30 asb.

pattern of alternate red and green checks. At no time is there a change in net (red plus green) luminance at *any* point of the stimulus field. As can be seen the appearance of a red-green checkerboard gives in a colour normal subject a contrast EP (red + green trace) that does not markedly differ from the EP's elicited either by the red checks or green checks alone. On the other hand the deuteranope gives no recordable EP's to the appearance of a red-green checkerboard, as could be expected.

Both the flicker fusion data to homogeneously modulated coloured fields and the EP data to red-green checkerboard stimulation point to the concept of separate colour coded contrast channels branching off before the colour interaction occurs. The colour interaction accounts to a large extent for the low frequency attenuation found both in EP and psychophysical studies.

CONCLUSION

In this paper we have pointed out that EP studies indicate that the human visual system handles stimuli in a different way depending on their characteristics. Since, in general, a stimulus contains features for which more than one processing channel is sensitive, great pains should be taken to design such stimuli that one feature dominates. The latter is the more important since all amplitude of

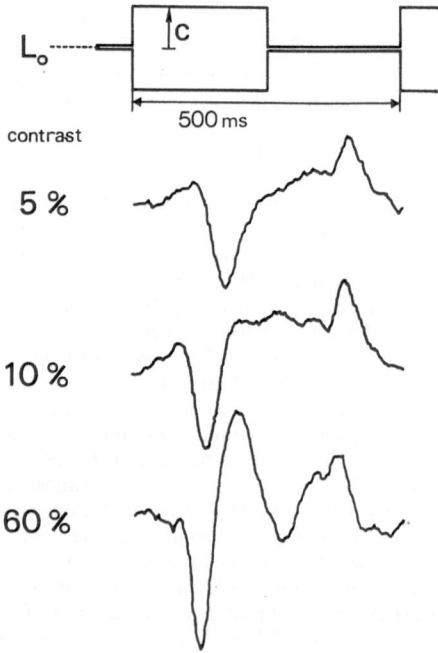

Fig. 14. Occipital responses (inion-vertex derivation) to an appearing-disappearing checkerboard with 10' checks as a function of contrast. Stimulation rate was 2.1 Hz, stimulus field subtended 2°; mean luminance is 3000 asb; binocular presentation.

response versus stimulus strength curves exhibit saturation. Hence, in a 'not-clean' stimulus the response to one feature may be taken over by that to another one, so that the amplitude response versus stimulus strength curve becomes ambiguous. Also to a 'clean' stimulus this problem can occur if the response contains components originating from different retino-cortical projections (JEFFREYS & AXFORD, 1972). A typical example of this can be found in Fig. 14 presenting the EP's to the appearance of a pattern with various contrasts. It shows that the first parts of these EP's do not depend much on contrast, whereas the last positive deflection becomes pronounced at high contrasts. With high presentation rates these components are mixed and the resulting picture is ambiguous. This forms a complication in the study of dynamic properties of contrast EP's.

ACKNOWLEDGMENTS

This work was supported by the Dutch Health Organization (TNO) and the Netherlands Organization for the Advancement of Pure Research (Z.W.O.).

REFERENCES

CAMPBELL, F. W. & MAFFEI, L. Electrophysiological evidence for the existence of orientation and size detectors in the human visual system. *J. Physiol. Lond.* 207: *635-652* (1970).
COBB, W. A., MORTON, H. B. & ETTLINGER, G. Cerebral potentials evoked by pattern reversal and their suppression in visual rivalry. *Nature (Lond.)* 216: *1123-1125* (1967).
ESTÉVEZ, O. & SPEKREIJSE, H. Relationship between pattern appearance-disappearance and pattern reversal response. *Experimental Brain Res.* 19: *233-238* (1974).
ESTÉVEZ, O. & SPEKREIJSE, H. A spectral compensation method for determining the flicker characteristics of the human colour mechanisms. *Vision Res.* 1974 (in press).
JEFFREYS, D. A. & AXFORD, J. G. Source locations of pattern-specific components of human visual evoked potentials. I. Component of striate cortical origin. *Exp. Brain Res.* 16: *1-21* (1972).
KUFFLER, S. W. Discharge patterns and functional organization of mammalian retina. *J. Neurophysiol.* 16: *37-68* (1953).
PADMOS, P., HAAIJMAN, J. J. & SPEKREIJSE, H. Visually evoked cortical potentials to patterned stimuli in monkey and man. *Electroenceph. clin. Neurophysiol.* 35: *153-163* (1973).
REGAN, D. Chromatic evoked potentials. from: The Visual System. Proceedings of the Ninth ISCERG Symposium, Brighton, 1971. Ed.: G. B. Arden. Plenum Press, pp. 171-187 (1972).
REGAN, D. & SPEKREIJSE, H. Electrophysiological correlate of binocular depth perception in man. *Nature* 225: *92-94* (1970).
REGAN, D. & SPEKREIJSE, H. Evoked potential indications of colour blindness. *Vision Res.* (in press) (1973).
RIGGS, L. A., JOHNSON, E. P. & SCHICK, A. M. L. Electrical responses of the human eye to moving stimulus patterns. *Science* 144: *567-* (1964).
RODIECK, R. W. & STONE, J. Analysis of receptive fields of cat retinal ganglion cells. *J. Neurophysiol.* 28: *833-849* (1965).
SCHELLART, N. A. M. & SPEKREIJSE, H. Dynamic characteristics of retinal ganglion cell responses in goldfish. *J. of Gen. Physiol.* 59: *1-21* (1972).
SHAPLEY, R. M. & TOLHURST, D. J. Edge detectors in human vision. *J. Physiol. Lond.* 229: *165-183* (1973).

Spekreijse, H. Analysis of EEG responses in man, evoked by sine wave modulated light. Dr. W. Junk Publishers, The Hague, pp. 166 (1966).

Spekreijse, H. Rectification in the goldfish retina: analysis by sinusoidal and auxiliary stimulation. *Vision Res.* 9: *1461-1472* (1969).

Spekreijse, H. & Norton, A. L. The dynamic characteristics of color-coded S-potentials. *J. of Gen. Physiol.* 56: *1-15* (1970).

Spekreijse, H., Norren, D. van & Berg, T. J. T. P. van den. Flicker responses in monkey lateral geniculate nucleus and human perception of flicker. *Proc. Nat. Acad. Sci. USA* 68: *2802-2805* (1971).

Spekreijse, H. & Tweel, L. H. van der. System analysis of linear and nonlinear processes in electrophysiology of the visual system. Proc. Kon. Ned. Akad. van Wetenschappen, Series C, 75: *77-106* (1972).

Spekreijse, H., Tweel, L. H. van der & Zuidema, Th. Contrast evoked responses in man. *Vision Res.* 13: *1577-1601* (1973).

Spekreijse, H., Estévez, O. & Tweel, L. H. van der. Luminance responses to pattern reversal. Xth ISCERG Symposium. Documenta Ophthalmologica Proceedings Series, Vol. 2, pp. 205-212 (1973).

Tomita, T., Kaneko, A., Murakami, M. & Paulter, E. L. Spectral response curves of single cones in the carp. *Vision Res.* 7: *519-531* (1967).

Tweel, L. H. van der & Verduyn Lunel, H. F. E. Human visual responses to sinusoidally modulated light. *Electroenceph. clin. Neurophysiol.* 18: *587-598* (1965).

Tweel, L. H. van der & Spekreijse, H. Visual evoked responses. In: The clinical value of electroretinography. Karger Basel, pp. 83-94 (1968).

Tweel, L. H. van der & Spekreijse, H. Signal transport and rectification in the human evoked response system. *Ann. N.Y. Acad. Sci.* 156: *678-695* (1969).

Wagner, H. G., MacNichol, E. F., Jr. & Wolbarsht, M. L. The response properties of single ganglion cells in the goldfish retina. *J. Gen. Physiol.* 43: *45-62* (1960)

Authors' address:

Laboratory of Medical Physics
University of Amsterdam
Herengracht 196
Amsterdam

284

VISUALLY EVOKED POTENTIAL METHODS
WITH CLINICAL APPLICATIONS

D. REGAN

(Staffordshire)

INTRODUCTION

There is a strong case for routinely recording evoked potentials (EP's) alongside ERGs when carrying out electrophysiological tests of vision. Evoked potentials can give information about central lesions that affect vision, whereas ERGs cannot; therefore, by comparing EPs and ERGs, in some cases a distinction between central and peripheral lesions can be made. Evoked potentials can test binocular functions. A further point is that, even for peripheral defects, EPs can provide information not available from ERGs (e.g. acuity) and vice versa.

Of course it is of the first importance to know which parameters to measure in any given disease. Given this knowledge the next problem is how to measure the required parameters. I therefore offer no apology for devoting most of this talk to discussing the how of evoked potential recording.

Two major problems in EP recording, especially in clinical applications, are (a) the slowness of EP procedures and (b) EP variability. To some extent, however, these problems are connected; thus an increase in speed may have the further advantage of reducing the effect of variability.

I will describe ways of attacking these two problems in two specific practical examples. These examples are (I) objective refraction, and (II) objective examination of visual fields. The problems of speed and variability are especially severe for EPs, but they also exist in ERG recording, so that my remarks also apply to ERGs.

OBJECTIVE REFRACTION BY EVOKED POTENTIAL RECORDING

Running Average Method

The electrophysiological recording method that I shall describe is based on Fourier analysis of the EEG. This is quite different from the well-known averaging or summation technique. Although it has been in use for almost as long as commercial averaging computers have been available (1–3) the Fourier analysis method* is comparatively unfamiliar. Nevertheless the method has the

---

* The Fourier analysis method is to obtain the various individual frequency components (harmonic components) of the EP by a cross-correlation process that is equivalent to narrow-

clinically-valuable advantage that it can be much faster than the averaging method.

Fourier analysis allows the EP to be presented as a moment-to-moment running average (1–3). Some time ago (1) I reported that, as a consequence, the result of changing a stimulus parameter can be seen immediately. For example the effect on EP amplitude and phase of changing the eye's state of chromatic adaptation can be seen at once (4). One result of pairing observations in this way is to reduce the effect of variability (4).

In one application, the 'running average' method can be used to measure the photopic spectral sensitivity of the eye as rapidly (roughly $1\frac{1}{2}$ hours) and as precisely (0.1 log units) as when conventional subjective methods are used (43).

This 'running average' presentation can also be used in measuring EP changes caused by changing the eye's refractive correction (6). Fig. 1 shows the effect on moment-to-moment EP amplitude of placing a trial lens before the patient's

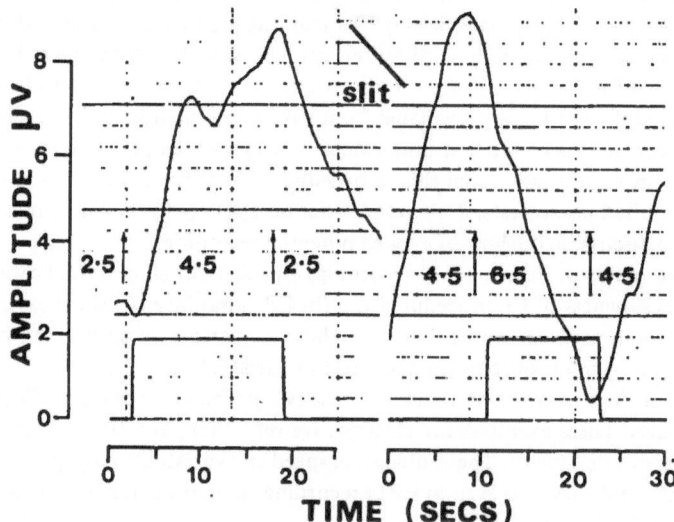

Fig. 1. Effect of changing refractive correction shown immediately by 'running average' display of evoked potential. The traces are plots of instantaneous EP amplitude (ordinates) versus time (abscissa). Optimal refractive correction is near –4.5D. The subject viewed a 7° pattern of 30% contrast, 20′ checks that exchanged places six times per second; 6 Hz EP component shown. From REGAN, D. (1973). Rapid objective refraction using evoked brain potentials. *Invest Ophthal.*, In press.

band filtering. Speed is obtained at the expense of information. This process gives latency (phase) information as well as amplitude information. When signals are very small, the filter bandwidth can be made narrow (e.g. 0.001 Hz, Reference 5 Fig. 5.12) so as to handle $0.1\mu v$ EEG signals. Alternatively with more favourable signal-to-noise ratios the filter bandwidth may be widened so as to increase speed. However, the important point here is that if the method provides all the information required (as established in preliminary experiments) then the increase in speed is 'free'.

The methods of Fourier analysis and averaging are compared in Reference 5, pp 233-242.

eye and then removing it. Adding a $-2.0D$ lens to a previously present $-2.5D$ lens caused EP amplitude to rise at once, while removing the lens caused an immediate fall of amplitude. However adding a further $-2.0D$ lens caused EP amplitude to fall at once.

The EP changes of Fig. 1 are analogous to a patient's immediate verbal responses 'that lens makes the pattern sharper' or 'that lens makes the pattern more blurred'.

Blurring, EP amplitude and check size

One pitfall here is the choice of check size for the stimulus pattern. Fig. 2A shows that the sharpest pattern gave the largest EPs when small (13') checks

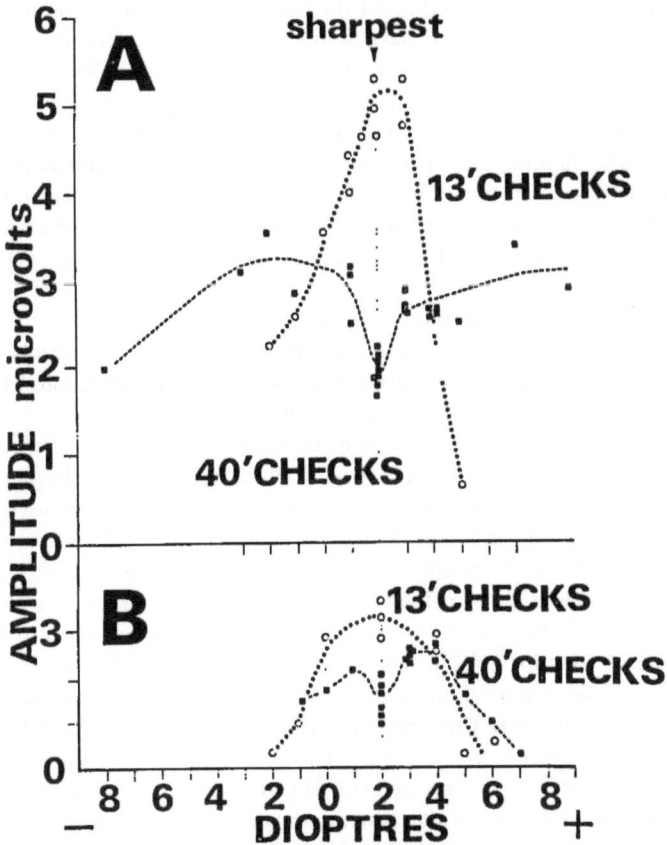

Fig. 2. A: The most sharply-accommodated pattern gives the largest EPs for small (13') checks but the sharpest focus gives a minimum amplitude for large (40') checks. B: Control experiment to show that an increase in stimulus field size due to blurring does not cause this effect. Subject viewed a 2° square pattern of checks that exchanged places 6 times per second. 6Hz EP component shown. From: REGAN, D. & RICHARDS, W. (1973). Brightness contrast and evoked potentials. *J. opt. Soc. Amer.* 63: *606-611.*

were used to stimulate the eye. This findings is not so obvious as it seems, since when larger (40′) checks were used the largest EPs were obtained for a blurred image that was substantially defocussed by between 1D to 6D; a sharp image gave a comparatively small response (7,8).

This potentially misleading effect may be due to the finite size of receptive fields. Large-check EPs would be a combination of responses to luminance and to contrast so that for sharply-focussed images the brightness and contrast EPs would cancel to some extent. Therefore, when the contrast EP is attenuated by blurring the total EP would increase and would not decrease until blurring is sufficient to attenuate the luminance EPs (8).

EP refraction in the presence of astigmatic plus spherical errors: grating method

Since SPEKREIJSE's demonstration of the effects of accommodation on pattern EPs (Reference 9, p. 131) there have been a number of descriptions of objective refraction using EPs elicited by patterned stimuli (10–13). Several of these reports, however, deal only with cases where astigmatism is negligible. One report which does treat the case of astigmatic combined with spherical errors uses a grating stimulus. (13). This method is to record EPs for different orientations of the grating pattern. The orientations that give maximum and minimum EP amplitudes are taken as the axes of astigmatism. Trial lenses are then inserted until maximum EP amplitude is obtained for each of these two orientations of the grating pattern.

Fig. 3 illustrates this method. Two plots of EP amplitude versus grating orientation are shown in Fig. 3A. Each point on the graphs was recorded separately. The dotted line was recorded with no cylindrical correction. The continuous line was recorded with optimal cylindrical correction.

Fig. 3 also illustrates three defects of associated with this use of grating stimuli. The first drawback (I) is that grating stimuli give smaller EPs than check stimuli. Consequently the procedure is slower when gratings are used rather than checks. The second drawback (II) is that the method confounds astigmatic errors of vision caused by optical errors of imaging with astigmatic errors of vision due to neural abnormalities. The continuous line of Fig. 3A shows that even when cylindrical correction was optimal, EP amplitude varied with the orientation of the stimulus grating. This effect was such that the grating orientation that gave the most blurred image in the uncorrected eye also gave the smallest EP after correction (6). This observation has recently been independently reported by FIORENTINI & MAFFEI (14). 'Neural astigmatism' (meridional amblyopia) was described many years ago (15, 16). It has recently been attributed to neural changes that arise in the visual pathway when optical astigmatism has been left uncorrected for too long (17–18). In addition, even the normal eye shows regular differences in its visual acuity for differently-oriented gratings (19).

The third drawback is that separate averaging of each reading is slow.

This last drawback, slowness, can be countered by continuously rotating the stripe pattern and arranging that the instantaneous value of EP amplitude is plotted versus the orientation of the stimulus bars. Fig. 3C shows such a plot,

288

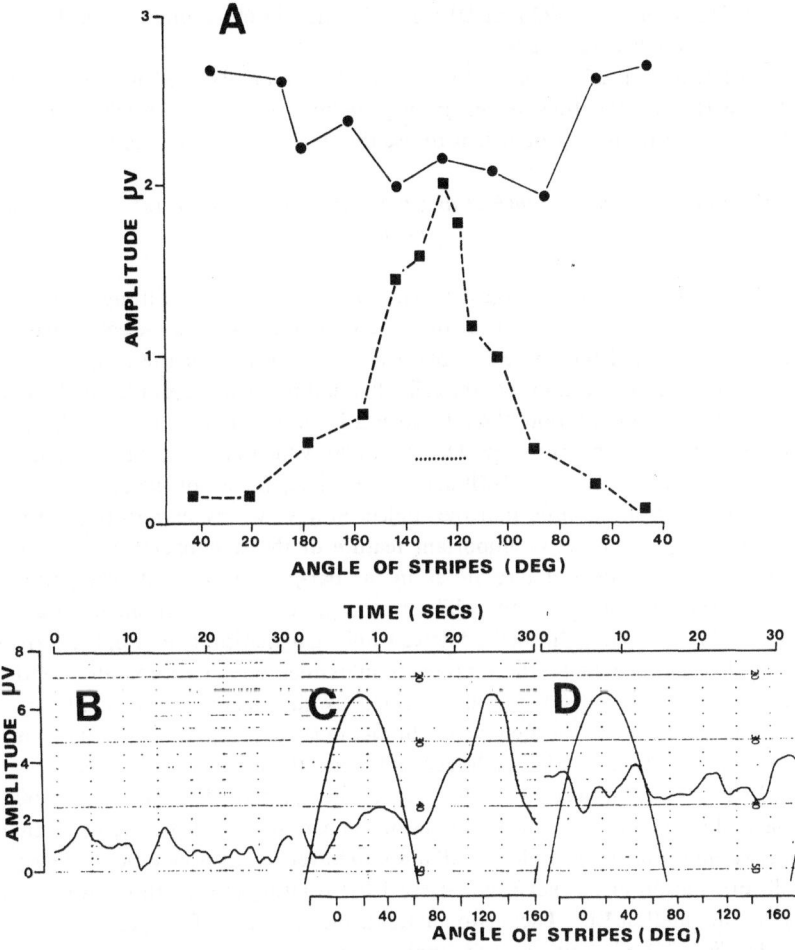

Fig. 3. Objective refraction by recording evoked potentials to a grating pattern of different orientations. *A*: EP amplitudes (ordinates) versus orientation of stimulus grating. Broken line recorded with no cylindrical correction, but with –2.0D sphere. Full line recorded with optimal cylindrical and spherical correction. Full line shows effect on EP of meridional amblyopia. Each point in *A* was recorded separately. Lower half of Fig. shows recordings obtained with faster method where stimulus grating was rotated continuously. *B*: shows noise level. *C* was without cylindrical correction. *D* was after optimal refractive correction. Ignore the smooth inverted 'U' lines. From: REGAN, D. (1973). Rapid objective refraction using evoked brain potentials. *Invest. Ophthal.*

recorded with no cylindrical correction; EP amplitude can be seen to vary markedly with grating orientation. Fig. 3D is a similar plot recorded after optimal cylindrical correction; EP amplitude now varied little with grating orientation. The rotating-grating plot of Fig. 3C is equivalent to the static-grating plot of Fig. 3A (broken line) and 3D equivalent to 3A (continuous line). However Fig. 3 (C and D) were obtained in 60 seconds, while Fig. 3A required roughly $1\frac{1}{2}$ hours.

Although a speed increase of some 90-fold can be obtained in this way, the defects (I) and (II) above of the grating method cannot be so easily overcome. One counter to these problems is to use the stenopaeic slit method.

EP refraction in the presence of astigmatic plus spherical errors: stenopaeic slit method

The stenopaeic slit method is to view a stimulus pattern through a narrow slit placed immediately in front of the cornea (20). The slit selects a narrow area of cornea. If the cornea is spherical, the sharpness of the image will not depend on slit orientation. On the other hand, if the sharpness of the image does depend on slit orientation, then the cornea is not spherical and this will result in an astigmatic retinal image. The slit angles which give the sharpest and the most blurred retinal images will define the principal axes of the cornea.

It is important to note that the subject may view any pattern (e.g. checks) while the slit rotates. An important feature of the stenopaeic slit method is that the pattern does not rotate as in the bar-pattern method. The pattern's orientation remains constant while its sharpness varies with slit orientation. Thus, the stenopaeic slit method detects only astigmatism due to optical errors. The defect (inherent to the grating-stimulus method) of confounding optical and neural astigmatism is, thus, avoided by the stenopaeic slit method*. A second advantage of the stenopaeic slit method is that since check patterns may replace bar patterns, EPs are larger and hence the procedure is faster.

In Fig. 4 the subject viewed a checkerboard pattern through a 1mm stenopaeic slit. The light and dark squares of the pattern exchanged places six times per second. Fig. 4A is a plot of EP amplitude versus slit orientation. Clearly, a slit orientation of 50° gave the largest EPs; rotating the slit through 90° then gave the smallest EPs. These two angles defined the axes of astigmatism.

In Fig. 4A each point on the graph was recorded separately. Fig. 4B shows a much faster way of obtaining the same data. In Fig. 4B the slit was continuously rotated at a rate of one revolution in 18 seconds. Fig. 4B shows plots of instantaneous EP amplitude versus slit orientation. Two replications are illustrated. Each plot in Fig. 4B was obtained in 18 seconds as compared with roughly $1\frac{1}{2}$ hour for Fig. 4A.

A more convenient way of displaying the data of Fig. 4 is illustrated in Fig. 5. In Fig. 4 EP amplitude is plotted in Cartesian Coordinates whereas in Fig. 5 it is plotted in polar coordinates so as to enable the directions of the axes of astigmatism to be seen more easily.

In Fig. 5 (A to E) the radial distance of any point from the origin gives EP amplitude while the orientation of the radius gives the orientation of the steno-

---

* A minor point is that some difficulty might be anticipated with the stenopaeic slit method in those (unfrequent) cases (Reference 20 pp. 276-278) where a large fraction of total cylindrical error is due to optical causes other than asphericity of the anterior surface of the cornea.

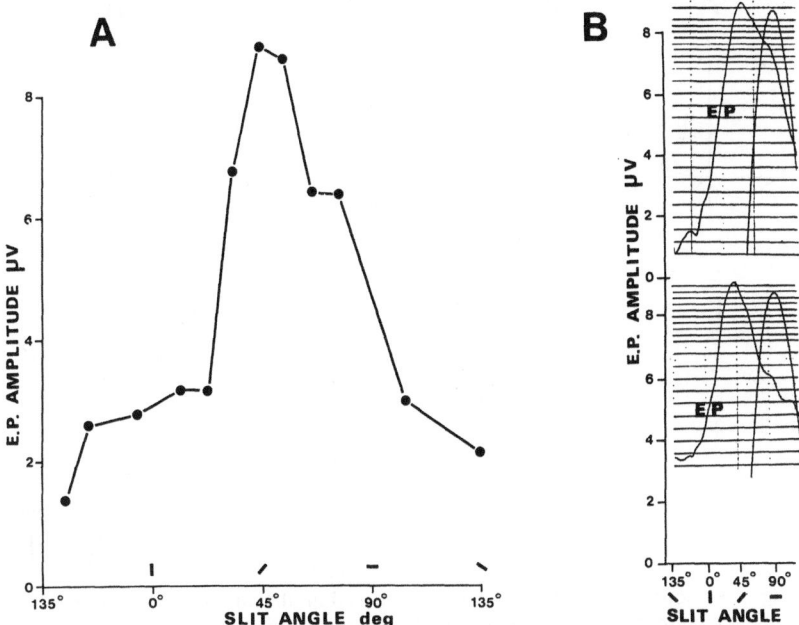

Fig. 4. Stenopaeic slit method of objective refraction: definition of axes of astigmatism. The subject viewed a checkerboard pattern through a narrow slit located immediately before the cornea. *A* is a plot of EP amplitude versus slit angle with no refractive correction. The slit angles that give maximum and minimum EP amplitudes give the directions of the axes of astigmatism. *B* shows two replications of this determination using a faster procedure in which the slit rotated continuously. Each of the traces in *B* was recorded in 18 seconds (ignore the regular sinewave traces in *B*). The stimulus was a 7° pattern of 30% contrast, 20′ checks that exchanged positions 6 times per second: 6Hz EP component shown. From: REGAN, D. (1973). Rapid objective refraction using evoked brain potentials. *Invest. Ophthal.*, In press.

paeic slit. Fig. 5 (G and H) show how radial angle in the graphs (Fig. 5G) relates to slit orientation (Fig. 5H).

Fig. 5 (A, B and C) are three replications that show similar data to Fig. 4B. Clearly, EP amplitude was maximum for a slit angle of 30°–50° and minimum (near zero) for a slit angle of 110°–140°. Fig. 5E is a similar plot obtained in 10 seconds. Fig. 5D was recorded after cylindrical correction and shows that EP amplitude was no longer affected by slit orientation. In this situation, subjective correction of astigmatism was also optimal. Fig. 5F is a 5 microvolt calibration.

Thus, Fig. 5 shows how the directions of the axes of astigmatism can be found within 10 seconds by using a rotating stenopaeic slit.

Refractive correction can be obtained by the method shown in Fig. 6. The subject gazed at the checkerboard pattern through a stenopaeic slit oriented parallel to one axis of astigmatism. In front of the slit was a lens whose power rhythmically oscillated once every 18 seconds. Fig. 6 shows plots of instanta-

291

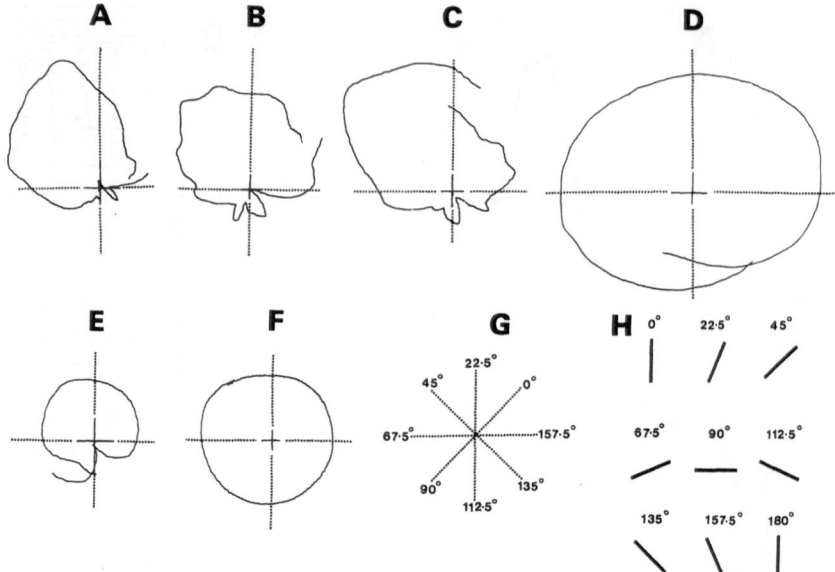

Fig. 5. Stenopaeic slit method of objective refraction: definition of axes of astigmatism. Similar data to that of Fig. 4 plotted in the more convenient form of polar coordinates. The radial distance to any point on a trace gives instantaneous EP amplitude, while the angle of the radius gives the instantaneous orientation of the slit. Three replications of similar data to that of Fig. 4B are shown in polar coordinates in *A*, *B* and *C*. Each plot took 18 seconds while the stenopaeic slit rotated through 180°. *E* shows a similar plot made in 10 seconds. *D* was recorded after astigmatism had been corrected. *F* – 5 micro-volt calibration. *G* shows slit angles as plotted in *A* to *F*. *H* shows corresponding physical orientations of slit. Thus *A*, *B*, *C* and *E* show maximum EP for slit angle of 30°–50° and near-zero EP for slit angles of 110°–140°. From: REGAN, D. (1973). Rapid objective refraction using evoked brain potentials. *Invest. Ophthal.*, In press.

neous EP amplitude versus instantaneous lens power. For one slit orientation, EP amplitude was maximal at a power of –4.5D. When the slit orientation was rotated through 90°, EP amplitude was maximal at a power of –2.0D. Thus the correction required along the axes of astigmatism was –4.5D and –2.0D respectively; these figures, taken in conjunction with the direction of the axes, define the required prescription lens.

Summarising this refraction procedure: (I) find the direction of the axes of astigmatism using the rotating slit method (this required 10 seconds); (II) find the correcting lens power with a stenopaeic slit set parallel to one axis (this required 18 seconds); (III) turn the slit through 90° and repeat (this required 18 seconds). Thus, this method is some 100 times faster than a comparable point-by-point procedure using an averaging computer.

292

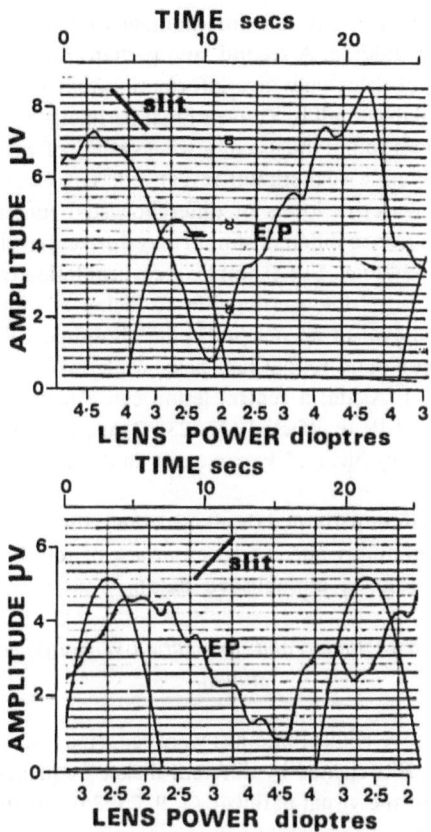

Fig. 6. Stenopaeic slit method of objective refraction: determination of cylindrical and spherical refractive corrections. The stimulus pattern was viewed through a stenopaeic slit set parallel to one axis of astigmatism (upper half of Fig.). A lens system was then placed in front of the slit and its optical power was continuously oscillated at a rate of one oscillation per 18 seconds. The trace shows how EP amplitude (ordinates) varied as a function of lens power (abscissae). EP amplitude was maximal for a power of –4.5D. In the lower half of the Fig. the stenopaeic slit was rotated through 90° and the experiment repeated. A power of –2.0D now gave maximum amplitude. These two lens powers and the direction of the axes define the required prescription lens. Ignore the smooth inverted 'U' lines. From: Regan, D. (1973). Rapid objective refraction using evoked brain potentials. *Invest. Ophthal.*, In press.

VISUAL FIELDS INVESTIGATION USING EPS: STIMULUS VARIETY

Clinical Findings

A patient's visual field can be investigated by evoked potential recording. At first sight such methods might seem to be no more than cumbersome and expensive forms of conventional perimetry or campimetry. However, there is a case for EP perimetry. One obvious application of objective EP methods is when subjective perimetry may fail, for example with uncooperative patients and with very young children. A second, and perhaps more important point is that EP tests of visual fields may give information that is either not so easily available or not available at all by conventional perimetry or campimetry. This latter possibility hinges round the use of a wide variety of visual stimuli.

It seems that different visual stimuli reveal different visual field losses that in turn may reflect selective losses of different visual functions. For central lesions, furthermore, EPs to different stimuli may differentiate between differently located cortical pathology. For example, a cortical lesion can abolish EPs to flicker of one frequency, while sparing EPs to flicker of other frequencies. In one case surgical removal of an occipital pole abolished EPs to 18Hz flicker stimulation of the ipsilateral retinal half-field, while leaving responses to 9Hz flicker unaffected (21). Again, a central lesion can attenuate 18Hz flicker EPs while leaving pattern EPs unaffected (22, 23). Thus, by comparing responses elicited by pattern and by flicker, EPs can assist in the detection and location of cortical lesions (5).

Furthermore, EPs to unpatterned (homogeneous) stimuli and EPs to patterned stimuli may be differently affected by an attack of retrobulbar neuritis (24) (MILNER, HERON & REGAN, unpublished data).

Eps to spatial-contrast stimuli and to spatially-unpatterned (homogeneous) stimuli.

Well before the above clinical findings were reported, basic research had already suggested that EPs elicited by different flicker frequencies reflected quite different properties of the visual pathway (2, 9, 25, 26). Furthermore, the Amterdam and other groups showed that EPs to patterned stimuli reflected different aspects of the visual pathway to those revealed by flickering an unpatterned patch of light (9, 25, 27–29).

The differences between spatial-contrast (pattern) EPs and EPs elicited by luminance changes are discussed elsewhere (Reference 30 and Reference 5 pp. 52–58). These differences include: (I) different distributions over the scalp of responses elicited by focal stimulation of upper and lower retinal half-fields and right and left half-fields (31–36). This suggests that contrast and luminance EPs have different cortical generators (33, 34); (II) the effect of stimulus repetition frequency (9, 28, 38); (III) the effects of blurring (7–10, 28).

Luminance-contrast and chromatic-contrast stimuli.

Luminance-contrast EPs elicited by a pattern of light and dark checks or stripes are not the only type of contrast EPs. There are also chromatic contrast EPs. These can be elicited by a pattern of equiluminant checks or stripes where alternate checks or stripes are of different colours (37, 38).

Fig. 7 shows EPs elicited by exchanging the colours of a pattern of red and green checks. A subject with normal colour vision gives clear EPs when viewing this stimulus (traces marked 'RED-GREEN'). However, SPEKREIJSE and I

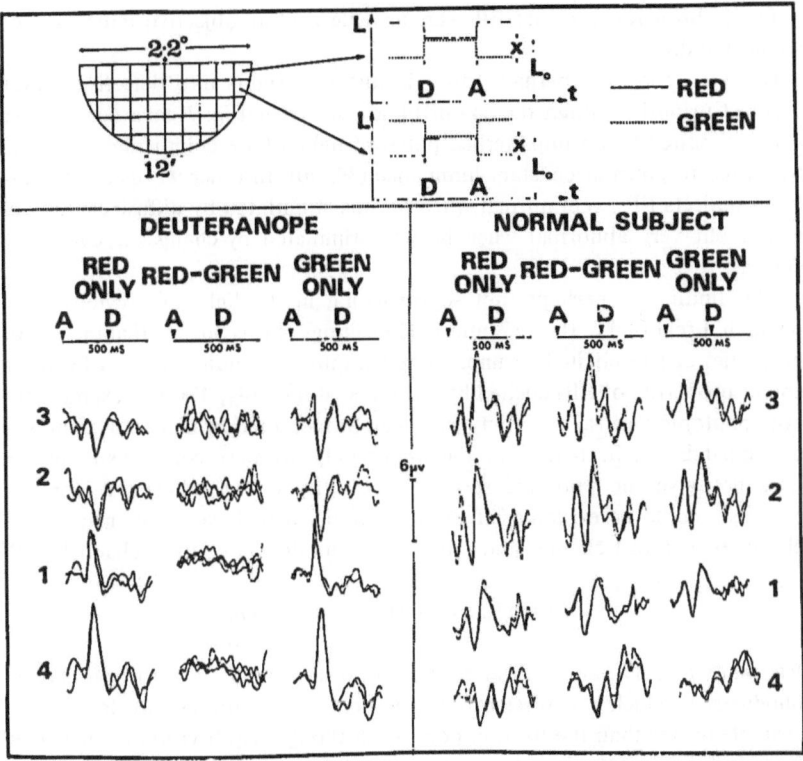

Fig. 7. Evoked potentials elicited by chromatic contrast stimulation in a normal and in a colour blind (deuteranopic) subject. The upper part of the Fig. shows the semicircular pattern that stimulated the lower visual half field. Each check emitted a mixture of red and green light. The stimulus was initially yellow and patternless, then abruptly changed into a pattern of equiluminant red and green checks (i.e. a change in chromatic contrast). The appearance of chromatic pattern gave clear EPs in subjects with normal colour vision, but no responses for a deuteranope (compare 'RED-GREEN' traces). However, clear EPs were recorded for both normal and deuteranopic subject when stimulated by either the red light only or by the green light only ('RED ONLY' or 'GREEN ONLY' traces). In this situation, for example, a patternless red semicircle changed into a pattern or bright and dark red checks (i.e. a change of luminance contrast). From: REGAN, D. & SPEKREIJSE, H. (1973). Evoked potential indications of colour blindness. *Vision Res.*, In press.

found that this stimulus gives no response for a colour blind (deuteranopic) subject (see 'RED-GREEN' traces in left half of Fig. 39).

Fig. 7. also shows that although the deuteranope gives no EPs to chromatic contrast, his EPs to luminance contrast are as clear as those for normal subjects. This can be seen by comparing the 'RED-ONLY' and 'GREEN ONLY' traces for deuteranope and normal. These EPs were elicited by the red or by the green light of the stimulus pattern, that is by patterns of bright and dark red checks or bright and dark green checks.

Thus, chromatic contrast EPs can provide a clear objective indication of colour blindness.

However, EPs can, perhaps, provide further insights into defective colour vision. Curiously enough the colour-blind subject of Fig. 7 gave normal EPs when stimulted by an unpatterned patch of light whose colour alternated between red to green at constant luminance (39, 40). In other words the colour-blind subjects EPs were normal when he was stimulated by diffuse changes of colour but very abnormal when he was stimulated by changes in chromatic contrast.

This finding is, perhaps, not so surprising in the light of previous basic research. I reported to the 1969 and 1971 meetings of this Society that the colour properties of EPs elicited by unpatterned stimuli were quite different from the colour properties of EPs elicited by patterned stimuli (41, 42). For example the eye's photopic spectral sensitivity curve can be measured by flickering an unpatterned patch of light: (41, 43) on the other hand, chromatic contrast stimulation does not give the photopic spectral sensitivity curve. Chromatic contrast responses could be explained if the human visual pathway contained both a chromatic contrast channel and colour-coded luminance contrast channels (38).

EPs to changes in stereoscopic depth.

RICHARDS (44, 45), and BEVERLEY and I (46) have reported a form of stereo-blindness in which a subject cannot see depth when objects are located for example nearer than the fixation point even though depth vision is unaffected for objects beyond the fixation point. Such a defect may involve the whole visual field or may be present in the form of stereoscotoma (Reference 47, see also Reference 48, pp 33 to 35). An important point here is that these defects of binocular depth perception can occur in the presence of normal visual acuity. RICHARDS has suggested that such a defects in stereoscopic depth perception, restricted to one hemisphere, could be a cause of squint (45).

Since SPEKREIJSE and I reported (49) that EPs were elicited by changes in retinal disparity (i.e. apparent depth) BEVERLEY and I have been trying to record objective differences to movements in depth for targets located (a) nearer and (b) beyond the fixation point. Fig. 8 shows such differences. This finding indicates that four different neural mechanisms are involved in seeing movement in depth. These four mechanisms handle movements directed towards and away from the eyes for objects located respectively (a) nearer and (b) beyond the fixation point (50). Furthermore, Fig. 8 indicates that EP recording offers an objective means of testing the integrity of these neural mechanisms and thus of investigating selective defects of binocular depth perceptions.

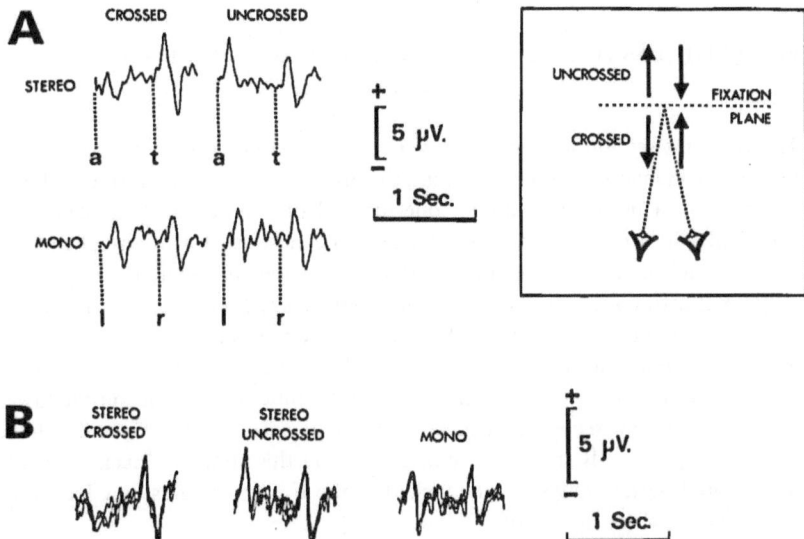

Fig. 8. Evoked potentials elicited by changes in retinal disparity (i.e. changes in stereo-scopic depth). The target was a 5° pattern of random dots whose central 2° appeared either to move in depth (stereo) or from side to side (mono). The four types of stimulus movement are illustrated in the insert. For crossed disparities, the targets remained in front of the fixation point; for uncrossed disparities the targets remained beyond the fixation point. *A*: In the stereo traces *a* means movement away from the eyes, and *t* movement towards the eyes. In the monocular (mono) control recordings, *l* indicates movement to the left and *r* movement to the right. Mono recordings are symmetrical, whereas stereo responses are asymmetric and depend both on the direction of move-ment in depth and on whether the target is in front of or behind the fixation point. *B*: Variability illustrated by three superposed traces. From: REGAN, D. & BEVERLEY, K. I. (1973). Electrophysiological evidence for the existence of neurons sensitive to the direction of movement in depth. *Nature*, In press.

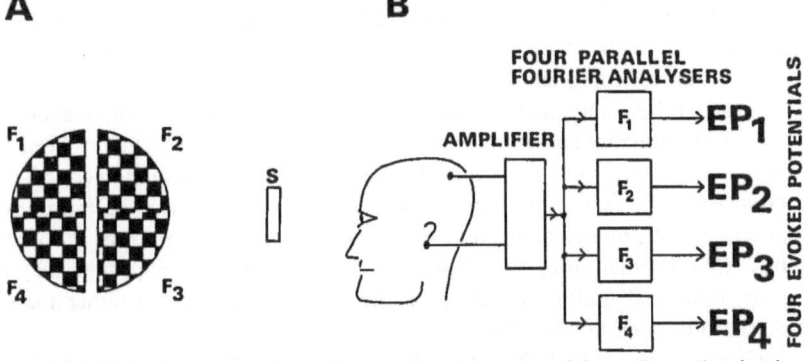

Fig. 9. Multiple-stimulus method of recording evoked potentials. *A* shows the circular checkerboard stimulus pattern. The subject gazes at the centre of the pattern. The black and white checks repetitively exchange positions, but the rate at which this occurs is slightly different in each quadrant of the pattern (F_1 Hz, F_2 Hz, F_3 Hz and F_4 Hz as indicated). *B* shows the subject gazing at the stimulus pattern S. Each EEG amplifier feeds four Fourier analysers, one locked to the F_1 Hz stimulus, one locked to the F_2 Hz stimulus and so on. Thus, four EPs are simultaneously recorded from each electrode. This method can be used with stimuli other than spatial patterns.

297

The previous section argued that a variety of different stimuli should be used in visual field investigation. Given that, the problems of speed and EP variability still remain. This section outlines one method of countering these problems. This multiple stimulus method (5, 22, 23, 51) can be used with any of the different stimuli used above, or even with combinations of different stimuli.

Fig. 9 illustrates, as an example, a four-channel system using pattern stimulation. The stimulus is illustrated in Fig. 9A. Each quadrant is a checkerboard pattern whose light and dark checks periodically exchange positions. The checks in the upper left quadrant exchange position F_1 times per second, in the lower right F_2 times per second and so on. The frequencies F_1, F_2, F_3 and $_4$ differ only slightly. Fig. 9B shows the subject viewing this stimulus. Each electrode feeds four Fourier analysers, one locked to the F_1 Hz stimulus, one locked to the F_2 Hz stimulus and so on.

In this way, four EPs are simultaneously recorded from each electrode.

The main feature of this method is to reduce the effect of EP variability. Variability is, to a large extent, common to all four EPs. Therefore the relation between the four EPs is much less affected by variability than if different retinal areas were separately tested.

VISUAL FIELD INVESTIGATION USING EP METHODS: CONGENITAL ABNORMALITIES OF VISUAL PROJECTION AND SQUINT.

Congenital abnormalities in the retino-geniculate and retino-cortical projections have recently been demonstrated. In most cases the misrouting of optic fibres is entirely from the temporal half-fields of the retina. In normal animals, fibres that originate in temporal retina do not cross at the chiasm; however, in abnormal animals a substantial proportion of temporal fibres do cross. As a result, each hemisphere receives an abnormally strong projection from the contralateral eye and an abnormally weak projection from the ipsilateral eye.

This abnormality has been associated with the albino gene, and has been reported in a number of species including cat, ferret, rat mouse and tiger. (52–58) GUILLERY et al. suggested that squint can be expected when the misrouting interferes with binocular fusion over an appreciable proportion of the visual field. (55). Furthermore, it has been proposed that the resulting squint may be a desirable and useful adaptation to the abnormal projection rather than a defect to be corrected (53, 59).

GUILLERY has raised the interesting question whether such congenital abnormalities of the visual projection occur in man. Certainly, human albinos often have visual problems including squint, reduced acuity and nystagmus. EPs offer a way of searching for an abnormal visual projection. The method of recording two EPs elicited by simultaneous stimulation of left and right visual half-fields, originally introduced to detect hemispheric imbalance in migraine, (22, 23, 51) is suitable for this purpose. In normal man, visual signals elicited by stimulation of left and right retinal half-fields excite EP generators in left and right hemispheres respectively. These EPs generated in the left and right hemispheres differ in topographical distribution and phase (polarity) (22, 23, 36). Although nystagmus created some difficulties, in preliminary experiments using pattern EPs I have found tentative evidence for abnormal visual projection in a human albino.

CONCLUSION

This talk discusses the notion of (I) using a wide variety of different stimuli so as to detect and locate discrete functional losses and pathology, and (II) deploying these stimuli in ways which yield the minimum information necessary and therefore allow maximum speed. However, it should be remembered that special-purpose rapid methods are special-purpose, and may be inflexible. Thus, one must be quite sure what one wishes to measure before designing the optimally rapid way of measuring it.

ACKNOWLEDGEMENTS.

This work was supported by Medical Research Council.
    I thank ROBERT F. CARTWRIGHT for invaluable technical support. I am grateful to HAZEL HENRY for assistance in preparing this manuscript.

REFERENCES

1. REGAN, D. A study of the visual system by the correlation of light stimuli and evoked electrical responses. Thesis, Lond. (1964).
2. REGAN, D. Some characteristics of average steady-state and transient responses evoked by modulated light. *Electroenceph. clin. Neurophysiol.* 20: *238-248* (1966).
3. REGAN, D. Apparatus for the correlation of evoked potentials and repetitive stimuli. *Med. Electron. Biol. Engin.* 4: *169-177* (1966).
4. REGAN, D. Evoked potentials and sensation. *Percept. Psychophys.* 4: *347-350* (1968).
5. REGAN, D. Evoked potentials in psychology, sensory physiology and clinical medicine, Chapman and Hall, Lond. and Wiley, New York (1972).
6. REGAN, D. Rapid objective refraction using evoked brain potentials. *Invest. Ophthal.*, In press (1973).
7. REGAN, D. & RICHARDS, W. Independence of evoked potentials and apparent size. *Vision Res.* 11: *679-684* (1971).
8. REGAN, D. & RICHARDS, W. Brightness contrast and evoked potentials. *J. opt. Soc. Amer.* 63: *606-611* (1973).
9. SPEKREIJSE, H. Analysis of EEG responses in man. Junk. The Hague (1966).
10. HARTER, M. R. & WHITE, C. T. Effects of contour sharpness and check size on visually evoked cortical potentials. *Vision Res.* 8: *701-711* (1968).
11. MILLODOT, M. & RIGGS, L. A. Refraction determined electrophysiologically. *Arch. Ophthal.* 84: *272-278* (1970).
12. DUFFEY, F. H. & RENGSTORFF, R. H. Ametropia measurements from the visual evoked response. *Amer. J. Optom.* 48: *717-728* (1971).
13. LUDLAM, W. & MYERS, R. R. The use of visual evoked responses in objective refraction. *Traps. N.Y. Acad. Sci.* 34: *154-170* (1972).
14. FIORETINI, A. & MAFFEI, L. Evoked potentials in astigmatic subjects. *Vision Res.* 13: *1781-1783* (1973).

299

15. MARTIN, G. Amblyopie astigmatique. Condition du développement parfait de la vision. *Bull. Soc. Francais d'ophtalmologie* 8: *217*-(1890).
16. MARTIN, G. Théorie et clinique de l'amblyopie astigmatique. *Ann. d'ocultistique* 104: *101* (1890).
17. FREEMAN, R. D., MITCHELL, D. E. & MILODOT, M. A. neural effect of partial visual deprivation in humans. *Science* 175: *1384-1386* (1972).
18. MITCHELL, D. E., FREEMAN, R. D., MILLODOT, M. & HAEGERSTROM, G. Meridional amblyopia: evidence for modification of the human visual system by early visual experience. *Vision Res.* 13: *535*-(1972).
19. TAYLOR, M. M. Visual discrimination and orientation. *J. opt. Soc. Amer.* 53: *763* (1963).
20. DUKE-ELDER, S. (Ed.) System of ophthalmology, Vol. 5, 1st Ed., London, Kimpton (1970).
21. MILNER, B. A., REGAN, D. & HERON, J. R. Theoretical models of the generation of steady-state evoked potentials, their relation to neuroanatomy and their relevance to certain clinical problems. 9th Internat. Symp. ISCERG, Brighton 1971. In: ARDEN, G. B. (Ed.) the visual system, Plenum Press, N. York (1972).
22. REGAN, D. & HERON, J. R. Clinical investigation of lesions of the visual pathway: a new objective technique. *J. Neurol. Neurosurg. Psychiat.* 32: *479-483* (1969).
23. REGAN, D. & HERON, J. R. Simultaneous recording of visual evoked potentials from the left and right hemispheres in migraine. In: background to Migraine, Heinemann, Lond., pp. 66-77 (1970).
24. HALLIDAY, A. M., McDONALD, W. I. & MUSHIN, J. Delayed visual evoked response in optic neuritis. *Lancet* 1: *982-985* (1972).
25. TWEEL, L. H. VAN DER & VERDUYN LUNEL, H. F. E. Human visual responses to sinusoidally modulated light. *Electroenceph. clin. Neurophysiol.* 18: *587-598* (1965).
26. REGAN, D. Chromatic adaptation and steady-state evoked potentials. *Vision Res.* 8: *149-158* (1968).
27. TWEEL, L. H. VAN DER & SPEKREIJSE, H. Signal transport and rectification in the human evoked-response system. *Ann. N.Y. Acad. Sci.* 156: *678-695* (1969).
28. COBB, W. A., MORTON, H. B. & ETTLINGER, G. Cerebral potentials evoked by pattern reversal and their suppression in visual rivalry. *Nature* 216: *1124-1125* (1967).
29. RIETVELD, W. J., TORDOIR, W. E. M., HAGENOUW, J. R. B., LUBBERS, J. A. & SPOOR, TH. A. C. Visual evoked responses to blank and to checkerboard-patterned flashes. *Acta Physiol. Pharmacol. Neerl.* 14: *259-285* (1967).
30. SPEKREIJSE, H., TWEEL, L. H. VAN DER & ZUIDEMA, TH. Contrast evoked responses in man. *Vision Res.* 13: *1577-1601* (1973).
31. TWEEL, L. H. VAN DER, REGAN, D. & SPEKREIJSE, H. Some aspects of potentials evoked by changes in spatial brightness contrast. Proc. 7th Internat. Symp. ISCERG, Istanbul, *1-12* (1969).
32. SPEKREIJSE, H., TWEEL, L. H. VAN DER & REGAN, D. Interocular sustained suppression: correlations with evoked potential amplitude and distribution. *Vision Res.* 12: *521-526* (1972).
33. JEFFREYS, D. A. Cortical source locations of pattern-related visual evoked potentials recorded from the human scalp. *Nature* 229: *502-504* (1971).
34. HALLIDAY, A. M. & MICHAEL, W. F. Changes in pattern-evoked responses in man associated with the vertical and horizontal meridians of the visual field. *J. Physiol.* 208: *499-513* (1971).
35. MICHAEL, W. F. & HALLIDAY, A. M. Differences between the occipital distributions of upper and lower-field pattern-evoked responses in man. *Brain Res.* 32: *311-324* (1971).
36. JEFFREYS, D. A. & AXFORD, J. G. Source locations of pattern-specific components of human visual evoked potentials – I. Component of striate cortical origin. II. Component of extra striate cortical origin. *Exp. Brain Res.* *1-21* and *22-40* (1972).
37. REGAN, D. & SPERLING, H. A. method of evoking contour-specific scalp potentials by chromatic checkerboard patterns. *Vision Res.* 11: *173-176* (1971).

38. REGAN, D. Evoked potentials specific to spatial patterns of luminance and colour. *Vision Res.* 13: *2381-2402* (1973).
39. REGAN, D. & SPEKREIJSE, H. Evoked potential indications of colour blindness. *Vision Res.*, 14: *89-95* (1974).
40. REGAN, D. An evoked potential correlate of colour: evoked potential findings and single-cell speculations. *Vision Res.* 13: *1933-1941* (1973).
41. REGAN, D. Colour vision and evoked potentials. 7th Internat. Symp. ISCERG, Istanbul (1969).
42. REGAN, D. Evoked potentials to changes in the chromatic contrast and to changes in the luminance contrast of checkerboard stimulus patterns. 9th Internat. Symp. ISCERG, Brighton, 1971. In: ARDEN, B. G. (Ed.) The visual system, Plenum Press, N. York (1972).
43. REGAN, D. An objective method of measuring the relative spectral luminosity curve in man. *J. opt. Soc. Amer.* 60: *856-859* (1971).
44. RICHARDS, W. Stereopsis and stereoblindness. *Exp. Brain Res.* 10: *380-388* (1970).
45. RICHARDS, W. Anomalous stereoscopic depth perception. *J. opt. Soc. Amer.* 61: *410-414* (1971).
46. REGAN, D. & BEVERLEY, K. I. Dynamic features of threshold and superthreshold depth perception. *Vision Res.* In press (1973).
47. RICHARDS, W. & REGAN, D. Visual fields for stereoscopic depth perception. *Invest. Ophthal.* 12: *904-909* (1973).
48. RICHARDS, W. Factors affecting depth perception. U.S. Air Force Report (AFOSR-TR-73-0439) pp. 28-35 (1973).
49. REGAN, D. & SPEKREIJSE, H. Electrophysiological correlate of binocular depth perception in man. *Nature* 225: *92-94* (1970).
50. REGAN, D. & BEVERLEY, K. I. Electrophysiological evidence for the existence of neurons sensitive to the direction of movement in depth. *Nature* 246: *504-506* (1973).
51. REGAN, D. & CARTWRIGHT, R. F. A. method of measuring the potentials evoked by simultaneous stimulation of different retinal regions. *Electroenceph. clin. Neurophysiol.* 28: *314-319* (1970).
52. GUILLERY, R. W. An abnormal retinogeniculate projection in Siamese cats. *Brain Res.* 14: *739-741* (1969).
53. GUILLERY, R. W. & KAAS, J. H. A study of normally and congenitally retinogeniculate projections in cats. *J. comp. Neurol.* 143: *73-101* (1971).
54. GUILLERY, R. W. An abnormal retinogeniculate projection in the albino ferret (Mustelafuro). *Brain Res.* 33: *482-485* (1971).
55. GUILLERY, R. W., AMORN, C. S. & EIGHMY, B. B. Mutants with abnormal visual pathways: an explanation of anomalous geniculate lamina. *Science* 174: *831-832* (1971).
56. HUBEL, D. H. & WIESEL, T. N. Aberrant visual projections in the Siamese cat. *J. Physiol.* 218: *33-62* (1971).
57. KALIL, R., JHAVERI, S. & RICHARDS, W. R. Anomalous retinal pathways in the Siamese cat: an inadequate substrate for normal binocular vision. *Science* 174: *302-305* (1971).
58. GUILLERY, R. W., SCOTT, G. L., CALTANACH, B. M. & DEOL, M. S. Genetic mechanism determining central visual pathways in mice. *Science* 179: *1014-1016* (1973).
59. BERMAN, N. & CYNADER, M. Comparison of receptive-fied organisation of the superior colliculus in Siamese and normal cats. *J. Physiol.* 224: *363-389* (1972).

Author's address:

Dept. of Communication
University of Keele
Staffordshire, ST 5 5 BG
England

LUMINANCE AND COLOR COMPONENTS IN THE V.E.R.

L. D. VAN HOEK

(Utrecht)

INTRODUCTION

The experiments briefly discussed in this paper were designed for the detection of components in the visual evoked response, associated with the luminosity processing and the color processing by the human visual system. We are mainly concerned with transient responses.

A set of responses is analysed by means of its principal components. Principal components are defined mathematically. They account for a maximum share of the power. The responses were reduced to 2-dimensional vectors. A configuration of response vectors informs us about the underlying processes. The configuration indicates a minimum number of differing processes, involved in the response generation. Sometimes it indicates directly the physiologically most relevant components.

A main difficulty in interpreting a response configuration is caused by non-linear effects. One type of non-linearity is the variation of latency of the responses and the components. In general, latency varies with the amplitude of the stimulus modulation. Non-linear effects distort the structure underlying a response configuration. On the other hand, non-linear effects are the only possible basis for an a posteriori definition of components.

EXPERIMENT 1

In this experiment the stimulus was a centrally fixated 4° field, modulated by a 1 c/s square wave between completely dark and 12 different luminances. These luminances ranged over 3.3 log. units from definitely scotopic conditions to photopic conditions. The responses exhibited a large apparant latency variation, amounting to 100 ms. We corrected for this variation. The result of a principal component analysis of the set of 'on'-responses is given in Fig. 1. In such a vectorial diagram vectorial length represents the r.m.s. amplitude of a response. The direction of a vector represents the shape of the response.

We observe a clustering of response shapes for the dimmest stimuli, as well as for the bright stimuli. These 2 shapes are significantly different. The non-linear behaviour of the response shape clearly indicates 2 ranges of the stimulus luminance, where different processes generate the responses. The processes may

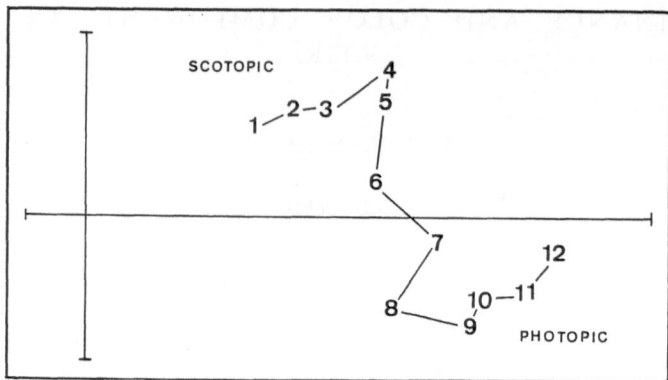

Fig. 1. Two-dimensional vectorial diagram of a set of 12 visual evoked responses to the onset of a circular centrally fixated 4° green stimulus field of the screen of a color television monitor with neutral density filters. The response vectors are denoted by the corresponding stimulus numbers 1-12, located at the end points of the vectors, starting from the origin. The origin is at the point of intersection of the principal coordinate axes. Stimulus luminances: st. 1, 0.004 cd/m²; st. 12, 8 cd/m²; 0.3 log. units difference between the subsequent stimuli. Dark surround. Binocular vision. Natural pupils. Adaptation before recording started. Differential derivation between 3 cm and 10 cm above inion at the midline of scalp. Averages of 800 individual responses of 4 separate sessions. 3 db bandpass 4.6-12 c/s. Time interval 80-480 ms after stimulus onset. Responses corrected for apparent latency differences. Accounted for 98.0% of power.

be indicated by the terms 'scotopic' and 'photopic'. Shape and corresponding process are given by a component with an arbitrary amplitude. Note that a scotopic and a photopic component can be defined a posteriori.

EXPERIMENT 2

The stimulus was a 1 c/s square wave green-red modulation. In stimulus 1 red was brighter than green. For stimulus 10 green was brightest. In the stimuli 5 and 6 green and red were about equally luminous. In the remaining stimuli 11 and 12 the luminance only was modulated. Analysis of the responses to the red-to-green transients results in Fig. 2. Apart from a slight variation of the amplitude, there is a clear variation of shape. The responses 5 and 6 have a minimum amplitude and a maximum apparent latency. We might state, that the point of folding of the trajectory near the responses 5 and 6 represents a response with no or a minimum contribution of 'luminosity'. So we can a posteriori define a color generated response and component. On the other hand, one might postulate, that the responses 11 and 12 represent a luminance-off and a luminance-on component respectively.

For the green-to-red responses a similar behaviour of the responses can be found. A striking difference was the increase of the amount of red relative to green in a luminosity match. This difference, the effect of color selective luminous adaptation being eliminated, was about 0.15 log. units of the ratio of the

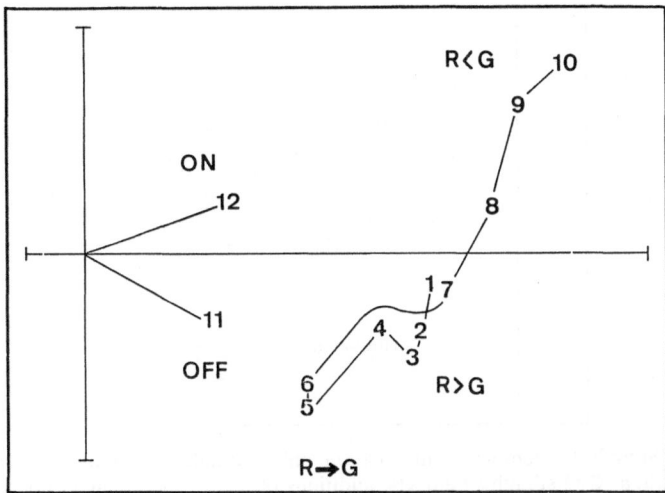

Fig. 2. Responses 1-10 to red-to-green transients of a centrally fixated 2° field in a white surround. Stimulus 1, red brighter than green. Stimulus 10, green brightest. The increment of the luminance difference between red and green is 8% of the mean luminance of the field (8 cd/m²). Stimulus 11 luminance-off transient of 16% of the yellow field. Stimulus 12 luminance-on transient. Averages of 1600 individual responses of 8 separate sessions. Bandpass 3.1-12 c/s. Time interval 100-480 ms after the transient. Accounted for 98.2% of power.

luminances of green and red. We ascribe this difference to interactions between the color modulation generated processes and the processes generated by luminance modulation. Possibly related features are a poor additivity of the color and luminance-off signals in the V.E.R. and some similarity of shape between the color response and the luminance-off response 11. For protanomalous subjects a better additivity of color and luminance associated components was found. We found no clear difference between the luminosity matches via the separate color transients for them.

EXPERIMENT 3

The stimulus field had various colors. For the stimuli 1–6 a small amount of the color of the background was added and subsequently removed by a 1 c/s square wave modulation. For the stimuli 7–12 the colors were added to backgrounds of differing colors. Apart from a luminance modulation, there were modulations of color in the latter stimuli. In view of the non-linearity of the response behaviour, we choose more than 1 amplitude of modulation for each type of stimulus.

Analysis of the set of responses results in Fig. 3. The response trajectories for the stimuli 1–6 lie close together. The responses to the stimuli with additional color modulations deviate from these pretty regularly. These observations can be generalized for more than 2 dimensions. The differences between the respon-

305

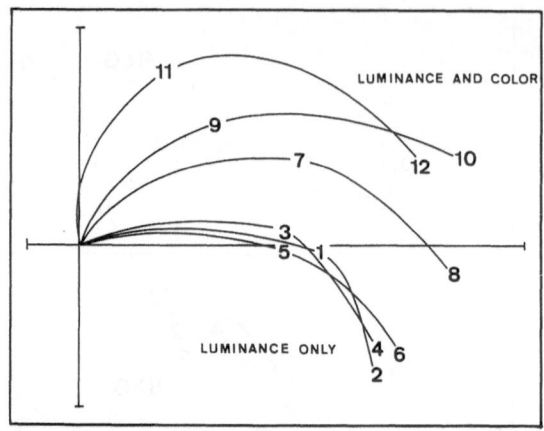

Fig. 3. Stimuli 1-6 luminance modulation only. Stimuli 7-12 luminance and color modulation. Odd stimulus numbers, additions of 5% of the luminance of the background. Even numbers 10% additions. Stimuli 1 and 2 addition of red to a red background. 3 and 4 green to green. 5 and 6 blue to blue. 7 and 8 red to yellowish green. 9 and 10 green to red. 11 and 12 blue to green. 2° centrally fixated stimulus field. Luminance of the background and the white surround 8 cd/m². Averages of 1600 individual responses of 8 separate sessions. Bandpass 3.7-12 c/s. Complete period of the responses analysed. Accounted for 89% of power.

ses 1–6 and the responses 7–12 can be related to the subjective color modulations of the stimuli. These differences can be seen as the result of superposition of 'color modulation components'. As there are no great color specific differences for the responses 1--6, luminosity processing presumably dominates in the generation of these responses. The variations of shape of the responses and the components, deduced from this diagram, can be seen as apparent latency variation mainly. So we found a correlate in the V.E.R. for color modulation in this and other similar experiments. Color modulation was a more appropriate stimulus factor for the analysis of the responses than the colors of the background or the addition.

Authors' address:

Depts. of Ophthalmology and
Physics, State University Utrecht.
F. C. Dondersstraat 65
Utrecht
The Netherlands

COLOUR VISION IN RHESUS MONKEY, STUDIED WITH SUBDURALLY IMPLANTED CORTICAL ELECTRODES

PIETER PADMOS & VIRGIL GRAF*

(*Soesterberg, The Netherlands*)

ABSTRACT

A set of nine electrodes (dimension of electrodes 0.1 × 0.3 mm) is chronically implanted on the subdural surface of the primary visual cortex of macaca mulatta. Responses to monochromatic, foveal light stimuli on various coloured backgrounds are recorded. On a white background the spectral sensitivity function shows three submaxima, like the functions SPERLING & HARWERTH (1971) found in behavioural experiments. From these results, and the chromatic adaptation experiments, it is evident that the responses reflect colour antagonistic interactions between cone systems. The extent to which these antagonistic interactions contribute to the electroretinographic response, is discussed.

Of the electrophysiological techniques used to study colour coding in the visual cortex two are currently very popular: Single nerve cells are studied with microelectrodes (GOURAS, 1972; DOW & GOURAS, 1973), and a mass response of the brain is recorded with scalp electrodes (e.g., CIGÁNEK & INGVAR, 1969; RIPPS & VAUGHAN, 1969; and KELLERMAN & ADACHI-USAMI, 1972/73). The technique presented here, with chronically implanted subdural electrodes has the advantage that it is possible to measure local graded reponses of the cortex (local VECP), while the measurement errors and sampling errors inherent to microelectrode studies are avoided. The local measurement of VECP avoids further the difficulty, encountered mainly with scalp electrodes on human subjects, of not knowing whether the potential is generated by the primary or secondary visual cortex.

This paper will show the spectral sensitivities at various white and chromatic backgrounds, recorded with surface cortical electrodes at the foveal projection projection of area 17.

METHODS

The data described here are from one male macaca mulatta (3 kg), which was verified with Vector-Retinography (PADMOS & NORREN, 1972) to have a normal scotopic and photopic spectral sensitivity (Fig. 1). Recently the results were

---

* On leave from Dartmouth College, Hanover, Nw. Hampshire, U.S.A.

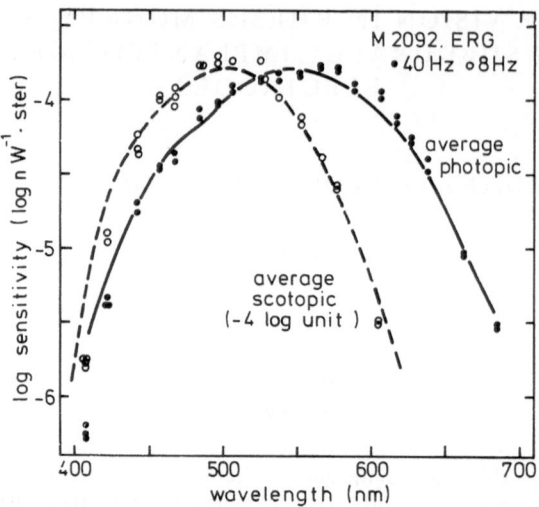

Fig. 1. Scotopic and photopic spectral sensitivity, measured with Vector-Retinography. Both sets of data points were measured with a 45 deg stimulus field, without background. In this and the following figures the ordinate refers to an absolute radiance scale (1 log nW. ster –1 = 1.2 log troland at 560 nm). The response criterion was 2 μV. The full drawn curve is the average monkey spectral sensitivity curve according to NORREN (1971), the dashed curve refers to unpublished data on the average monkey scotopic curve.

confirmed partially on other individuals of the same species. The monkey had a sheath of epoxy resin, with nine stainless steel surface electrodes (0.1 × 0.3 mm uninsulated surface), implanted subdurally over the foveal projection area of primary visual cortex (technique modified after HUGHES & MAZUROWSKI, 1959) which is in the monkey exposed to the parieto-temporal skull. The distance between electrodes was 3-8 mm. A centrally placed stainless steel bone screw served as a reference electrode (code nr. 14).

The *preparation* of the animal is described in detail in another paper presented at this symposium (NORREN & PADMOS, 1974). The animal was paralyzed, artificially respirated and anaesthetized with 70% N_2O in O_2, combined with 0.2-0.3% Halothane. To protect the cornea and correct for accommodation errors the monkey was fitted with contact lenses.

The basic *optical system* is described previously (NORREN & PADMOS, 1973). It consists of a Xenon light source, a double beam light path with narrow band interference filters in the stimulus path, and broad band colour filters (red: Schott RG630; yellow: Schott OG550; blue: Schott BG18 + Wratten 47; purple: Wratten 35) in the adaptation beam. For the present experiments the adaptation and stimulus beam were combined in a laboratory-built ophthalmoscope-stimulator, which made possible to direct stimulus spots onto the macular area. The position of the stimulus with respect to the fovea was known with an accuracy better than 20 min. of arc. Standard stimulus diameter was

5 deg of arc, the adaptation beam subtended 12 deg of arc. An electro-me-chanical shutter provided flashes of 300-500 ms at a repetition time of 700-1000 ms.

The *measuring system* consisted of a differential preamplifier, a passband amplifier (5-200 Hz) and an averaging computer (CAT).

RESULTS

In Fig. 2 the response waveform and spectral sensitivity are given for mono-chromatic stimuli superimposed on a steady white background of 3000 td. The on and off responses are similar in shape, but the spectral sensitivities of respectively the on and off responses show small but systematic differences (compare full line and broken line). For comparison a human psychophysical spectral sensitivity curve is given, which is recorded under the same stimulus conditions. The electrophysiological response criterion was 50 μV from first negative to second positive peak.

Figs. 3A and B give the spectral sensitivities (from a neighbouring electrode) on several coloured backgrounds. The foveal receptor primaries (at corneal level) are also given (dashed lines). The Red (R) and Green (G) primaries are human data from Vos & WALRAVEN (1971). For the macaque Blue (B) primary the data is from NORREN & PADMOS (1973).

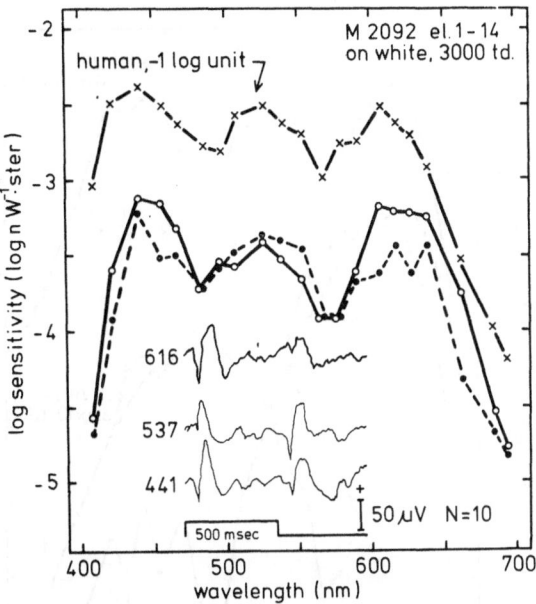

Fig. 2. Spectral sensitivity (average of 3 measurements) on a white background of 12 deg., 3000 td. Stimulus 5 deg., centered on the fovea. The response criterion was 50 μV. ——O—— = on-sensitivity, – – ●– – = off-sensitivity. The upper curve is a human psychophysical curve obtained under the same stimulus conditions. The psychophysical criterion was detection of the flash on the steady white background.

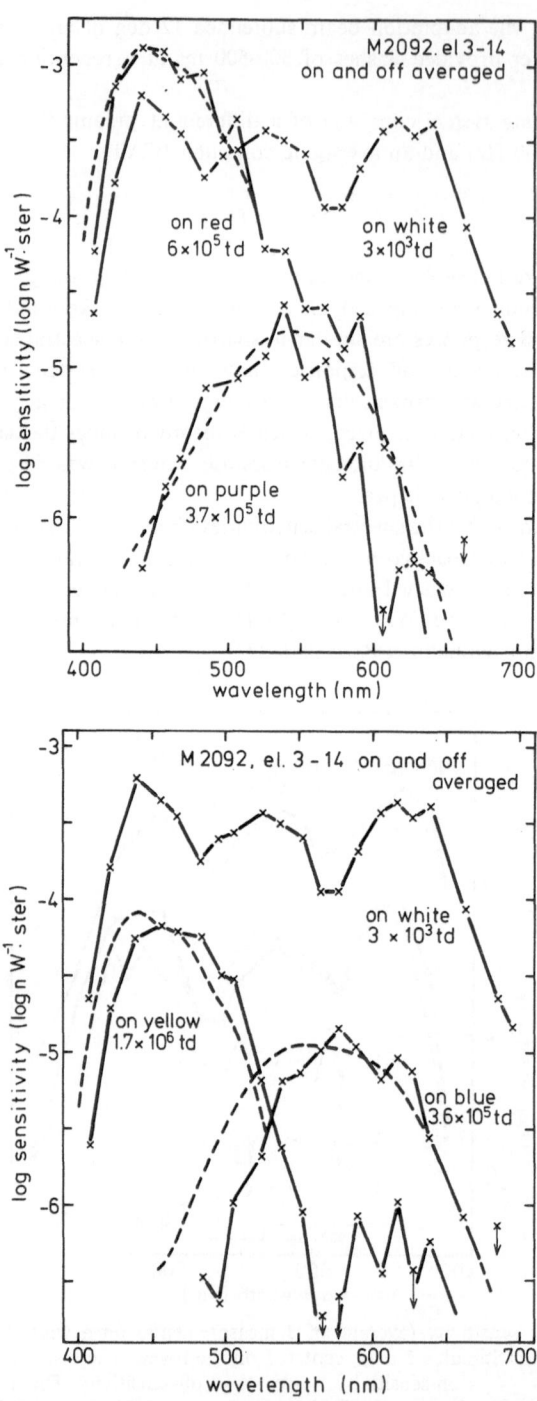

Fig. 3A, B. Spectral sensitivities on various coloured backgrounds. The on- and off sensitivities are averaged. The other conditions are similar to those of Fig. 2.

The B mechanism fits reasonably well the sensitivities recorded on red and yellow backgrounds. The curves on blue and purple backgrounds are definitely narrower than the respective R and G mechanisms.

On the white background a peak sensitivity is present at about 610 nm, whereas the peak sensitivity on a blue background is shifted towards the peak of the R mechanism ($\sim$ 565 nm at corneal level). Likewise the 525 nm peak on white background shows a similar but smaller shift towards the 540 nm G-peak when measured on a purple background.

Although there sometimes is evidence that two electrodes at neighbouring place have different spectral sensitivities, we were seldom able to record systematic interelectrode differences. Electrode shunting by subdural fluid may be a cause. However, note that Figs. 2-3 are from monopolar recordings, i.e. an active cortical electrode versus the central reference electrode (code nr. 14). Common cortical activity may obscure local activity. Fig. 4 shows a bipolar recording between electrodes 1 and 7, which were 6 mm apart, but both in the foveal projection area. The resulting spectral sensitivity has no apparent B input, in fact it could be fitted with the absolute value of a linear subtraction of R and G spectral sensitivity curves.

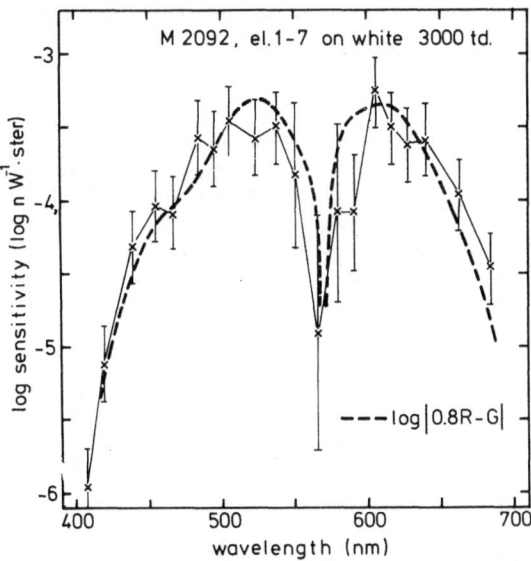

Fig. 4. Bipolar recording of spectral sensitivity on a white background. Average of 3 measurements. Standard deviation is given by vertical bars. Similar conditions as in Fig. 2. The dashed curve is the absolute value of a linear subtraction of weighted R and G mechanisms.

311

The results on a white background have certain features in common with the previous VECP work of CAVONIUS (1965), CIGÁNEK & INGVAR (1969) and SIEGFRIED (1971), who also found more or less enhanced blue and red sensitivities, in more or less comparable recording situations. Recently KELLERMAN & ADACHI-USAMI (1972/73) studied chromatic adaptation of the human VECP and in their paper the curves on a blue-green and purple background indeed are narrower than respectively the R and G fundamental mechanisms proposed by VOS & WALRAVEN (1971). KELLERMAN & ADACHI-USAMI do not present spectral sensitivity on a white background.

The present results are very similar to the behavioural data on monkeys, obtained by SPERLING & HARWERTH (1971). The latter authors assume that the spectral sensitivity on a white background is caused by antagonistic interaction of the R and G receptor mechanisms. The shifting of the 610 nm peak towards shorter wavelengths during blue adaptation indeed makes the idea of antagonistic R-G interaction likely. Our Fig. 4 illustrates this point more clearly.

Studies on single cells have forwarded the basic assumption that antagonistic interaction between receptor systems is a necessary condition for colour perception. Excitation is characterized by an on-discharge, inhibition is followed by an off-discharge. Although differences in on and off spectral sensitivity are small (Fig. 2), the systematically greater sensitivity at light-on, for the short and long

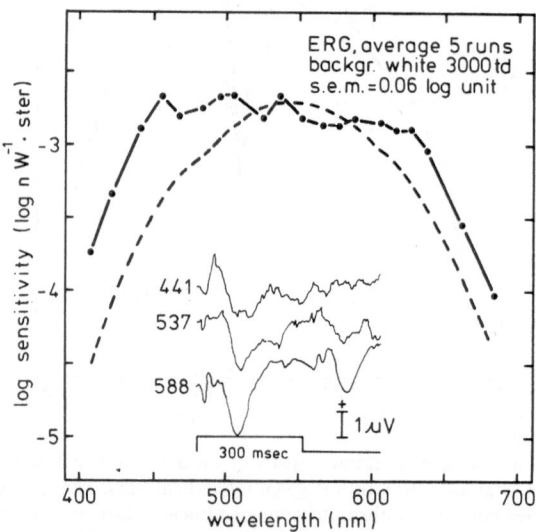

Fig. 5. ERG recording of spectral sensitivity. Average of 5 recordings from 3 monkeys. Stimulus: duration 300 ms, repetition time 700 ms, field width 45 deg, Maxwellian view. Adaptation: white 3000 td, 75 deg. Criterion: 1 μV peak to peak for on-response. The dashed curve is the average monkey photopic spectral sensitivity as measured with Vector Retinography.

wavelength peak again points toward antagonistic interactions of receptor systems (see also GOURAS, 1972).

Since it is known that antagonistic R-G interaction is present at the retinal ganglion cell level, one may ask whether colour opponency can be detected with electroretinography. An indication in this direction is given in Fig. 5. Whereas at high frequencies the large field ERG spectral sensitivity is similar to WALD's (1945) extrafoveal curve (NORREN, 1971), at low frequencies (300 ms flash, repetition time 700 ms) the curve broadens. Since the background light subtends a large angle (75 deg.) and is strong enough (3000 td) to suppress all rod activity, the higher sensitivity at short wavelengths must reflect enhanced B activity. The shoulder on the long wavelength part of the curve can only be explained, like before at the cortical recordings, by the contribution of antagonistic R-G interaction to the ERG. Therefore, either the Müller cells receive antagonistic input from R and G, or at these lower frequencies the ganglion cells contribute to the ERG response.

Concluding, we state that:
- antagonistic interactions between receptor systems and thus colour vision mechanisms, are very evident in local VECP recordings on monkeys.
- the primate ERG also shows evidence, at lower frequency stimulation, for a relatively weak contribution from antagonistic R-G systems.

REFERENCES

CAVONIUS, C. R. Evoked response of the human visual cortex: Spectral sensitivity. *Psychon. Sci.* 2: *185-186* (1965).

CIGÁNEK, L. & INGVAR, D. H. Colour specific features of visual cortical responses in man evoked by monochromatic flashes. *Acta Physiol. Scand.* 76: *82-92* (1969).

DOW, B. M. & GOURAS, P. Color and spatial specificity of single units in rhesus monkey foveal striate cortex. *J. Neurophysiol.* 36: *79-100* (1973).

GOURAS, P. Color opponency from fovea to striate cortex. *Invest. Ophthalmol.* 11: *427-434* (1972).

HUGHES, J. R. & MAZUROWSKI, J. A. Studies on the supracallosal mesial cortex of unanaesthetized, conscious mammals. *Electroenc. clin. Neurophysiol.* 11: *447-458* (1959).

KELLERMAN, F. J. & ADACHI-USAMI, E. Spectral sensitivities of colour mechanisms isolated by the human visual evoked response. *Ophthal. Res.* 4: *199-210* (1972/73).

NORREN, D. V. Macaque photopic spectral sensitivity. *Vision Res.* 11: *1175-1177* (1971).

NORREN, D. V. & PADMOS, P. Human and macaque blue cones studied with electro-retinography. *Vision Res.* 13: *1241-1254* (1973).

NORREN, D. V. & PADMOS, P. Halothane retards dark adaptation. Proc. XIth ISCERG symp., September 1973, Bad Nauheim, Germany, This volume-(1974).

PADMOS, P. & NORREN, D. V. The vector voltmeter as a tool to measure electroretino-gram spectral sensitivity and dark adaptation. *Invest. Ophthalmol.* 11: *783-788* (1972).

RIPPS, H. & VAUGHAN, H. G., Jr. The spectral sensitivity of evoked potentials from the retina and cortex of nocturnal and diurnal monkeys. *Vision Res.* 9: *895-907* (1969).

SIEGFRIED, J. B. Spectral sensitivity of human visual evoked cortical potentials: a new method and a comparison with psychophysical data. *Vision Res.* 11: *405-417* (1971).

SPERLING, H. G. & HARWERTH, R. S. Red-green cone interactions in the increment-threshold spectral sensitivity of primates. *Science*, N.Y. 172: *180-184* (1971).

Vos, J. J. & Walraven, P. L. On the derivation of the foveal receptor primaries. *Vision Res.* 11: *799-818* (1971).

Wald, G. Human vision and the spectrum. *Science*, N.Y. 101: *653-658* (1945).

Authors' address:

Institute for Perception TNO
Kampweg 5
Soesterberg
The Netherlands

RESPONSES TO SPECTRAL LIGHT STIMULI RECORDED IN TECTUM OPTICUM OF THE FROG

H. SCHEIBNER, MURIEL BEZAUT & W. HUNOLD

(Bad Nauheim)

ABSTRACT

Retinal ganglion cells classified by MATURANA et al. as members of class I and III were investigated by means of extracellular micro-electrode recording in the optic tectum of the frog Rana esculenta. Light stimulation was performed by the method of stimulus substitution.

Results:
Class I could be divided into four subclasses: 1) neurons with a univariant spectral sensitivity function analogous to GRANIT's photopic dominator; 2) neurons with a spectral sensitivity function exhibiting one break in the short wavelength region; 3) neurons with a spectral sensitivity function exhibiting one break in the long wavelength region; 4) neurons with a spectral sensitivity function exhibiting one break in the short wavelength region as well as one break in the long wavelength region.
Class III neurons showed a univariant spectral sensitivity function throughout, analogous to GRANIT's photopic dominator. The results of class I point to the possibility that the frog can see stationary colour contrast.

In the waterfrog, Rana esculenta, there exists a projection of the retina onto four layers of axonal terminals in the optic tectum. While the ganglion cells are distributed randomly in the retina, they appear partitioned in the tectum in the form of four classes (cf. SZÉKELY, 1973). The various classes can be distinguished by the depth of their layers from the tectum surface, and, above all, by functional criteria.

We would like to report on investigations on class I and class III. LETTVIN and his co-workers (MATURANA et al., 1960, LETTVIN et al., 1959, 1961) termed the neurons of class I 'sustained edge detectors' and the neurons of class III 'changing contrast detectors'. Our aim was to subdivide the existing partition of neurons with the help of spectral radiation stimuli and find out whether or not the frog possesses a neurophysiological basis for a colour vision.

APPARATUS AND METHODS

Fig. 1 shows the apparatus schematically. The optical stimulator consists of two paths, which originate from two xenon 150 Watt lamps. The two beams are superimposed by a beam splitting cube, they then pass a fixed 90 degree prism (M), a pivoted plane mirror (Mirror), a concave mirror, and are finally directed into the right eye of the frog.

In both beams there are polarizing filters, P_I and P_{II}, before the superimposing cube. They produce linearly polarized light in planes at right angles to each other. A polarizing filter (A) acts as an analyser. This analyser may be in one of two fixed positions, which differ by a rotation of 90 degrees. In the one position, its plane of polarization is parallel to the plane of P_I, in the other position it is parallel to the plane of P_{II}. Within 60 milliseconds, the analyser can be rotated from one position to the other. In this way, a smooth intensity transition from one beam to the other can take place without any interruption or doubling of the radiant flux. For extracellular recording of impulse discharges, platinum-iridium alloy micro-electrodes after WAGNER et al. (1960) were inserted into the left tectum.

Photic stimulation was as follows: Two stimuli of different wavelengths were released according to the following time pattern: firstly, the analyser (A, Fig. 1) was in such a position that a 'test stimulus' could pass; after 3.5 s, the analyser was turned by 90 degrees, so that a 'reference stimulus' could pass; four seconds later (i.e. 7.5 s from the onset of the stimulus), the analyser was turned once more by 90 degrees so that the test stimulus could pass once more; 1.5 s later the shutter closed. The duration of the whole stimulation amounted, thus, to $(3.5 + 4 + 1.5)\,s = 9$ seconds. This stimulus pattern was repeated at intervals of one minute. Our attention was particularly directed to the stages 3.5 s and 7.5 s after stimulation onset, where stimulus substitution took place. Here, we distinguish two possibilities:

a. For a certain flux ratio of the two successive stimuli, no new discharge of the neuron is initiated. Following DONNER & RUSHTON (1959), we call this event a 'silent substitution', and chose this non-appearance of discharge as an equivalent criterion of colour match.

b. Whenever a stimulus is replaced by the following one, a new discharge always occurs. This we took to indicate the lack of silent substitution.

For those wavelengths for which a silent substitution occurs we defined the following spectral sensitivity function $S_q(\lambda)$

$$S_q(\lambda) = \frac{I_o(\lambda_r)}{I(\lambda)}$$

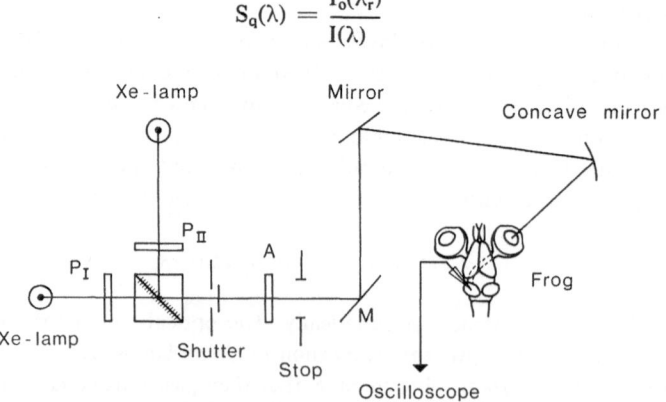

Fig. 1. Scheme of the experimental set up. P_I, P_{II}: polarizers, A: analyser; M: fixed 90 degree prism, the other elements are fully designated.

wherein $I_o(\lambda_r)$ means the flux of the reference stimulus (constant in wavelength), and $I(\lambda)$ means the flux of the test stimulus (variable in wavelength). The value of $I_o(\lambda_r)$ was chosen one log unit above the absolute threshold and kept constant. $I(\lambda)$ is determined as that value for which silent substitution occurs. All fluxes are expressed as relative numbers of light quanta per second. According to these measures, our sensitivity functions are quantum based action spectra.

If a silent substitution can by no means be brought about, a description by means of a connected sensitivity function is not possible. In general, however, a different reference wavelength may be found that can be silently substituted. Thus, disconnected parts of sensitivity functions are obtained. With a slight modification of RUSHTON's concept of univariance (RUSHTON, 1972; SCHEIBNER & SCHMIDT, 1969), we call a transducing system 'univariant', if it exhibits a connected invariant spectral sensitivity function. If a transducing system exhibits a disconnected spectral sensitivity function, it is in any case not univariant. The 'breaks' that separate the parts of the sensitivity function in these cases are wavelength intervals, where, according to the chosen criterion, no sensitivity is defined.

RESULTS

Fig. 2 shows a class I neuron with a univariant sensitivity function. The arrow indicates the reference wavelength λ_r. According to the definition, the sensitivity at such wavelengths λ_r (or alternatively at the test wavelengths approximately equal to them) has the value one, and so the logarithm is zero. This curve means that every wavelength could be silently substituted by any reference wavelength, in this case of 500 nm.

Fig. 3 shows a class I neuron with a break in the sensitivity function in the short wavelength region. Silent substitution in the short wavelength region was possible only by a reference wavelength in the same region, but not by a reference wavelength taken from the long wavelength region, and vice versa. Similarly, Fig. 4 shows a class I neuron exhibiting a break in the long wavelength region; finally Fig. 5 shows a class I neuron exhibiting a break in the short wavelength region as well as a break in the long wavelength region. In summary, we could subdivide class I in four subclasses of neurons, one class with a

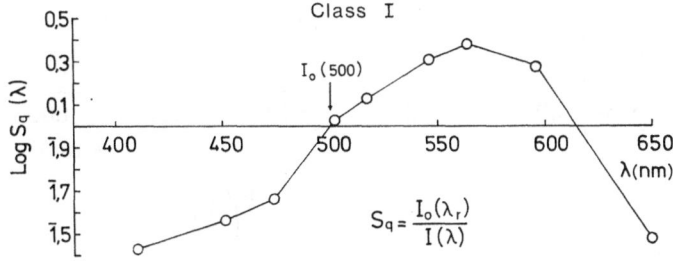

Fig. 2. Spectral sensitivity function of a univariant neuron of class I.

univariant spectral behaviour, three subclasses with various different kinds of non-univariant spectral behaviour.

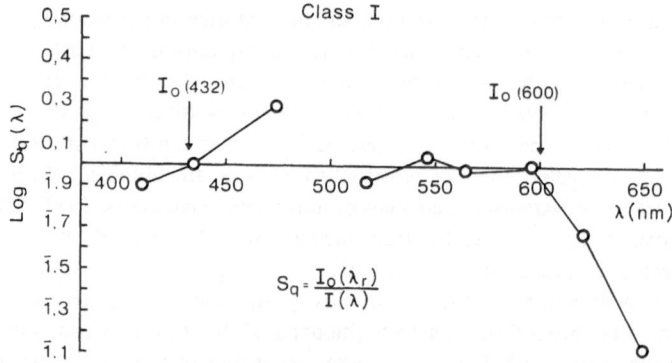

Fig. 3. Spectral sensitivity function of a class I neuron exhibiting one break in the short wavelength region.

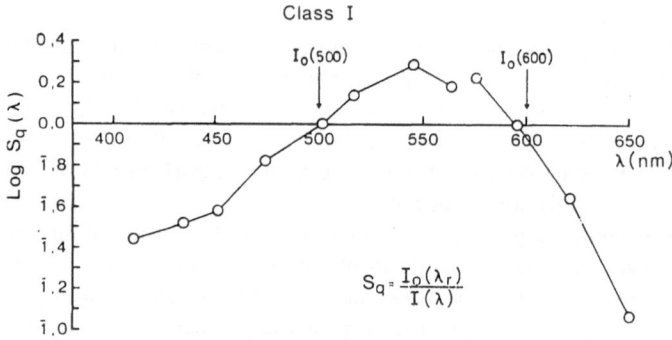

Fig. 4. Spectral sensitivity function of a class I neuron exhibiting one break in the long wavelength region.

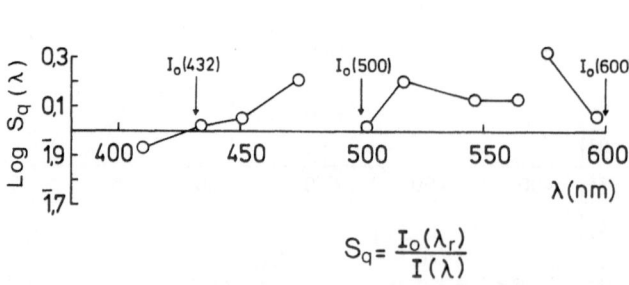

Fig. 5. Spectral sensitivity function of a class I neuron exhibiting one break in the short wavelength region, as well as one break in the long wavelength region.

318

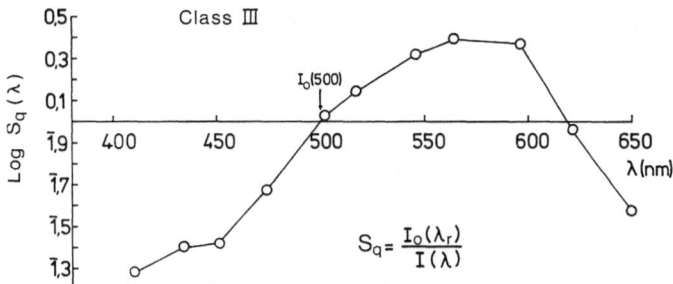

Fig. 6. Spectral sensitivity function of a class III neuron. All neurons of this class investigated so far showed this univariant behaviour.

Fig. 6 shows a neuron of class III exhibiting a univariant sensitivity function. Only this type could be found for class III.

DISCUSSION

Those neurons of class I and class III which could be silently substituted throughout the spectrum (Figs. 2, 6) and we call therefore 'univariant' show a spectral sensitivity function in good agreement with curves reported by GRANIT in 1942. GRANIT called the underlying mechanism 'photopic dominator'. A univariant response behaviour necessarily comes forward, if a mechanism is fed by only one visual pigment, in man e.g. by rhodopsin during night vision. But the converse need not be true: a univariant response behaviour need not be subserved by only one photopigment. It is very likely that the ganglion cells showing univariance are nevertheless fed by more than one visual pigment. REUTER & VIRTANEN (1972) argue that the two types of cones – absorbing maximally at 575 nm and 502 nm (LIEBMAN & ENTINE, 1968) – make up the photopic dominator. REUTER & VIRTANEN (1972) recorded from the frog dominator-like retina sensitivity functions of class I similar to ours, but unlike our results, no dominator-like sensitivity functions of class III.

Besides univariant neurons, class I contains neurons with one or two breaks in the sensitivity curves (Figs. 3, 4, 5). Here, we can draw a cogent conclusion: if it is true that a single visual pigment leads to a univariant sensitivity function, then non-univariance necessarily means that not only one visual pigment contributes to the output of this neuron.

The type of breaks found in the short wavelength region is in a good agreement with results of SCHEIBNER & BAUMANN (1970) as well as REUTER & VIRTANEN (1972), whereas the break in the long wavelength region seems to be a new result for the frog. It is, however, compatible with the visual pigments present in the frog's retina (LIEBMAN & ENTINE, 1968). Our results on class I suggest that the neural processing in the frog's retina and tectum includes colour. They point to a neurophysiological basis of a trichromatic colour vision in the frog. Behavioural studies seem to indicate a dichromatic colour vision in the frog. (BIRUKOW, 1949; THOMAS, 1965; CHAPMAN, 1966). The question remains whether and how the frog makes use of its neurophysiological disposition.

319

ACKNOWLEDGEMENT

We would like to thank WALTER KLEIN for designing and constructing the timing apparatus.

REFERENCES

BIRUKOW, G. Die Entwicklung des Tages- und Dämmerungssehens im Auge des Grasfrosches. *Z. vergl. Physiol.* 31: *322-347* (1949).

CHAPMAN, R. M. Light wavelength and energy preferences of the bull frog: evidence for colour vision. *J. Compar. Physiol. Psychol.* 61: *429-435* (1966).

DONNER, K. O. & RUSHTON, W. A. H. Retinal stimulation by light substitution. *J. Physiol.* 149: *288-302* (1959).

GRANIT, R. Colour receptors in the frog's retina. *Acta physiol. scand.* 3: *137-151* (1942).

LETTVIN, J. Y., MATURANA, H. R., McCULLOCH, W. S. & PITTS, W. H. What the frog's eye tells the frog's brain. *Proc. IRE* 47: *1940-1951* (1959).

LETTVIN, J. Y., MATURANA, H. R., PITTS, W. H. & McCULLOCH, W. S. Two remarks on the visual system of the frog. In: Sensory Communication ed. by W. ROSENBLITH, MIT Press, Cambridge, Mass (1961).

LIEBMAN, P. A. & ENTINE, G. Visual pigments of frog and tadpole (Rana pipiens). *Vision Res.* 8: *761-775* (1968).

MATURANA, H. R., LETTVIN, J. Y., McCULLOCH, W. S. & PITTS, W. H. Anatomy and Physiology of Vision in the frog (Rana pipiens). *J. Gen. Physiology* 43: Supplement, *129-175* (1960).

REUTER, T. & VIRTANEN, K. Border and colour coding in the retina of the frog. *Nature* 239: *260-263* (1972).

RUSHTON, W. A. H. Visual pigments in Man. In: Handbook of Sensory Physiology. Vol. VII/1, ed. by H. J. A. DARTNALL. Springer-Verlag, Berlin, Heidelberg, New York (1972).

SCHEIBNER, H. & SCHMIDT, B. Zum Begriff der spektralen visuellen Empfindlichkeit mit elektroretinographischen Ergebnissen am Hund. *A. v. Graefes Arch. Ophthal.* 117: *124-135* (1969).

SCHEIBNER, H. & BAUMANN, CH. Properties of the frog's retinal ganglion cells as revealed by substitution of chromatic stimuli. *Vision Res.* 10: *829-836* (1970).

SZÉKELY, G. Anatomy and synaptology of the optic tectum. In: Handbook of Sensory Physiology Vol. VII/3 Part B, ed. by R. JUNG. Springer-Verlag, Berlin, Heidelberg, New York (1973).

THOMAS, E. Untersuchungen über den Helligkeits- und Farbensinn der Anuren. *Zool. Jahrbuch* 66: *129-178* (1956).

WAGNER, H. G., McNICHOL, E. F. JR. & WOLBARSHT, M. L. The response properties of single ganglion cells in the goldfish retina. *J. gen. Physiol.* 43: Supplement *45-62* (1960).

Authors' address:

Max Planck Institute
W.G. Kerckhoff Institute
D 6350 Bad Nauheim
B.R.D.

STUDY OF CLINICAL INTEREST OF THE VISUAL EVOKED RESPONSES OBTAINED BY FOCAL STIMULATION FOLLOWING THE EYE MOVEMENTS

J. Cl. HACHE, P. DUBOIS & P. FRANCOIS

(*Lille*)

The clinical application of the study of the visual evoked potentials by means of a focal stimulation of a retinal area poses very difficult problems.

These difficulties have already been described by Professor HENKES and VAN LITH at the the tenth ISCERG Symposium of the last year.

Our work confirms their results and tries to provide certain explanations.

METHOD DESCRIPTION

Our device has been described at the IX Symposium of ISCERG. Basically it consists of a perimeter composed of a bowl with a one meter radius, with a device for the detection of the eye movements. We followed the suggestion of HENKES to use his contact lens.

It is possible to obtain a depression between the lens and the cornea which fixes it strongly on the eye. Its weight and the contact of the eyelids lessen the eye-ball movements and this is very useful in our system. We have equipped this lens with a microphotodiode which emits in the infrared (wavelength:1 micron). The image of this photodiode is formed on a photosensitive matrix made of 1024 elements. The position of the eye is then sent to a computer every two milliseconds. The computer places two stepping motors which send the light spot of stimulation towards the cupola, so as it may be always facing the same retinal point.

Because of the geometry of the system, the size of the spot cannot exceed 2 degrees and the studied field is limited at the central field (30 degrees). We use white or red spots of 1000 apostilbs on a blue or white photopic background. The E.R.G. and the V.E.R. are processed by the computer.

CLINICAL STUDY

Like many others, we hoped to obtain an objective perimetry from the V.E.R. We were first concerned by the response to macular stimulations.

At the present time, after 256 or 512 white two degrees central stimulations, we obtain for a normal patient an evoked response usually between 1 and 2 microvolts. But as soon as there is an alteration of the central vision (maculopathy or optic neuritis) the response cannot be recognized out of the noise.

Concerning the paramacular areas, it is necessary to obtain 1024, or even 2048 stimulations to obtain a registrable response (1μv). This needs 8 minutes for each retinal studied point.

The S/N quotient is too small to quantify in this way an alteration of the macular or paramacular areas. So we can confirm the idea of HENKES & VAN LITH who think that the evoked potentials do not enable an electro-perimetry. The clinical reliability of the evoked response to focal stimulations does not seem sufficient to justify its use. With these methods of global red stimulations, (658 nanometers as ALFIERI & SOLE) we obtain an evoked response which reflects rather well the quality of the central vision.

CONDITIONS TO OBTAIN FOCAL V.E.R.

With the preceding findings in mind, we tried to determine the conditions necessary to obtain registrable potentials for a located stimulation of *at least* two degrees.

On account of the small number of nervous fibres activated by such a stimulation (except in the macular area) and with the classic methods of averaging by summation, it is necessary to have more than 2500 stimulations to get a noise lower than 0.2 microvolt and an evoked response higher than 1μ volt (S/N = 50 at least). This requires a very long time: between 10 and 20 minutes for a point.

It is not possible for the patient to maintain such long fixation and this justifies the use of stimulation following the eye movements.

This system is much more useful in case of central scotoma. At the present time it is clinically difficult to achieve because the depression contact lens can become dangerous if it is worn too long. Also, we are not sure that the statistical properties of the signal (specially the stationarity) can be maintained during the examination. Of course, all these difficulties do not exist with the E.R.G.

CONCLUSION

In spite of the use of an assessed stimulation, the clinical interest of the focal V.E.R. cannot be proved.

As HENKES, VAN LITH and collaborators, we think that only Electroretinography can be actually useful at the present time.

However, all this may change in a near future. It may become possible to make servomechanism for a system without needing a contact lens for the collection and processing of signal. In this field, the use of lock-in amplifiers proposed by Dutch authors poses an interesting new approach.

CONTRIBUTION TO OBJECTIVE PERIMETRY BY MEANS OF THE VER

W. MÜLLER, E. HAASE, W. HÖHNE, E.SCHMÖGER &
G. HENNING

(Erfurt)

We still remember the interesting statements of Prof. HENKES at the IV. Congress of the European Society of Ophthalmology. We studied them carefully and agree with him in the fundamental points. But in spite of all hesitations, it is necessary that a large number of investigator groups deal with this problem. If we are convinced that the cortical reaction represents a light stimulating reaction and that the retina has its representation in the occiput, then it must be possible to derive an individual reaction when stimulating different retinal areas. In our opinion, objective perimetry by means of VER is finally a question of methodology, not of principle.

The first figure shows the block diagram of our examination device.

We describe in short three essential considerations of our team.

1. We developed a stimulation device as we assumed that it is an important prerequisite for investigations of objective perimetry. It is an hemisphere having a diameter of 1.5 m. The inner side is white.

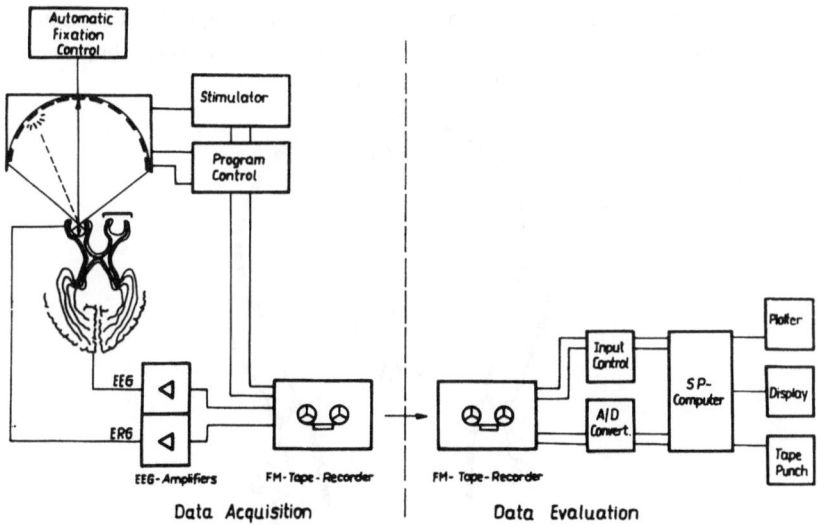

Fig. 1. Block diagram. Method of objective perimetry by means of VER

323

It shows a diffuse background-illumination that can be varied between dark and 20 lx.

Conversion to background-illumination with blue light is under development. The stimulation device provides 50 stimulation points, each of which is equipped with xenon flash tubes allowing discharge energies of 0,05 to 2.0 Ws. The maximum opening of each stimulation point is 8 mm, but it may be reduced by providing circular stops in front of it. Arbitrary filters can be employed as well. A specially developed electronics device permits to call each stimulation point separately or in a programmed circuit. Flash frequency is continuously variable up to a maximum of 7 Hz; a statistical generator is under development. The number of flashes per stimulation point can be varied between 1 and 10000.

An essential possibility to keep the scattered light fraction to a minimum is to put the background-illumination and the respectively selected flash brightness into a certain relation, since the problem of scattered light certainly is a question of this relation.

2. As long as there is no automatic signal recognition available, a derivation method keeping the temporal stress on the person under investigation within reasonable limits has to be developed empirically. We have determined that at a 3-Hz frequency, 50 flashes per stimulation point are sufficient and that a minimum 15 to 20 stimulation points should be called during a session. That means an examination period of abt. 6 minutes for the patient. The majority of patients could maintain a sufficiently exact fixation, during this period. We record 3 derivation channels for each examination i.e. unipolar 2 channels, bipolar 1 channel (Figure 2).

This is a minimum demand due to the technical possibilities available (capacity of magnetic tape recorder and computer). Examination is carried out without previous adaptation to the dark. The only adaptation occurs during the time when the electrodes are arranged in a room having a brightness of 10 lx. Dilation o the pupils was not applied.

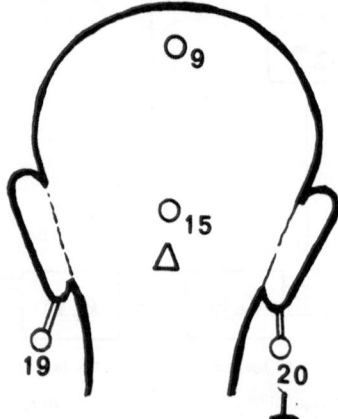

Fig. 2. Arrangement of electrodes

3. Here, too, we must say: as long as there is no automatic signal recognition available, we are forced to assess the data supplied by the computer (mean-value curve), i.e. the Yes-No decision in case of the signal under discussion is not solved by the computer; the computer only improves the signal-to-noise ratio; the decision with the highly variable curves is left to the investigator. That certainly is the weakest point of this method.

The following fact has proved to be a criterion for evaluation: if there is no positive potential during the 80 to 120 millisecond period and if these findings can be detected at least in two of the three channels, we assume that this is a 'No' decision and record this value as not seen, i.e. as scotoma. We leave to the discussion whether this procedure can be justified. In our opinion Z. NAKAMURA & W. R. BIERSDORF apply similar criterion for evaluation. For the purpose of control, we note at each stimulation point whether the test subject has recognized the light flash.

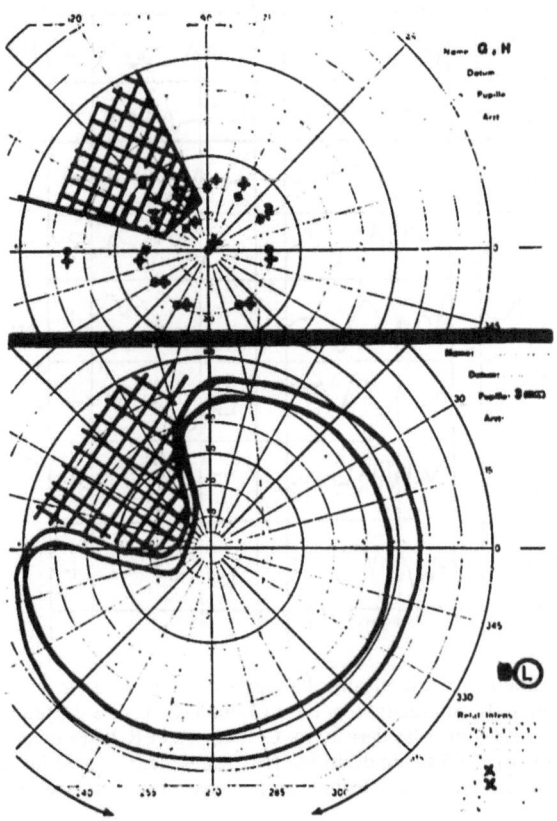

Fig. 3. The figure shows the visual field of the patient H. G., as determined by the Goldmann perimeter. This eye shows a failure in the upper nasal quadrant. For comparison, the visual field determined by VER. The results are highly similar.

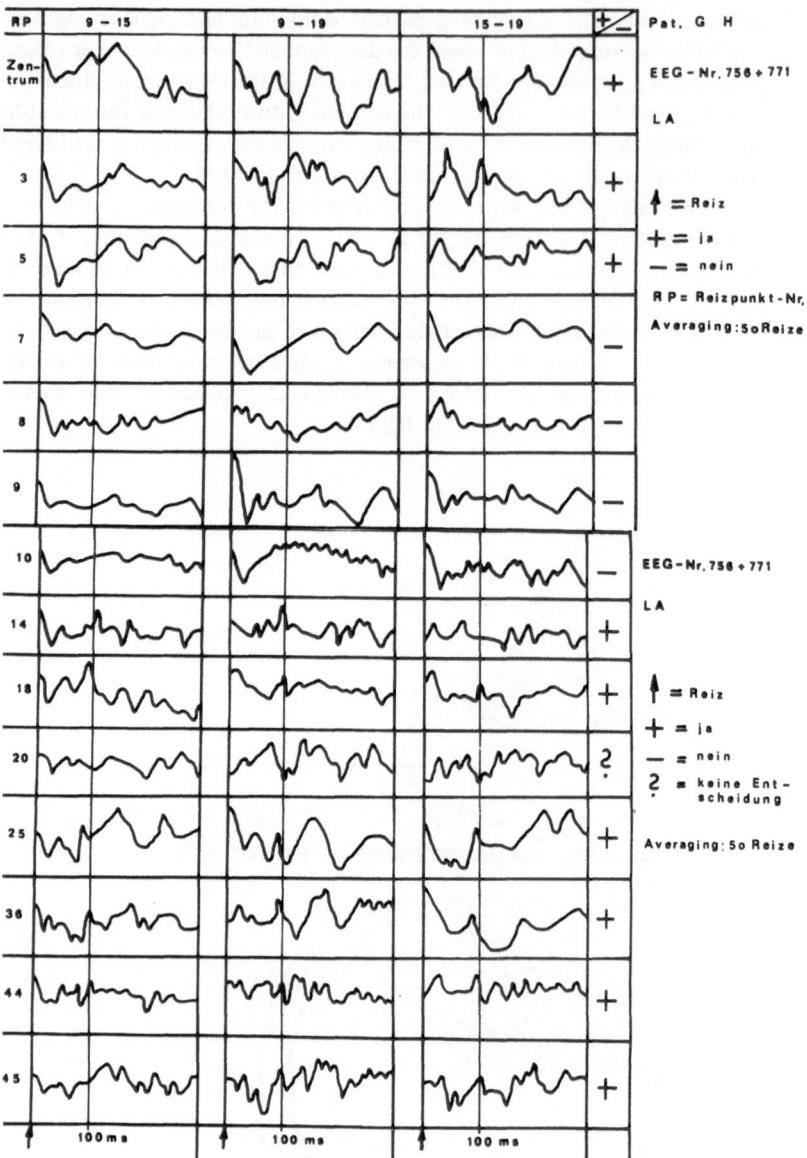

Fig. 4. Representation of the mean-value curves during analysis of the visual field by VER. Column 1: Stimulation points. Column 2: VBR 9-15 bipolar derivation. Column 3: VER 9-19 unipolar derivation. Column 4: VER 15-19 unipolar derivation. Column 5: contains our Yes-No decision. 'No' means: During a period from 80 to 120 ms no clearly positive potential can be detected in 2 channels at least.

326

We are at a state of our experiments where we are still conscious of the fact that our greatest success at present is when the visual field determined by us approaches the subjective, conventional one. Under the aspect listed by us, we believe we can detect coarse failures, such as central scotomas, hemianopsias or quadrant failures, in abt. 80 % of the cases. We are sure that the program for automatic signal recognition prepared by us will be of major importance for the evaluation of our work and that we can possibly make the so-called objective visual field a little more objective.

The last figures show derivation result. The left-hand visual field of a 49-year female patient after hypophysectomy. The figure at first shows the subjectively obtained failure, then the results of the VER derivation entered into the visual field scheme. This not very large failure of the visual field, not being centrally located, can be detected by our method. The following figure shows the mean-value curves obtained from which we made our Yes-No decision.

Authors' address:

Augenklinik der
Medizinischen Akademie Erfurt
Nordhäuser Strasse 74
Erfurt 50
D.D.R.

A STIMULATOR FOR ELECTRORETINOTOPOGRAPHY

W. M. C. AARTS, H. E. HENKES, G. H. M. VAN LITH & J. MEININGER

(Rotterdam)

ABSTRACT

In order to register the electroretinotopogram (ERTG) as a measure for local retinal sensitivity, a stimulator has been developed able to present light stimuli with a flicker frequency of 40 Hz at any point within the 90° visual field of the eye. Size and luminance of the test light can be varied. Stray light effects are suppressed by applying a 30° adaptation field around the test light. Positioning of the stimulus is done with an easy to operate coordinating table, the output of which steers an electronic position servo system.

The results are promising, but a number of problems still have to be solved before the instrument can be fully accepted for clinical use.

INTRODUCTION

In 1973 van Lith & Henkes introduced the term electroretinotopography (ERTG) for the determination of the local retinal sensitivity by means of the flicker ERG. To apply this method for clinical purposes, a reliable stimulator had to be build. With such a stimulator it must be possible to present light stimuli of variable size, luminance and flicker frequency at any point of the retina within 90° of the visual field. The discomfort to the patient had to be minimal. The registration of an ERTG in one meridian of the visual field should take only a few minutes, if the stimulator is easy to operate with a logical and simple display.

With the electroperimeter of Beinhocker et al. (1966) as well as in Hache's experiments with a Tübinger perimeter test stimuli are presented in a hemisphere. Using hemispheres, stray light effects from the test light may easily become unacceptably high. For this reason we abandoned the hemisphere principle. It appeared that an adaptation field with a diameter 2 or 3 times the stimulus diameter was sufficient to suppress stray light effects and to guarantee obtaining reliable local responses. As a consequence, with a stimulus of 10° an adaptation field of at least 30° has to be applied. This means that both adaptation field and test light have to be moved in the visual field.

---

* This project was carried out together with the laboratory of measurement and control, department of mechanical engineering of the Delft University of Technology, the Netherlands.

It is rather difficult technically to move a 30° illuminated field around the eye. The main problem is to minimize inaccuracy as a result of lateral eye movements, which can only be done by establishing a large distance between the stimulation field and the eye. Consequently, the dimensions of the field will also be large.

A solution has been chosen, with which the stimulus is moved virtually in the visual field by a rotating mirror in front of the eye. A great advantage is that the adaptation field and the test light can be installed in a fixed position and light conditions can be changed relatively easy. The rotating mirror is semi-transparent, in order to use the visual axis for fixation and fixation control. The latter is very important for knowing whether the right spot on the retina is stimulated. For the following description of the instrument see Figures 1 and 2.

On the opaque screen (S) a stimulus is projected by a halogen incandescent

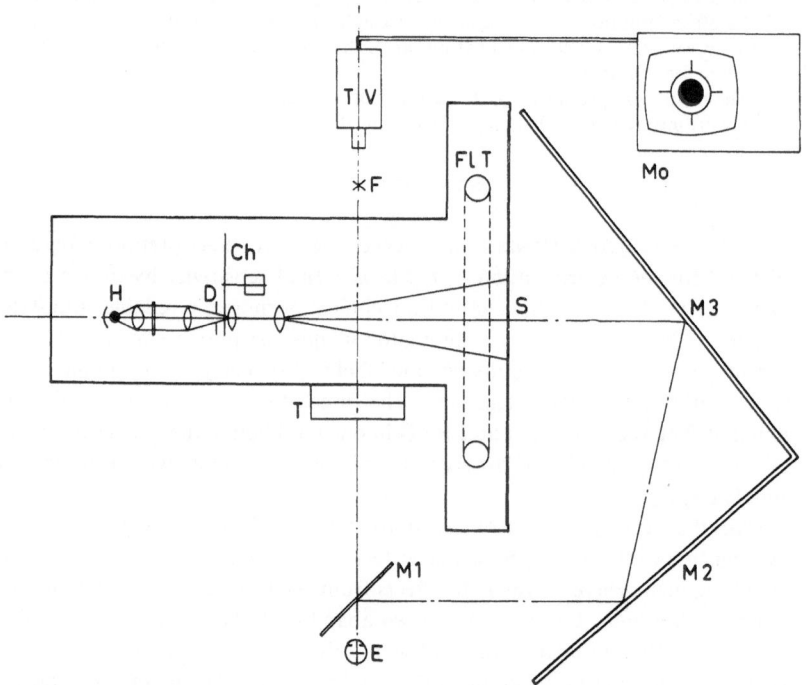

Fig. 1. Principle of the method for ERTG stimulation.

H: Halogen light source. M_1: Semi transparent, rotating mirror.
D: Diaphragm M_2, M_3: Fixed mirrors
Ch: Chopper   F: Fixation light
S: Opaque screen   E: Eye.
Fl T: Fluorescent ring tube   T: Platform.
TV: Television camera   Mo: Monitor.
                        See also Fig. 2.

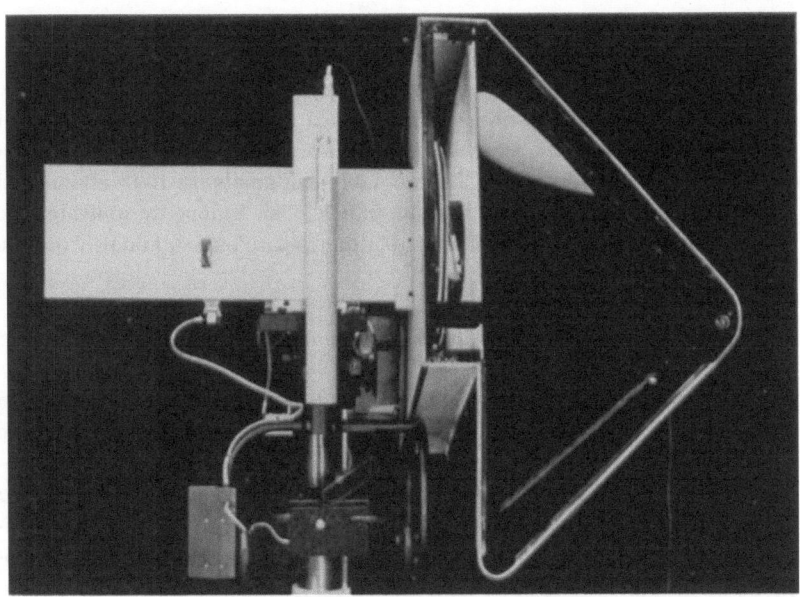

Fig. 2. Stimulator for electroretinotopography. See also Fig. 1.

lamp (H). The optical system contains a diaphragm (D) and a chopper (Ch) to interrupt the stimulus. The stimulus area can be changed from 5° to 10° and has a maximum luminance of 1700 cd/m², which can be lowered with neutral density filters. On the same screen a white adaptation field of 30° is created with a fluorescent ring tube (FlT) (Philips 40 Watt, colour 34), which produces a luminance of 35 cd/m². Via the fixed mirrors M_2 and M_3 and the rotating semi-transparent mirror M_1 the stimulus can be positioned at any point in the 90° visual field of the eye (E). Rotation of the latter occurs around two mutual perpendicular axes which are also perpendicular to the visual axis EF. Through the semi-transparent mirror the eye has to fix on the fixation light F.

DETAILS

Central adjustment

The instrument is designed for clinical use. Therefore, it is important that the cooperation of the patient for central adjustment of the eye is not required. Figure 1 shows how the fixation of the patients' eye is controlled by TV and monitor. For central adjustment the picture of the eye has to be placed in the centre of a target on the monitor screen.

Therefore, the stimulator is put on a platform (T) on which it can be moved in three mutually perpendicular directions. Whenever, during measurement, the monitor shows a lateral eye movement, central adjustment can be restored immediately.

Stimulus

Two kinds of stimulation can be applied with the instrument. The first is the projection of a diaphragm on an uninterrupted adaptation field. Influence of eye movements is reduced, since the stimulus always finds a place on the retina of the same state of adaptation. The second type is an almost 100% modulated stimulation with a surrounding adaptation field. This is done by applying tube diaphragms of different sizes (5° and 10°) that separate the stimulus from the adaptation field.

Positioning of the stimulus

The semi-transparent mirror is suspended in a double framework and moved with two independently operated stepping motors. Steering of the stepping motors occurs with an electronic position servo system, the feedback potentiometers being on the rotation axes of the mirror. The input of the servo system comes from an electronic coordinating table. Figure 3 shows that perimetric field maps, as are commonly used in psychophysic perimetry, can be applied on this table. The point in the visual field that has to be stimulated is indicated with a high resistance pen. The coordinates of this point are electronically detected by a wire screen lying underneath, and transferred to the position servo system. The wire screen is designed in such a way that it transforms the

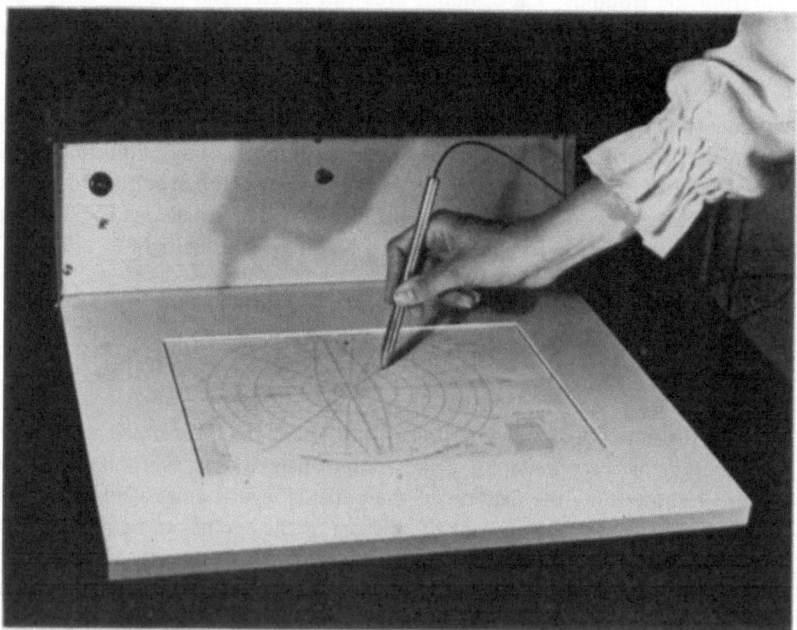

Fig. 3. The electronic coordinating table, on which perimetric visual field maps can be used to indicate the point that has to be stimulated.

polar coordinates of the visual field map to the coordinates with which the stimulus is moved. With the coordinating table the stimulus can easily be piloted around the 90° visual field.

Control desk

Figure 4 shows that the stimulator is operated form a control desk. It consists of (from bottom to top): the coordinating table; the TV monitor (Sony Telelookie); a key board to operate the light conditions and the central adjustment; two lock-in amplifiers (PAR 117, PAR 126/127) for the signal processing; and the position servo system (Omnistep, spec.)

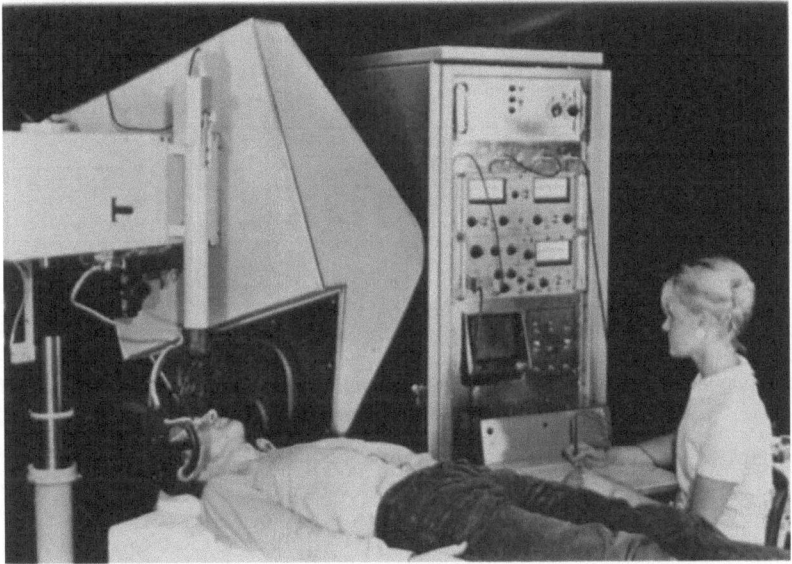

Fig. 4. The stimulator for electroretinotopography in use. See text for description.

PROCEDURE

The stimulus consists of a 10° test field of white light with a luminance of 300 cd/m², or a 5° test field with a luminance of 520 cd/m². The flicker frequency is 40 Hz. The ERG signal is led off from the cornea with a Henkes contact lens electrode, the reference electrode being at the ear lobe. After amplification of the signal by the lock-in amplifiers (band pass of the pre-amplifier 10-100 Hz, time integration constant 10 seconds) the ERTG amplitude and phase angle are registered on a two channel X-time writer.

The curves of Figure 5 show an ERTG in the horizontal meridian of a normal subject. A 10° stimulus is moved in steps of 10° from 40° eccentricity at the nasal side to 40° at the temporal side of the visual field (upper curve). The lower curve is made in the opposite direction.

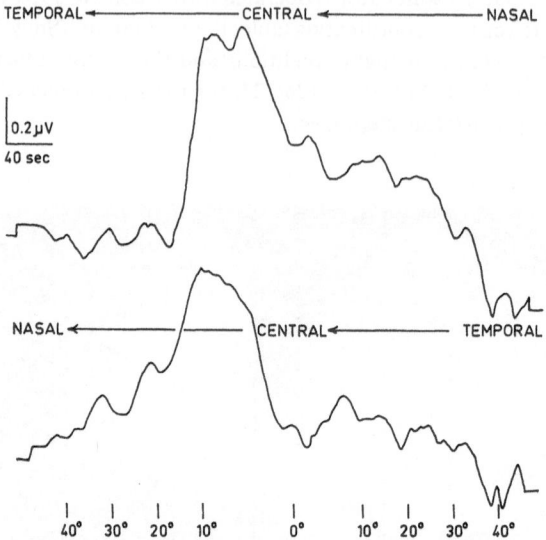

Fig. 5. ERTG of the horizontal meridian in the visual field of a normal subject after stimulation with a 10° stimulus. Stimulus luminance is 300 cd/m². The vertical bars indicate the moment the stimulus is moved to the next position.

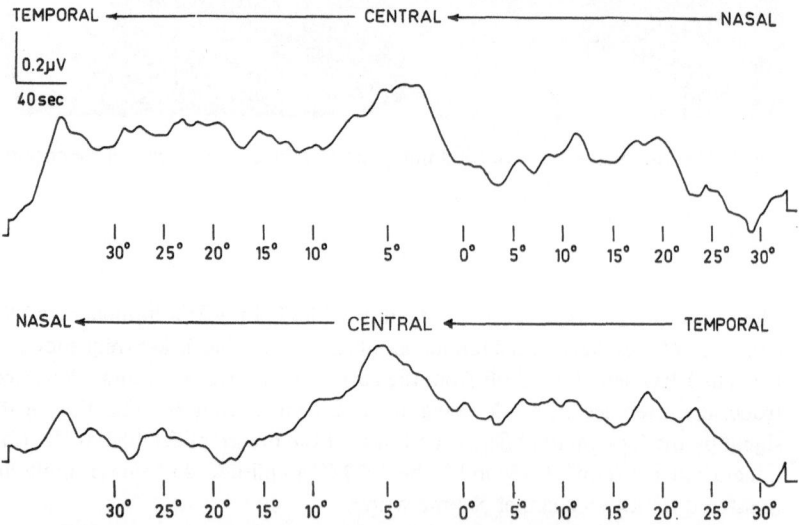

Fig. 6. ERTG of the horizontal meridian in the visual field of a normal subject after stimulation with a 5° test light. Luminance 520 cd/m².

The curves of Figure 6 show an ERTG of the same meridian after stimulation with a 5° test light. The amplitude is rather low. It cannot be improved by a higher stimulus luminance, since stray light effects become already apparent. The curves show no distinct difference in amplitude between separate points in the periphery.

DISCUSSION

The stimulating conditions of the described instrument are not yet sufficiently tried out to compete with the results previously reported by VAN LITH & HENKES (1973). The ratio between test light and adaptation light is very critical. When too low, no response is registered. When it is too high, stray light effects tend to dominate the responses. Also the fitting of the contact lens is quite critical with local stimulation; the slightest air bubble can influence the ERTG considerably.

The electronic coordinating table turned out to be of significant importance for the manageability of the instrument. The time to measure 9 points of a meridian can be limited to less than 10 minutes.

Maybe the fact that the patient can lie down and relax with a good head support contributed to a better fixation than was expected. With the stimulator it is not possible to test more than one point in the visual field at a time.

REFERENCES

BEINHOCKER, G. D., BROOKS, P. R., ANFENGER, E. & COPENHAVER, R. M. 'Electroperimetry', IEEE Trans. on Bio-Med. Eng. *BME* 13/1: *11-8* (1966).

BOYCE, P. R. Monocular fixation in human eye movement (1966).

HACHE, J. CL., DUBOIS, P. BERTOLACCI, G., VETU, E. & MALVACHE, N. New method of stimulation for the study of photoreceptors.

HENKES, H. E. & VAN LITH, G. H. M. Electroperimetry. Proc. 10th ISCERG Symp. Doc. Ophthal. Proc. Ser. 3: *245-251* (1973).

VAN LITH, G. H. M. & HENKES, H. E. Electroretinotopography (ERTG). Proc. 10th ISCERG Symp. Doc. Ophth. Proc. Ser. 3: *253-259* (1973).

NIEUWKERK, L. R. Writing tablet for converting current handwriting in two electrical signals. To be published in Tijdschrift van het Nederlands Electronica en Radio Genootschap (1973).

PADMOS, P. & VAN NORREN, D. VECTOR voltmeter as a tool to measure ERG spectral sensitivity and dark adaptation. Rep. No IZF 1972-4. Soesterberg, Inst. for Reception RVO/TNO (1972).

STOUTENBEEK, P., VERDUYN LUNEL, H. F. E. & VAN DER TWEEL, L. H. Some factors influencing the frequency response of the human ERG. *Doc. Ophth.* 18: *508-514* (1964).

Authors' address:

Eye Hospital
Erasmus University
Rotterdam
The Netherlands

THE HUMAN VISUAL EVOKED RESPONSE: INTEREST AND LIMITS OF ITS STUDY IN CLINICAL PRACTICE

C. BIANCHI & G. LAURI

(Bollate & Monza)

The study of the VER is without doubt very important in ophthalmological clinical practice. But, both for the continuous progress of techniques and equipments, and for the many aspects of VER behaviour which have not yet been fully explained, we think that this test is carried out less frequently than its usefulness might suggest.

For about two years we devoted ourselves to the clinical application of the VER in the hospital of Monza, attempting to make the method quicker by simplifying it, without altering the credibility of the responses in view to make the test fit to the requirements of routine hospital service. Nevertheless, the test remains long and rather complicated to carry out; besides, it involves the use of an averaging computer for the responses. This, together with the difficult interpretation of the responses in many cases, constitutes the main obstacle to widespread use of the test which is absolutely innocuous and not disagreeable to the patient, even if he is either very young or uncooperative.

METHOD

The subject is placed in an arm-chair facing a wall painted an uniformly light colour in a very quiet room illuminated by means of 20-25 Lux lamp. He is given about 20 minutes to adapt himself to the surroundings. In the meantime the electrodes (non polarizable silver disks, ∅ 5mm.) are placed and connected. A monopolar recording is placed 1-2 cm. above the inion, a reference electrode is connected to one ear lobe, a ground wire to the other.

The stimulus light source is placed in front of the subject at one meter's distance; the stimulated surface is about 20°. Stimuli are produced with 0,25 J., Xenon flashes, 0,7-1 Hz. frequency. The flicker is interrupted every 20-50 flashes. The length of the intervals between trains of stimuli varies from 5 to 30 seconds. Monochromatic stimulation is carried out with a red filter (660 nm., transmission factor 10%).

The stimulus triggers the beginning of the sweep. The collected potentials, after pre-amplification, pass into amplifiers with 0,1-100 Hz. band pass. Then, the signal goes on to an averaging computer which – after a pre – arranged number of stimuli (generally 100) – projects an averaged curve of all the responses on an oscilloscope, with 200 memory points.

337

The analysis time is settled in 500 seconds.

The response can be photographed, memorized, reversed on a magnetic tape, and then reproduced.*

RESULTS

Fig. I shows the response in a normal subject; we have marked the parameters we took into consideration. The response is divided in three segments:

I. Period of latency and first positive wave (up to about 130 seconds)

II. Negative -positive biphasic complex (up to 300 seconds)

III. Late oscillatory potentials (up to 500 seconds)

Table No. I shows the data we collected both from normal subjects and subjects with pathological conditions.

The table shows the number of subjects examined, the average amplitude with standard error of responses to red and white stimuli, both for the first and second segments, and the percentage of response amplitude of the affected eye in comparison with the good eye. In fact, we think that in clinical practice this datum should be taken into consideration, because a direct comparison with averaged values obtained from normal subjects is more problematic, considering the large number of variables that may come into play. In this report, we expound only data concerning the peak to peak amplitude of the first and second segments, in response to both red and white stimuli.

Our results are largely superimposable to those already reported by several

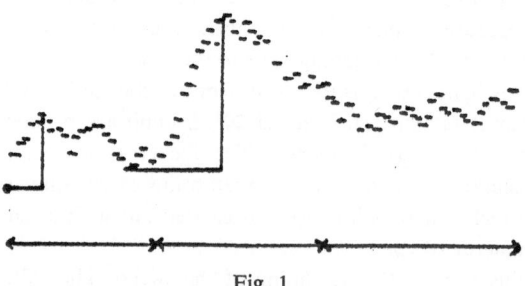

Fig. 1.

* Some other characteristics of the MEDELEC equipment we used are described in C. BIANCHI, V. DE-MOLFETTA, G. LAURI: L'averaging nella valutazione degli artefatti indotti da vari tipi di elettrodi oculari sulla risposta elettroretinografica. *Ann. Ott. Cl. Oc.*, XCVII, 6: *225-231*, 1971.

TABLE 1 Light V.E.R. Amplitude (μV.)

	1st segment		2nd segment	
	white st.	red st.	white st.	red st.
Normal (70 pt.)	7.00 ±1,152	6,25 ±1.046	13,56 ±1,264	14,04 ±1,435
Optic neuropathies (16 pt.)				
normal eye	7,14 ±1,203	7,20 ±1,392	11,85 ±1,654	13,75 ±2,32
affected eye	4,00 ±0,395	3,34 ±0,330	7,20 ±0,959	6,39 ±0,605
a/n	0,54	0,46	0,65	0,46
Macular diseases (8 pt.)				
normal eye	7,25 ±0,853	4,66 ±0,333	13,75 ±0,946	12 ±1,525
affected eye	4,70 ±0,803	4,89 ±0,873	8,50 ±1,144	8,33 ±1,154
a/n	0,64	1,06	0,62	0,69
Retinitis pigmentosae (8 pt.)				
affected eye	6,25 ±0,573	5,43 ±0,341	9,55 ±0,735	10,00 ±0,718
Strabismic amblyopia -eccentric fixation- (21 pt.)				
normal eye	6,25 ±0,321	5,58 ±0,611	10,83 ±2,167	11,55 ±1,72
affected eye	5,78 ±0,926	5,41 ±0,894	11,56 ±1,016	11,28 ±2,347
a/n	0,93	0,98	1,06	0,95
Cataracts (26 pt.)				
normal eye	6,05 ±2,118	4,78 ±1,458	10,00 ±2,077	9,01 ±1,051
affected eye	5,06 ±1,831	5,41 ±2,056	10,01 ±2,037	10,03 ±2,156
a/n	0,83	1,15	1,00	1,11

authors (1, 2, 3, 7, 10, 12, 14, 15, 18, 19). For example, in strabismic amblyopia with eccentric fixation, the response is within standard limits, except for a very small bilateral amplitude reduction without meaning. Even in senile cataract the VER of the affected eye is practically the same as in the other eye (these cases have been chosen among patients who regained good visual acuity after surgery.)

Even in retinitis pigmentosa, the alterations of the VER were often very small, although the visual field was sometimes reduced to less than 10°, visual acuity and colour vision were endangered, and ERG showed small or absent response even after averaging technique. (Tab. 2).

The discrepancy between the VER and the other functional tests may depend on the fact that under our examining conditions the response is mostly due to the activity of the photopic system (light-adaptation, stimuli of high intensity, wide response to red); moreover, several authors have already pointed out that the VER is predominantly connected with the activity of the photopic system (7, 9, 10, 20, 21).

However, it is not very easy to explain why, even when using the same equipment, the stimulus which does not produce any retinal response, then succeeds in evoking a much wider potential at the cortical level.

Still more questionable was the interpretation of the VER in optic neuropathies and macular diseases.

TABLE 2 RETINITIS PIGMENTOSAE

Name	Eye	Visual acuity	Visual field	E.R.G. (μV.) a	b	Light V.E.R. (μV.) 1st segment white	red	2nd segment white	red
1 C.L.	RE	4/10	tubular 10°	extinct		4	5	10	5
	LE	7/10	tubular 10°	extinct		4	5	10	5
2 D.A.	RE	7/10	tubular 8°	extinct		3	3	9	9
	LE	7/10	tubular 8°	extinct		5	4	10	10
3 M.R.	RE	m.m.	tubular 8°	extinct		6	6	4	9
	LE	m.m.	tubular 8°	extinct		6	6	4	9
4 S.C.	RE	9/10	anular scotoma	20	25	8	8	10	9
	LE	9/10	anular scotoma	20	25	9	6	10	9
5 P.V.	RE	10/10	anular scotoma	70	110	6	6	9	12
	LE	10/10	anular scotoma	60	130	10	8	13	11
6 C.I.	RE	5/10	costriction of visual	10	10	4	4	11	9
	LE	8/10	field (bilateral)	10	15	3	4	6	10
7 C.G.	RE	9/10	constriction of visual	30	60	9	6	14	13
	LE	8/10	field (bilateral)	30	60	9	6	14	13
8 R.A.	RE	3/10	tubular 15°	extinct		7	5	9	13
	LE	3/10	tubular 15°	extinct		7	5	9	13

In the optic neuropathies examined by us, the VER was greatly altered, showing highly reduced amplitude and increase in latency. The alteration was very precocius and had a course which was not in agreement with that of the other functional tests. For example, in one case, we found a visual acuity of 6/10 in the affected eye with the VER reduced to 50% compared to the good eye; in another case, the visual acuity was 2/10 with a VER reduced to 80% (a value, which, in the normal subjects we examined, falls within the physiological variations between one eye and the other). (Fig. 2).

Still larger is the discrepancy between the range of scotomas of the visual field (measured by means of Goldmann perimeter and Friedmann analyzer) and the size of the VER. Not only does a central scotoma alter the VER more than an eccentric one, but small or relative central scotomas sometimes reduce the VER more than large or absolute central scotomas. In one third of the cases we examined, in spite of the presence of a scotoma even extensive in the affected eye, or of a scotoma more extensive and deep than in the other eye, the

340

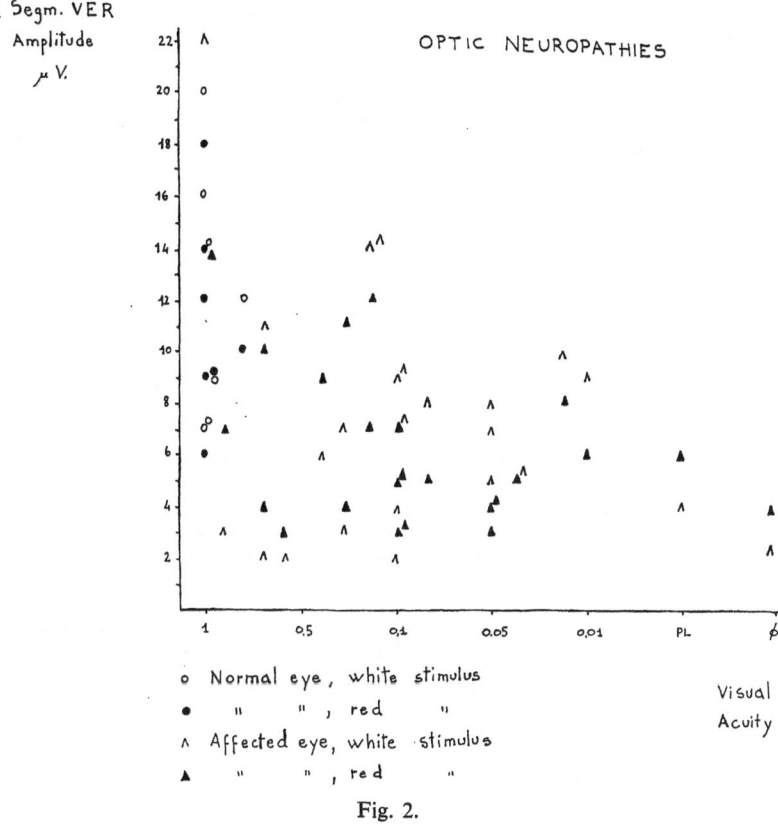

II Segm. VER
Amplitude
μV.

OPTIC NEUROPATHIES

o Normal eye, white stimulus
• "   " , red   "
Λ Affected eye, white stimulus
▲ "   " , red   "

Visual
Acuity

Fig. 2.

potentials were like those of the fellow eye, or even wider (Fig. 3).

As for colour vision (Fansworth 100 Hue Test), we have noticed the same discrepancy in the behaviour of the VER. Finally, in macular disease where we expected a strong reduction of the VER, our results were often uncertain. The alteration of the VER was often small; in fact while visual acuity, visual field and colour vision were severely endangered, the affected eye often succeeded in evoking cortical potentials with an amplitude up to 70% in comparison with the good eye (Fig. 4-5).

Even in a case of highly developed toxoplasmic chorioretinitis with a big macular scar covering more than 1 disk diameter, the VER was larger than in the good eye. We strongly doubt that in some of the subjects we examined, if the fundus had not been explorable, we would have succeeded in suspecting the existence of a macular lesion through the study of the VER, even if – as we have already stated – under our examining conditions they seem to depend mostly on photopic activity.

In conclusion, we think we can state that in our clinical practice the study of the VER usefully integrates with the tests of visual function already in use, but cannot substitute for any of them; it is very useful indeed, in non-co-opera-

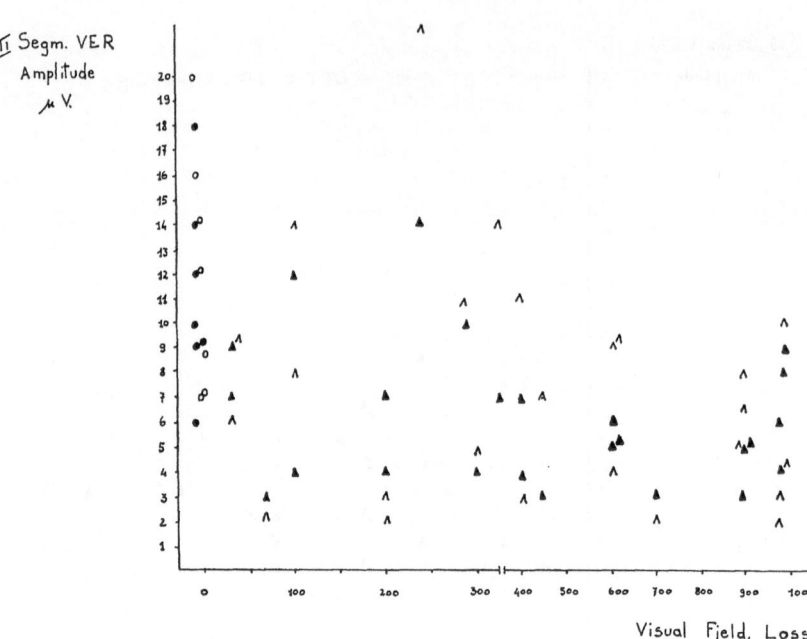

Fig. 3.

MACULAR   DISEASE

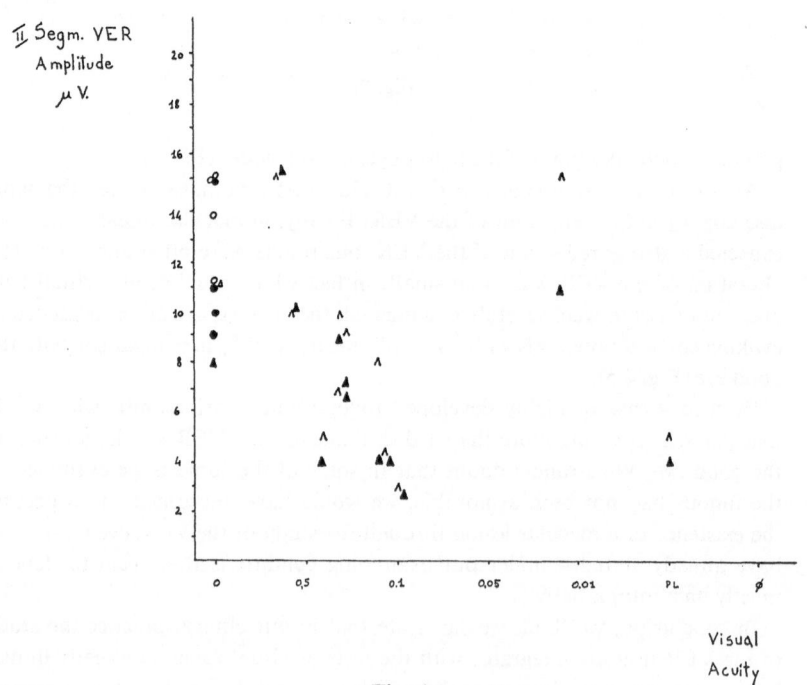

Fig. 4.

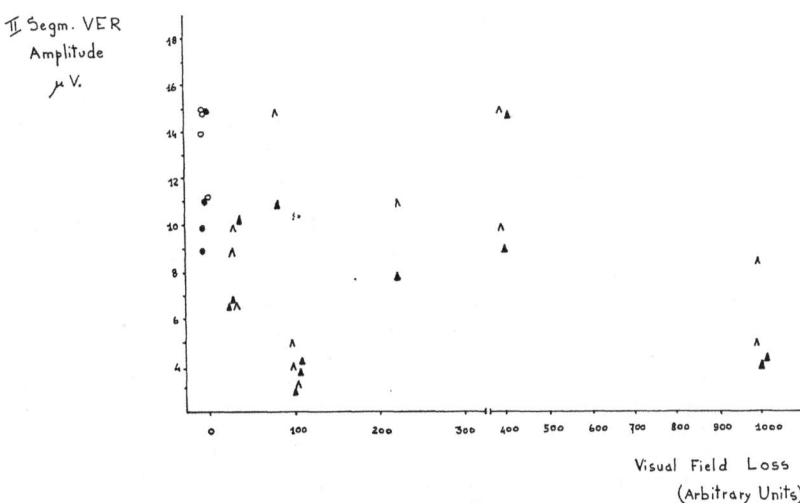

Fig. 5.

ting subjects (children, simulators); however, the interpretation of the results is often difficult and uncertain. In practice, the study of the VER allows us to discriminate only alterations of certain importance, if the response can be compared with the response of the good eye.

In our opinion, for a future wider use in clinical practice we must find a better method of stimulation and adaptation, and a more selective standard of response evaluation, ones more fit for separating normal responses from pathological ones.

REFERENCES

1. AUERBACH, E. & ROWE, H. The 'good' eye in unilateral retinitis pigmentosa. *Ophthalmologica* 155: *98* (1968).
2. VAN BALEN, A. T. M. & HENKES, H. E. Recording of the occipital lobe response in man after light stimulation. *Brit. J. Ophth.* 44: *449* (1960).
3. VAN BALEN, A. T. M. & HENKES, H. E. Attention and amblyopia. An electroencephalographic approach to an ophthalmological problem. *Brit. J. Ophth.* 46: *12* (1962).
4. BEHRMAN, J., NISSIM & ARDEN, G. B. A clinical method for obtaining visual evoked responses. in: Arden – The visual system – Neurophysiology, Biophysics, and their Clinical Applications. pag. 199, Plenum Press (1972).
5. BURIAN, H. M. & JACOBSON, J. H. Clinical electroretinography. Pergamon Press (1966).
6. COPENHAVER, R. M., BEINHOCKER, G. D. & PERRY, N. W. jr. Visual evoked retinal and occipital potentials. *Doc. Ophth.* 18: *473* (1964).
7. COPENHAVER, R. M. & PERRY, N. W. jr. Factors affecting visually evoked cortical potentials such as impaired vision of varying etiology. *Inv. Ophth.* 3: *665* (1964).
8. DAWSON, W. W., PERRY, N. W. jr. & CHILDERS, D. G. Variations in human cortical response to patterns and image quality. *Inv. Ophth.* 11: *789* (1972).
9. DE VOE, R. G., RIPPS, H. & VAUGHAN, J. H. G. Cortical responses to stimulation of the human fovea. *Vis. Res.* 8: *135* (1968).

10. FISHMAN, R. S. & COPENHAVER, R. M. Macular disease and amblyopia; the visual evoked response. *Arch. Ophth.* 77: *718* (1968).
11. GÉRIN, P. Les potentiels évoqués occipitaux. in Paufique L. Ophtalmologie. Ed. Med. Flammarion, Paris (1968).
12. HAUT, J., BERNARD, J. A., LIMON, S., TRIKI, M. F. & SOWINSKA, S. L'intéret des potentiels évoqués visuels dans les atteints traumatiques du nerf optique. *Bull. Soc. Ophth. France* 71: *549* (1971).
13. JACOBSON, J. H., HIROSE, T. & SUZUKI, T. S. Simultaneous ERG and VER in lesions of the optic pathways. *Invest. Ophth.* 7: *279* (1968).
14. JAYLE, G. E., BÉRARD, P. V., TASSY, R. F., & DE RANSART-FERRERO J. Potentiels évoqués occipitaux chez le suject normal et en pathologie ophtalmologique. *Revue O.N.O.* 43: *78* (1971).
15. JAYLE, G. E., TASSY, A., DE RANSART-FERRERO, J. & BÉRARD, P. V. Valeur pratique des potentiels évoqués visuels (PEV). Année Thér. et Clin. en Ophtalmologie (1972).
16. VAN LITH, G. & HENKES, H. E. Local scotopic responses in ERG and VER. in: ARDEN – The visual system – Neurophysiology, Biophysics, and their Clinical Applications. pg. 237 Plenum Press (1972).
17. PERDRIEL, G., FONTAINE, M., ARON, J. J., CHEVALERAUD, D. & LEBLANC, M. Electroretinogram and evoked occipital potentials in blindness cases in children. Symp. ISCERG, pg. 78 (1970).
18. PERRY, N. W. Jr. & CHILDERS, D. G. The human visual evoked response. Thomas Ed. (1969).
19. RAVAULT, P., GERIN, P., DAVID, C. & MUNIER, F. Valeur fonctionelle du nerf optique et potentiels évoqués moyens occipitaux. *Arch. Ophth.* 26: *641* (1966).
20. SCHREINEMACHERS, H. P. & HENKES, H. E. Relation between localized retinal stimuli and the visual evoked response in man. *Ophthalmologica* 155: *17* (1968).
21. SHIPLEY, T. The visually evoked occipitogram in strabismic amblyopia under directview ophthalmoscopy. *J. Ped. Ophth.* 6: *97* (1969).

Authors' address:

G. LAURI
Ospedale Civile
S. Gerardo dei Tintori
Divisione Oculistica
Monza
Italy

C. BIANCHI
Ospedale Civile
Divisione Oculistica
Bollate
Italy

THE AVER IN OPHTHALMOLOGY

S. KOROL

(Geneva)

ABSTRACT

The clinical value of the AVER has been investigated in 85 patients (163 eyes) with chorioretinal degenerations and 156 patients (287 O.N.) with optic nerve diseases.

We have studied the AVER in 287 pathologic optic nerves (156 patients) and 163 eyes (85 patients) with chorio-retinal alterations. All cases presented have had complete ophthalmic examinations. The investigations have included ERG and EOG.

METHOD

The AVER was recorded in a monopolar derivation 3 cm above the inion on the midline, one ear lobe used as reference and other as the ground.

Full field white stimulation in light adapted state (Grass PS-2 photo-stimulator) was obtained at a rate of 2 c/sec.

We employed a preamplifier Tektronix 122 with a bandwidth of 50/0,2 Hz. and a time constant of 1 second.

128 responses were averaged by a computer 'Biomac 1000' (Data Labor, London) with a sweep time of 160 msec.

The AVER was recorded after separate monocular stimulation from each eye.

The late potentials of the AVER which follow this primary response have not been considered in our measurements.

We have compared the latency and amplitude parameters of normal and pathologic groups.

Fig. 1 shows the method of measuring latency and amplitude, Table I shows the statistical mean and standard deviation of our normal group obtained from 20 normal subjects between ages 18 and 35 years old.

Our criteria for evaluation:

a. *latency:* normal or pathologic in comparison with the statistical mean and standard deviation of the normal group;

b. *amplitude:* if one response is normal (17,85 μV ± 5,7 μV) we consider a diminution of more than 50% of the other response as pathologic; if both

345

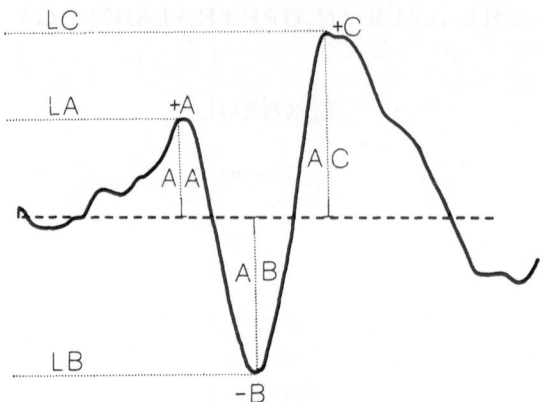

Fig. 1. Method of measuring latency and amplitude. Positive wave A, negative wave B and positive wave C. LA: A wave peak latency. LB: B wave peak latency. LC: C wave peak latency. AA: A wave amplitude. AB: B wave amplitude. AC: C wave amplitude.

TABLE 1

Statistical mean and standard deviation of our normal group (20 subjects). LA: A wave peak latency (msec). LB: B wave peak latency (msec). LC: wave peak latency (msec). AA: A wave amplitude (μV) 2×. AB: B wave amplitude (μV) 2×. AC: C wave amplitude (μV) 2×.

	$\bar{X}$	S
L A	53,92	4,33
L B	81,86	4,21
L C	108,56	7,14
A A	15,00	4,44
A B	35,48	12,21
A C	14,17	7,55

responses are affected, we arbitrarily consider 5 μV as borderline between normal and pathologic response.

c. *response extinct:* no AVER was recordable within the limits of our technique.

I. *AVER in optic nerve pathology*

Table II shows the AVER in pathologic states of the optic nerve. The photopic averaged ERG was normal in all cases. We can point out these differences:

346

TABLE II
AVER in optic nerve pathology

DIAGNOSIS	Number of optic nerves (287)	AVER		LATENCY		AMPLITUDE	
		extinct (60)	present (227)	normal	patholo-gical	normal	patholo-gical
1. Acute retrobulbar neuritis (M.S.)	40	3	37	2	35	3	34
2. Chronic retrobul-bar neuritis (MS)	39	2	37	16	21	8	29
3. Papillitis	38	3	35	11	24	2	33
4. Papilloedema	12	–	12	12	–	7	5
5. Tumoral compression	17	5	12	8	4	2	10
6. Traumatic injury	4	3	1	1	–	–	1
7. Optic atrophy	76	31	45	39	6	2	43
8. Hereditary optic atrophy	6	5	1	1	0	0	1
9. Anomalies of the optic disc	5	–	5	4	1	1	4
10. Toxic nevropathy	50	8	42	32	10	3	39

A. *Acute retrobulbar neuritis*: (40 O. N.).
Table III shows the statistical mean and standard deviation in 40 cases with retrobulbar neuritis.
– latency pathologic (94,5 %), 35 of 37 cases;
– amplitude pathologic (91.8 %), 34 of 37 cases;
– response extinct (7,5 %), 3 of 40 cases.

TABLE III
Statistical mean and standard deviation in cases with acute retrobulbar neuritis.
Legend idem table I.

	$\bar{X}$	S
L A	81,80	14,23
L B	119,93	18,32
L C	147,85	20,42
A A	11,21	6,57
A B	18,39	6,63
A C	7,63	7,21

B. *Resolved retrobulbar neuritis* (2 months to 1 year post neuritis): 39 O.N.
- latency pathologic (56,7 %), 21 of 37 cases with AVER presents;
- amplitude pathologic (78,3 %), 29 of 37 cases with AVER presents;
- response extinct (5,1 %), 2 of 39 cases.

Comment: The latency and amplitude are pathologic in the acute stage.

The amplitude remains pathologic more often than the latency in the resolved cases.

C. *Papillitis* (38 O.N.)
- latency pathologic 68,5 %, 24 of 35 cases;
- amplitude pathologic 94,2 %, 33 of 35 cases;
- response extinct 7,8 %, 3 of 38 cases.

D. *Papilloedema* (12 O.N.)
- latency pathologic 0 %, 0 of 12 cases;
- amplitude pathologic 41,7 %, 5 of 12 cases;
- response extinct 0 %, 0 of 12 cases

Comment: The difference of AVER latency in papillitis and papilloedema is not yet statistically significant and should not be considered criteria for the differential diagnosis.

E. Toxic neuropathy (alcohol, Myambutol, Trichlorethylene, metabolic): 50 O.N.):

- latency pathologic 13,3 %, 6 of 42 cases with AVER presents;
- amplitude pathologic 92,8 %, 39 of 42 cases with AVER presents;
- response extinct 16 %, 8 of 50 cases.

Comment: acute retrobulbar neuritis usually has a pathologic latency.

Toxic and metabolic optic neuropathy have pathologic latency less frequently.

F. In cases of *prechiasmal syndrome* (8) due to compression of optic nerve from aneurysm and tumor, the AVER was valuable in localization and evaluation of surgical treatment.

G. *Optic nerve atrophy* (glaucoma, vascular accident, post traumatic, post surgical and idiopathic (76 O.N.):
- latency pathological 13,3 %, 6 of 45 cases with present AVER;
- amplitude pathologic 95,5 %, 43 of 45 cases with present AVER;
- response extinct 40,7 %, 31 of 76 cases.

Comment: In atrophy from the above class the latency was more often normal, while the amplitude was generally pathologic in those cases having a response. In medico-legal evaluation of optic nerve atrophy the AVER has an important role as an objective test and should be included with the visual field, visual acuity and fundus examination to judge the functional activity of the optic nerve.

H. In cases of *hereditary optic atrophy* and anomalies of the optic disc there are insufficient cases to comment.

The AVER in chorio-retinal pathology.

Table IV shows our results in chorioretinal pathology. The same criteria were used for evaluation as in the previous cases.

The first group shows alteration of the scotopic system (Table IV: 1 to 6). The AVER was present in 71,7% of our cases. When there was pathology in the scotopic system and associated macular degeneration the AVER was generally extinct.

In the group with alteration of the photopic system (Table IV: 7 to 9) we found:
a. macular degeneration and aquired pathology of the macula (inflammatory process) (43 eyes);
   the AVER is extinct in 4 cases of 43 (9,4%);
   the AVER is present in 39 cases of 43 (90,6%);
   the latency is pathologic in 8 of 39 cases (20.5%) (AVER present);
   the amplitude is pathologic in 36 of 39 cases (89.5%). (AVER present).
b. diffuse photopic dysfunction (14 eyes):
   The AVER is extinct in 10 of 14 cases (71.9%).
   the AVER is present in 4 of 14 cases (28,1%).

DISCUSSION

The AVER is of objective value in the clinical diagnosis of acute retrobulbar neuritis, optic nerve atrophy and compression of the optic nerve.

In our study of chorioretinal pathology we find that the photopic system contributes a larger portion of the AVER than the scotopic system.

The AVER is of clinical importance in that it can be made part of the ophthalmic examination and must be interpreted in the context of the whole clinical examination.

We consider our results significant within the limits of our technique, which is simplified and the testing time limited to about 15 minutes for practical reasons.

REFERENCES

ADAMS, W. L., ARDEN, G. B. & BEHRMAN, J. Responses of human visual cortex following excitation of peripheral retinal rods. *Brit. J. Ophth.*, 53: *439-452* (1969).
AUERBACH, E. Clinical application of bioelectrical test. In: BALLANTYNE, A. J. & MICHAELSON, I. C.: Textbook of the fundus of the eye. Edinburgh, London, E. et S. Livingstone, 512-542 (1970).
BERGAMINI, L. & BERGAMASCO, B. Cortical evoked potentials in man. Springfield, CHARLES C. THOMAS (1967).

TABLE IV

Diagnosis	Number of eyes (163)	AVER extinct	AVER present	Latency		Amplitude	
				N	P	N	P
1. Retinitis pigmentosa	33	14	19	11	8	6	13
2. Central, pericentral, inverse pigmentary retinopathy	18	1	17	6	11	10	7
3. Sector pigmentary retinopathy	10	2	8	8	0	3	5
4. Unilateral pigmentary retinopathy	1	1	0	0	0	0	0
5. Fundus flavimaculatus	22	8	14	12	2 (14,2%)	10	4
	92	26 (28,3%)	66 (71,7%)				
6. Fundus albipunctatus (Lauber)	8	0	8	8	0	5	3
7. Cone dysfunction and diffuse posterior pole degenerations	14	10 (71,9%)	4	4	0	2	2
8. Macular degeneration	28	2 } 4	26 } 39	19	7	3	23
9. Macular inflammatory process	15	2 } (9,4%)	13 } (90,6%)	12	1	0	13
10. Leber's congenital amaurosis	4	3	1	0	1	0	1
11. Choroideremia	2	2	0	0	0	0	0
12. Gyrate atrophy	2	0	2	2	0	0	2
13. Sex-linked juvenile retinoschisis	2	0	2	0	2	0	2
14. Albinism	4	2	2	2	0	0	2

350

CARR, R. E. The night-blinding disorders. In: Electrical responses of the visual system. FRICKER, S. J. (Ed.). *I.O.C.*, 9 (No 4): *971-1003* (1969).

CHILDERS, D. G. & PERRY, N. W. Analysis of simultaneously recorded visual evoked retinal (ERG) and cortical potentials (VER). In: Advances in electrophysiology and pathology of the visual system. 6th ISCERG Symp. Leipzig, Thieme, *139-149* (1968).

COPENHAVER, R. M. & PERRY, N. W. Factors affecting visually evoked cortical potentials such as impaired vision of varying etiology. *Invest. Ophthal.*, 3: *665-673* (1964).

DE HAAS, J. P. An electro-ophthalmological study of affections of the optic pathway. *Doc. Ophthal.* 31: *251-399* (1972).

FEINSOD, M. & AUERBACH, E. The electroretinogram and the visual evoked potential in two patients with tuberculum sellae meningioma before and after decompression of the optic nerve. *Ophthalmologica* (Basel), 163: *360-368* (1971).

FISHMAN, R. S. & COPENHAVER, R. M. Macular disease and amblyopia (The visual-evoked response). *Arch. Ophth.*, 77: *718-725* (1967).

FRANCESCHETTI, A., FRANÇOIS, J. & BABEL, J. Les hérédodégénérescences chorio-rétiniennes. Rapport S.F.O. Paris, Masson et Cie (1963).

JACOBSON, J. H., TATSUO, H. & TAKASHIA, S. Simultaneous ERG and VER in lesions of the optic pathway. *Invest. Ophthal.*, 7: *279-292* (1968).

KOROL, S. & STANGOS, N. Les potentiels évoqués corticaux dans les affections du nerf optique. *Oto-Neuro-Ophthal.*, 44: *387-394* (1972).

BABEL, J., STANGOS, N., SPIRITUS, M. & KOROL, S. Dégénérescences chorio-rétiniennes du pôle postérieur. *Bull. Mém. Soc. Franç. Ophthal.* 85: *479-494* (1972).

KOROL, S. Les potentiels évoqués visuels (PEV); (Etude clinique et expérimentale). Thèse, Genève (1973).

PERRY, N. W. & CHILDERS, D. G. The human visual evoked response method and theory. Springfield, I11., CHARLES, C. THOMAS Ed. (1969).

PLANE, C. Potentiels évoqués visuels chez le sujet normal et dans les atteintes du nerf optique. Thèse Clermont-Ferrand (1969).

Authors' address:

Clinique universitaire d'ophtalmologie de Genève (prof. J. BABEL)
22 rue Alcide Jentzer
1205 (GE)

351

PATTERN STIMULI FOR CLINICAL ERG

THEODORE LAWWILL, MD*

(Louisville)

ABSTRACT

Electrophysiological studies on six patients with different types of retinal disease have been presented. These cases are used to illustrate the effectiveness of the alternating bar pattern ERG in detecting electrophysiological dysfunction when it is limited to the macular and paramacular area.

INTRODUCTION

Macular electroretinography has been attempted by several investigators. (1-3) Previous techniques have generally involved suppression of the peripheral retina with intense light while stimulating the central retina with even more intense light. Scattered light has continued to be a problem with these techniques, causing the response to be recorded from the entire retina rather than from the area directly stimulated.

In 1964, RIGGS, JOHNSON, & SCHICK (4) reported a technique of stimulation which has proven capable of eliminating much of the problem of stray light. Other investigations (JOHNSON, RIGGS, & SCHICK) (5) have shown that this stimulus evokes a response almost exclusively from the photopic system. Work in our laboratory over the last several years has shown us that we can reliably record ERG's from retinal areas as small as five degrees with this method of stimulation.

METHODS

The uniqueness of the technique lies in the stimulus system. A pattern which has alternating dark and light bars is projected onto the retina (Fig. 1). These bars are periodically reversed in position, thus the light bars become dark and the dark bars become light. This shift constitutes the stimulus.

The stimulus pattern contains an equal number of dark and light bars. Therefore, the shift in the pattern causes no change in the total amount of light

*From the Department of Ophthalmology, University of Louisville, School of Medicine. The work was supported in part by grant No. EY00412, of the National Eye Institute, National Institutes of Health and a Fight For Sight Grant-In-Aid No. G-386.

Fig. 1. Pattern which is viewed by the patient. The center fixation dot contains a small red light. The bar width can be varied from 20 minutes to 2½ degrees. The diameter of the entire pattern can be varied from 5-18 degrees. The intensity difference between the dark and light bars is 1.5 log units.

entering the eye. Thus, the peripheral retina receives a constant amount of scattered light and is not stimulated by the shift of the pattern.

The stimulus is of relatively low effective contrast and the ERG is recorded from a small area, resulting in a signal of less than 10 μV. It is necessary to computer-average several responses in order to obtain a readable result. It is also necessary in the clinical situation to do extensive editing prior to averaging the responses. At present editing is performed with an analog device which in turn controls the computer averaging process. Measuring the response requires a template method to be sure that ERG and not artifact is measured. There are many electronic details and internal controls in this system which we do not have time to discuss.

The patients are optically corrected with lenses in front of the contact lens electrodes for our studies have shown that with a one degree bar refraction must be within ± 1 diopter to achieve maximum response. There is a small red light in the center of the field for fixation.

I became interested in applying the alternating bar technique to clinical cases when I first saw it used by Dr. John Armington in 1966. I felt that it might prove a better objective technique for evaluating the function of the central retina, since most clinical macular defects affect an area larger than the anatomical macula, but often less than the entire retina.

We frequently see a child with questionable ophthalmoscopic changes in the macular region and possibly reduced visual acuity without other evidence of organic disease. I felt that if this technique were developed, it might provide a better method of evaluating and categorizing the macular degenerations.

354

Our data shows that this technique does in truth reflect the functional status of the macular area, and we are using it to evaluate clinical patients.

Figure 2 shows the data which can be obtained from a well-trained and highly cooperative subject. This figure shows an intensity series for a single subject with a bar width of 20 minutes and a field size of 22 degrees. In this case the threshold is approximately 20 ft. L for a readable signal.

There are two reversals of the pattern in each trace, one shortly after the beginning of the trace and one toward the end of the trace. The symmetry of these two responses reflects the accuracy with which the optical system is operating. This duplication also provides split half analysis for validation of the presence or absence of a response. Unfortunately, data on clinical patients does not tend to be as easily readable.

Figure 3 shows the actual data for the 20 minute bar and the straight line

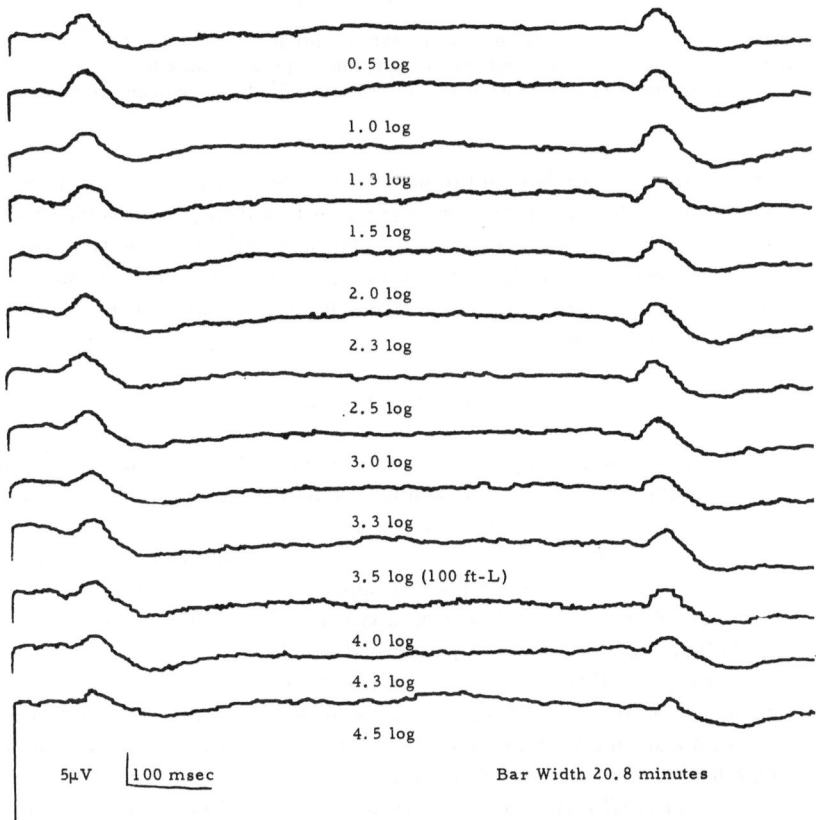

Fig. 2. Bar pattern ERG's for a single subject with field size 22 degree and bar width 20.8 minutes. This data is plotted separately in Figure 3. There are two responses evident in each trace.

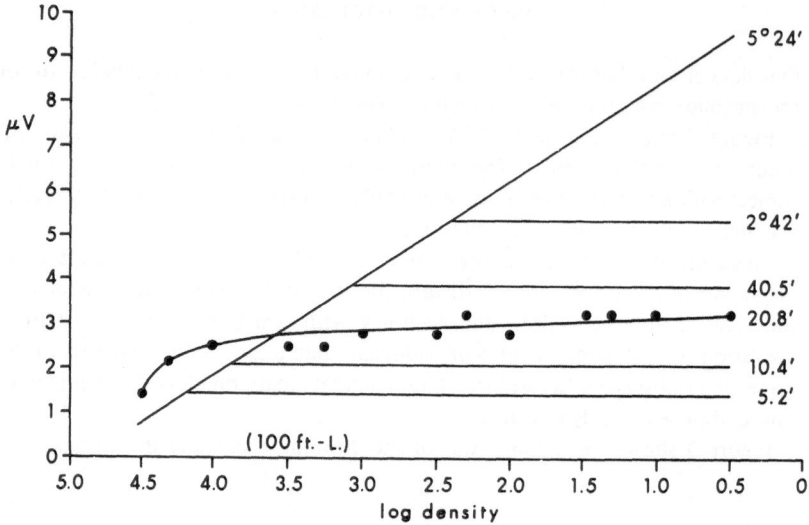

Fig. 3. A graph of the actual data of b-wave amplitude vs. intensity of the light bars for 20.8 minute wide bars, and the straight line approximations for five other bar widths. The data is from a single subject using a 22 degree diameter pattern.

approximations of the intensity response curves for other bar widths. Part of the explanation for the shape of these curves is that there is a constant 1.5 log difference in intensity between the dark and light bars: as intensity increases contrast decreases. Also, the response saturates at a lower intensity with the narrower bar patterns, because defects in the optical media reduce contrast more for the finer patterns.

CLINICAL DATA

We have now examined approximately 60 patients with this method along with the conventional flash method. Examples comparing the bar pattern ERG and the photopic and scotopic flash ERG in several patients will be given here.

Figure 4 shows the fundus photograph of a 30 year old woman who has an old macular scar secondary to toxoplasmosis. The visual acuity in this eye is 20/300. The fellow eye is normal with a visual acuity of 20/20. Figure 5 shows the photopic, scotopic, and bar pattern ERG's for each eye. The first tracing (P) represents an ERG using a deep red flash on top of a white background illuminated at 10 ft. L. The response is completed in the first one-third of the trace with a small a-wave and a b-wave with prominent oscillatory potentials. The other two-thirds of the trace represent movement artifact after the flash. The second trace (S) represents the dark adapted flash ERG. In this case, movement artifact distorts the second one-half of the trace. The bar pattern ERG marked M5 represents the results with a pattern 18 degrees in diameter made up of black and white bars approximately $2\frac{1}{2}$ degrees in width. The shifting base

356

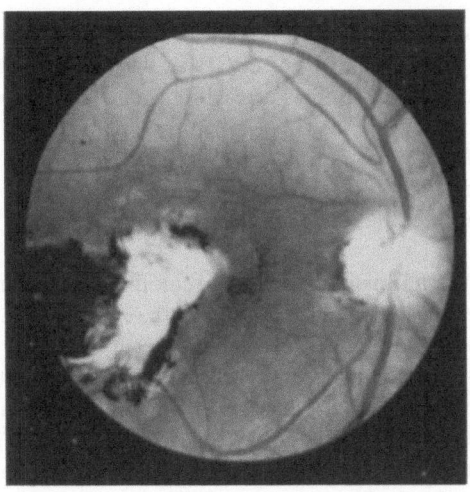

Fig. 4. Fundus photograph of the patient (L.C.) whose ERG responses are shown in Figure 5. The macular scar is secondary to toxoplasmic chorioretinitis. The visual acuity in this eye is 20/300.

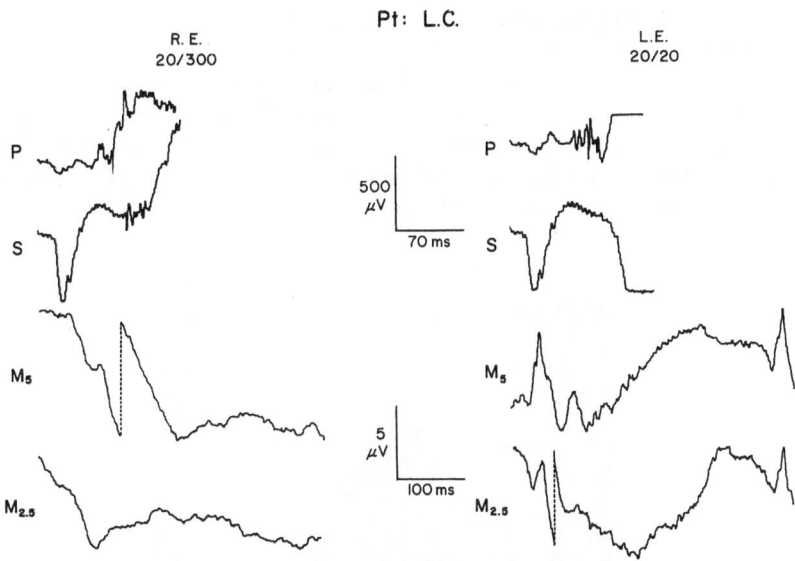

Fig. 5. The electroretinographic responses of a patient (L.C.) with a large macular scar in one eye. The responses for each eye marked (P) are photopic responses produced by a red flash on top of a background illumination of 10ft. L. The response is complete in the first 60 msec and the remainder of the trace is only eye movement artifact. The responses marked (S) are scotopic responses elicited by a single bright flash after 30 minutes dark adaptation. The traces marked (M5) are bar pattern responses produced with an 18 degree field of 2½ bars. The traces marked (M2.5) are produced by 1 degree bars. The traces are 500 msec in length. There are two responses in each trace, one at the beginning and one at the end.

357

line and increase in artifact over the trained subjects is readily evident. We have shifted the first and second half of the traces when there was a large base line shift so that the two small areas at each end of the trace, which include the ERG, can be easily seen.

The normal left eye has normal bar pattern ERG's. There is a small a-wave with a prominent b-wave at the beginning and at the end of each trace. The second trace marked M2.5 is the response for a bar width of approximately 1 degree.

This patient has normal photopic and scotopic flash electroretinograms for the two eyes, while the bar pattern ERG in the right eye is almost extinct and the bar pattern ERG in the left eye is large. In this case the bar pattern ERG detects this gross macular defect more efficiently than the photopic ERG.

The second patient is a 36 year old woman whose visual acuity is 20/100 in each eye. We feel that the appearance of this fundus picture (Fig. 6) most closely resembles choroidal sclerosis. Our electrophysiological findings (Fig. 7) show a low normal photopic flash electroretinogram in each eye, a normal scotopic flash electroretinogram in each eye, and a bar pattern electroretinogram which is approximately one-third to one-half of normal amplitude. It appears that in this case we have a patchy reduction of visual function in the macular area with preservation of some of the photopic components. Therefore, we feel that this is not basically a retinal degeneration but is of vascular or choroidal origin. The bar pattern ERG in this case parallels the photopic flash ERG.

The next case is an eleven year old girl whom we originally tested before we had the bar pattern electroretinogram available for clinical use. On original testing we were forced to report that we could not find evidence of retinal degeneration because her flash ERG and EOG findings were normal, although she reported visual acuity of 20/50 in each eye. Eighteen months later we

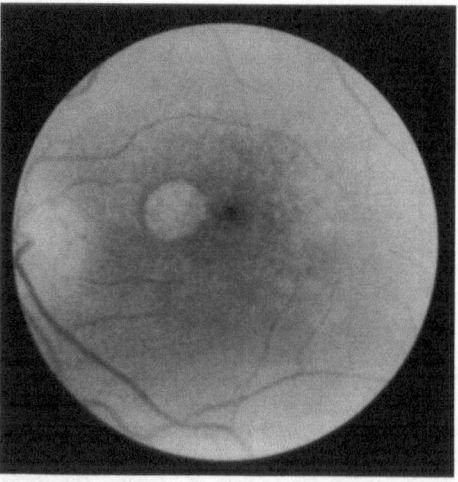

Fig. 6. Fundus photograph of a patient (S.M.) with choroidal sclerosis. Visual acuity is 20/100 in this eye. The opposite fundus is similar in appeareance.

Pt: S.M.

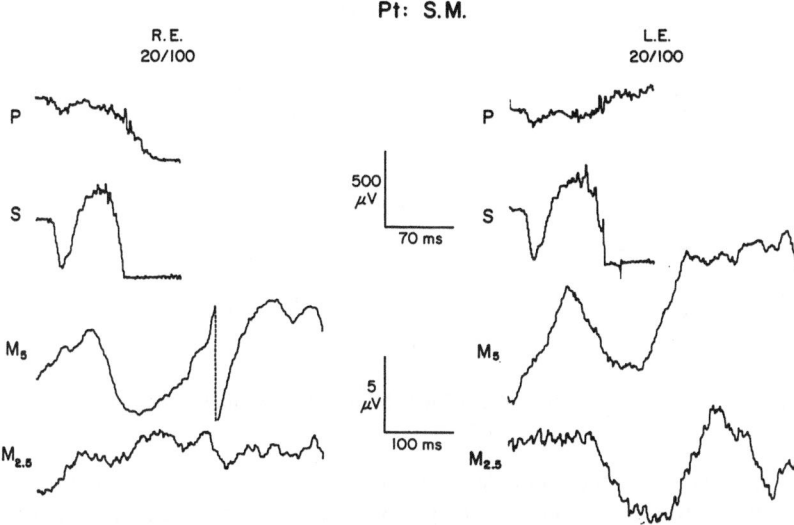

Fig. 7. The ERG responses of patient S.M. The key is similar to that in Figure 5.

retested the patient at which time she still had high normal photopic and scotopic flash electroretinograms. The patient was very cooperative and we were able to record an almost artifact-free bar pattern ERG. By this time, the fundus had begun to show very mild pigmentary changes in the foveal area (Fig. 8). Figure 9 shows a normal photopic and scotopic flash ERG for each eye with a totally absent bar pattern. So, in this patient, with visual acuity reduced to only 20/50 and with a normal flash ERG, there is an extinct bar pattern ERG. We believe that this represents definite evidence of retinal degeneration and rules out malingering which we had previously suspected.

The patient whose fluorescein fundus photograph is shown in Figure 10 has been classified as having flavimaculatus. Her visual acuity is 20/200 in each eye.

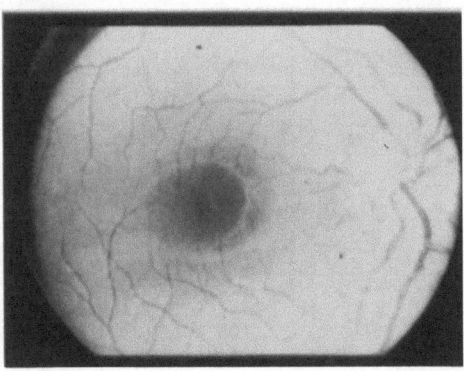

Fig. 8. Fundus photo of a patient (C.N.) showing very mild pigmentary changes in the central macula. The opposite macula is less visibly affected.

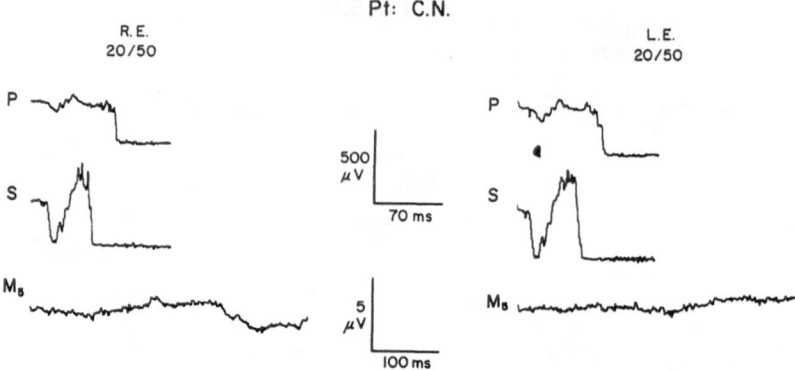

Pt: C.N.

R.E.
20/50

L.E.
20/50

P

S

M₅

500
μV

70 ms

5
μV

100 ms

Fig. 9. The ERG responses of patient C.N. The key is similar to that in Figure 5.

Figure 11 shows the photopic b-wave to be reduced in each eye and the bar pattern ERG to be extinct in the right eye and reduced to a trace in the left eye. In this disease the entire photopic system appears affected, but in this case the central area in particular is severely affected as shown by the extinct bar pattern ERG.

The last case is that of a 60 year old man who has noted nightblindness and loss of visual field. On examination, he has a constricted visual field and bone spicule pigmentation in the mid periphery. Flash type photopic and scotopic electroretinograms are all but extinguished, while the bar pattern ERG's are consistently present and approaching normal amplitude (Fig. 12). This implies that the loss of electrical response occurs in the same area as the loss of visual field in some types of retinitis pigmentosa.

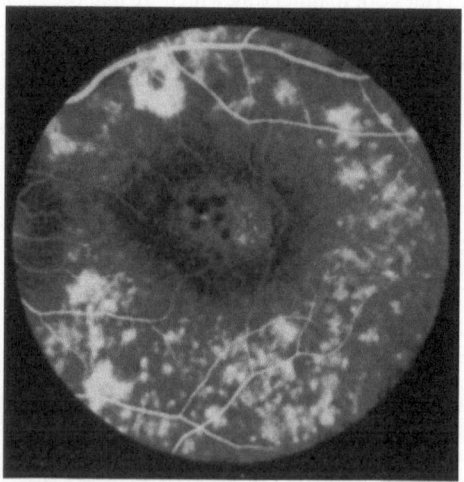

Fig. 10. The fluorescein fundus photograph of a patient (A.S.) with fundus flavima-culatus. The opposite eye is similarly affected.

360

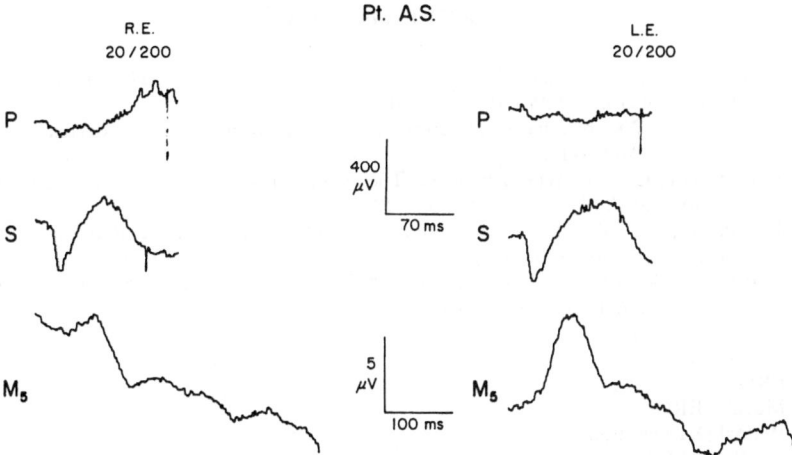

Fig. 11. The ERG responses of patient A.S. The key is similar to that in Figure 5.

We have noted in some cases of macular degeneration that the entire photopic system is affected causing a decrease in the flash photopic response as well as the bar pattern response. But, there are also cases of macular degeneration where the usual tests for the photopic system are normal and the bar pattern ERG is abnormal.

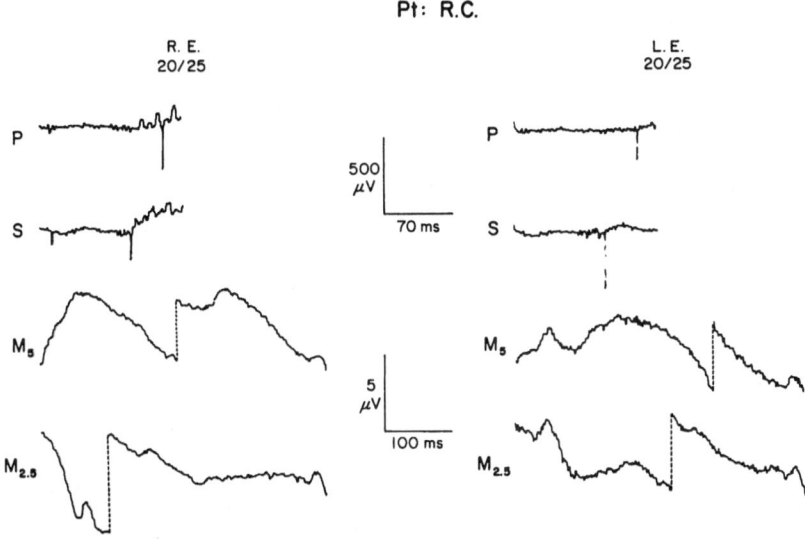

Fig. 12. The ERG responses of a patient (R.C.) with a form of retinitis pigmentosa whose fundus picture shows typical bone spicule pigmentation and whose dark adaptation curve shows only a photopic limb and whose fields are constricted to approximately 15 degrees in each eye. The key is similar to that in Figure 5.

REFERENCES

1. ARMINGTON, J. C., TEPAS, D. I., KROPFL, W. J. & HENGST, W. H. Summation of retinal potentials. *JOSA* 51: *877* (1961).
2. BIERSDORF, WM. & DILLER, D. Local electroretinogram in macular degeneration. *AJO* 68: *296-303* (1969).
3. BRINDLEY, G. S. & WESTHEIMER, G. The spatial properties of the human electroretinogram. *J. Physiol.* 179: *518-537* (1965).
4. JOHNSON, E. P., RIGGS, L. A. & SCHICK, A. M. Photopic retinal potentials evoked by phase alternation of barred pattern. *Vis. Res.* Supp. II *75-91* (1966).
5. RIGGS, L. A., JOHNSON, P. E. & SCHICK, A. Electrical responses of the human eye to moving stimulus patterns. *Science* 144: *567* (1964).

Key Words:
ERG
Macular ERG
Retinal Degeneration
Bar Pattern ERG

Author's address:

301 E. Walnut Street, Louisville
Kentucky 40202, USA

362

INTEREST OF MONOPOLAR LEADS IN VISUAL
EVOKED RESPONSES OF LATERAL
HOMONYMOUS HEMIANOPSIA

D. SAMSON-DOLLFUS, A. POULIQUEN, D. LEVILLAIN
& M. ROGLER

(Rouen)

ABSTRACT

19 patients with hemianopsia have been chosen for this study because of (1) the rather precise diagnosis and (2) the recordings of VER with monopolar and bipolar leads.

Abnormal responses have been recorded in each case. But they were different: complete lack of response on the occipital lead, abnormal response and/or response in phase with the central lead.

A beginning of correlation between the neuroanatomical and clinical findings has been discussed.

INTRODUCTION

The topography of visual evoked responses, (VERs) has been described by some people (1-2-3-5-7-8-11-12). Others have pointed out the importance of the topography in homonymous lateral hemianopsia (H.L.H) (4-9-10-13). We shall try to show that the monopolar leads have to be compared to the bipolar leads if we want to have a good idea of the topography of these responses.

MATERIAL AND METHODS

19 cases suffering of H.L.H or double hemianopsia have been recorded. A GOLDMANN campimetry was performed when their clinical state allowed it. Neurological examinations, electroencephalograms, arteriographies, brain operations and in 3 cases anatomically verified brain showed various but rather well – defined aetiologies.

The stimulus until now has usually been a flash of 0,3 joules of energy. More recently, we have used checkerboard patterns.*

Two montages have been chosen and are successively recorded. The first one is right and left bipolar centro-occipital leads and right and left monopolar central and occipital leads. The second one concerns the frontal leads and the mid-line.

---

* The problems of checkerboard pattersn and of the midline responses will not be discussed here.

The common reference is either the chin or either of the two-ears. Some tests have shown that both of these references are similar. However it seems that the chin is the best reference and it has been proved (7) that in a few cases the ear is able to record the last part of the visual evoked response.

Eighty responses to the visual stimuli are computed, either by a conventional averager (MOPEV Saip-Alvar) or by a small computation on PDP 8. This last method allows us to average also the 200 milliseconds before the stimulus and it is very useful to know how great the noise is and to differentiate some poor responses that are difficult to recognize. We compute only the responses which are not disturbed by the eye movements = a simple analog device eliminates the responses when they arrive at the same time as a large eye movement. This method permits us to obtain a good fixation of the glaze.

<h2 style="text-align:center">RESULTS</h2>

The VERs have been compared to the VERs of normal subjects. The symmetry or dyssymmetry of the response are appreciated by comparisons between the bipolar and monopolar leads.

They may be observed on the occipital leads or central leads or both of them. In this last case, they can be in phase or not.

Out of these 19 patients, 8 have shown the same asymmetry with monopolar and bipolar leads. But 11 patients have had different results with the two types of montages. Several explanations can be given for this fact.

1. The response is obviously asymmetric on the bipolar leads. The monopolar leads demonstrate that an occipital *and* a central response exist, in fact. But they are in phase, and that explains the appearance of inactivity in the bipolar record. (Fig. 1).
2. The response can be symmetric on the bipolar leads (Fig. 2). The monopolar leads show that, in fact, there is no response on the occipital lead, but a response on the central electrode of the damaged hemisphere.

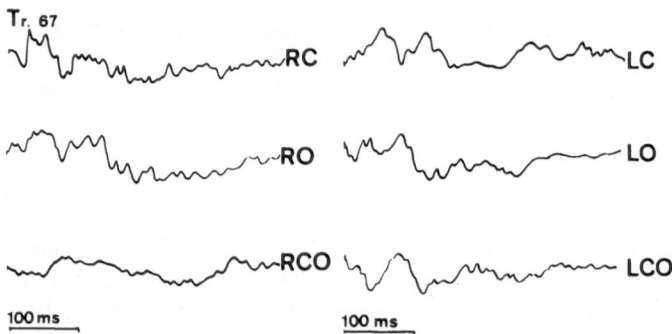

Fig. 1. The bipolar leads show an obvious asymmetry. The monopolar leads reveal that on the right hemisphere there exists an abnormal response on the occipital lead, but it is in phase with the central one. This patient suffered of a large softening of the brain with interruption of the optic tracts but the calcarine was partially normal.

364

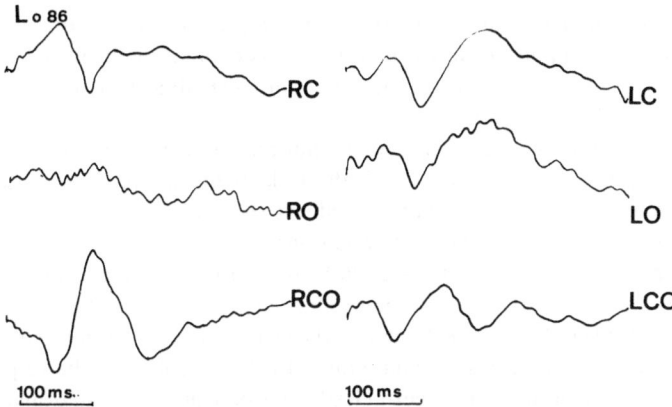

Fig. 2. Asymmetry of the responses: on the right hemisphere the response comes from the central lead and not from the occipital one. On the left hemisphere, the response is abnormal but exists on the occipital lead. The patient had a double hemianopsia. Anatomical verification showed a complete destruction of the calcarine fissure on the right hemisphere and interruption of the optic tracts. On the left hemisphere, the optic tracts were also interrupted but the calcarine was partially normal.

If we mixed the results of the bipolar and of the monopolar leads, we determine four different types of abnormalities:

a. There is no response on occipital and central leads (3 cases): a cerebral blindness which has partially improved; a patient with a very probable ischaemic parietal lesion and some peduncular symptoms, and a patient with a post-traumatic hemianopsia and aphasia.

b. There is no occipital response but a central response (5 cases). One patient had a complete destruction of the calcarine (anatomically verified brain). One had a stenosis of the bifurcation of the right carotid, two had sylvian vascular brain damage, and the last one had, very probably, a vascular disease of the vertebrobasilar territory.

c. There is an occipital response. But, it is a very abnormal one, slower and/or of very little amplitude (5 cases). Two thrombosis of the carotid one parieto-occipital tumor, one temporal astrocytoma and probably a right posterior cerebro-vascular lesion.

d. The occipital responses exist, but they are in phase with the central responses (7 cases). There, anatomically verified brains have shown a sylvian softening of the brain with an interruption of the optic tracts, but the calcarine is partially intact. Two of the other cases were thrombosis of the carotid; one case was a complete sylvian softening of the brain and the last one a very probable an embolism in the sylvian artery.

DISCUSSION

In spite of the disparity of these cases, it is possible to point out the anatomically verified brains. They show that when there is a complete lack of response

365

on the monopolar occipital lead, there is a complete destruction of the calcarine fissure. At the opposite, when the calcarine is completely or partially normal, an occipital response can exist. This one is often an abnormal one and it can be in phase with a central response.

It is possible to compare these anatomically verified cases with the clinical ones, because in the clinical cases, the lack of the occipital response with a preservation of a central response, confirms the clinical symptoms which were very often cortical blindness or vertebrobasilar lesions. But, the existence of abnormal responses have been seen in hemianopsia and stenosis or thrombosis of the carotid, or in temporal tumours, or sylvian softening of the brain.

Two problems have to be discussed: the lack of occipital response opposite to the existence of a central response and also the problem of the responses in phase between occipital and central leads. It is difficult to give an explanation of these facts, but it is possible to think that they show the existence of the association ways. It may be that these ways are more important when the optic tracts are partially or totally distroyed.

SUMMARY

It seems quite obvious that the monopolar leads are very important to recognize the asymmetry of the responses in hemianopsia. This method can be helpful for the topographic diagnosis and may be explain some paradoxal responses recorded by bipolar methods.

BIBLIOGRAPHY

BLATT, S. & OFFNER, F. Distribution of visual evoked responses of man. *Electroenceph. Clin. Neurophysiol.* 20: *p. 96* (1966).
BOURNE, J. R., CHILDERS, D. G. & PERRY, Jr. N. W. Topological characteristics of the visual evoked potentials in man. *Electroenceph. Clin. Neurophysiol.* 30: *423-436* (1971).
CONTAMIN, F. & CATHALA, H. P. Réponse électrocorticale de l'homme normal éveillé à des éclairs lumineux. Résultats obtenus à partir d'enregistrements sur le cuir chevelu à l'aide d'un dispositif d'intégration. *Electroenceph. Clin. Neurophysiol.* 13: 6: *674-694* (1961).
CRIGHEL, E. & BOTEZ, M. I. Photic evoked potentials in man in lesions of occipital lobes. *Brain* 89: *311-316* (1966).
GASTAUT, H., REGIS, H., LYAGOUBI, S., MANO, T. & SIMO, L. Comparison of the potential recorded from the occipital, temporal and central regions of the human scalp, evoked by visual, auditory, and somato-sensory stimuli. *Electroenceph. Clin. Neurophysiol.*, Suppl. 26: *19-28* (1967).
JAYLE, G., ETASSY, A. F., FERRERO, J. & CORNAND, A. Un cas de cécité cérébrale avec conservation du potentiel évoqué visuel. *Rev. Otoneurophtalmo* 43, 5: *229-231* (1971).
LEHTONEN, J. B. & KOIVIKKO, M. J. The use of a non cephalic reference electrode in recording cerebral evoked potentials in man. *Electroenceph. Clin. Neurophysiol.* 31: *154-156* (1971).
LESEVRE, N. & REMOND, A. Potentiels évoqués par l'apparition de patterns. Effet de la dimension du pattern et de la densité des contrastes. *Electroenceph. Clin. Neurophysiol.* 32: *593-604* (1972).
LEVILLAIN, D., POULIQUEN, A., ROGLER, M. & SAMSON-DOLLFUS, D. Potentiels évoqués

visuels dans 16 cas d'hémianopsies latérales homonymes: Etude électroclinique. *Revue d'E.E.G.* Tome 2, 3: *299-301* (1972).

OOSTERHUIS, H. J., PONSEN, L., JONKMAN, E. J. & MAGNUS, O. The average visual response in patients with cerebrovascular diseases. *Electroenceph. Clin. Neurophysiol.* 27: *23-24* (1969).

REMOND, A. & LESEVRE, N. Distribution topographique des potentiels évoqués visuels occipitaux chez l'homme normal. *Rev. Neurol.* 112: *317-330* (1965).

SAMSON-DOLLFUS, D. & LEVILLAIN, D. Premiers résultats de l'étude des potentiels évoqués visuels dans 57 cas d'épilepsie. *Revue d'E.E.G.* 1: *434-437* (1971).

VAUGHAN, H. G., KATZMAN, R. & TAYLOR, J. Alterations of visual evoked responses in the presence of homonymous defect. *Electroenceph. Clin. Neurophysiol.* 16: *345-361* (1963).

Authors' address:

Laboratoire d'Explorations Neurologiques
Hotel Dieu
76038 Rouen (Cedex)
France

MEAN VISUAL EVOKED POTENTIALS IN HEMIANOPSIA

J. FAIDHERBE, G. LENNES & M. JOACHIM

(Liège)

In this paper, we are going to describe two methods of measuring the dissymmetry of the mean evoked visual potentials. We are going to define two indices of dissymmetry.

Then, in order to test the efficiency of these two indices, we are going to use them to compare a group of normal subjects with a group of subjects suffering either from quadranopsia or from hemianopsia. For this latter group of subjects, the two hemispheres must, of course, work differently.

Our records are made from eight electrodes symmetrically located on the two hemispheres. These electrodes are numbered from 1 to 8, going from right to left.

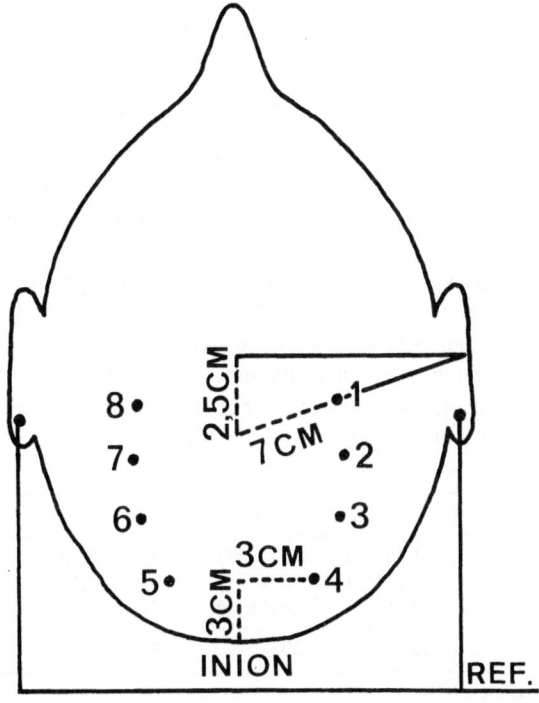

Fig. 1.

The stimulation takes place in the middle of the period of analysis, which is equal to 1024 ms.

The interval between two stimulations is equal to 2400 ms. Thus, the summed activity corresponding to the first part of the period of analysis may be considered to be spontaneous. The potentials are sampled every 2 ms, so that at the end of the summation process, each electrode gives rise to a sequence of 512 values. The first part of such a time series corresponds to the spontaneous activity preceding the stimulation, the second part corresponds to the activity recorded after the stimulation: it constitutes the observed evoked response.

In this paper, we will consider only this last part and more precisely the values recorded between the 60th and the 260th ms after stimulation, for one may wonder if the values recorded immediately after the stimulation are not essentially made up from spontaneous activity.

In order to build our first index of dissymmetry, called δ_V, we need the variances of the eight time series.

The variance is a measure of spread. It measures the dispersion of the sampled values around their mean. Roughly speaking, a time series showing high peaks will be characterized by a large variance. On the other hand, a time series for which the sampled values are nearly constant will be characterized by a small variance.

For each subject studied, we have calculated eight variances denoted by V_1, V_2, ..., V_8, the subscript referring to the rank of the electrode from which the time series has been recorded.

The expression for the index δ_V is as follows:

$$\delta_V = (\frac{V_1}{V_8} + \frac{V_8}{V_1}) + (\frac{V_2}{V_7} + \frac{V_7}{V_2}) + (\frac{V_3}{V_6} + \frac{V_6}{V_3}) + (\frac{V_4}{V_5} + \frac{V_5}{V_4})$$

Each bracket corresponds to a pair of electrodes symmetrically located on the two hemispheres. Let us suppose now that we are studying a perfectly symmetric subject, whose two hemispheres are responding rigorously in the same way.

Then $V_1 = V_8$, $V_2 = V_7$, $V_3 = V_6$, $V_4 = V_5$ and the value of δ_V will be exactly equal to 8. It may be easily demonstrated that whether $V_1 > V_8$ or whether $V_8 > V_1$, and so on ..., δ_V will be greater than eight.

We have calculated the value of the index δ_V for our 24 normal subjects, for our 9 quadranopsia cases and for our 7 haemianopsia cases. Here are the average values for our three groups and the ranges:

TABLE 1

Groups	$\delta_V \leqslant 8,71$	$\delta_V > 8,71$		mean	range
Normal	16 (67%)	8 (33%)	24	8,63	8,0 to 9,6
Quadranopsic	3 (33%)	6 (67%)	9	12,17	8,1 to 23,0
Hemianopsic	1 (14%)	6 (86%)	7	12,25	8,4 to 15,9
	20	20	40		

Median value of δ_V : 8,71
Median test: N : Q + H : $\chi_c^2 = 5,10$ (P <0,050)

370

As might be expected, the disease cases are characterized on the average by higher values of δ_V than the normal people. In order to see if the observed differences are statistically significant, we have calculated the median value of δ_V for our 40 subjects and we have applied the median test. The differences turn out to be statistically significant at the 5% level. So, it seems that δ_V is an acceptable index of dissymmetry.

In order to build our second index of dissymmetry, called D, we need the coefficients of determination between our eight time series.

The coefficient of determination is equal to the square of the correlation coefficient. In order to denote these coefficients, we need two subscripts.

For instance r_{ij} is the correlation coefficient between the two time series recorded respectively from the electrodes of rank i and of rank j. Similarly, K_{ij} is the corresponding coefficient of determination.

Here, we recall the well known relations between these coefficients:

$$r_{ij} = r_{ji} \qquad r_{ii} = 1$$
$$K_{ij} = K_{ji} \qquad K_{ii} = 1$$

Each subject may be characterized by 28 coefficients of determination. The problem is now to summarize all this information, so as to be able to discriminate efficiently between our 3 groups of subjects. The solution of this problem rests upon the following theoretical considerations.

Let us study a perfectly symmetric subject.

For such a person,

the eight time series is identical to the first

the seventh time series is identical to the second

the sixth time series is identical to the third.

the fifth time series is identical to the fourth.

Then, if we calculate the coefficients of determination of each of these eight series with a fixed time series, for instance that of rank i, we must have the following 4 relations between these coefficients:

$$K_{i8} = K_{i1} \quad K_{i7} = K_{i2} \quad K_{i6} = K_{i3} \quad K_{i5} = K_{i4}$$

That is the theory. But, what is found in practice? And, are the findings identical for our three groups?

A part of the answer to these questions is given by Figure 2. In this figure, i is equal to 1 and the coefficients of determination are average values calculated for each of our three groups. Along the horizontal axis we find the second index of K and along the vertical axis, the value of K.

As far as the normal subjects are concerned, we see that on the average:

K_{18} is nearly equal to K_{11}, is a good image of K_{11}

K_{17} is nearly equal to K_{12}, is a good image of K_{12}

K_{16} is nearly equal to K_{13}, is a good image of K_{13}

K_{15} is nearly equal to K_{14}, is a good image of K_{14}

Thus, in the normal cases, the theory is approximately verified. The right part of the graph is nearly a mirror image of the left part.

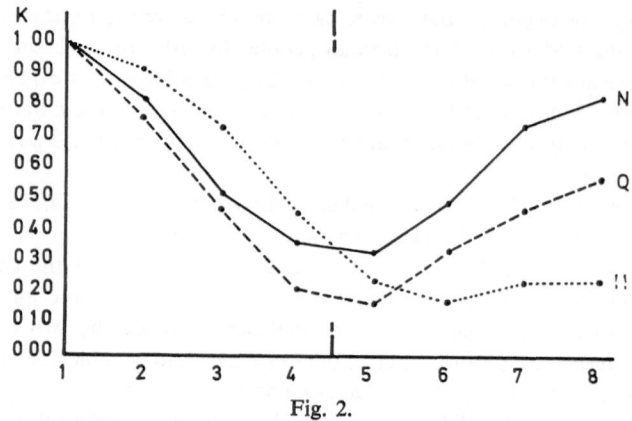

Fig. 2.

But, when we pass from the normal subjects to the quadranopsic and from the quadranopsic to the hemianopsic subjects, we observe that the image is getting worse and worse.

These findings have consequently led us to the definition of our second index of dissymmetry, D. This index is simply the sum of the differences between the individual object coefficients and their images. Or, to put it in other terms, the index D opposes the coefficients of determination relative to electrodes lying on the same hemisphere (for instance K_{11}, K_{12}, K_{13}, K_{14}) to those relative to electrodes lying on different hemispheres (for instance K_{18}, K_{17}, K_{16}, K_{15}).

The contribution of figure 2 to the index D is as follows: Contribution to D:
$1 - K_{18} + K_{12} - K_{17} + K_{13} - K_{16} + K_{14} - K_{15}$
Of course, similar results are observed when i is equal to 2, 3, ..., 8.

When all these contributions are summed, we arrive then at the following expression for D
$$D = (1 - K_{18} + K_{12} - K_{17} + K_{13} - K_{16} + K_{14} - K_{15}) + (K_{78} - K_{28} + K_{68} - K_{38} + K_{58} - K_{48})$$
$$+ (1 - K_{27} + K_{23} - K_{26} + K_{24} - K_{25}) + (K_{67} - K_{37} + K_{57} - K_{47})$$
$$+ (1 - K_{36} + K_{34} - K_{35}) + (K_{56} - K_{46}) + (1 - K_{45})$$
Each of the 28 coefficients is mentioned once and only once in this formula.

Just as we did for our first index, we have calculated the value of D for every subject.

TABLE 2.

Groups	D $\leqslant$ 1,97	D > 1,97		mean	range
Normal	19 (80%)	5 (20%)	24	1,72	0,6 to 5,2
Quadranopsic	1 (11%)	8 (89%)	9	5,09	1,3 to 11,8
Haemianopsic	0 (0%)	7 (100%)	7	9,13	3,0 to 13,3
	20	20	40		

Median value of D : 1,97
Median test: N : Q + H : $\chi_c^2 = 17,60$ (P <0,001)

As might be expected, the disease cases are characterized on the average by higher values of D than the normal people. The differences are very highly significant. Moreover, there seems to be a natural order between the three groups, the quadranopsia cases appearing to be intermediate between normal cases and haemianopsia cases.

If one considers simultaneously these two indices and if, for instance, the values of D are plotted along an horizontal axis and the values of δ_v along a vertical axis, each individual will be represented by a point in the plane.

The points corresponding to our normal subjects are clustering in the lower left part of the plane while those corresponding to the disease cases are scattered in the upper right part. A border line may easily be drawn between the normal subjects and the disease cases.

Authors' address:

Institut L. Fredericq
17 Place Delcour
B 4000 Liège
Belgium

A QUANTITATIVE EVALUATION OF THE VECP IN OPTIC NEURITIS.

G. H. M. VAN LITH & G. T. M. MAK

(Rotterdam)

ABSTRACT

In a group of 31 patients with optic neuritis, visually evoked potentials have been determined with luminance stimuli both in the acute stage and during the recovery period. In the acute stage, local stimuli or low luminance stimuli usually reveal no response, while high luminance total retinal stimulation can produce a response. During the recovery period, in between the stage of absent cortical responses and the stage of a more or less clear response, rhythmic discharges could be observed.

Blockage of the electric signals and non-uniform conduction velocities of the electric signals are most likely to explain the alterations of the evoked potentials.

INTRODUCTION

It is well-known from the literature that in optic neuritis the electroretinogram (ERG) is normal, while the amplitudes of the visually evoked cortical potentials (VECPs) are lowered (HIROSE & JACOBSON, 1968; VAN LITH, 1971) and their latency time increased (HALLIDAY et al. 1972; ADACHI-USAMI et al. 1972/1973). As compared to the psychophysical functions, the VECPs are generally more disturbed, remaining abnormal longer during the recovery period (DE HAAS 1972; HALLIDAY et al. 1972; ADACHSI-USAMI et al. 1972/1973). In spite of this fact, it may be that some relation exists between psychophysics and evoked potentials, when we suppose that all the symptoms of optic neuritis are caused by the same demyelination process. Such a relation can only be established when we are able to determine the VECPs quantitatively. Measurement of the amplitudes is not very profitable in view of the great variations that occur in normal individuals (JONKMAN, 1967). Measurement of the latency time would be preferable (VAUGHAN & KATZMAN 1964; ADACHI-USAMI et al. 1972/1973). For several reasons, however, we did not use this method.

JONKMAN (1967) describes the latencies in optic neuritis as less disturbed than the amplitudes. Secondly, and more often than not, no measurable responses are obtained in the acute stage, so that latencies cannot be measured. Even when there is a small response, it may be difficult through the variability of the wave-form to determine which peak to take for the latency measurement. Finally, our flash frequency of 4 cps appeared to be too high for latency measurements. This is especially true in optic neuritis where latency is lengthened. The exam-

375

ination time per patient being fairly long a lower flash frequency could hardly be applied.

We have tried to obtain a quantitative estimation of the VECPs by altering the stimulus conditions and the electrode positions. This set-up was chosen for two reasons, viz. the various stages which optic neuritis may show, and the absent VECPs which may occur even with almost normal psychophysical functions.

- In optic neuritis there may be a serious loss of vision. Visual acuity is markedly reduced and large parts of the visual field may be lost.
- In less serious cases there is an absolute or relative central scotoma with a more or less lowered visual acuity. The patient often says that central vision is blurred, as in a fog.
- Occasionally no alterations can be found with routine examination methods. The affected eye sees everything somewhat darker than usual. Visual acuity is normal or lowered somewhat, but is strongly reduced after placing a filter in front of the eye.

The loss of retinal sensitivity, which may even be a loss of light perception, is possibly due to a blockage of the electric signals in the optic nerve. With this assumption, the absence of the VECPs can easily be explained, too. The reduction of visual acuity after light filtering may then be the result of a relative barrier. With a high light intensity the barrier is broken. This hypothesis provided us with the reason to vary light intensity. As a central scotoma may be the only loss in the visual field, both total and local stimulation have been applied.

Somewhat difficult to understand with the assumption of a blockage of the signals is the loss of contrast sensitivity, which may be the reason for the blurred vision. This can easily be understood when we suppose that through demyelination within the optic nerve a leakage between the nerve fibres exists. Such a leakage, too, may result in a non-recordable VECP. Through leakage the evoked potentials will spread over the occipital lobe, causing an iso-electric field, which will be larger the more leakage there is. It goes without saying, that from bipolar leads, positioned over the iso-electric area, an evoked potential cannot be expected, while with a monopolar lead from the iso-electric field referential to a neutral point, viz. the earlobe, at least some response has to be present. If an iso-electric area exists, then it must be possible to determine its size by using electrodes at different places over the occipital lobes. This was the second aim of our investigation.

The absence of the VECPs may also be explained, when through inflammation or edema in the optic nerve, differences in conduction velocities occur. In that case, the electric signals from the illuminated retina will not reach the occipital cortex at the same time, but one after the other. This, too, may result in the responses levelling out. The combination of decreasing VECPs amplitudes together with increased latency times favours the latter supposition.

The light source was a Xenon arc, with a chopper, a diaphragm and neutral density filters in the lightbeam. The stimulus was a 20 msec blocksignal, presented with a frequency of 4 cps and a delay of 20 msec after the start of the sweep of the averager. Local macular stimulation of 5° and 8° and total retinal stimulation were applied. Maximum test light luminance was 4 log asb. All the experiments have been carried out under photopic conditions. Light adaptation was obtained with a bright blue background of 90° visual angle. Without the blue filter (cinemoid 20) luminance of the adaptive field was 3.3. log asb.

At first the electrodes were placed according to the EEG 10%-20% system. As these distances were rather large, later on an electro-ophthalmological 5%-10% system was applied. The electrodes were positioned in the midline from 5% above the inion on up to 30% (CPZ) above the inion in steps of 5%. For the bipolar registration, all measurements have been done from the 5% electrode position, so from 5% to 10% above the inion (in the figures drawn at the 10% position), from 5% to 15% (drawn at the 15% position) and so on (see Figure 1). The referential registrations have been made from the various electrode positions over the inion always to the earlobe.

The pupils were dilated and ERGs were always measured together with the VECPs. After amplification (time constant 1 sec, high frequency filter 75) 300 responses have been averaged with a CAT-computer.

RESULTS

The results of two patients will be discussed, which are representative for the whole group of 31 patients we examined in this way. As most patients have also been examined during the recovery period, the total number of examinations amounts to 84.

Figure 1 represents the results of a 25-year old woman in an acute stage of optic neuritis. Visual acuity was 2/60; the lower half of the visual field was lost. With a 2 log asb global stimulation the VECPs were absent both in the bipolar and referential leads. Local stimulation did not reveal a response either. With a 4 log asb global stimulation, a small evoked response is seen in the bipolar leads. This response is higher, the greater the distance between both electrodes. The latter finding may favour the leakage hypothesis. In the referential leads several peaks can be observed. The first peak cannot be a response of the stimulus just presented, as the latency time would be too short. It is probably triggered by the foregoing stimulus. These peaks, giving the impression of rhythmic discharges, are also present in Figure 2, both in the bipolar and the referential leads. In this stage, which was a fortnight after that shown in the first figure, visual acuity was again 1.0, while the visual field was normal. In the bipolar leads with the 4 log asb illumination a more or less clear evoked response can be recognized. From a comparison of Figures 1 and 2, it appears that the use of so many electrode positions for the detection of an iso-electric field, did not reveal positive results. Where the responses are absent in Figure 1,

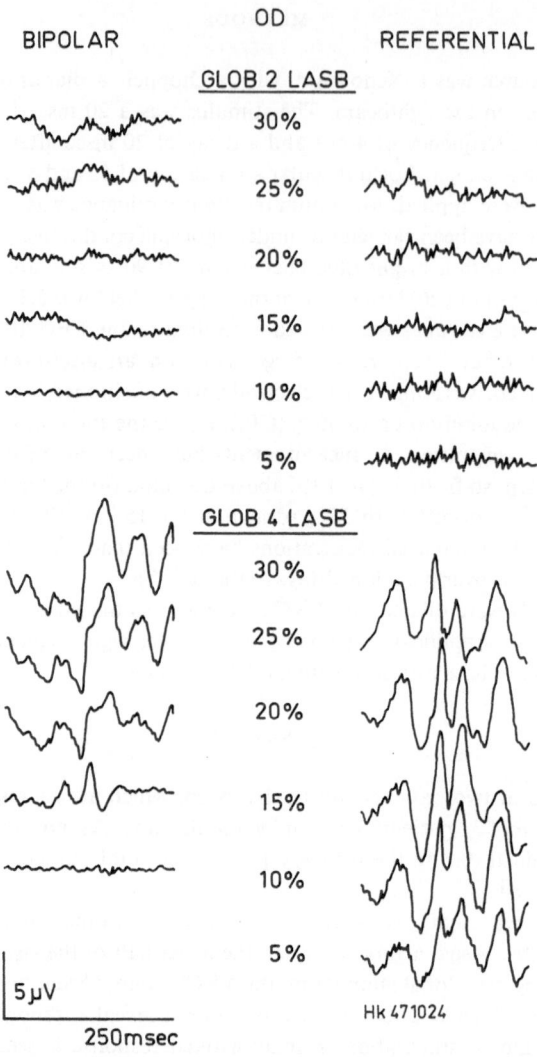

Fig. 1. VECPs in the acute stage of an optic neuritis obtained with global retinal stimulation of 2 log asb (upper recordings) and of 4 log asb (lower recordings). For description of the bipolar and referential leads see text.

some response is seen in all leads of Figure 2. This observation and the absence of a response not only in the bipolar, but also in the monopolar leads of Figure 1 are in contradiction to the leakage hypothesis. Therefore, in the next figures not all these leads are displayed.

It was only 10 months later that the cortical responses became the same as those of the normal eye (Figure 3). During that time the responses gradually increased after an intermediate stage of rhythmic discharges. A survey is given

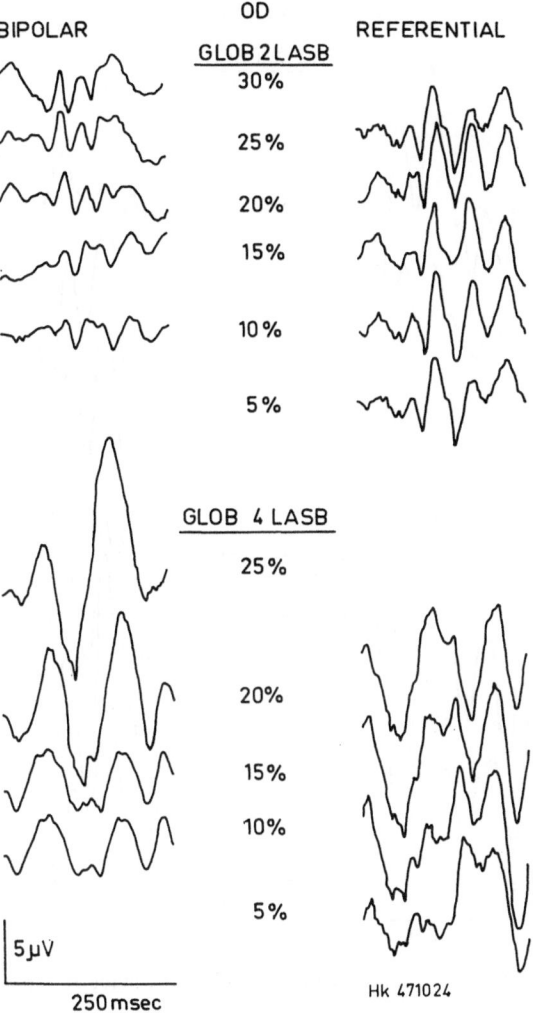

Fig. 2. VECPs of the same patient as in Figure 1, made a fortnight later, when visual acuity and visual field were normal again.

in Figure 4 in which only one bipolar lead (5%-15%) and one referential lead (5%-earlobe) is drawn. The moment a response was obtained with global stimulation, local stimulation (Sept. 15) was applied.

Data of another patient are shown in Figures 5, 6 and 7. In the acute stage visual acuity was 2/10. Local stimulation revealed almost no response, global stimulation with 2 log asb only a very small response, while after 4 log asb stimulation a rhythmic discharge was obtained.

The patient recovered rather quickly. During the next examination, 15 days later, visual acuity was again 10/10, the visual field being normal (Figure 6).

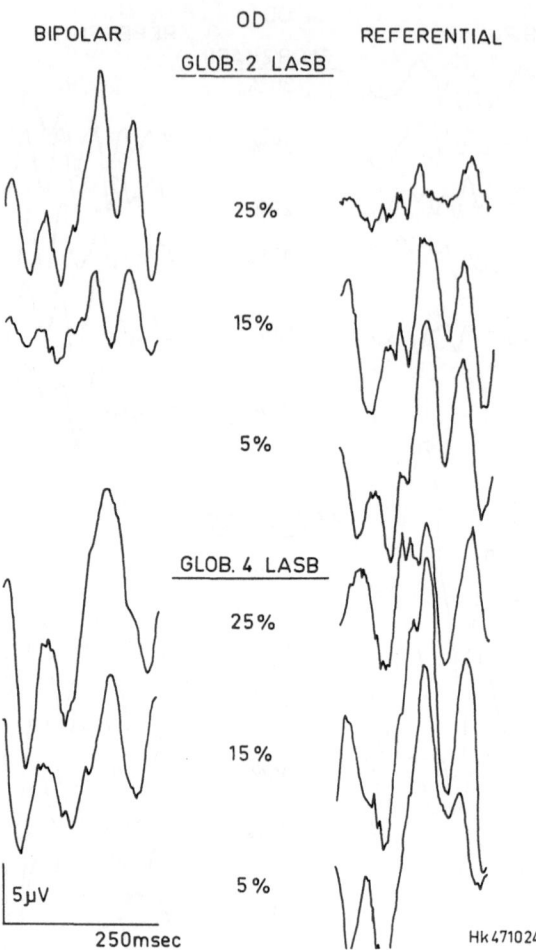

Fig. 3. VECPs of the same patient as in Figure 1, made 10 months later.

Clear, but low responses were obtained from the bipolar leads. After local stimulation the responses were higher than after total stimulation. This is seldom seen. More often during the recovery period, the bipolar leads produce clearer responses than the monopolar leads. In the latter, rhythmic discharges are seen.

The patient had a new attack 10 days later. Visual acuity was again reduced to 2/10, the visual field was even worse in comparison with that after the first attack (Figure 7). Bipolar responses became much lower again, especially those after local stimulation. It is unusual that the referential leads show a clearer response than the bipolar leads. They are even clearer when compared to the rhythmic discharges of Figure 6.

All 31 patients were first examined as soon as possible in the acute stage. A

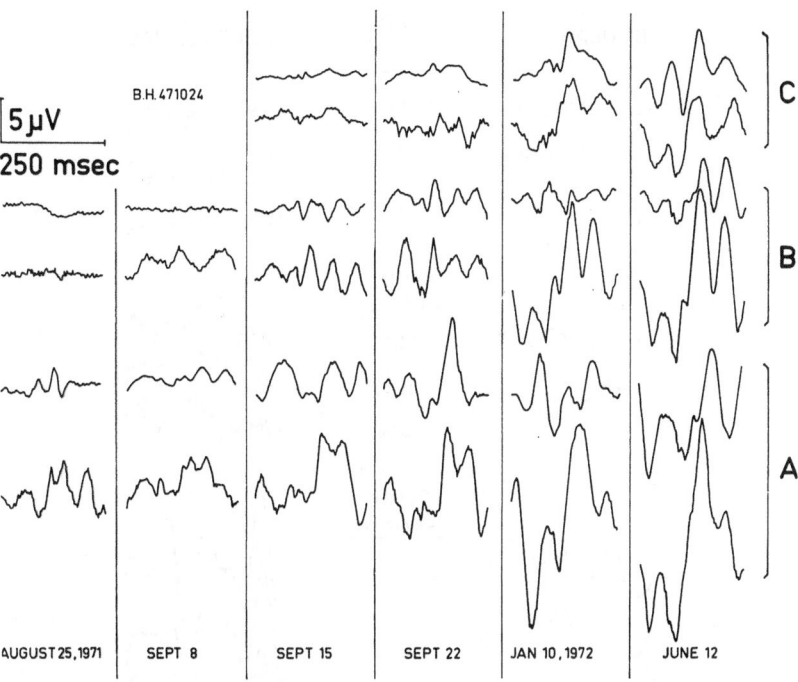

5 μV
250 msec

B.H. 471024

C

B

A

AUGUST 25,1971 | SEPT 8 | SEPT 15 | SEPT 22 | JAN 10,1972 | JUNE 12

Fig. 4. Survey of the examinations, done in the patient of Figures 1, 2 and 3. A: global stimulation of 4 log asb, B: global stimulation of 2 log asb, C: 10° macular stimulation of 3 log asb. Upper recording of each pair is a bipolar lead (5%-15%), the lower recording of each pair a referential lead (5% earlobe).

survey of the results of the first examination and those of later examinations during the recovery period is given in Table 1. In the acute stage the VECPs are more often absent after local stimulation than after global stimulation; of the latter, the responses obtained with low stimulus luminance are more disturbed than those following a high stimulus luminance. During the recovery period these differences are levelled.

TABLE 1

Presence (higher than 2 muV) or absence (lower than 2 muV) of the VECPs in optic neuritis.

stimulus	acute stage 31 exam.		recovery period 53 exam.	
macular	present	absent	present	absent
	4	27	26	27
total				
2 log asb	13	18	42	11
4 log asb	27	4	50	3

381

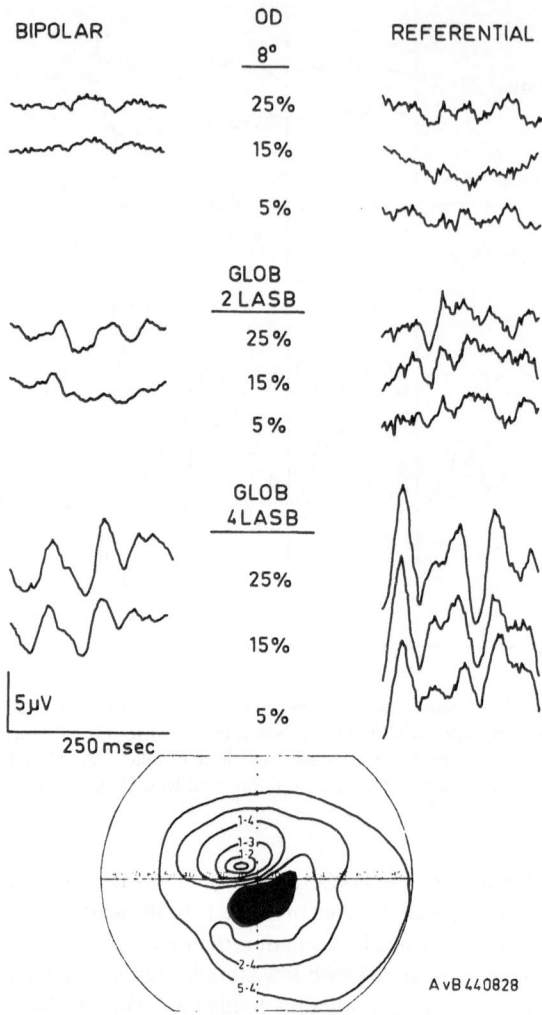

Fig. 5. VECPs in the acute stage of an optic neuritis in another patient.

DISCUSSION

From the investigation of this group of patients, it became clear that the great number of electrode positions applied, did not contribute essentially to the diagnosis. An iso-electric area which should become smaller during the recovery, was not found. On the other hand, bipolar and referential recordings often reveal different results. Therefore, it is advisable to use at least one of both leads. Otherwise, some phenomena, especially the stage of the rhythmic discharges, are not observed.

Comparison of the results with local and global stimulation demonstrates

382

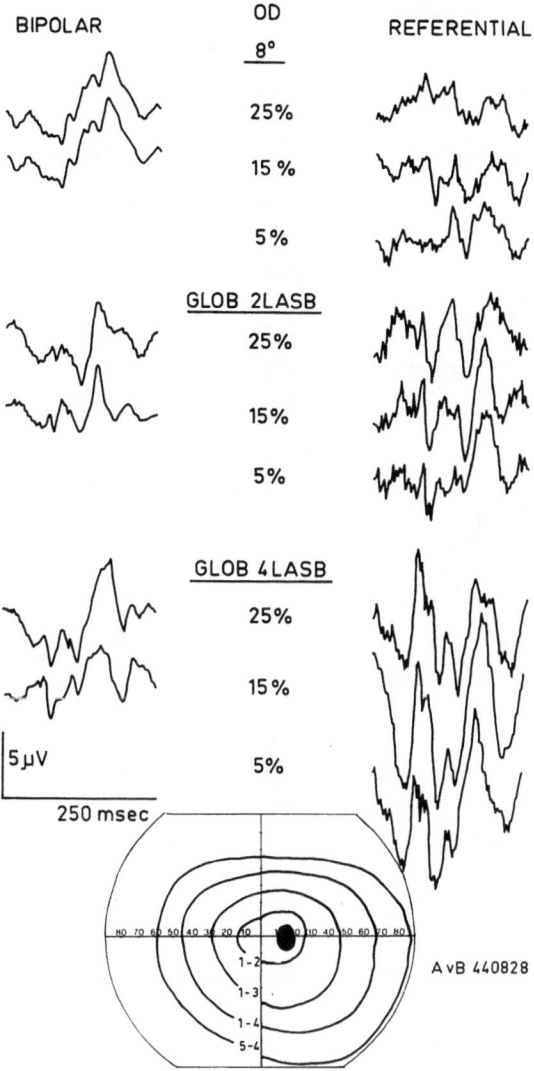

BIPOLAR OD REFERENTIAL
8°
25%
15%
5%

GLOB 2LASB
25%
15%
5%

GLOB 4LASB
25%
15%
5%

5 μV
250 msec

A vB 440828

Fig. 6. idem, 5 days later.

that the diagnosis of a neuritis may be missed, if only global stimulation is applied. Even in the acute stages, 27 of 31 patients produced reasonable VECPs with the global high luminance stimulation. The measurement of amplitudes or latencies is then the only way to inform us of the existence of a pathological process. Due to their great variability these measurements are less reliable, especially in cases of bilateral optic neuritis, when the results of the affected eye cannot be compared with those of an unaffected eye in the same person (ADACHI-USAMI et al. 1972/1973).

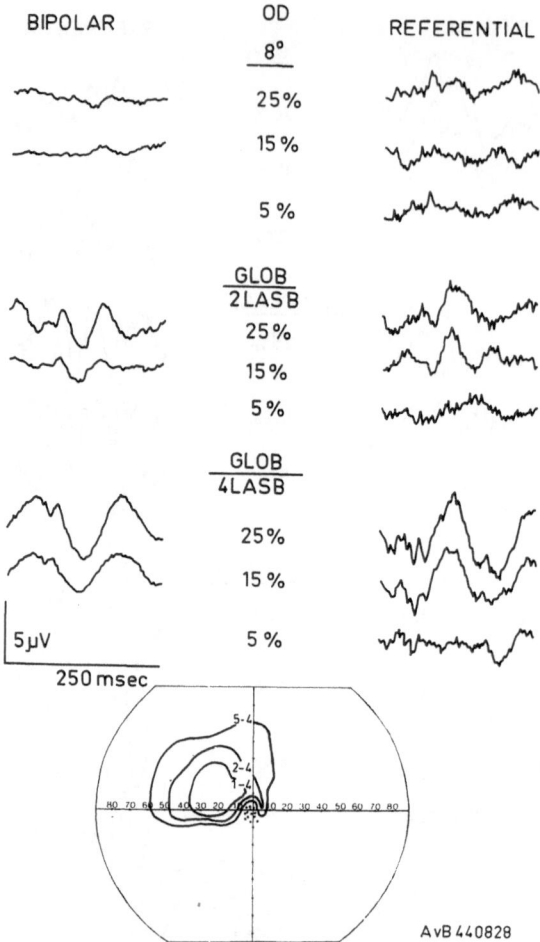

Fig. 7. idem, 9 days later, after a new attack.

The nature of the rhythmic discharges we often saw during the recovery period, between the stage of an absent response and the moment a response is present, is still vague. HIROSE & JACOBSON (1968), reviewing literature in this regard, describe three types of rhythmic VECPs in normal subjects after bright light stimuli. The luminance, with which we found rhythmic VECPs in optic neuritis, was much lower. The frequency was generally between 15 and 20 cps. It may be a photic driving of the α-rhythm or a harmonic component of the α-rhythm. As this reaction is not always seen during the whole analysis time (see Figure 2, 2 log asb illumination), it seems to us more of an actual discharge than a photic driving. Lower stimulus frequencies have to be used to differentiate between both suppositions. If it is an actual discharge, it may be a split wave, as NAMEROW (1970) suggested for the broad somatosensory evoked potentials in multiple sclerosis.

No indications have been found to support the leakage hypothesis. There-fore, we incline more towards the two other explanations for the lowered VECPs. The blockage hypothesis is supported by the fact that high luminance stimuli may produce a response, while low luminance stimuli do not. In favour of the supposition that different conduction velocities of the electric signals levelled out the VECPs, is the observation that absent VECPs may be present together with restored psychophysical visual functions. Blockage and non-uniform conduction velocities are also assumed to be the cause of absent somatosensory evoked potentials (HALLIDAY & WAKEFIELD 1963; NAMEROW 1968). From the experiments of McDONALD (1970) it appears that the degree of demyelination determines whether conduction blockage or conduction slowing exists.

We may suppose that in the acute stage of optic neuritis, when even light perception is lost, a real blockage of the electric signals occurs, and that in less severe cases or during the recovery different conduction velocities are responsible for the absent VECPs. In accordance with this hypothesis are the increased latencies of the VECPs after low frequency stimuli (ADACHI-USAMI et al. 1972/1973) and the phase-shifts of the steady-state VECPs after high frequency stimulation (HALLIDAY 1972). In the less severe cases or after the acute stages, when evoked potentials are present again, only these phenomena will provide us with information. In this regard, application of pattern stimulation is of great importance for further quantitative evaluation, since HALLIDAY (1972) found the pattern evoked responses more disturbed, as compared to the flash evoked responses.

As pattern evoked responses, however, can be lowered for so many other reasons, such as refractive errors and media opacities, we are of the opinion that an abnormal evoked potential obtained with ordinary luminance stimulation is more reliable than an abnormal potential obtained with pattern reversal stimulation. Therefore we prefer luminance stimulation for the acute stage of optic neuritis.

REFERENCES

ADACHI-USAMI, E., KELLERMAN, F. J. & MAKABE, R. VER threshold in different stages of optic neuritis. Ophthal. Res. 4: 284-297 (1972/73).

HAAS, J. P., DE. An electro-ophthalmological study of affections of the optic pathway. Thesis Rotterdam. Den Haag, Junk (1972).

HALLIDAY, A. M. & WAKEFIELD, G. S. Cerebral evoked potentials in patients with dissociated sensory loss. J. Neurol. Neurosurg. Psychiat. 26: 211-219 (1963).

HALLIDAY, A. M., McDONALD, W. I. & MUSHIN, J. Delayed visual evoked response in optic neuritis. Lancet II: 982-985 (1972).

HIROSE, T. & JACOBSON, J. H. Combined recording of the electroretinogram (ERG) and visual evoked occipital response (VER) in lesions of the visual pathways. In: Advances in electrophysiology and -pathology of the visual system; Proc. 6th Iscerg Symp. Erfurt (1967); ed. by E. SCHMÖGER, p. 125-138. Leipzig, Thieme (1968).

JONKMAN, E. J. The average cortical response to photic stimulation. Thesis Amsterdam. Den Haag, Trio (1967).

McDONALD, W. I. & SEARS, T. A. The effects of experimental demyelination on conduction in the central nervous system. Brain 93: 583-598 (1970).

NAMEROW, N. S. Somatosensory evoked responses in multiple sclerosis patients with varying sensory loss. *Neurology* 18: *1197-1204* (1968).

NAMEROW, N. S. Somatosensory recovery functions in multiple sclerosis patients. *Neurology* 20: *813-817* (1970).

VAN LITH, G. H. M. The combined use of the macular electroretinogram (M-ERG) and the visually evoked response (VER). *Ophthalmologica* 162: *208-212* (1971).

VAUGHAN, H. G. Jr. & KATZMAN, R. Evoked response in visual disorders. *Ann. N.Y. Acad. Sci.* 112: *305-319* (1964).

Authors' address:

Eye Hospital, Erasmus University
Rotterdam
The Netherlands

VECPS IN PATIENTS WITH GLAUCOMA

H. J. M. ERMERS, L. J. DE HEER & G. H. M. VAN LITH

(Rotterdam)

INTRODUCTION

In a group of 40 patients with open angle glaucoma, we compared the visual functions and the anatomy of the optic disc with the visually evoked cortical potentials (VECPs). As the VECPs are mainly a reflection of the central part of the visual field (VAN HOF et al., 1960; RIETVELD et al., 1965; DE VOE et al., 1968), our attention concerning the visual functions was mainly paid to the influence on the VECPs of lowered visual acuity, central sensitivity loss or peripheral visual field defects. In one part of the group the VECPs have been provoked with pattern reversal stimulation, while the other part of the group was examined with flash stimulation, the latter including both local macular and total retinal stimulation. So far as we know, no systematical investigation of glaucoma patients has been published up to now.

METHODS

Only those patients were selected for this examination, who had no other eye diseases. Moreover, they had open angle glaucoma, so that pupils could be dilated. For the flash evoked responses, pupils were always dilated up to about 8 mm. For the pattern reversal responses pupils were not dilated, while the best possible refraction was made. Intra-ocular pressure during the examination was always lower than 25 mm. mercury. When necessary Diamox was administered. For the flash evoked responses the ball-stimulator as described by VAN LITH et al. (1973) was applied. Both ERG and VECPs have been made under photopic conditions (blue background) with total retinal and a 10° local macular stimulation. Flash frequency was 4 per second. Maximum flash intensity was 1 Joule and could be lowered with neutral density filters in steps of 0.5 log unit.

For the pattern reversal a projector with checkerboard slide has been used with a total field amount of 30° and a check size of 1°. Movement of 4 per second was obtained with a constantly moving mirror in front of the projector. Without neutral density filters the luminance of the white fields was 1.6 log ft-L and of the black fields 0.4 log ft-L.

The ERG was led off with a Henkes contact lens. For the VECPs electrodes

387

were positioned in the midline 5% 15% and 25% above the inion. One bipolar derivation from 5%-25% and one referential derivation from 15% to the earlobe was used. Band pass of the amplifier was 0.015-500 Hz. After amplification 300 responses for the VECP and the macular ERG (M-ERG) were averaged; for the global ERG 30 flashes were sufficient.

Visual fields shown in the figures were made according to the Goldmann technique.

RESULTS

Only some examples, which are representative for the whole group we have examined up to now, will be discussed.

In Figure 1 the results of 2 glaucoma patients are shown. Those of the left eye are of a patient with a good visual acuity, a good visual field, and no excavation of the optic disc. Those of the right eye are of a patient with a deep central excavation, a great peripheral visual field defect, small loss of central sensitivity and a good visual acuity. The upper recording of each pair is a bipolar lead, while the lower recording is a referential lead. The amplitudes of the normal left eye are about 15 muV after total retinal stimulation and

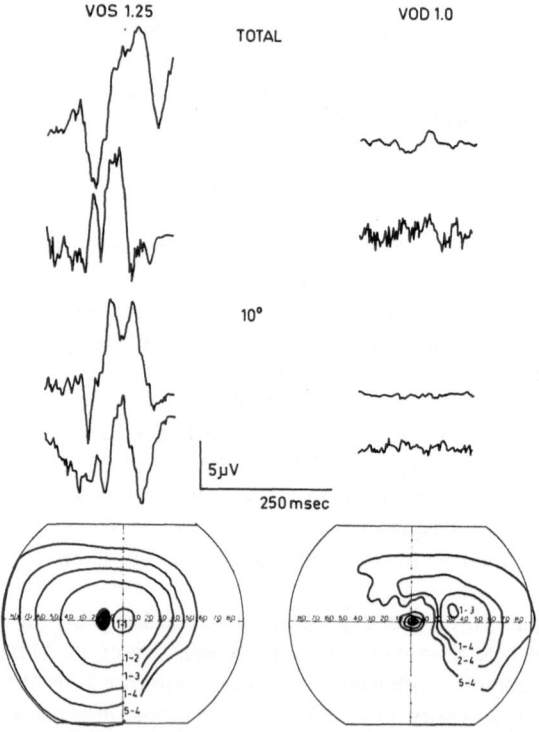

Fig. 1. VECP's of 2 glaucoma patients; the upper pair of recordings obtained with total retinal stimulation, the lower pair with 10° macular stimulation.

388

about 10 muV after 10° macular stimulation. The responses of the right eye are almost absent.

In all the next figures only the results of one patient per figure will be shown. We have chosen those patients that have clear differences between both eyes, preferably when one eye was normal, to make the comparison as simple as possible.

The patient in Figure 2 displays a left eye with a good visual acuity and only a small defect in the visual field around the optic disc, while the other eye has a low visual acuity and a peripheral as well as a central loss in the visual field. The central sensitivity is only one log unit lowered. Although the psychophysical functions of the left eye are rather good, the cortical responses are markedly lowered. Those of the right eye are almost absent in the 10° stimulation and hardly detectable in total stimulation.

The patient in Figure 3 has been stimulated both with flash light and with pattern reversal. The visual acuity of both eyes is normal. The left eye has also a normal visual field, while the right eye has some small paracentral scotomas. The VECPs after flash stimuli of the left eye are rather good, viz. in the bipolar lead about 10 muV, in the referential lead about 5 muV. Those of the right eye are clearly lower, especially in the referential lead. From the pattern stimulation, one period is shown. The amplitudes in the bipolar lead of the left eye are approximately 15 muV, those in the referential lead are about 20 muV. The VECPs of the right eye are obviously reduced.

In the visual fields of Figure 4, both eyes show small paracentral scotomas. The central sensitivity of the left eye is normal, that of the right eye is half a

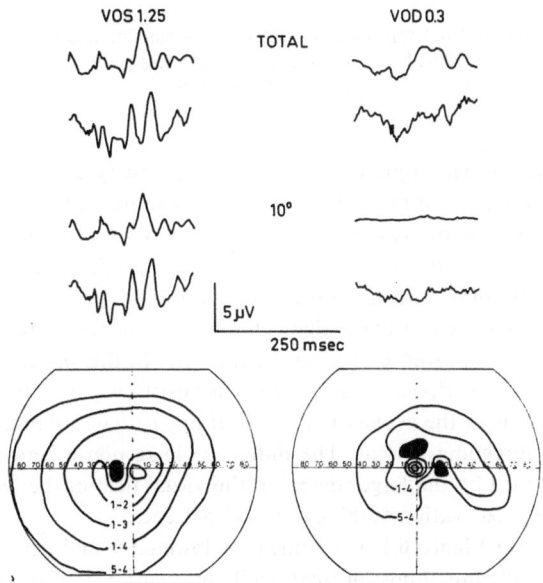

Fig. 2. Flash VECP's of a glaucoma patient.

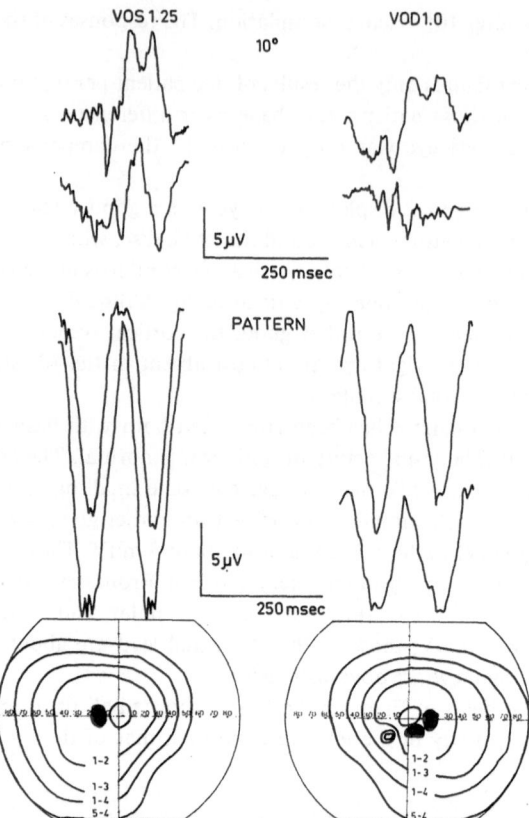

Fig. 3. Flash light and pattern reversal VECP's of a glaucoma patient. The upper pair of recordings were obtained with 10° macular stimulation, the lower pair with pattern reversal stimulation.

log unit lowered. This difference in central sensitivity is also reflected in a difference of the pattern evoked responses. As compared to the results of the foregoing patient, both eyes show low responses. We are not sure if this is an individual variation, or caused by the paracentral scotomas or due to the excavation of the optic disc that is present in both eyes.

The results obtained in the patient of Figure 5 are very interesting as they clearly show the importance of central sensitivity. In this patient, especially in the left eye, a large peripheral visual field defect exists, while central sensitivity is good. The results of the evoked potentials of this patient are much better than those of the foregoing patient. The difference in response between both eyes may be explained by the larger defect in the visual field of the left eye and by the fact that the excavation of this eye was also deeper.

The patient in Figure 6 has a somewhat lowered visual acuity. The visual fields peripherally are almost normal, while the central sensitivity is normal in the right eye and only half a log unit lowered in the left eye. In spite of the small

390

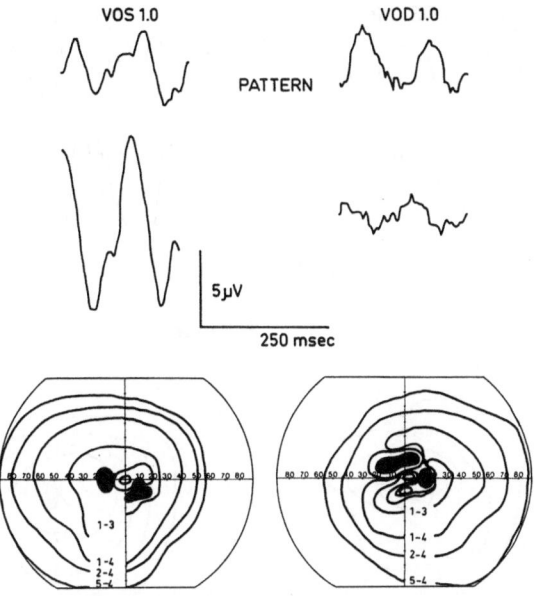

Fig. 4. Pattern evoked VECP's of a glaucoma patient.

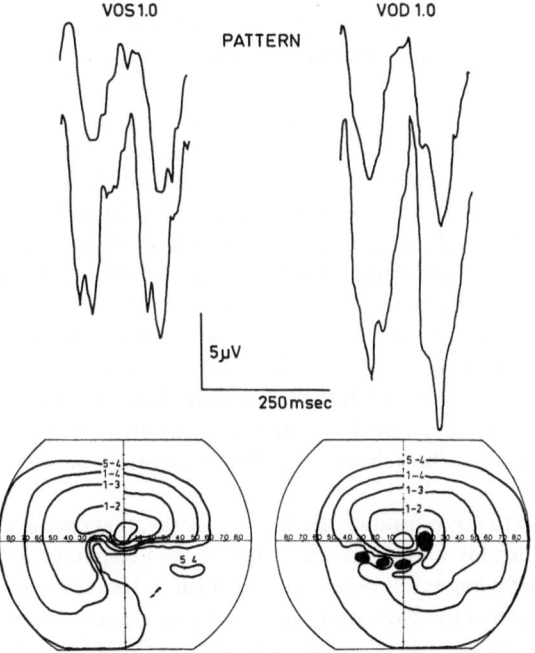

Fig. 5. Pattern evoked VECP's of a glaucoma patient.

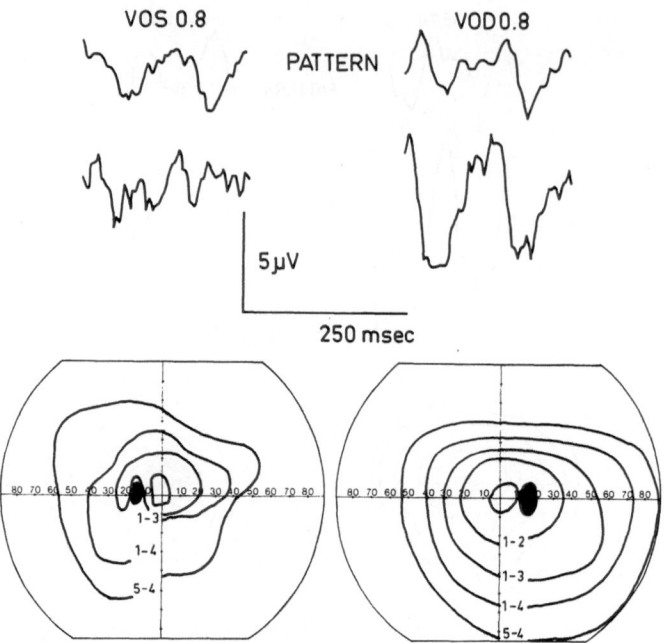

Fig. 6. Pattern evoked VECP's of a glaucoma patient.

loss in the central sensitivity, the evoked potentials are very small. This patient, however, also has deep excavations of both eyes.

In conclusion, we may deduce from the results of the examination of the 40 patients that in glaucoma, there is no apparent relation between visual acuity and the amplitude of the evoked potentials. The evoked potentials decline much sooner than the visual acuity. Peripheral field defects are also not so important in determining the height of the cortical responses. This is reasonable as the evoked potentials are known to rise mainly from the central retinal area (OGUCHI & VAN LITH, 1974). Central sensitivity in the visual field seems to be the main factor. As shown in the last patient, however, it is not the only one. This patient combines a small loss in central sensitivity with very low responses, the latter being possibly related to the deep excavations present.

In relation to this central sensitivity we may say, that central sensitivity loss of more than one log unit always gives low evoked responses. If the central sensitivity is half a log unit lowered, then the evoked responses may or may not be lowered. Depth of the excavation will than be the second main factor.

In the future we will pay more attention to the relation between the light stimulation and the pattern stimulation, and to the relation between the evoked

392

potentials, the depth of the excavation of the optic disc and the peripapillary choroidal circulation.

REFERENCES

DE VOE, R. G., RIPPS, H. & VAUGHAN Jr., H. G. Cortical responses to stimulation of the human fovea. *Vision Res.* 8: *135-147* (1968).

RIETVELD, W. J., TORDOIR, W. E. M. & DUYFF, J. W. Contribution of fovea and para-fovea to the visual evoked response. *Acta Physiol. Pharmacol. Neerl.* 13: *330-339* (1965).

OGUCHI, Y. & VAN LITH, G. H. M. Contribution of the central and peripheral part of the retina to the VECP under photopic conditions. To be published in *Doc. Ophthal. Proc. Ser.* 1974.

VAN HOF, M. W. Open-eye and closed-eye occipito-cortical response to photic stimulation of the retina. *Acta Physiol. Pharmacol. Neerl.* 9: *443-451* (1960).

VAN LITH, G. H. M., MEININGER, J. & VAN MARLE, G. W. Electrophysiological equipment for total and local retinal stimulation. In: Xth Iscerg Symposium, Los Angeles 1972; ed. by J. T. PEARLMAN. *Docum. Ophthal. Proc. Ser.* 3: *213-218* (1973).

Authors' address:

Eye Hospital, Erasmus University
Rotterdam
The Netherlands

393

ERGS AND NOISE:
DETECTION PROBABILITY, TIME AND AMPLITUDE
ERRORS*

STEPHEN J. FRICKER, M. D. & JAMES J. SANDERS, III

(Boston)

ABSTRACT

The effect of background noise on a waveform is to change it in a manner which to some extent depends upon statistical parameters of the signal and the noise. When the signal-to-noise ratio is low the signal may be masked by the noise so that it is not detected most of the time, that is the probability of detection is close to zero. As the signal-to-noise ratio increases, the probability of detecting the signal increases. This process can be described by a curve of probability of detection as a function of signal-to-noise ratio. Measurements of the amplitude and implicit time of the signal have ranges of errors associated with them which also depend upon the signal-to-noise ratio, tending to be large when the signal-to-noise ratio is low, and decreasing as the signal-to-noise ratio improves. These general concepts can be readily applied to electroretinography measurements, and some model ERG and noise waveforms are described and compared with live recordings. The model system is used to obtain measurements of the probability of detection and of the time and amplitude errors which occur at different signal-to-noise ratios. Some techniques are discussed for estimating these effects in practical cases.

INTRODUCTION

Electrophysiological measurements often involve the examination of a signal waveform in the presence of a noise background. When the noise is small compared with the signal, its effect can be ignored to a considerable extent. However as the signal decreases relative to the noise, the signal characteristics can be modified significantly. The first point of concern is whether a signal is considered to be present or not. If it is thought to be present, how large is it, and when does it occur in relation to the stimulus?

In non-biological systems the characteristics of the signal waveform can be specified quite closely, and the noise characteristics often can be well defined. In such cases a number of theoretical and practical approaches have been devel-

* From the Howe Laboratory of Ophthalmology, Harvard Medical School, Massachusetts Eye and Ear Infirmary. This study was supported in part by the United States Health Center Grant No. EY00292, the General Research Support Grant No. FRO5485 from the National Institute of Health, and Research Grant No. EY00885-01 from the National Institute of Health, United States Public Health Service.
Reprint requests to STEPHEN J. FRICKER, M.D., Howe Laboratory of Ophthalmology, Massachusetts Eye and Ear Infirmary, 243 Charles Street, Boston, Massachusetts, 02114.

395

oped in order to deal with the problem of reliability of detection (or probability of detection), and the possible errors to be expected in amplitude and time measurements (LAWSON & UHLENBECK, 1950 and CARLSON, 1968). An application of these basic principles to biological measurements is needed in order to give a firmer understanding of the inherent limitations of such measurements, and to provide a rational approach to possible improvement in techniques. For example, in the literature there are many reports of electroretinogram recordings which by inspection are grossly influenced by noise, and yet where various amplitude and timing measurements are quoted as if they can be made very accurately. The problems becomes particularly important when abnormal signal waveforms are encountered, as often these are much reduced in amplitude while the noise characteristics remain basically unchanged. This report illustrates how the problem can be approached experimentally in order to better define the errors involved. References are made to clinical electroretinography studies as one of the areas where the basic principles often can be applied in a relatively simple manner.

For signals which are pulse-like in nature, a useful parameter is that of the peak signal amplitude, measured from a zero baseline. Noise has to be handled differently however, as it is necessary to consider the frequency spectrum and the root-mean-square (RMS) magnitude of the noise. The mean-square noise level describes the total power of the noise, while its frequency spectrum shows how this power is distributed at different frequencies. The signal-to-noise (S/N) ratio then may be defined as the ratio of the peak signal voltage to the root-mean-square noise voltage. Because of the large range encountered, this ratio often is given in decibels (decibels (db) = 20 $\log_{10}$ (Voltage Ratio)).

A somewhat different concept of the signal and noise is obtained by considering their autocorrelation functions (LANGE, 1967 and LEE, 1960). In simplified terms, the autocorrelation function at zero time delay gives the mean-square value of the function, and hence allows the RMS value to be calculated. Also the Fourier transform of the autocorrelation function yields the frequency power spectrum of the signal.

SIGNAL CHARACTERISTICS

Figure 1a shows four successive sweeps of photopic electroretinograms with a relatively large S/N ratio. (The recordings were made under normal room illumination levels with the subject in his normal light-adapted state, using a white electronic flash stimulus as described in reference 6.) The sweep duration is 100 milliseconds and the bandwidth of the recording system is 625 Hertz (Hz). An average peak signal amplitude can be measured, and the position of the peak of the signal estimated to give its implicit time. Both of these measurements will have some uncertainty associated with them because of the noise level.

Figure 1b gives consecutive sweeps of some different photopic electroretinograms at a much lower S/N ratio. The sweep duration and frequency bandwidth are the same as for Figure 1a. An improvement in the S/N ratio is obtained by

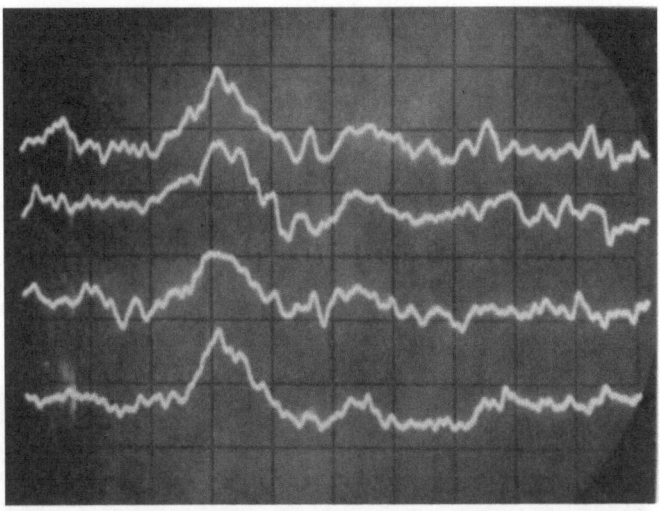

Fig. 1a. Photopic ERGs (large). 4 successive 100 msec sweeps at 1/sec. Vertical scale 0.5 volts/large division (Voltage Gain 6000).

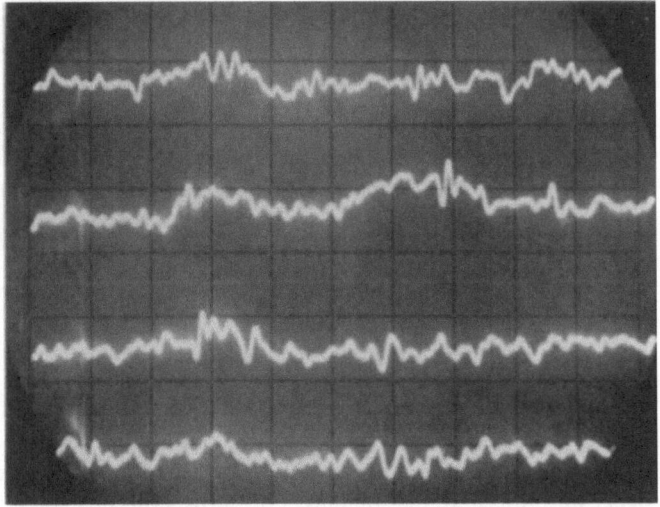

Fig. 1b. Photopic ERGs (small). 4 successive 100 msec sweeps at 1/sec. Vertical scale 0.5 volts/large division (Voltage Gain 6000).

summing 128 sweeps, as shown in Figure 1c, also for a baseline of 100 milliseconds.

In order to study the problem experimentally, the signal to be detected was modelled by a single sinusoidal pulse, as shown in Figure 2. The total pulse duration was set at 50 milliseconds, and the sweep width at 200 milliseconds. The ratio of the signal width to sweep width obviously may influence the signal

397

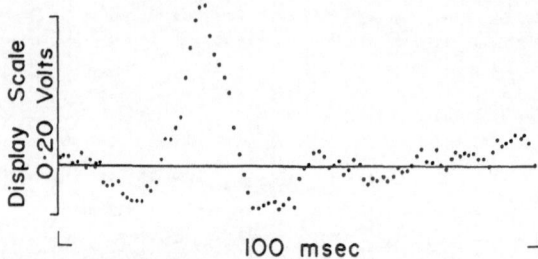

Fig. 1c. Waveform obtained by summation of 128 consecutive 100 msec sweeps of the small photopic ERGs shown in Fig. 1b.

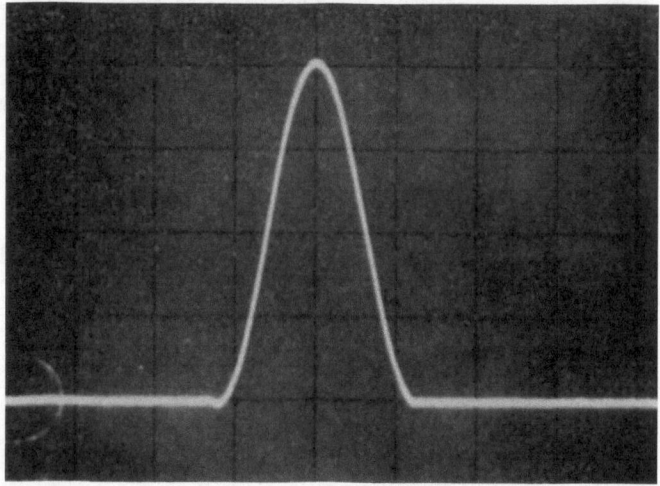

Fig. 2. Model waveform for ERG. 50 msec base width, 200 msec sweep, waveform center at 4 divisions.

detection characteristics, as may the vertical gain settings on the oscilloscope presentation. These parameters were chosen so as to give a relatively normal appearing trace. Another factor to be considered is that of the time of occurrence of the signal with respect to the stimulus. For the experimental conditions, the signal was set to occur anywhere across the 2 to 9 centimeter portion of a 10 centimeter trace. That is, within this region, there was no *a priori* knowledge of where the signal would appear.

NOISE CHARACTERISTICS

For test purposes it was convenient to use an electronic noise generator to model the noise background. From experience it has been found that the general appearance of actual noise on an oscilloscope presentation, and its frequency power spectrum, often can be modelled reasonably well by taking

398

uniform spectrum Gaussian noise (e.g. from a Hewlett-Packard noise generator no. 3722A) with a bandwidth of 500 Hz and passing the noise through a low-pass filter with a single pole at 10 Hz. The lower tracings in Figures 3a-3e show different recordings of this noise on 200 millisecond sweep presentations.

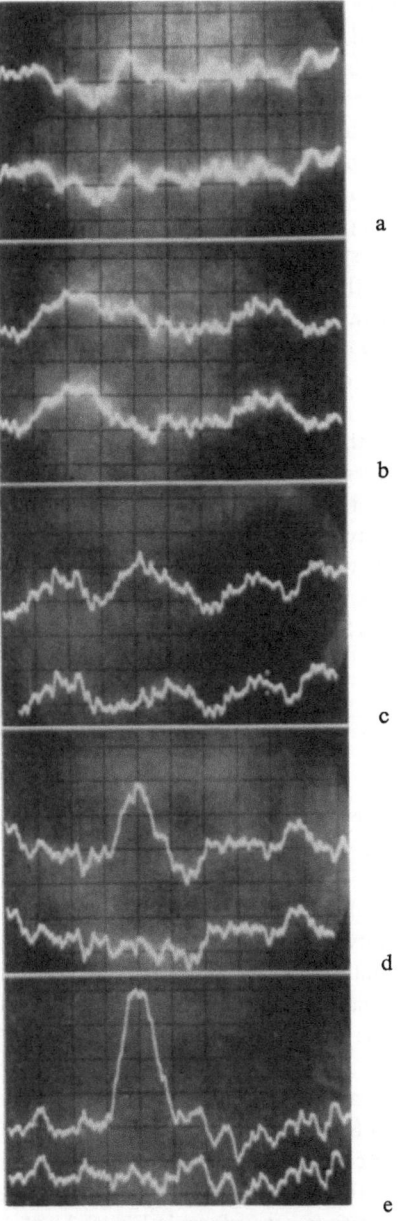

Fig. 3. Model Signal and Noise waveforms: (i) Signal and Noise superiorly, and (ii) Noise only inferiorly. The signal is always centered at 4 divisions. 3a. S/N = 0 db; b. S/N = 4 db; c. S/N = 8 db; d. S/N = 14 db; e. S/N = 20 db.

399

The single sinusoidal pulse was added to the specified noise waveform so as to give a specific 'peak signal' to 'RMS noise' (S/N) ratio. The frequency spectrum of the noise overlaps that of the signal, so that when the peak signal amplitude is equal to the RMS noise voltage (0 db S/N ratio) the signal usually will be missed. When the signal peak is 10 times the magnitude of the RMS noise voltage (20 db S/N ratio) the signal is very evident. Figures 3a-3e show typical sweep presentations at S/N ratios of 0, 4, 8, 14 and 20 db. The top trace always has the combined signal and noise, with the signal centered at 4 centimeters on the graticule, while the lower trace shows the noise only.

The observer was presented with combined signal and noise displayed on an oscilloscope with a storage screen (Hewlett-Packard 141A). The signal waveform was known to the observer, but its amplitude was varied in 2 decibel steps in a random manner. The 'implicit time' also was varied in a random manner between the 2 and 9 divisions of the 10 division scale of the trace. The observer's first task was to determine if a signal was present or not. If he thought it was present, he gave an estimate of the time (distance) to the peak of the signal and an estimate of the peak amplitude. This was carried out for 200 tests for each of three observers, two of whom were expert observers with a considerable background in detection theory, while the third observer was familiar with the general principles involved but had a limited background in the subject. The experimental results were analyzed to give estimates of the probability of detection of the signal, as well as the errors in amplitude and timing of the detected signals at the various S/N ratios.

EXPERIMENTAL RESULTS

1. Probability of Detection

The probability of detection was plotted versus the S/N ratio to give the curves shown in Figures 4a-4d for the three observers and the total combined results for all three. At a S/N ratio of 0 db it is seen that the probability of detection is approximately 0.1, while for a S/N ratio of 16 to 20 db the probability of detection increases to unity essentially. The point at which the signal is detected 50% of the time (probability of detection = 0.5) occurs at a S/N ratio of slightly greater than 8 db, that is at a point where the peak signal amplitude is approximately 2.5 times the magnitude of the RMS noise level. Figure 3c illustrates one particular sweep for these conditions, with the signal which is centered at 4 centimeters on the trace being evident when the top sweep is compared with the bottom sweep. At a S/N ratio of 14 db or more, as in Figures 3d and 3e, there is almost complete certainty of detection. However, the signal characteristics still are affected by the noise, as seen by comparing the waveforms in Figures 3d and 3e with the noise-free waveform in Figure 2.

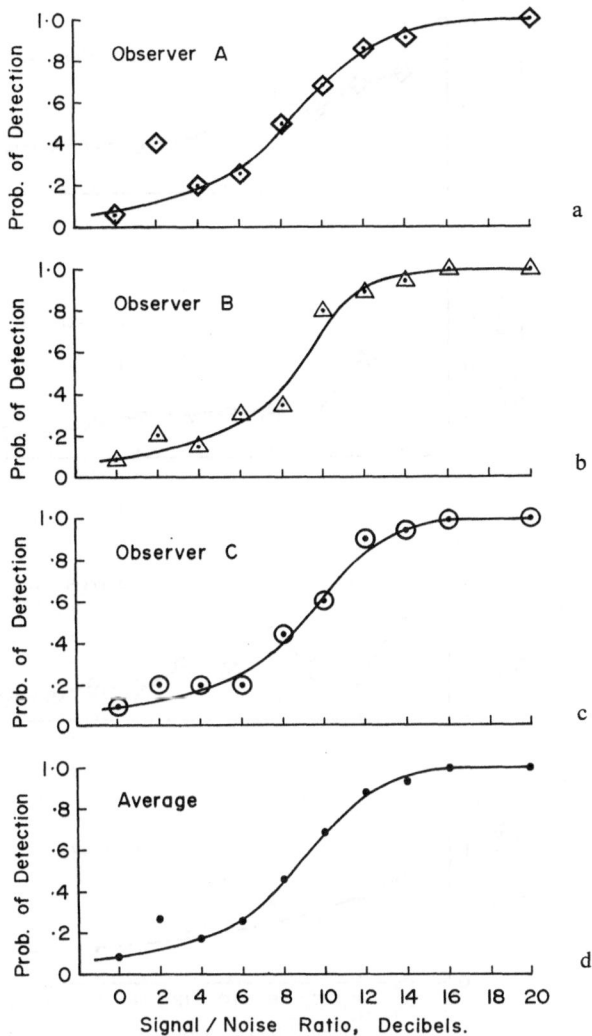

Fig. 4. Probability of Detection versus S/N ratio. 4a. Observer A; b. Observer B; c. Observer C; d. Average of above 3.

2. Delay Errors

The difference between the experimental observation of the delay time and the known delay time gives the delay error. The mean delay error is close to zero, and the standard deviation of the delay error distribution may be used to describe the expected error. This was computed for different S/N ratios for each of the three observers, and the average combined results also were obtained. These results are shown in Figures 5a-d. The ordinate represents the root-mean-

401

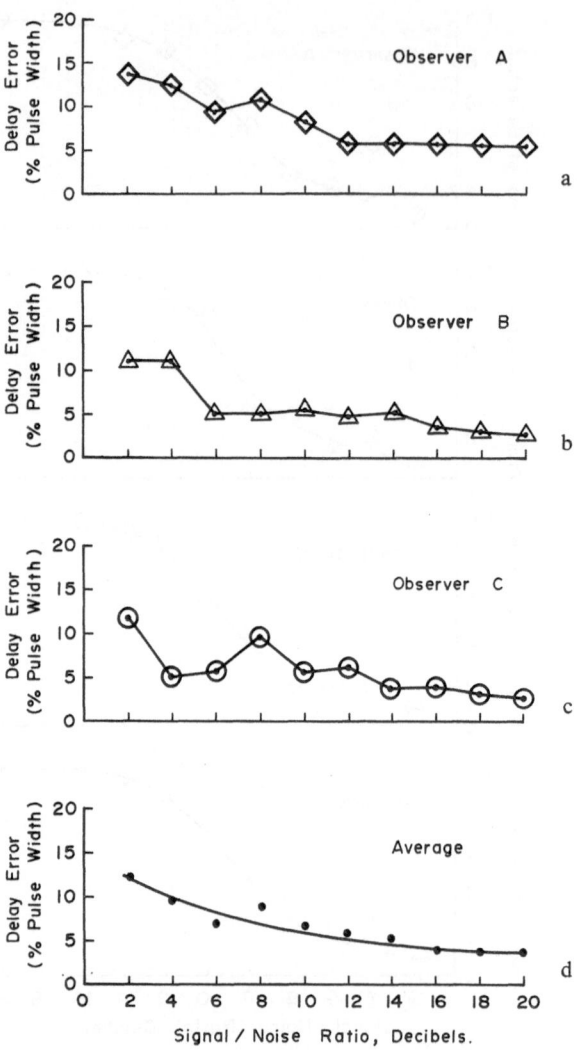

Fig. 5. Delay Error (as % of total Pulse Width) versus S/N ratio. 5a. Observer A;
b. Observer B; c. Observer C; d. Average of above 3.

square delay error (the standard deviation) as a percentage of the total pulse
width (50 milliseconds).

3. *Amplitude Errors*

The average values of the measured signal amplitudes at prescribed S/N ratios
were plotted against the actual amplitudes on log/log paper, Figure 6. At the
lower S/N ratios there is a distinct tendency to overestimate the average signal
amplitude, by factors of approximately 100% or more in the case of the least

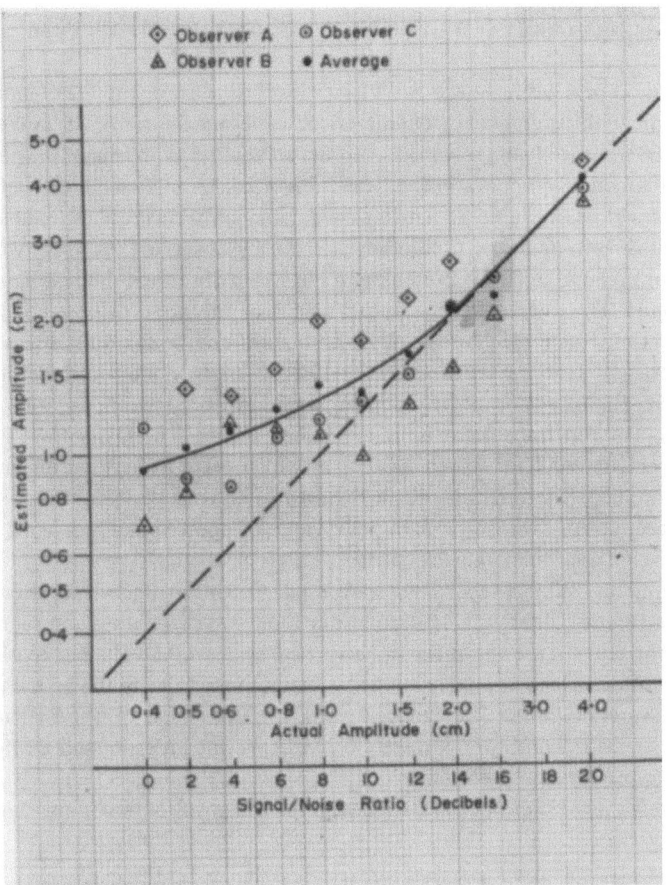

Fig. 6. Estimated Signal Amplitude versus Actual Signal Amplitude, combined plot.

experienced observer. Although the amplitude distributions are not 'normal' distributions in the mathematical sense, their standard deviations were calculated and used to give a measure of the spread of the distribution. For example, for observer A, at a S/N ratio of 8 db, the standard deviation is 0.39 centimeters. As the actual pulse height is 1 centimeter, the normalized standard deviation is 0.39. At 20 db S/N ratio, the normalized standard deviation is 0.16.

For S/N ratios larger than 20 db, the effect of the noise may be estimated by taking its RMS value as a measure of the standard deviation to be expected when measuring the peak amplitude. For example, at a S/N ratio of 30 db, with a peak signal amplitude of 4 centimeters, the RMS noise value is 0.126 centimeters, and the normalized value of the standard deviation is 0.031.

One method of measuring the RMS noise level is to use a true RMS-indicating voltmeter, with its frequency characteristic covering the range of interest for the actual measurements involved. Another method is by means of the autocorrelation function computation, as mentioned earlier. Often neither of these methods will be available, in which case a reasonably accurate estimate can be obtained directly from an oscilloscope screen by observing the trace when no signal (or no large signal) is present, and the sweep duration is increased to 10 to 30 seconds. The average peak-to-peak height of the noise display is approximately 5 times the RMS noise level. (A number of approximations are involved; see references 1 and 2.) Examples for two different model noise spectra are shown in Figure 7 for a DC-coupled system with a sweep duration of 30 seconds. The top trace is for noise as defined earlier. The lower trace is for a noise spectrum which is flat to 500 Hz, at which point a sharp cutoff low-pass filter is applied. The vertical scale in Figure 7 is 0.5 volts per centimeter, so that each trace has an average peak-to-peak value of approximately 1 volt, or an RMS level of approximately 0.2 volts.

When actual subject recordings were used, various artifacts may occur. For example Figure 8a shows a 10 second duration sweep for the same signal and noise shown in Figure 1a, at the same vertical scale of 0.5 volts per centimeter. The spikes occurring at approximately 1 second intervals are the actual photopic electroretinograms. The average peak-to-peak value of the artifact-free portion of the trace is approximately 0.3 volts, giving an estimated RMS noise level of approximately 0.06 volts.

Figure 8b is a 33 second duration sweep for the low S/N recording shown in

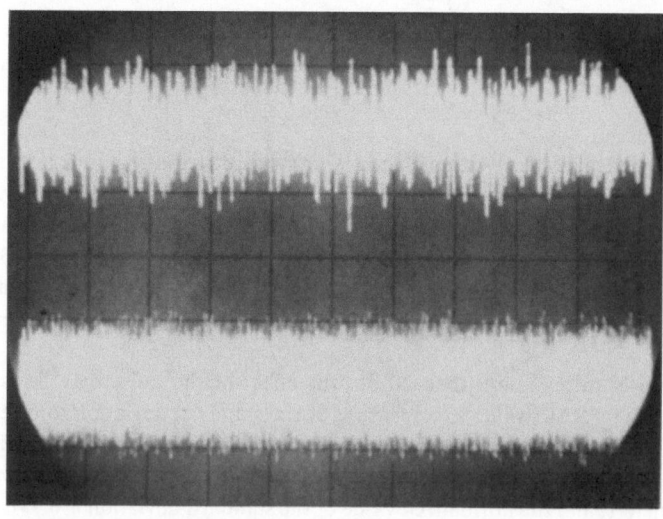

Fig. 7. 30 sec sweep of 'noise'. Top trace: Noise as used in tests. Lower trace: Noise with essentially flat frequency spectrum to 500 Hz. Vertical scale 0.5 volts/division.

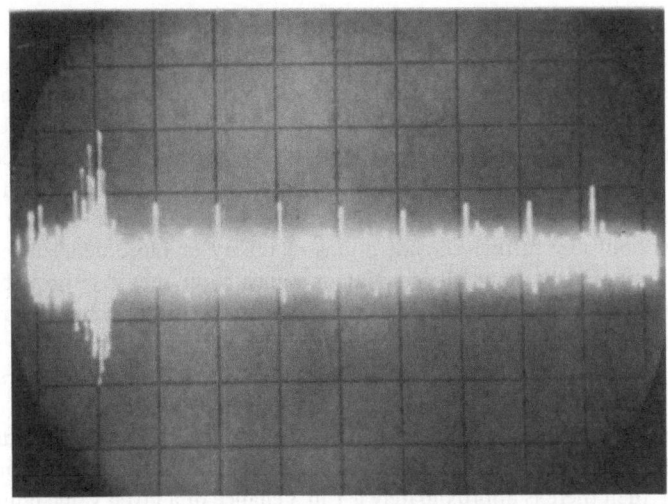

Fig. 8a. 10 sec sweep display of ERG and Noise. (Same test as shown for Fig. 1a). Vertical scale 0.5 volts/division.

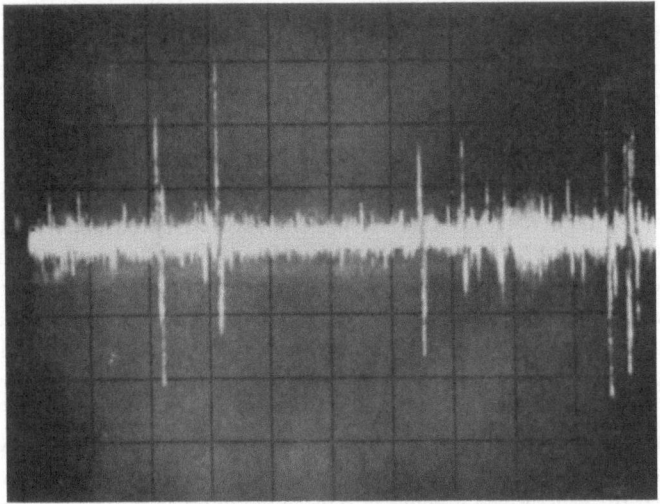

Fig. 8b. 33 sec sweep display of ERG and Noise. (Same test as shown for Fig. 1b). Vertical scale 0.5 volts/division.

Figure 1b. If the artifacts are ignored, the peak-to-peak value is approximately 0.25 volts, that is the RMS noise level is approximately 0.05 volts. It is not evident from Figure 1b what the actual signal level is, as it cannot be defined from these traces alone, but from the average signal in Figure 1c its display level (peak from baseline) is approximately 0.15 volts. Hence the S/N ratio for the unprocessed sweeps would be approximately 3, or 9.5 db, and the recordings can be compared with the experimental model traces of Figure 3c.

405

The first and most important question to be answered obviously is whether a signal is present or not. For the display conditions described, the curves show that at S/N ratios of approximately 8 db, the probability of detection becomes 0.5. It is useful to keep in mind the characteristics of the trace shown in Figure 3c for a S/N ratio of 8 db, for if actual recordings appear at all similar to this, then without any further considerations of theory or more detailed measurements it should be remembered that one may be at the 50% probability of detection point, and that conclusions to be drawn from such measurements must necessarily have little significance on a statistical basis.

If a signal is thought to be present, one must then consider the errors which may occur in the time and amplitude measurements. Useful measures to keep in mind here relate to properties of the 'normal' Gaussian statistical distribution (SOKAL & ROHLF, 1969). If the standard deviation (s) of this distribution is known, then there is approximately a 1 in 3 chance of a given value falling outside the range of ± 1 standard deviation from the mean, and a 1 in 20 chance of being outside the range ± 2 times the standard deviation from the mean.

From Figure 5a the standard deviation of the delay distribution at a S/N ratio of 8 db is approximately 10%. Thus there is 1 chance in 3 that a delay time estimate will be in error by more than ± 5 milliseconds. Alternatively one may state that there is a 95% chance that any delay time estimate will be in error by less than ± 10 milliseconds. The problem may be approached in a different manner by defining limits for the measured time delay, and then determining the S/N ratio necessary in order to achieve this accuracy. For example, for a 95% chance that the delay measurement should be within ± 3 milliseconds (± 2s) of the actual mean value, the standard deviation must be 1.5 milliseconds. This is 3% of the total pulse width of 50 milliseconds. Hence from Figures 5b and 5c, a S/N ratio of approximately 20 db is needed. For the less experienced observer, it is evident that such accuracy could not be achieved without increasing the S/N ratio to large values, beyond the range tested.

The amplitude measurements show that at low S/N ratios large errors may occur in the estimated signal amplitude. As the probability of detection becomes less than 0.5, details of the actual errors become irrelevant. At higher S/N ratios, for example 20 db for observer A, the normalized standard deviation is 0.16, as described previously. The actual pulse amplitude is 4 centimeters on the screen, and therefore the actual standard deviation is 0.64 centimeters. Application of the above estimates gives 1 chance in 3 that the measured amplitude will be outside the range of 3.36 to 4.64 centimeters. For 95% confidence limits, the possible range of signal amplitudes will be approximately 2.7 to 5.3 centimeters. If closer limits are required then larger S/N ratios must be obtained. As mentioned previously, for S/N ratios greater than approximately 20 db, the effect of the noise can be estimated by taking its RMS value as the standard deviation to be expected for measurements of the peak amplitude. Thus at 30 db S/N ratio, the standard deviation for a 4 centimeter pulse is approximately 0.13 centimeters. Consequently there is a 95% probability of the amplitude being in the range 3.74 to 4.26 centimeters, i.e. approximately $\pm 5\%$ accuracy.

In practice such high S/N ratios often are not obtained from direct single response recordings. The use of averaging techniques becomes most appropriate in such circumstances. Without entering into details regarding a number of assumptions, it may be recalled that averaging N sweeps increases the S/N ratio by the square root of N. Thus if N = 100, the S/N ratio increases by a factor of 10, or 20 db. This is particularly convenient when dealing with relatively small photopic electroretinograms, as for example in Figure 1b. Typically the S/N ratio of a single sweep may be in the 0 to 10 db range, so that an increase of 20 db moves the S/N ratio into the 20 to 30 db range. This takes the signal out of the range where measurements are basically worthless statistically, into the range where reasonable accuracy can be expected with some degree of confidence.

It is clear that in any actual measurement, the above mentioned detection probability and error estimates can be applied only in an approximate manner, and in effect one is in the position of having to know the results before being able to apply such estimates. While this is not too satisfactory philosophically, in practice a possible procedure might be as follows:

1. The noise RMS level is estimated or measured as described above.
2. Some test waveforms are obtained. If they are large enough to minimize the effects of the noise, that is the probability of detection is essentially unity, then an average signal amplitude can be estimated fairly quickly, and the possible errors in the amplitude and delay derived as above. If these errors are acceptable little more need be done. If they are not acceptable then the appropriate amount of averaging must be carried out in order to increase the S/N ratio to a level sufficient to decrease the errors to the desired amount.
3. If the test waveforms are small, irregular, or possibly not even detectable, then signal averaging is used in order to try to detect a signal. This will then allow a second estimate of the proability of detection, signal amplitude and delay, and the errors associated with this averaged signal may then be considered. If the results are not satisfactory then theoretically more averaging may be carried out to further improve the S/N ratio.

An alternative practical procedure is to use signal averaging for each test, with a limited number of possible modifications. For large signals, this may be more processing than really is required, but it does provide increased confidence levels.

The extent to which such improvements can be carried out in actual biological tests is limited of course. Patient cooperation is one factor, and the length of the test is another. The question of the basic repeatability of the responses forms another large unknown factor. Consequently one may be left with a less than optimum S/N ratio, and thus have a reduced probability of detection and the possibility of significant errors in the estimates of signal amplitude and time delay. These possible errors should be kept in mind when statements are made regarding the signal characteristics and in arriving at any clinical conclusions.

ACKNOWLEDGEMENT

The authors wish to thank DR. DAVID G. COGAN for his continued support and encouragement during the course of this work.

REFERENCES

LAWSON, J. L., & UHLENBECK, G. E. Threshold Signals, MIT Radiation Lab Series, Volume 24, New York, McGraw Hill (1950).

CARLSON, A. B. Communication Systems. An Introduction to Signals and Noise in Electrical Communication, New York, McGraw Hill (1968).

HELSTROM, C. W. Statistical Theory of Signal Detection, 2nd edition, New York, Pergamon Press (1968).

LANGE, F. H. Correlation Techniques, New Jersey, D. Van Nostrand Co., Inc. (1967).

LEE, Y. W. Statistical Theory of Communication, New York, John Wiley & Sons, Inc. (1960).

FRICKER, S. J. Application of synchronous detector techniques for electroretinographic studies in patients with retinitis pigmentosa, *Investigative Ophthalmology* 10: *329-339* (1971).

SOKAL, R. R. & ROHLF, F. J. Biometry, San Francisco, W. H. Freeman and Co. (1969).

Key Words
Signal-to-noise ratio
Detection probability
Delay error
Amplitude error
Electroretinography

Authors' address:

Howe Laboratory of Ophthalmology
Harvard University Medical School
Massachusetts Eye and Ear Infirmary
Boston, Massachusetts 02114

COUPLED ELECTROPHYSIOLOGICAL AND COLOUR FLUOROGRAPHIC STUDIES AS A PART OF THE ANATOMICAL DIAGNOSIS OF RETINOPATHIES

R. ALFIERI, P. SOLÉ & DANIELLE RIGAL

(Clermont – Ferrand)

The main procedures involved in the electrophysiological investigation of the visual tract are (ALFIERI et al., 1970):

1. the electroretinogram (ERG) which demonstrates the activity of the photo-receptors and bipolar cells; this examination conducted in monochromatic light (SOLE, 1965) makes it possible to study individually the photopic system in red stimulation (ERG-r) and the scotopic system in blue stimulation (ERG-b);

2. the visual evoked response (VER) which, in our point of view, essentially reflects the permeability of the visual pathways from the 'optic nerve' link to the 'visual cortex'. Such an examination carried out in monochromatic light (PLANE, 1969 and RIGAL, 1970) allows an individual study of the conduction systems: the macular ones (central cones) in red stimulation (VER-r) on the one hand, and the extramacular ones (peripheral cones and rods) in blue stimulation (VER-b) on the other hand.

The results of these electrophysiological examinations may be summed up as a four-digit binary number (RENAUD, 1972 and ALFIERI et al., 1972): each digit (1 where normal, 0 where pathological) representing, from left to right respectively, the ERG-r, the ERG-b, the VER-r and the VER-b. By assuming the integrity of the retroretinal visual pathways, we will thus obtain a binary translation of the electrophysiological nosology of retinopathies as presented by us in Pisa in 1970:

1. photopic retinopathies: either merely central ones (1101: the ERG-r is normal since the central cones, in a comparatively small number, are electrically negligible at the retinal level; conversely, the VER-r is extinguished as it corresponds selectively to the central conduction and to the cortical projection of the macula), or global photopic retinopathies (0100: the ERG-b alone is normal, indicating rod activity);

2. scotopic retinopathies (1011: the ERG-b alone is pathological, showing rod deficiency; this is the complementary aspect of global photopic retinopathies);

3. combined retinopathies, either peripheral only (0010: the VER-r is normal, which proves that the macula is unimpaired), or global (0000: the whole complex is pathological).

However these two ERG and VER examinations alone are not sufficient to

409

obtain in every case a truly anatomical diagnosis of retinopathies as they explore but the nerve elements, and then in a global way only. This is the reason why we decided to couple to ERG and VER electro-oculography (EOG) and colour fluorescein angiography (CFA) aimed at investigating the trophic elements. EOG will make it possible to study the 'pigment epithelium – external part of photoreceptors' area, both in its generator function (basic value of the potential) which will be impaired in destructive lesions, and in its function as impedance (potential variation as a function of luminance) which will be impaired in exudative lesions. CFA makes it possible to study the 'choroid – retinal vessels' area, both in its morphology (chrono-evolution of the fluorescent embolus) which will be altered in angiomatoses, and in its permeability (abnormal fluorescence in terms of time and space) which will be altered in angiopathies; moreover, as opposed to electrophysiology which yields global data only, CFA proves valuable to help discern isolated impairments.

I. PROCEDURE

A. ERG and VER

The procedures used for both examinations have already been described at previous ISCERGs, particularly the physical parameters which were detailed in 1972 in Los Angeles.

B. EOG

The physical recording procedure has been derived from the technique developed by HENKES et al. (1968): each vertical deflection on the oscillogram represents the potential variation observed between two electrodes placed on the inner and outer canthus of the eye during a horizontal eye movement of about 55° arc; but two peculiarities must be noted: every minute we record four consecutive movements, which minimizes artefact variations, and on the oscillogram deflections are perceptible in one direction only, starting from the iso-electric datum (downwards for the right eye, upwards for the left one). The physiological recording procedure is derived from the one used by ARDEN et al. (1962): results may be expressed as the ratio of maximal deflection in light adaptation (LA) to minimal deflection in dark adaptation (DA); however we allow ten minutes for pre-adaptation to the dark and start recording (first 4-deflection group) at the tenth minute which becomes zero time; we then keep on recording once per minute for ten minutes of light adaptation followed by ten minutes of dark adaptation.

C. CFA

We use the technique developed by SHIKANO & SHIMIZU (1968) and by MATSUI et al. (1969). The excitation filter used is a 32 magenta Kodak Wratten which lets through the short exciting wavelengths and also the red with which we may

410

study the choroid since it is but slightly absorbed by pigment epithelium. The stopping filter is a 56 green Wratten Kodak filter which lets through medium fluorescence wavelengths and also the red reflected by the choroid. An I.V. solution of 12.5 grams of fluorescein for a 100 cm³ solution is the fluorescent substance injected. Photographic recordings are made at last rate in order to detect the appearance of the fluorescent embolus in the fundus, then follow its progress: 1. first, at choroid level where a fluorescence will appear if the pigment epithelium is transparent, either organically (anatomical destruction: 'window effect') or functionally (no pigment: albinism); 2. then at retinal level where the arterial, capillary and venous systems will get impregnated.

II. RESULTS

They are detailed in chronological order according to the anatomical structure initially injured: pigment epithelium or chorioretinal vascular system.

A. Pigment epithelium

1°/ Observation 1: Marius Pag..., 62.

ERG: orange Wratten filter and VER: red interferential filter (Fig. 1): global bilateral photopic impairment.

EOG (Fig. 2): very low base value, remaining stationary during successive light and dark adaptations, for the right eye and the left eye, as well.

CFA (Fig. 3): choroid vessels become visible.

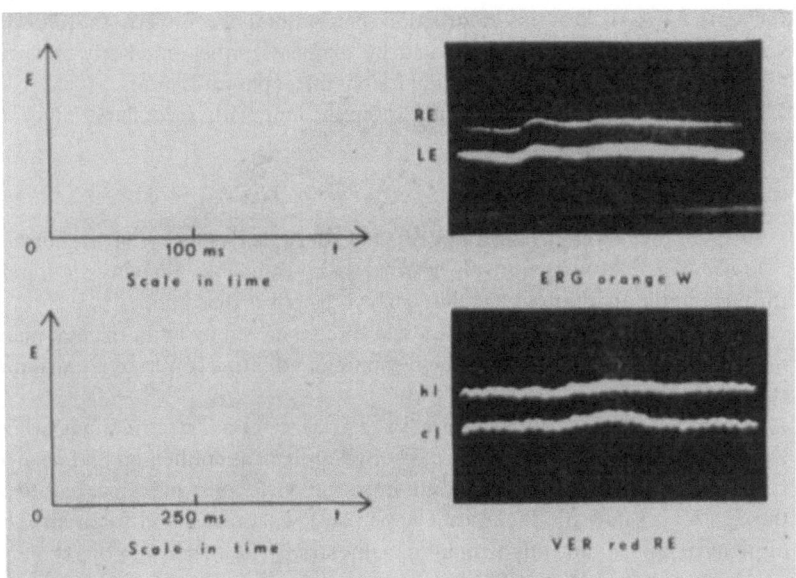

Fig. 1, 4, 7 and 9. E: variation in potential; t: time. RE: right eye; LE: left eye; W: Wratten; hl: homolateral; cl: controlateral.

411

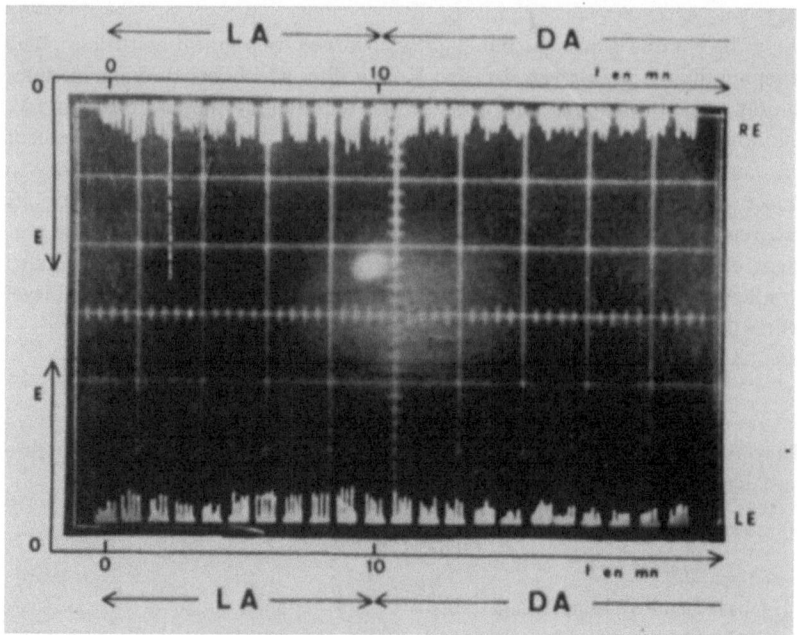

Fig. 2, 5 and 10. E: variation in potential; t: time; LA: light adaptation; DA: dark adaptation.

Interpretation: the nearly extinguished EOG indicates that the 'electric sources' are injured, which we relate to a wide-spread destruction of the pigment epithelium; CFA makes this destruction perceptible: we discern the choroid vessels which are normally concealed by pigment epithelium; lastly as is revealed by ERG and VER, these initial lesions affect photoreceptors.

Diagnosis: initial atrophy of pigment epithelium with secondary injury to peripheral and central cones.

2°/ Observation 2: André Lib..., 28.

ERG: orange Wratten filter and VER: red interferential filter (Fig. 4): normal.

EOG (Fig. 5): comparatively normal base value but remains stationary throughout the adaptations, for the right eye as well as the left one.

CFA (Fig. 6): the macula appears as a disc separated by an horizontal plane into a fluorescent upper area at the beginning and into a lower area remaining constantly opaque.

Interpretation: stationary EOG reveals the presence of an 'electric shunt' which we ascribe to an exudation occurring between pigment epithelium and near-by structures; this exudation is inferred from the lower opaque area perceived through CFA; now the fluorescent upper area will correspond to an atrophy of pigment epithelium; this atrophy remains strictly localized, and this explains why it does not affect the EOG base value; lastly, normal ERG and VER tend to indicate that discharge occurs on the choroid side of pigment epithelium.

Diagnosis: vitellus-shaped disc at pseudohypopyon stage.

412

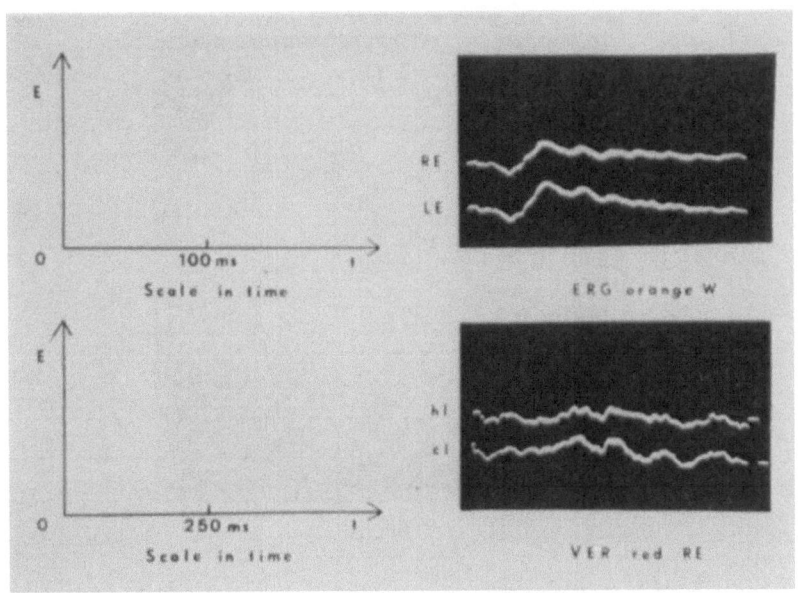

Fig. 4.

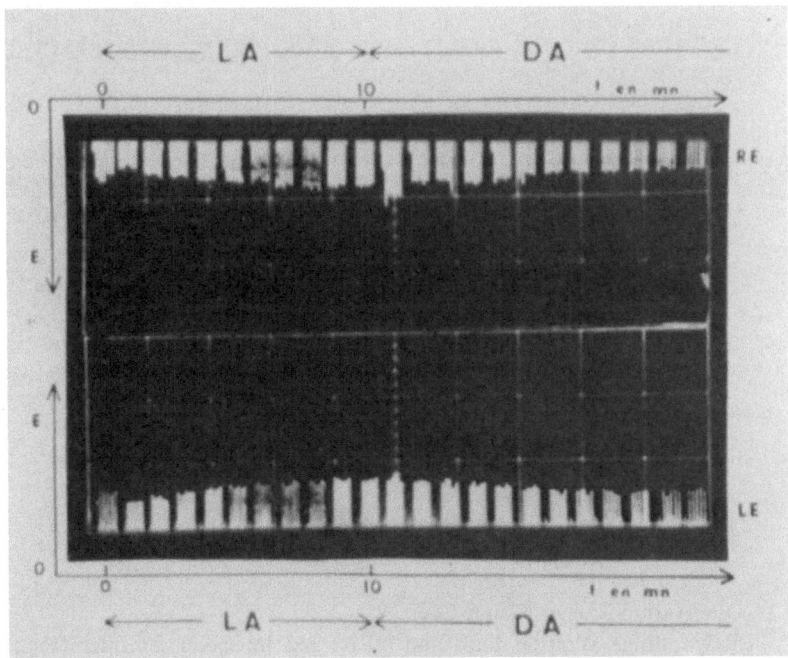

Fig. 5.

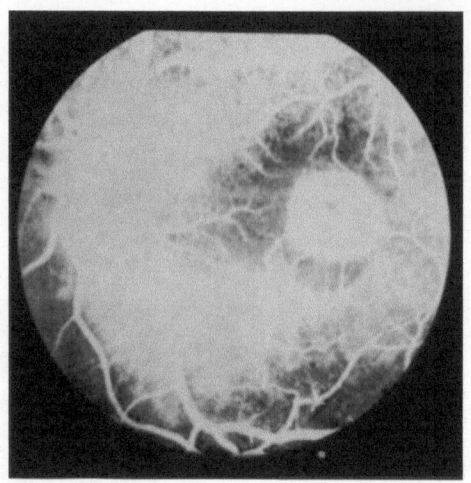

Fig. 6.

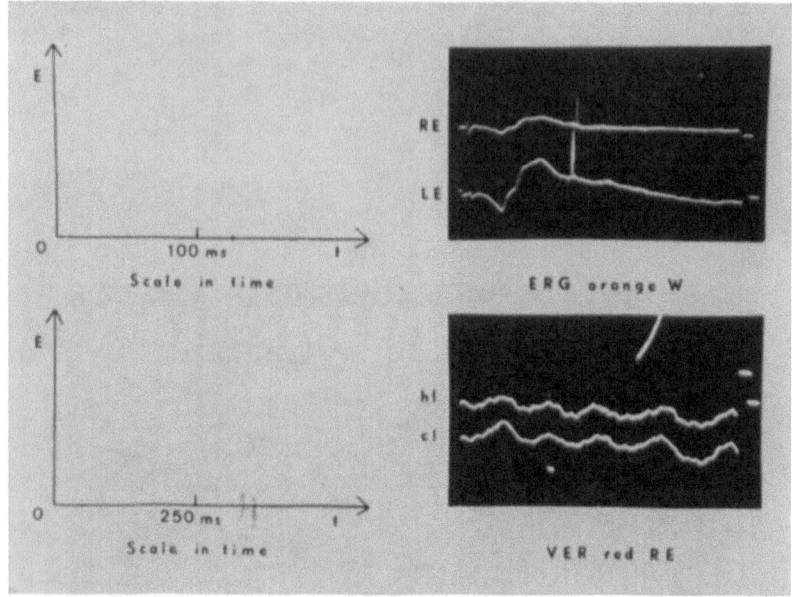

Fig. 7.

B. Chorioretinal vascular system

1°/ Observation 3: Jean-Claude Gre..., 9.

ERG: orange Wratten filter and VER: red interferential filter (Fig. 7): global photopic impairment of right eye.

EOG: not carried out.

414

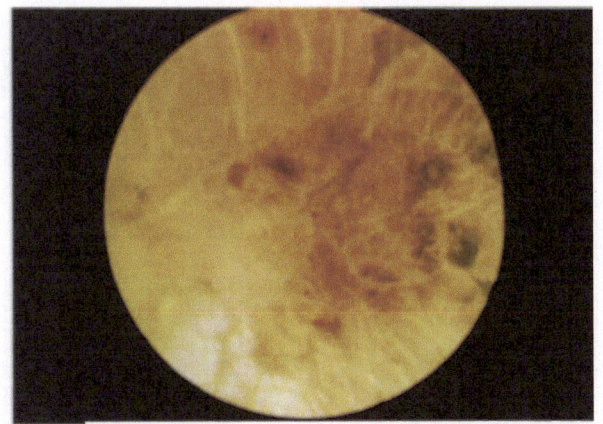

fig. 3

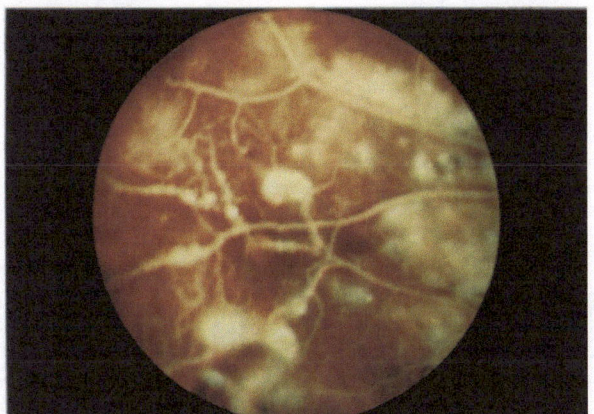

fig. 8

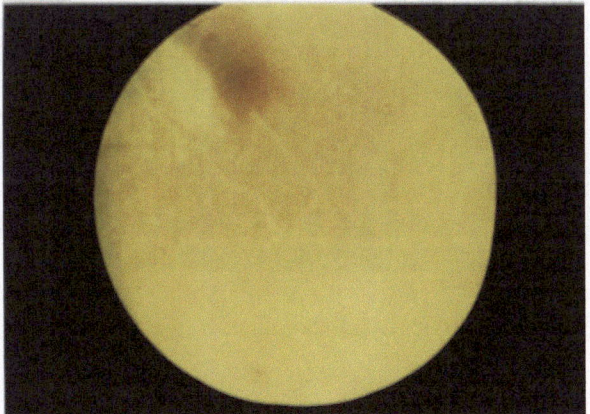

fig. 11

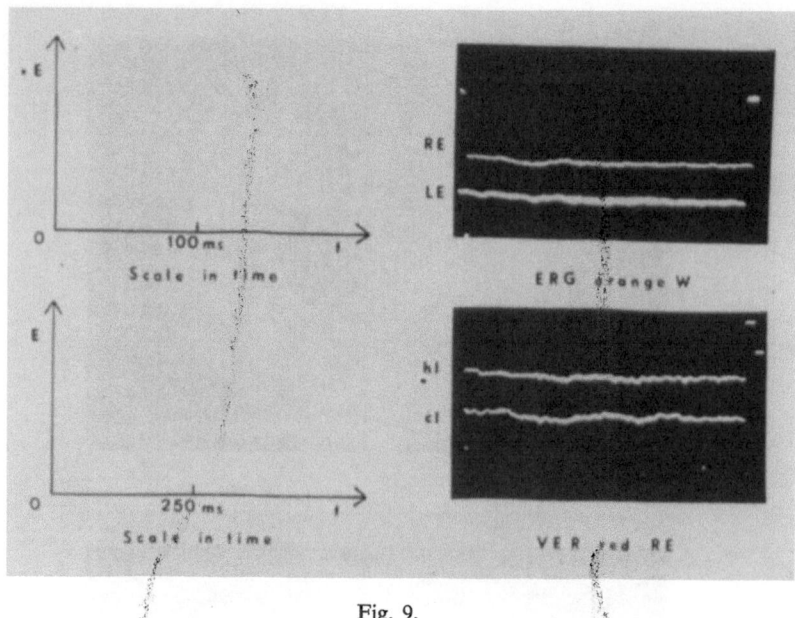

Fig. 9.

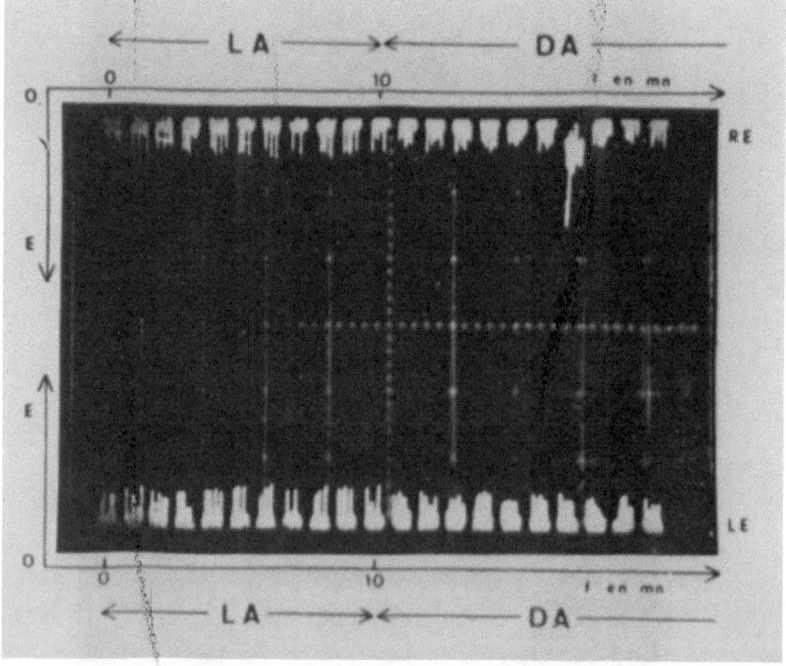

Fig. 10.

CFA: on the one hand it shows for the right eye a highly fluorescent vascular tumor at the macula, on the other hand (Fig. 8) it shows enlarged retinal vessels with aneurysms, vessel tangles and parietal deterioration.

Interpretation: CFA makes it possible to link up photopic impairment to 'vascular malformative etiology'.

Diagnosis: right retinal angiomatosis with secondary injury to peripheral and central cones.

2°/ Observation 4: Jeanne Ney..., 65.

ERG: orange Wratten filter and VER: red interferential filter (Fig. 9): extinguished right and left.

EOG (Fig. 10): nearly extinguished, both on the left and the right.

CFA (Fig. 11): shows several retinal micro-aneurysms with retinal haemorrhage along with major vessel extravasation.

Interpretation: through CFA we may connect the combined sensorial impairment with a 'vascular degenerative etiology'; also the extinguished EOG indicates how severe the lesions are which affect the whole chorioretina.

Diagnosis: last stage diabetic retinopathy.

III. CONCLUSIONS

The interest of this coupled exploration lies in the fact that it allows a proper clinical anatomical diagnosis as each examination explores one structure selectively:

1. ERG: photoreceptors and bipolar cells
2. VER: central cones and macular bundle
3. EOG: pigment epithelium and its interfaces
4. CFA: chorioretinal vascular system.

REFERENCES

ALFIERI, R., RIGAL, D. & SOLE, P. Electrophysiological nosology (ERG and VER) of retinopathies. In: Symposium on electroretinography; Proc. 8th ISCERG Symp. Pisa 7-12 Sept. 1970., p. 305. Pisa, Pacini (1972).

ALFIERI, R., SOLE, P. & RENAUD, P. Boolean notation for ocular electrophysiology (ERG and VER) and dioptric factors. In: Doc. Ophthal. Proc. Series, Vol. 2, 10th ISCERG Symp. Los Angeles 20-23 Aug. 1972., p. 181. The Hague, Junk (1973).

ARDEN, G. B., BARRADA, ADEL & KELSEY, J. H. *Brit. J. Ophth.* 46: *449* (1962).

HENKES, H. E., DENIER VAN DER GON, J. J., VAN MARLE, G. W. & SCHREINEMACHERS, H. P. *Brit. J. Ophth.* 52: *122* (1968).

MATSUI, K., OKA, Y. & MATSUI, T. *Acta Soc. ophthal. jap.* 73: *653* (1969).

PLANE, C. Potentiels évoqués visuels chez le sujet normal et dans les atteintes du nerf optique. (Thèse de médecine, Clermont-Ferrand, 1969).

RENAUD, P. Etude comparative pré- et post-opératoire de l'électrorétinographie et des potentiels évoqués visuels dans la cataracte. (Thèse de médecine, Clermont-Ferrand, 1972).

RIGAL, D. Potentiels évoqués visuels chez l'enfant normal et dans les troubles de la fonction visuelle. (Thèse de médecine, Clermont-Ferrand, 1970).

SHIKANO, S. & SHIMIZU, K. Atlas of fluorescence fundus angiography. Philadelphia, Saunders (1968).

SOLE, P. Electrorétinographie théorique. (Thèse de médecine, Clermont-Ferrand, 1965).

Authors' address:

Faculty of Medicine
Clermont-Ferrand
France

EXAMINATION UNDER GENERAL ANAESTHESIA OF CHILDREN WITH DEFECTIVE VISION (1969-1972).

C. P. LEGEIN, H. E. HENKES & A. Th. M. VAN BALEN

(Rotterdam)

ABSTRACT

A survey is given of 134 children with impaired vision which were examined under general anaesthesia during a four year period (1969-1972).

INTRODUCTION

From all children with impaired vision who came to the outpatient-department in the four year period 1969-1972, 134 children were hospitalized for evaluation or confirmation of diagnosis under general anaesthesia. Most of the children were sent by ophthalmologists, a few by neurologists and paediatricians.

In general the children were hospitalized for 2 or 3 days. On the second day the examination under general anaesthesia took place.

A surgery room is prepared for this purpose one morning a week. As a full ocular examination complete with electrodiagnostic procedures and eventually extended with fundus photography and echography is very time-consuming, not more than 2 children are examined on one day. Three children were examined two times so 137 examinations were done.

METHODS

To get maximal mydriasis atropine and Mydriaticum (R) eyedrops were instilled.

Atropine orally was given as premedication. As anaesthetics were used a mixture of O_2; NO_2 and Halothane (max. 1,5 %) gas.

Ocular examination was done by at least two experienced ophthalmologists; if needed fundus photographs were taken.

For ERG-recording 'low-vac' ERG contact lenses (Henkes-type) were used. The VER was recorded (monopolar) with one electrode placed in the midline above the inion.

For scotopic ERG-recordings single blue light flashes – frequency 1/sec – with neutral density filters were used, after dark adaptation for 15 minutes. For the photopic ERG: single red light flashes – frequency 4/sec – after and under bluelight adaptation for 5 minutes, were used.

419

In general, the VER-recordings were made with photopic stimulation. All signals are averaged by a CAT-computer, and recorded on an X-Y plotter.

If more information was needed, an EOG-registration was made by the special developed apparatus which produced sine-wave movement of the eyes. In one case echography was done.

RESULTS

Table 1: Most of the children were under two years of age. In the older children examination without anaesthesia had failed because of poor cooperation.

patients	
age	number
< 1	38
1 – 2	40
2 – 3	12
3 – 5	21
> 5	23
total	134

Table 2: ERG and VER recordings were made from all children. In 48 children an EOG-recording was made and from 28 children photographic documentation was done.

examinations	patients
E.R.G./V.E.R.	137
E.O.G.	48
fundusphotography	28
ECHO	1

Table 3: The children were divided in 3 groups:
– Group I: (unexplained) impaired vision of one or both eyes. Totally 106 patients; from 48 of them the diagnosis was expected.
– Group II: Children who came for pre-operative examination.
– Group III: Patients referred by neurologists and paediatricians where visual problems were not dominating the clinical picture.

Table 4: Gives a summary of Group I. For the surveyability the final diagnosis is not split up in details. In cases of hereditary familiar retinal diseases or obvious symptoms or signs the diagnosis was often expected.

($\pm$) means that abnormalities could be found. In 6 cases no final diagnosis

420

TABLE 3

		patients
group 1	impaired vision	108 (48 diagnosis expected)
group 2	preoperative examination	18
group 3	on request of other disciplines (neurology, paediatrics)	8

TABLE 4

GROUP I : IMPAIRED VISION

final diagnosis	ERG scot	ERG phot	VER	patients total	patients diagnosis expected
Leber, amaurosis congenita	−	−	−	19	9
tapeto-retinal dystrophies	−	+(±)	+	13	10
cone dysfunctions (achromatopsia)	+(±)	−	+(scot)	7	3
non retinal (visual pathways)	+	+	−	15	5
no abnormality found (psychomotor retardation)	+	+	+	10	
mixed group (connatal anomalies, retrolental fibroplasia, nystagmus, etc.)				38	21
no diagnosis (relation between history, examination and electro-diagnostic results not clear)				6	
				108	

could be made because the relation between history, examination and electrodiagnostic results was not clear.

Table 5: Group II: In some cases of proven Rubella infection we found signs of a retinopathy (±). When VER-recordings were negative operation was not adviced.

Table 6: Group III: In 4 patients we could not detect any abnormality of the visual system. In 4 patients the visual system was affected; one patient proved to be a Leber amaurosis congenita, which diagnosis was not expected.

TABLE 5

GROUP II : PRE OPERATIVE EXAMINATION

diagnosis	ERG		VER	number
	scot	phot		
congenital cataract	+(±)	+	+	12
	+	+	–	3 (2 micro-ophthalmos)
traumatic cataract	+	+	+	1
	–	–	–	1
vitreous opacity (P.A.: retinoblastoma)	– (also echo)	–	–	1
				18

TABLE 6

GROUP III : ON REQUEST OF NEUROLOGY/PEDIATRICS

diagnosis	ERG	VER	number
hypobetalipoproteinaemia	–	–	1
leucodystrophy	–	–	1
psychomotor retardation	+(–)	+(–)	2 (1 Leber am.cong.)
mixed	+	+	4 (no abnorm. found)
			8

COMMENT

In our opinion it is essential for the parents (genetic advice) and for the education of the visually handicaped child that an early diagnosis is made. In general, this examination is proposed when the child is half a year old, to exclude a delayed development of the visual system.

EOG-results are not mentioned as the value of EOG-recording in diagnosis and prognosis is under study and will be reported later.

A follow-up study is essential for the evaluation of this study. We planned a follow-up study for the next years focused on subjective testing (visual acuity, colour vision etc.) to get a better understanding of the correlation between the results of the objective examination at an early age and the visual state of the grown-up child.

REFERENCES

FONTAINE, M. Les cécités de l'enfance. Paris, Masson (1969).
HENKES, H. E. & LEGEIN, C. P. Electrodiagnostic procedures in the blind and partially sighted young child. *Int. Ophthal. Clinics* 9: *921-933* (1969).

SCHAPPERT-KIMMIJSER, J. & HENKES, H. E. Amaurosis congenita (Leber). *Arch. Ophthal.* 61: *211-218* (1959).

Authors' address:

Eye Hospital
Erasmus University
Rotterdam
The Netherlands

COMPLEXITY OF P_{III}, AS MANIFESTED BY LIGHT ADAPTATION

H. BORNSCHEIN & L. WÜNDSCH

(Vienna)

ABSTRACT

Isolated rabbits' bulbs respond to light stimuli with a negative deflection (P_{III}) keeping the same amplitude for many hours. At least two subcomponents may be distinguished using d.c. and r.c. amplification. As shown in former experiments poisoning the carbohydrate metabolism reduces al subcomponents by about the same amount. In the present experiments, however, the ratio of the subcomponents may be changed by light adaptation, the slow subcomponents being reduced more severely than the fast ones. The difference is statistically significant and proves inhomogenity of P_{III}.

The negative component of the electroretinogram (P_{III} of GRANIT) commonly is considered of receptor origin since BROWN & WIESEL (1961) and BROWN (1968). Already 1953 NOELL has shown that P_{III} may be differentiated in an early component and a late one characterized by different sensitivity towards chemical agents. In 1965 BÖCK, BORNSCHEIN & HOMMER have demonstrated (in rabbit and man) P_{III} not only surviving enucleation of the eye but increasing its amplitude during the first eight hours after enucleation and maintaining rather high constant amplitudes for more than 24 hours (in a cooled oxygenated glucose-rich medium); a small negative potential persisted for at least 5 days. BORNSCHEIN & VON LÜTZOW (1965) have made use of simultaneous r.c. and d.c. amplification in two channels to show that surviving P_{III} of enucleated eye bulbs may be differentiated. Surprisingly enough, four blocking agents of the carbohydrate metabolism have not shown any significant difference in the velocity of their poisoning effect on P_{III}. In the present study the same method of differentiation of P_{III} was used. Sensitivity to different levels of light adaptation served as criterion to decide about the homogenous origin of the subcomponents.

METHODS

Experimental animals were 5 rabbits (about 2 kilograms body weight) anesthetized by urethane (2,0 g/kg b.w.). After one hour of dark adaptation the eye bulbs were stored in cold oxygenated glucose Ringer solution for 8 hours; this interval has been proved to be optimum for recording isolated negative potentials of stable high amplitudes during several hours (Böck et al., 1965; BORN-SCHEIN & VON LÜTZOW, 1965). Thereafter, the bulbs were mounted between two Ag-AgCl-electrodes in an oxygenated moist chamber (at room temperature) as described by Böck et al. (1964).

Two white light sources were used: 1. Test stimulus (Xenon arc): 60 degrees diameter, 200 nt intensity, 0,2 s or 0,1 s duration. 2. Adaptation stimulus (incandescent light): 120 degrees diameter, different intensities (0,031 nt up to 8 nt, neutral density filters of the NG series, Schott), 30 s duration.

Amplification and recording of the ERGs were performed by Cardiopan + RC preamplifier (Liechti) combined with DC amplifier (J. F. Tönnies). Recording was done in 3 channels (and traces):
1. ERG, d.c. amplification; 2. ERG, r.c. amplification, time constant 1 s; 3. Stimulus.

Procedure: After recording the ERG of the bulb in dark adaptation the retina was light adapted for 30 s. Then the ERG was recorded by superimposing test stimulus to adapting stimulus. Immediately afterwards the adapting light was switched off. Thereafter, test stimuli were presented in the dark every two minutes. When it was beyond doubt that the original amplitudes were restituted, the experiment was continued with another background intensity.

RESULTS

Fig. 1 presents original recordings with different adaptation levels: in the upper trace (d.c. amplification) fast and slow components are included, in the middle trace (r.c. amplification) the fast ones are predominating. In these records it is obvious that light adaptation reduces the amplitude of the d.c. amplified

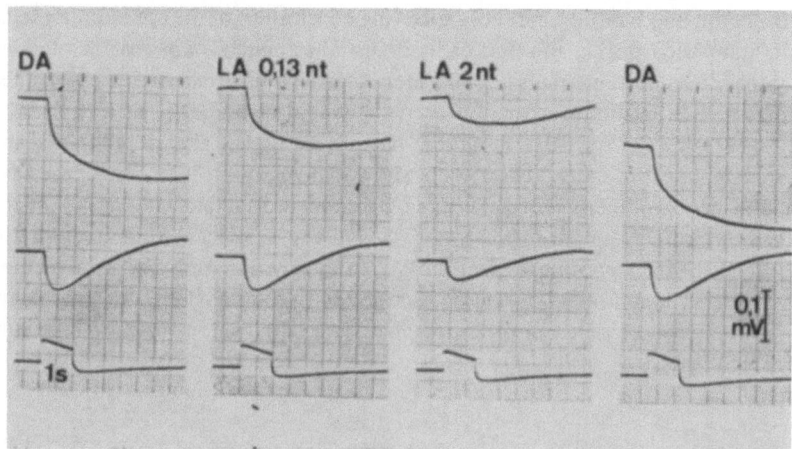

Fig. 1. ERG of eye bulb of rabbit, 8 hours after enucleation, negative component P_{III} only surviving. Upper trace: d.c. amplified; middle trace: r.c. amplified (time constant 1 s); bottom trace: light stimulus (200 nt, 1 s). From left to right: preparation dark adapted, light adapted to 0.13 nt, light adapted to 2 nt, after 2 min of dark adaptation. Calibration (0.1 mV) in the lower right corner.

426

negative response more than that of the r.c. amplified potential. Readaptation to darkness restitutes previous amplitudes within 2 minutes (right records).

The Table contains measurements and calculations of all experiments. In the left two columns the P_{III} amplitude of the dark adapted bulbs d.c. and r.c. recorded are listed. In the next column the ratios of each pair (r.c./d.c.) are calculated. The following columns show the corresponding values for different levels of light adaptation. The number of experiments differs for each group. The last column contains a statistical calculation (t-test for matched pairs); the corresponding ratios in light- and dark-adaptation were compared and the error probabilities (p) were listed. With exception of adaptation to a background of 0.063 nt all differences proved to be significant, even highly significant with a background of 2.0 nt.

Fig. 2 shows graphically how the results depend upon the intensity of light adaptation (means and errors of the means). The graph includes one measurement with 8 nt light adaptation (at the utter right side circle between brackets); it represents only one experiment (too bright intensities were avoided to exclude irreversible effects); no statistical evaluation, therefore, could be made with this intensity.

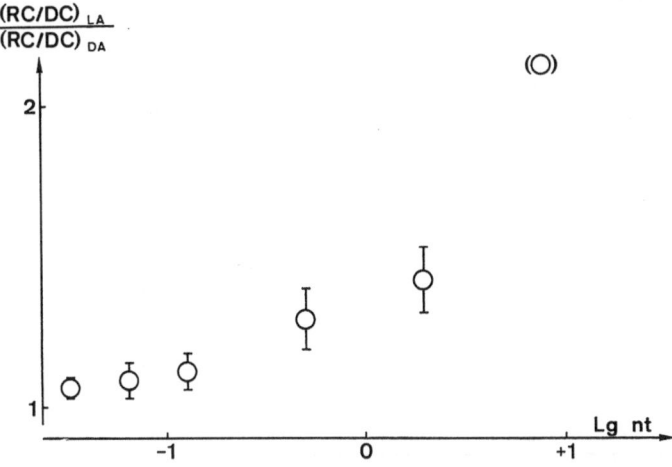

Fig. 2. Effect of adaptation level (abscissa) on composition of P_{III} (ordinate); the composition is mathematically defined by compound fraction of 4 values (RC = r.c. amplified amplitude; DC = d.c. amplified amplitude; each of this ratios measured in light and dark adaptation, symbolized by suffixes LA and DA). Means (circles) and Error of Means (vertical bars).

DISCUSSION

By d.c. amplification (time constant infinite) fast and slow subcomponents are measured, by r.c. amplification (time constant 1 s) predominantly the faster ones are traced. The statistical difference of the ratios of amplitudes in different states of adaptation is consistent with the assumption of complexity of P_{III}.

Dark adaptation			Light adaptation				Significance of difference between ratios D.A.-L.A.; found error of probability (p)
Amplitude μV		Ratio r.c./d.c.	Intensity	Amplitude μV		Ratio r.c./d.c.	
d.c.	r.c.			d.c.	r.c.		
144	76	.53	.031 nt	120	70	.58	
130	67	.52		110	60	.55	< .05
105	78	.74		90	70	.78	
135	71	.53	.063 nt	100	64	.64	
135	70	.52		135	70	.52	< .30
95	65	.68		75	55	.73	
130	70	.54	.125 nt	85	56	.66	
123	66	.54		75	46	.61	
85	55	.65		80	50	.63	
125	85	.68		95	70	.74	
100	70	.70		90	65	.72	< .05
105	78	.74		105	75	.71	
137	68	.50		45	30	.67	
108	40	.37		50	22	.44	
85	31	.36		50	20	.40	
115	64	.56	.50 nt	70	42	.60	
120	61	.51		50	34	.68	
102	72	.71		65	50	.77	
142	69	.49		15	13	.87	< .05
108	38	.35		27	12	.44	
90	32	.36		30	14	.47	
110	62	.56	2.0 nt	30	24	.80	
110	62	.56		30	20	.67	
125	85	.68		60	50	.83	
100	65	.65		55	45	.82	< .001
110	83	.75		65	60	.92	
107	38	.36		10	7	.70	
88	32	.36		13	8	.62	
86	30	.35	8.0 nt	4	3	.75	– –

This, at first sight, seems not surprising. The conclusion, however, may be stressed for two reasons.

First of all, P_{III} is sometimes interpreted as *the* receptor potential. In the present experiments by a rather simple technique (without any use of micro-electrodes) the complex nature of P_{III} became evident. By intraretinal recording from different retinal layers combined with use of aspartate as recommended by SILLMANN, ITO & TOMITA (1969) a splitting of P_{III} may be demonstrated. Using this technique in mammals 3 different components have been discriminated by HANITZSCH (1973).

Furthermore, it seems interesting that blocking of carbohydrate metabolism failed in identification of different P_{III} subcomponents (BORNSCHEIN & VON LÜTZOW, 1965), whereas light adaptation proved to be a valuable tool in the same kind of simple preparation.

The present experiments don't tell anything about the nature of fast and slow parts of P_{III}. A possible explanation may be derived from the results of CERVETTO & MACNICHOL (1972) indicating a feedback on the photoreceptor from horicontal cells. If, however, complexity of P_{III} were simply a matter of photopic and scotopic receptors it could be decided in a rather simple way by further experiments using monochromatic instead of white light.

ACKNOWLEDGEMENT:

Technical assistance of Mr. W. HÖFLER and Mr. H. WIENER is thankfully acknowledged.

REFERENCES

BÖCK, J., BORNSCHEIN, H. & HOMMER, K. *Vision Res.* 4: *609-626* (1964).
BÖCK, J., BORNSCHEIN, H. & HOMMER, K. *v. Graefes Arch. Klin. exp. Ophthal.* 168: *264-289* (1965).
BORNSCHEIN, H. & VON LÜTZOW, ASTRID. *v. Graefes Arch. Klin. exp. Ophthal.* 168: *455-467* (1965).
BROWN, K. T. *Vision Res.* 8: *633-677* (1968).
BROWN, K. T. & WIESEL, T. N. *J. Physiol.* 158: *257-280* (1961).
CERVETTO, L. & MACNICHOL, E. F. *Science* 178: *767-768* (1972).
HANITZSCH, RENATE. *Vision Res.* 13: *2093-2102* (1973).
NOELL, W. K. Studies on the Electrophysiology and the Metabolism of the Retina. Proj. No. 21-1201-0004 Rep. No. 1 (1953).
SILLMAN, A. J., ITO, H. & TOMITA, T. *Vision Res.* 9: *1435-1442* (1969).

Authors' address:

Institute of General and Comparative Physiology
University of Vienna
A-1090 Vienna
Austria

429

MECHANISM OF ACTION OF
ω-HYDROXYLHEXYLPYRIDONE-2 ON THE ERG

K. A. HELLNER & K. K. GAURI

(Hamburg)

ABSTRACT

We can say that OH-AAD seems to have a direct effect on the retinal function. Most probably these effects are due to an interaction of the biological formed aldehyde of the OH-AAD with the non-active site on the opsin molecule.

Whereas a single injection of 175 mg/kg ω-hydroxylhexylpyridone-2 (in the following called OH-AAD) leads in mice to increment of the b-wave amplitudes and also accelerates the rate of dark adaptation in mice, no effect could be traced in rat after this treatment (GAURI et al., 1972/1973). On the other hand in vit-A deficient rats after 8 weeks of deprivation the OH-AAD afforded an effective protection against the loss of retinal sensitivity. This was judged from the ERG threshold determinations. From this result it was concluded that the OH-AAD was substituting for vit-A in rhodopsin (GAURI et al., 1973).

In the present experiments the effect of OH-AAD is studied in animals where the vit-A depletion was continued up to 28 weeks. The results of these experiments in which the vit-A-depletion was carried out beyond the 8th week are shown in Fig. 1. As is seen from this diagram, the threshold in the deprived rats continuously increased depending upon the time of depletion. The amplitudes diminish progressively; whereas in corresponding vit-A deficient rats fed with 25 mg/kg/day OH-AAD the increment of the threshold, as well as the accompanying loss of the b-wave amplitude, is slower. At all times during these investigations they lie between the normal and the depleted rats.

To study the direct effect of OH-AAD in vit. A deficient rats, three 28 weeks depleted rats obtained a single injection of 175 mg/kg 18 hours before the ERG recording. The mean of the threshold and the reincrement of the b-wave amplitudes is compared with those determined 48 hours before the injection (Fig. 2). Evidently, in vit-A deficient rat a single injection of OH-AAD is capable of increasing both the retinal sensitivity as well as the increment of the b-wave amplitudes.

Results with the mice:

Originally we found that the treatment of 175 mg/kg of our pyridone derivatives increases the reincrement of the b-wave after bleaching, starting 4 hours post injection. The effect of the drug kept increasing during 24 hours and

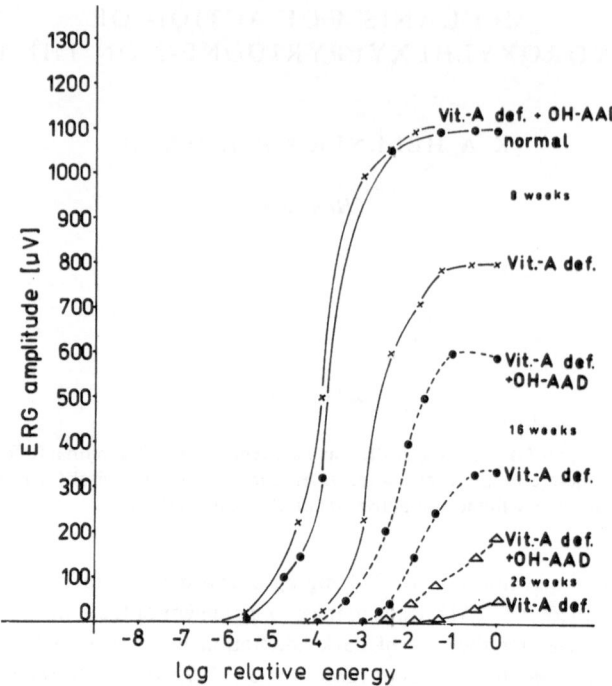

Fig. 1. Effect of 25 mg/kg/day oral treatment of OH-AAD in vit-A deficient rats as a function of time of depletion period of 8-28 weeks (black dots + solid line = normal rat; crosses and solid line = 8 weeks vit-A depletion; black dots and interrupted line = 16 weeks of vit-A depletion; triangles = 28 weeks of vit-A depletion). Both the lower thresholds and the higher amplitudes were found in vit-A depleted animals fed with OH-AAD.

then it started to decline. No effect, what so ever on the ERG was present 36 hours after the injection (HELLNER & GAURI). While repeating these experiments with mice, however, the original results could not be reproduced. A thorough examination led to the following results:

1. No activity of the pyridone compound can be detected in mice of about 3 months age.
2. Mice of 6 months show an activity as in the original experiments.
3. In old mice of about 18 months age the drug is without effect on the ERG. In these animals, from histological studies, it was found that retinal degeneration persist. (Fig. 3).

The ERG of mice decrease from more than 1,0 mV to 0,1 mV progressively with age.

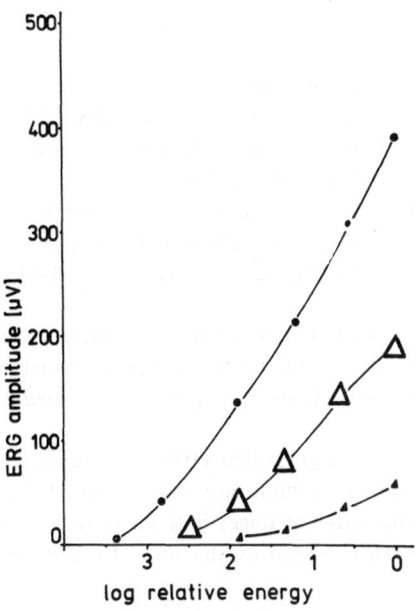

Fig. 2. Effect of a single intraperitoneal injection of 175 mg/kg OH-AAD in 28 weeks vit-A depleted rats. (black triangle = vit-A depleted rat; open triangle = vit-A depleted rat fed with 25 mg/kg/day OH-AAD; block dots = vit-A depleted rat injected with 175 mg/kg 18 hours before ERG).

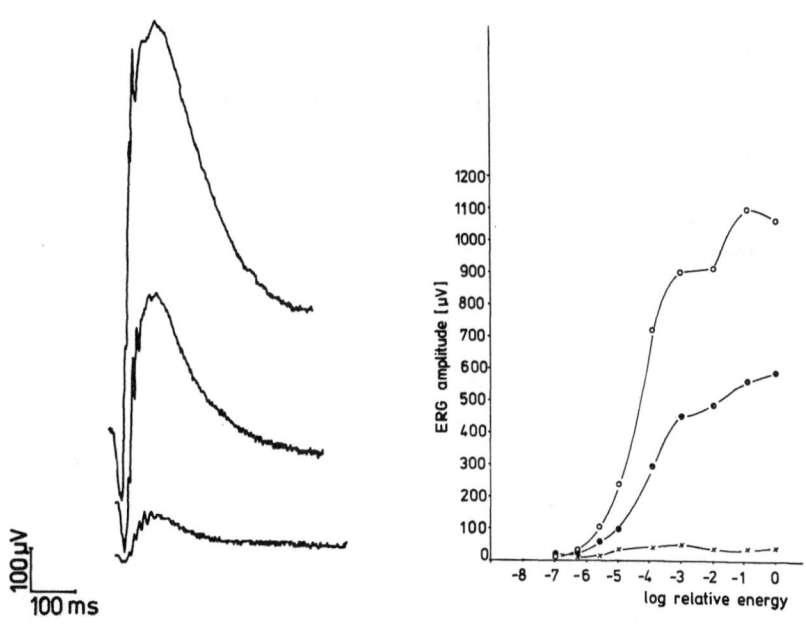

Fig. 3. ERG determinations of mice as a function of their age. Progressive loss of the amplitudes from young (3 months) to adult (6 months) and old mice (14 months).

From these results we can conclude that:

a. with regard to the experiments with rats, OH-AAD can not completely replace the retinal function of vit-A, but it clearly protects the animals against the progressive loss of retinal sensitivity.

Two modes of the protective action of OH-AAD in rats are suggested:

Firstly, the biologically formed aldehyde of the pyridone compound stabilizes the rhodopsin most probably by reacting at the non-active sites of the rhodopsin molecule.

Secondly, it releases the bound vit-A as is concluded from the growth and physiological function of the treated depleted animals as a function of the time of depletion. Results of these growth experiments will be published later.

b. The results with mice suggest that OH-AAD shows effects on the ERG of animals which show a medium amount of retinal degeneration, as is the case with the 6 months old mice; it is ineffective in mice which show no retinal degeneration or which exhibit almost complete degeneration of the retina.

REFERENCES

GAURI, K. K., HELLNER, K. A., RICKERS, J. & WATANABE, I. Effect of N-Hexylpyri-done-2 on the mouse electroretinogram. *Ophth. Res.* 4: *265-269* (1972/73).

GAURI, K. K., HELLNER, K. A., RICKERS, J. & WATANABE, I. Effect of alcohol-dehy-drogenase activators on the mouse ERG. Doc. Ophthal. Proc. Series Vol. 2, X. ISCERG Symposium, 119-124 (1973).

HELLNER, K. A. & GAURI, K. K. Uber die Wirksamkeit von Alkoholdehydrogenase-Effektoren im Tierexperiment. Ber. Dtsch. Ophthal. Ges. 1972 (in press).

Authors' address:

Univ. Augenklinik
2000 Hamburg 20
Martinistr. 52

ERG AND DIAGNOSIS OF ENCEPHALIC DEATH
CLINICAL FINDINGS AND EXPERIMENTAL DATA

G. MACK, A. LOBSTEIN, J. M. MANTZ, J. D. TEMPE & P. KARLI

(Strasbourg)

The diagnostic value of electroretinographic changes in retinal ischaemia due to local causes is well established. But retinal functions may also be altered by an ischaemia due to partial or complete failure of the brain circulation. This is the case in patients in a state of so-called 'overcoma' or encephalic death in whom survival is maintained through circulatory and respiratory assistance (MOLLARET et all., 1959). The diagnosis of the latter state is not an easy one, and various clinical, angiographic and electrophysiological criteria have been used. This had led us to try to assess the diagnostic value of the ERG in cases of overcoma. In each patient the state of the brain circulation was evaluated by an indirect method: determination of the arm-to-retina circulation time by fluorescence retinal angioscopy. Our clinical findings are compared with results obtained in experiments in which rats were submitted to anoxia by stopping the ventilation of the lungs.

METHODS

Thirty-six patients have been studied: 31 patients were really in a state of over-coma, as proven by the fatal outcome; the 5 others proved to be comatose patients with a more or less profound and more or less lasting decerebration. It must be stressed that patients in a state of overcoma need uninterrupted care. Therefore, only a brief electroretinographic exploration can be performed, and the state of visual adaptation is often quite different from one case to another. The ERG was recorded with a portable pen-recorder having a time constant of 1 second. The photic stimulation was achieved with flashes of an energy of 0,3 joule and a duration of 150 microseconds. A Wratten-filter n°26 was used for red-light stimulations.

The arm-to-retina circulation time (A.R.C.T.) was measured by the method devised by NOVOTNY & ALVIS (1961). A fluorescein solution of 20 per cent (4 ml) was injected fairly rapidly through a catheter inserted into an antecubital vein as far as the axillary vein. The A.R.C.T. is the interval between the beginning of injection and the first appearence of fluorescence at the disc, as observed with a modified ophthalmoscope (fluoroscope according to Amalric). The normal values are 8-14 seconds in the recumbent position. The A.R.C.T. becomes prolonged if the carotid arterial flow is obstructed. It provides indirect evidence of delayed circulation time to the brain (GOTHAM et al., 1962). The test is a harmless one and can be used in comatose patients. In all our patients, the systemic blood pressure was not lower than 100 mm Hg.

As regards the experiments performed on rats, the techniques used have been described in detail elsewhere (MACK & KARLI, 1973). But the main points may be briefly recalled. The animal is curarized and artificially ventilated. The control ERG is recorded on an oscilloscope (Amplior II Alvar) following a dark adaptation period of 15 minutes. At the same time, the EEG, the bioelectrical activity of the lateral thalamus (through a stereotaxically implanted electrode) and the EKG are recorded in order to obtain base-line values. During the periods of arrest as well as of resumption of the artificial ventilation, the EEG, the thalamic activity and the EKG are recorded continuously, the ERG being recorded every 15 seconds.

RESULTS

1. Clinical findings

In the 31 patients with overcoma, the A.R.C.T. varied greatly, from normal values (12-14 seconds) up to 2-3 minutes (the A.R.C.T. was below 30 seconds in 20 patients, among whom 6 had entirely normal values). In contrast with this wide range of findings as regards the A.R.C.T., the ERG was deeply altered in every case. An important reduction of the b-wave amplitude in response to a flash of white light was found regularly (Fig. 1), and this reduction (below the isoelectric line) points to a severe anoxia of the inner layers of the retina. When flashes of red light were used, a reduction of the b-wave down to or below the isoelectric line was found only in those cases in which the A.R.C.T. exceeded 1 minute (Fig. 2).

In the 5 comatose patients with decerebration, the A.R.C.T. never exceeded 21 seconds. The ERG was repeatedly recorded in each one of these patients,

NORMAL ERG   **ERG In CASES of OVER – COMA**

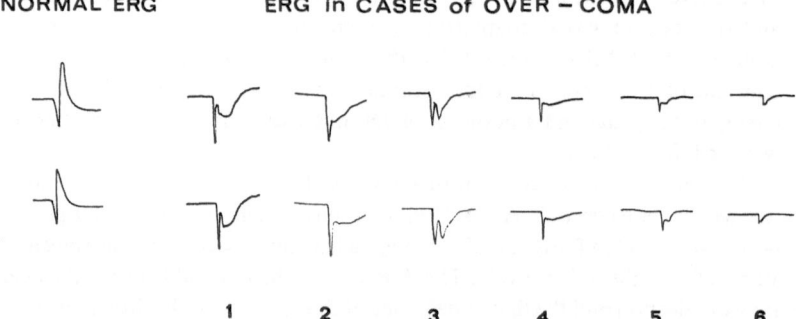

1   2   3   4   5   6

Fig. 1. ERGs recorded in 6 patients with encephalic death (in cases 1, 2, 3 and 4 the arm-to-retina circulation time was less than 30 seconds; it exceeded 1 minute in cases 5 and 6).

436

white
stimulation

red
stimulation

r.e.

< 30"

r.e.

> 60" r.e.

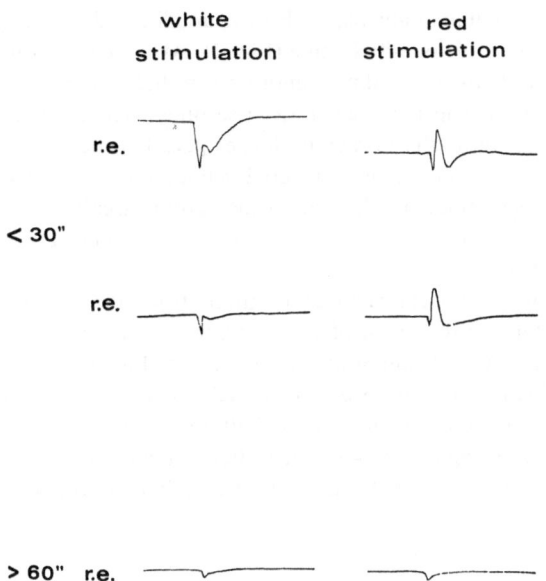

Fig. 2. ERGs recorded from the right eye (r.e.) in 3 patients with encephalic death (in two cases, the arm-to-retina circulation time was less than 30 seconds; in the third case, it was over 60 seconds).

and we never found the kind of severe alteration of the b-wave which appears to be typical of the patients with encephalic death (Fig. 3).

NORMAL ERG   ERG in CASES of COMA with DECEREBRATION

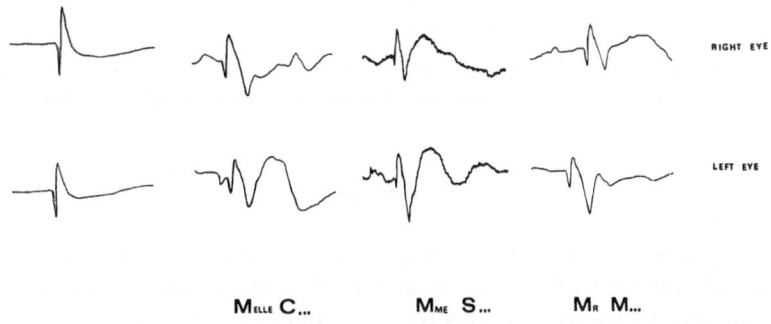

RIGHT EYE

LEFT EYE

M$_{ELLE}$ C...   M$_{ME}$ S...   M$_R$ M...

Fig. 3. ERGs recorded in 3 comatose patients with decerebration.

437

2. *Experimental data*

During the first minute of anoxia, the b-wave amplitude decreases progressively to about one/third of its initial value (Fig. 4). At the end of this minute, the cortical activity (EEG) has almost entirely vanished, whereas a spontaneous thalamic activity is still recorded. Fifteen seconds later, the thalamic activity disappears in its turn; the b-wave no longer goes beyond the isoelectric line, whereas the a-wave still remains unaltered. About 3 minutes after the arrest of the artificial ventilation, the damage to the cardio-vascular system is irreversible. It takes 6 to 7 minutes of anoxia to provoke a complete vanishing of the a-wave of the ERG.

The electrophysiological changes resulting from the anoxia are entirely reversible as long as the arrest of the ventilation is not prolonged beyond 3 minutes. Following resumption of the ventilation (Fig. 5), the a-wave of the ERG is the first potential to recover its initial amplitude (within no more than 60 seconds). A spontaneous thalamic activity reappears about 2 minutes later; an EEG is recorded again 3 to 4 minutes after resumption of the ventilation. It takes at least another minute for the b-wave amplitude to recover in its turn its initial value.

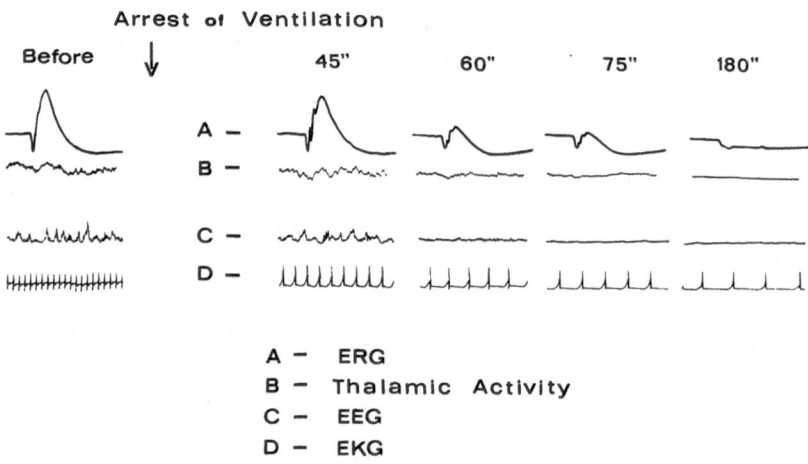

Fig. 4. ERG, spontaneous thalamic activity, EEG and EKG recorded in a curarized rat before and at various times following arrest of the artificial ventilation.

DISCUSSION

In the group of patients studied, there was no close correlation between the A.R.C.T. and the ERG: a severely altered ERG was in some cases on a par with an equally severely altered A.R.C.T.; but in some other cases, the altered ERG was on a par with a subnormal or even normal A.R.C.T. This absence of

438

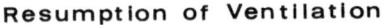

Resumption of Ventilation

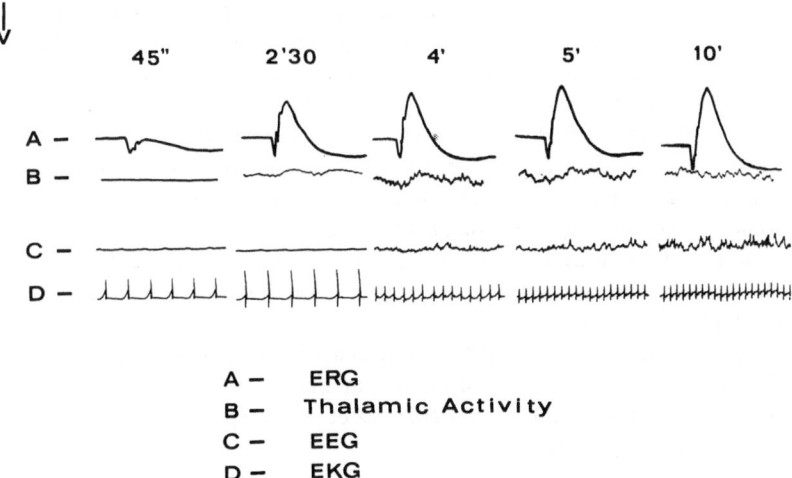

| | 45" | 2'30 | 4' | 5' | 10' |

A — ERG
B — Thalamic Activity
C — EEG
D — EKG

Fig. 5. Same animal as in Fig. 4, at various times following resumption of the artificial ventilation.

correlation between the A.R.C.T. and the ERG is due to the fact that an irreversible alteration of retinal functions may have been provoked by a more or less prolonged arrest of the systemic circulation before the circulatory and respiratory assistance has established anew subnormal or even normal A.R.C.T. Thus, it appears that in comatose patients, the A.R.C.T. can hardly give much information as to whether or not the transient arrest of the systemic circulation has produced irreversible damage to the brain. On the contrary, an important depression of the b-wave (the latter reaching no longer the isoelectric line) appears to be a much better criterion for the diagnosis of encephalic death: a fatal outcome occurred every time such a deeply altered ERG had been recorded; on the other hand, an almost normal ERG was regularly recorded in those patients that would recover from their comatose state.

Considering that it is often difficult to record the ERG in comatose patients under well-controlled conditions and that a control record prior to the coma is rarely, if ever, available for a precise quantitative assessment of the pathological changes, the mere morphological alteration (b-wave no longer reaching the isoelectric line) is a convenient criterion for the diagnosis of encephalic death. It is only in the late stages of retinal anoxia and in relation with an important increase of the A.R.C.T. that such a morphological alteration of the ERG is observed also with flashes of red light. This provides a still more reliable sign of encephalic death.

In the rat as well as in the human patient, the anoxia affects the b-wave of the ERG long before it starts affecting the a-wave; in either case, the inner layers of the retina are more sensitive to anoxia than the outer ones. A difference between our clinical and experimental findings consists in that an important reduction of the b-wave amplitude may in the human patient already be the sign of an irreversible alteration of both retina and brain, whereas in the rat the ERG as well as the EEG may recover entirely despite a complete vanishing of the b-wave, as long as the a-wave amplitude is not reduced by more than 30 per cent of its initial value.

When the rat is artificially ventilated with pure oxygen, its resistance to anoxia shows a twofold increase: a complete recovery of the bioelectrical potentials is still possible following an arrest of the' ventilation for 6 to 7 minutes. The more or less lasting continuance of retinal responses observed in some patients following the fatal circulatory collapse might well result from such an enhanced resistance to anoxia due to the conditions of the respiratory assistance.

To conclude, we may report the interesting case of a comatose patient whose EEG was flat for more than 24 hours, but whose ERG remained almost un-altered during that period of time (MANTZ et al., 1971). Today, this patient has recovered in every respect.

REFERENCES

GOTHAM, J. E., GILROY, J. & MEYER, J. S. Studies of cerebral circulation time in Man. Normal values and alterations with cerebral vascular disease and tumour in arm-to-retina circulation times. *J. Neurol. Neurosurg. Psychiat.* 25: *292-302* (1962).

MACK, G. & KARLI, P. ERG et diagnostic de la mort cérébrale: étude expérimentale chez le Rat. *C.R. Soc. Biol. Paris* 1973 (in press).

MANTZ, J. M., TEMPE, J. D., JAEGER, A., KURTZ, D., LOBSTEIN, A. & MACK, G. Silence électrique cérébral de vingt-quatre heures au cours d'une intoxication massive par 10 g de Pentobarbital. *Presse Médicale* 79: *1243-1246* (1971).

MOLLARET, P. & GOULON, M. Le coma dépassé. *Rev. Neurol.* 101: *3-15* (1959).

NOVOTNY, H. R. & ALVIS, D. L. A method of photographing fluorescence in circulating blood in the human retina. *Circulation* 24: *82-86* (1961).

Authors' address:

Institut de Biologie Médicale
Clinique Ophthalmologique et Service de Réanimation de la Faculté de Médecine
Strasbourg
France

O₂ DEPENDENCE OF THE B-WAVE IN THE ISOLATED PERFUSED MAMMALIAN EYE

GÜNTER NIEMEYER

(Zürich)

If, after enucleation of a cat eye the ophthalmociliary artery is canulated and perfused with an appropriate medium, the functional state of the retina can be maintained for many hours (GOURAS & HOFF, 1970; NIEMEYER & GOURAS, 1973a). This technique has been published elsewhere (GOURAS & HOFF, 1970; NIEMEYER, 1973a). The isolated and perfused feline eye has proved to be a preparation eminently suitable for the application of four major investigative techniques: 1. an analysis of the electroretinogram (ERG) under various *in vitro* conditions (NIEMEYER, 1973b; NIEMEYER & GOURAS, 1973b, HOFF & GOURAS, 1973), 2. intracellular recording at various layers of the retina (NIEMEYER & GOURAS, 1973 a + b; NIEMEYER, 1973a), 3. iontophoretic dye injection into single cells (NELSON, V. LÜTZOW-KAFKA & GOURAS, 1973), and 4. analysis of the fine structure of the *in vitro* retina (REMÉ & NIEMEYER, 1973). In this particular communication we report the successful use of the *in vitro* perfused eye as a means of determining some of the perfusion parameters that influence the amplitude of the b-wave of the ERG.

In a previous, preliminary study, it was reported, that there was an apparent inter-relation between the b-wave amplitude and the flow rate of the perfusion medium (NIEMEYER, 1973b). Consequently, experiments have been extended to include a comparison of the influence of haemoglobin-free perfusates of different levels of oxygenation. These data are presented and discussed below.

The preliminary experiments indicated that the b-wave of the ERG obtains its energy from the perfusate. An example to illustrate this point is shown in Figure 1. The figure shows a time series of ERGs taken at the cessation of the perfusion flow and at subsequent 4 second intervals. The resulting signals are electrically superimposed on the oscilloscope screen. After about 50 seconds, it appears that the available energy of the perfusate in the organ has been consumed and the b-wave has practically no sensible amplitude.

Further, a remarkable diminution of the amplitude of the b-wave appears, if the flow rate of the perfusion is decreased gradually, as illustrated in Figure 2. Similarly, an increase of the flow rate usually increases the ERG response to a given stimulus. Such an experiment is graphically demonstrated in Figure 3, where the solid curves represent amplitude-intensity functions of the b-waves for a perfused eye (solid curves). For comparison, the mean of response amplitudes for 3 *in vivo* cat eyes, as obtained under virtually identical stimulus

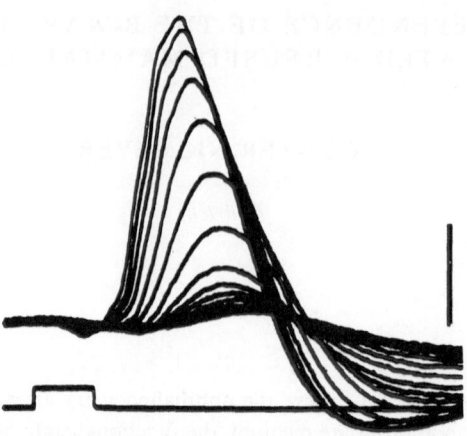

Fig. 1. Electroretinograms recorded from the cornea of the dark adapted isolated cat eye following complete cessation of the perfusion. Responses to a 20 msec pulse (lowermost trace indicates the photocell's response) of monochromatic light (581 nm), which was delivered prior to and every 4th second after the circulatory arrest. Calibration: 200 μV.

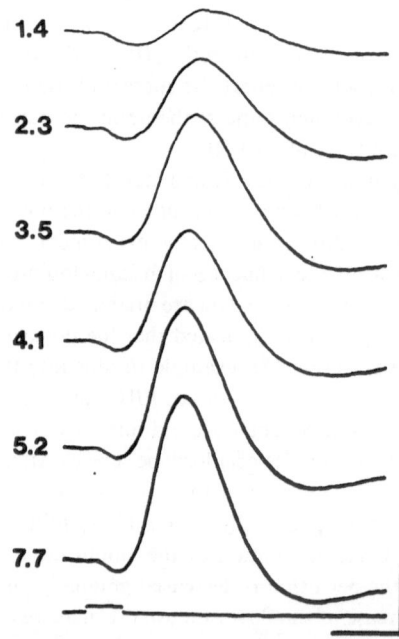

Fig. 2. ERGs from the dark adapted isolated cat eye at various flow rates of perfusion. The numbers indicate the flow rates in ml/min. The stimulus was a 20 msec pulse of monochromatic light (620 nm), marked in the lowermost trace. Calibration: 40 msec and 200 μV.

442

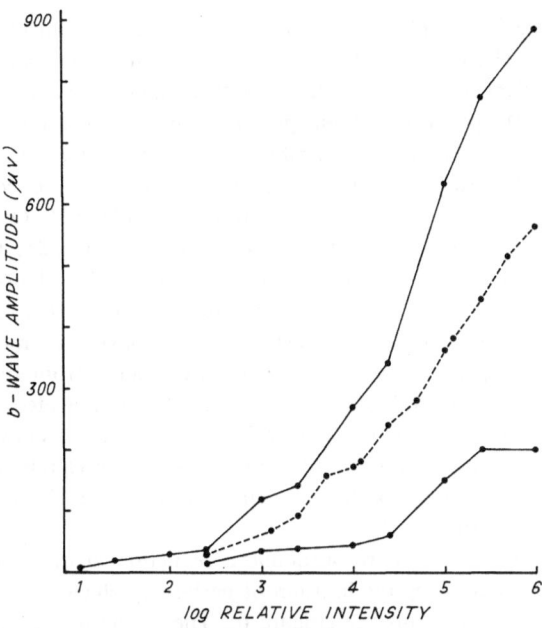

Fig. 3. Amplitude-intensity functions from ERGs, obtained in *in vivo*, eyes and from *in vitro* preparations at two different flow rates of perfusion. Dashed line, mean of b-wave amplitudes from 3 cat eyes, recorded *in situ*. Upper curve (solid line), b-wave amplitudes of ERGs recorded from a perfused eye at a flow rate of 8 ml/min, lowermost curve (solid line), b-wave amplitudes from the same preparation obtained at a low flow rate (2.9 ml/min). The stimulus was a 20 msec pulse of 620 nm monochromatic light in all three experimental conditions.

conditions, are shown (dashed curve). By this it is demonstrated, that at high flow rates of the perfusate, b-wave amplitudes higher than normal can be elicited. This *pari passu* increase of the ERG of the perfused eye with increasing flow rate is shown in figure 4 for 7 experiments. It was further noted, that the relationship between changes in flow rate and relative b-wave amplitudes was of the following form: firstly, at low flow rates, the rate of change of relative amplitude of the b-wave with respect to incremental change in flow rate is approximately constant. However, at higher flow rates the value of the constant diminishes and the curves tend to be asymptotic to a line parallel to the flow axis. Secondly, the initial rate of change of b-wave amplitude with respect to flow is extremely rapid. In Figure 4B, the data of Figure 4A have been horizontally displaced to emphasize the above points.

The question arose, whether this peculiar feature was due to variations in oxygen supply to the retina, particularly since the oxygen carrying capacity of the haemoglobin-free perfusate is some 2 orders of magnitude less than that of the blood (KNIGHT, pers. comm.). Several gas mixtures of varying O_2 fraction were prepared for oxygenating the perfusate. The concentration of CO_2 (5%), the pressure and the duration of gas insufflation were maintained constant. These 3 factors play an important role in the experiments, since derivations of the pH from an average value of 7.4 could occur and influence the excitability of the retina (WINKLER, 1972). It should be mentioned here, that loss of CO_2 from the perfusion system produced an increase in the pH and in turn decreased the ERG amplitude in pilot experiments. The gas mixtures used in the experiments presented here were 1. standard gas mixture, containing 95 % O_2 and 5 % CO_2, 2. reduced oxygen mixture, containing 65 % O_2, 5 % CO_2 and 30 % N_2, and 3. low oxygen mixture, containing 35 % O_2, 5 % CO_2 and 60 % N_2. The final mean oxygen partial pressures obtained in the perfusates were 1.) 426 mm Hg for the standard gas mixture, 2.) 340 mm Hg for the reduced oxygen gas mixture, and 3.) 239 mm Hg for the low oxygen gas mixture.

In a typical experiment, when perfusion was switched from a highly oxygenated medium (based on 95 % O_2) to a moderately oxygenated medium (65 % O_2), the b-wave amplitude was reduced within seconds, as shown in Figure 5. After having perfused with the '65 % O_2' medium for 11 minutes, the highly oxygenated standard perfusate was delivered again and the ERG recovered well within about 10 minutes.

A similar, but much more pronounced reduction in the amplitude of the b-wave was produced by the infusion of perfusate, which had been insufflated with the 35 % O_2 gas mixture (Figure 6). The amplitude of the b-wave was reduced to about one tenth of the control and recovered well after switching back to the standard medium, but in a slower time course compared to the previous experiment.

The latencies of the a- and b-waves were not significantly affected by variations in either the flow rate or the oxygenation of the perfusate. However, it

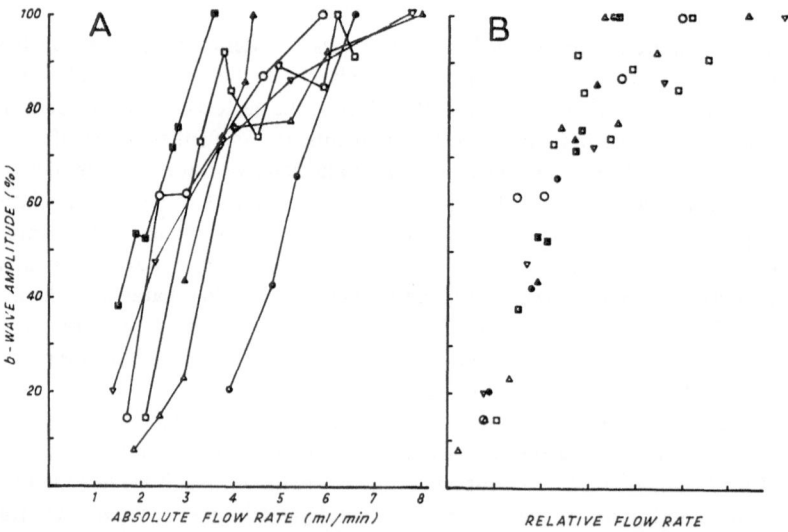

Fig. 4. A, relative b-wave of the ERG, plotted versus absolute flow rate of perfusion from 7 experiments. In B, these curves have been horizontally displaced.

444

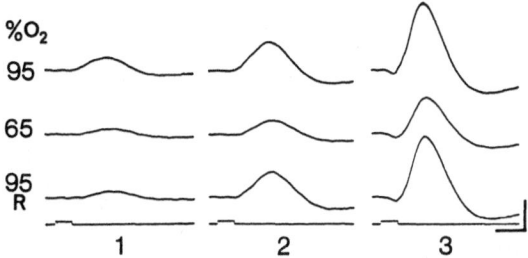

Fig. 5. ERGs from a perfused cat eye at standard and at moderate oxygenation of the perfusate. The O_2 content of the oxygenating gas mixture is indicated on the left side; the 65% O_2 recordings (middle row of signals) were obtained 10 minutes after the change of the perfusate. 95R (lower row of signals) indicates the recovery in presence of the standard perfusate which had been oxygenated with a 95% O_2 gas mixture following the application of the less oxygenated perfusate (65% O_2) for a period of 11 min. The numbers at the bottom indicate the Log of relative light intensity of the stimulus. The flow rate in the experiment shown in Figures 5 to 8 was kept at 4 ml/min. Calibration 40 msec, 200 μV.

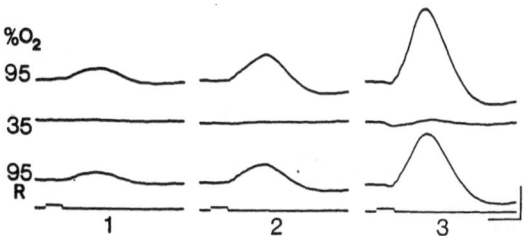

Fig. 6. ERGs from the perfused cat eye, from which the signals in figure 5 were recorded, at standard (95% O_2) gas mixture and at much lower (35% O_2) gas mixture-oxygenation of the perfusate. 95 R, intensities, and calibration as in legend to Figure 5.

was noted, that there was a temperature dependency, which is currently under investigation.

The general relationship between b-wave amplitude, photic stimulation, and degree of oxygenation is shown quantitavely in Figures 7 and 8.

The dependence of the b-wave amplitude upon the two parameters of the perfusate, i.e. flow and oxygen concentration can be approximated to a single parameter, the oxygen mass flow rate, i.e. the number of grams of O_2 per minute entering the organ. In the example shown in Figure 9, a high concentration-low flow situation (upper curve) is contrasted with a low concentration-high flow regime (lower curve) under conditions of equal stimuli. Under these virtually different conditions the responses appear to be very similar in amplitude, shape and time course.

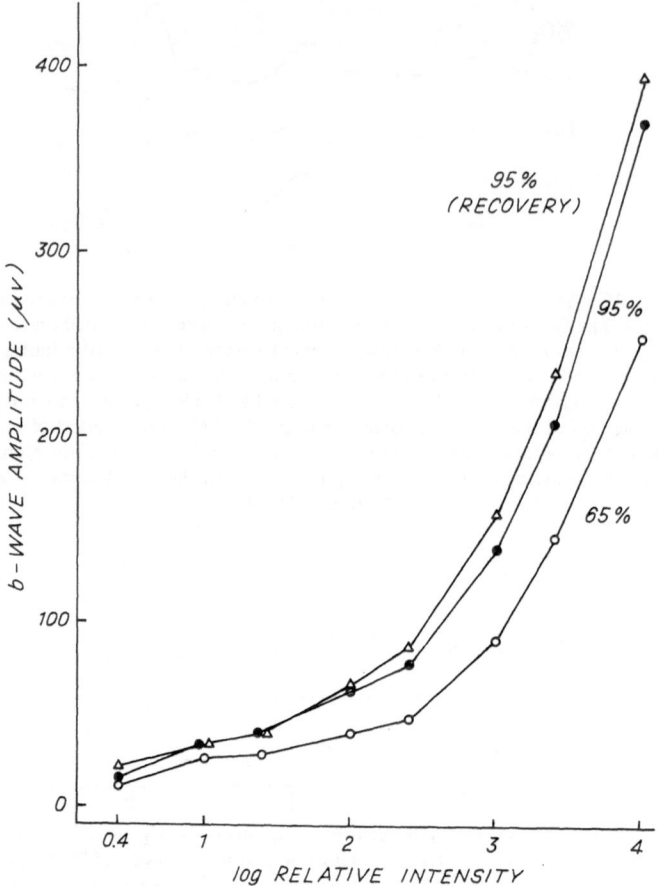

Fig. 7. Amplitude-intensity functions of the b-wave of the ERG corresponding to the oxygen-deprivation experiment illustrated in Figure 5. (●) data from initial recordings under standard oxygenation; (○), data obtained 10 min. after perfusion with moderate hypoxia (65% O_2 gas mixture) of the perfusate; (△), recovery under perfusion with standard medium.

CONCLUSIONS

The *in vitro* eye has permitted the analysis of low concentration oxygen dependence for the b-wave of the ERG. In particular, it has been shown, that the flow rate of, and the oxygen concentration in, the perfusate are determining factors. To a close approximation, it is apparent, that the b-wave of the ERG is strongly influenced by the oxygen mass flow rate. It is stressed, however, that this study has been performed under conditions of controlled pH and temperature, factors which also have a marked effect on the ERG.

446

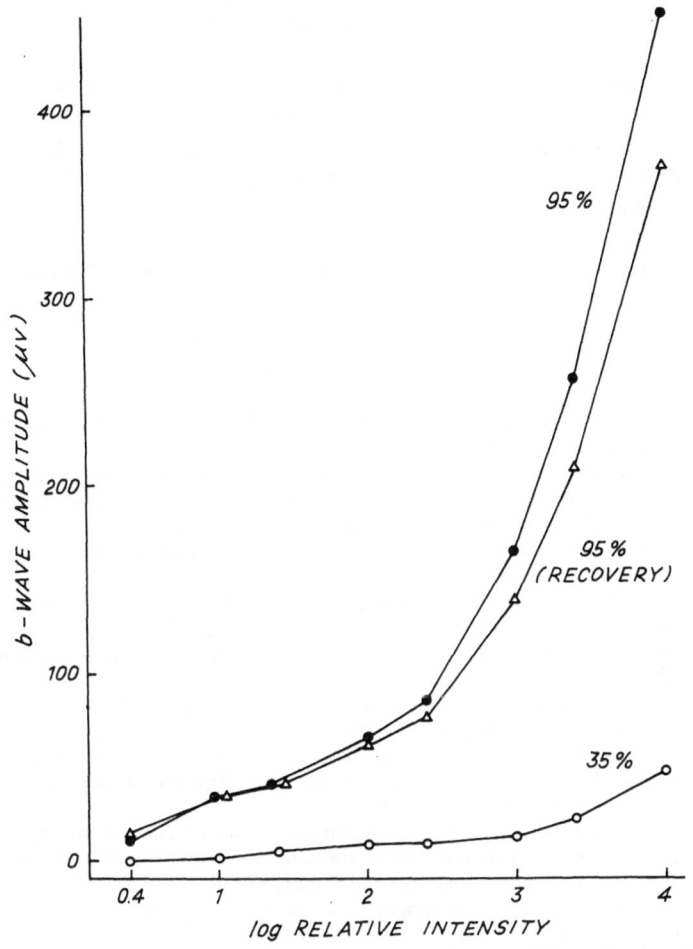

Fig. 8. Similar experiment to that illustrated in Figure 7, but with application of more severe hypoxia (○), obtained by insufflation of the perfusate with the 35% O_2 gas mixture. The recovery (△) reached amplitudes in the range of the control (●).

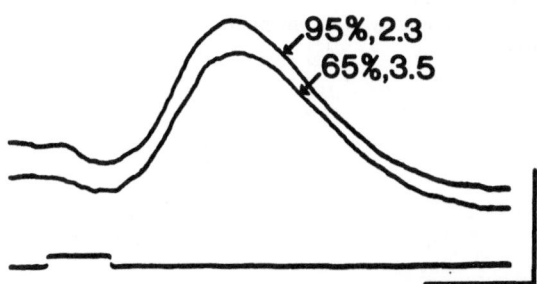

Fig. 9. ERG from an isolated eye under standard oxygenation and low flow rate (2.3 ml/min) of the perfusate (upper curve) in comparison to the ERG elicited by the same stimulus, at lower oxygenation, but at higher flow rate (3.5 ml/min) of the perfusate (lower curve). Calibration 40 msec, 200 µV.

ACKNOWLEDGEMENTS

I should like to thank Prof. R. WITMER for his generous support throughout this study, and Dr. C. KNIGHT for the most stimulating and valuable discussions we had during the preparation of the manuscript. Mrs. M. MÄRKLIN provided excellent technical assistence during this study, Miss. U. BUCK kindly helped with pO_2 measurements, and I thank as well Mr. H. R. MÄRKLIN for his help in building the modified perfusion chamber.

This study was supported, in part, by the Hartmann Müller-Foundation, Zürich.

REFERENCES

GOURAS, P. & HOFF, M. Retinal functions in an isolated perfused mammalian eye. *Invest. Ophthal. 9: 388-399* (1970).

HOFF, M. & GOURAS, P. Tolerance of mammalian retina to circulatory arrest. Proc. 10th Symp. ISCERG 1972, Docum. Ophthal. Proc. Series Vol. 2: *57-63* (1973).

KNIGHT. C. J. University of Zürich. Personal communication.

NELSON, R., v. LÜTZOW-KAFKA, A. & GOURAS, P. Unpublished results, personal communication.

NIEMEYER, G. Intracellular recording from the isolated perfused mammalian eye. *Vision Res.* 13: *1613-1618* (1973a).

NIEMEYER, G. ERG dependence on flow rate in the isolated and perfused mammalian eye. *Brain Res.* 57: *203-207* (1973b).

NIEMEYER, G. & GOURAS, P. Rod and cone signals in S-potentials of the isolated perfused cat eye. *Vision Res.* 13: *1603-1612* (1973a).

NIEMEYER, G. & GOURAS, P. The perfused mammalian eye as a preparation for electrophysiological studies. Proc. 10th Symp. ISCERG. Docum. Ophthal. Proc. Series, Vol. 2: *261-268* (1973b).

REMÉ, CH. & NIEMEYER, G. Retinal finestructure and function of the isolated and perfused mammalian eye. Presented at the Symposium on the application of electron microscopy to ophthalmic anatomy and pathology. Glasgow, Sept. 20-21 (1973).

WINKLER, B. S. The electroretinogram of the isolated rat retina. *Vision Res.* 12: *1183-1198* (1972).

Authors' address:

Neurophysiology Laboratory
Department of Ophthalmology, Kantonsspital
Rämistrasse 100
8006 Zürich/Switzerland

THE FAST OCULAR DIPOLE OSCILLATION*

J. HENNIG, R. TÄUMER & D. PERNICE

(Freiburg)

The initial behaviour of the ocular dipole moment (ODM) to a step stimulus has been described by ASERINSKY, KRIS, KOLDER, ARDEN and TÄUMER.

KOLDER (1966) has excited fast oscillations of the ODM with square waves of a period time of 2.2 min. In our paper we will describe the differentiation of the components of ODM to a step stimulus by the 'resonance' method.

We measured the beginning of the dipole oscillation following a luminance step from 0.2 to 2000 asb with a time resolution of 1/sec (Fig. 1). That means the person makes eye movements of 40° each second for a period of 10 min or 15 min. In the upper curve (Fig. 1a) the response to a light step is shown. The maximum of the main oscillation occurs at 9 min. At the beginning of this curve, there are some irregularities. This 'fine structure' is composed of two quick processes: At the 10th sec there is a well pronounced peak – the on-peak (pk^h) – with an amplitude of $+ 14\%$ above the Base Level (BL). At the 40th sec a minimum (n_1^h) of $- 7\%$ (beneath the BL) is seen. In the rising part of the curve after 3,5 min a small depression occurs (n_2^h).

Following a step to darkness (Fig. 1b) the minimum of the main oscillation is reached after 12 min. At the beginning a first elevation to $+ 10\% (p_1^d)$ of the BL occurs at the 40th sec. This elevation has disappeared by the 80th sec.

In order to differentiate the single components of this step response, we stimulated the system with an exponential sinus (like TÄUMER et al., 1974). In Fig. 2 the response of the system to some of the frequencies is shown. The amplitude of stimulation is 4 log units. The sinus had a period time of 1.5, 2.5 and 3.5 min. We found the maximal amplitude at a period time of 2.5 min.

Fig. 3 shows the amplitude and the phase behaviour of the system in relation to the different sinus frequencies. The upper curve shows the amplitude behaviour with a flat maximum at the period time of 2.5 min. The lower curve shows the phase behaviour between a period time of 1 and 3 min. The phase comes down from $+ 210°$ to $+ 40°$, which means an amount of about 180°. The fastest change occurs at a period time of about 2 min. This amplitude and phase behaviour is typical for a highly damped oscillating system. So we found another oscillation of the ocular dipole with an 'eigenfrequency' of 2.5 min. This fast wave is responsible for most of the irregularities at the beginning of

* Supported by the Deutsche Forschungsgemeinschaft SFB 70.

449

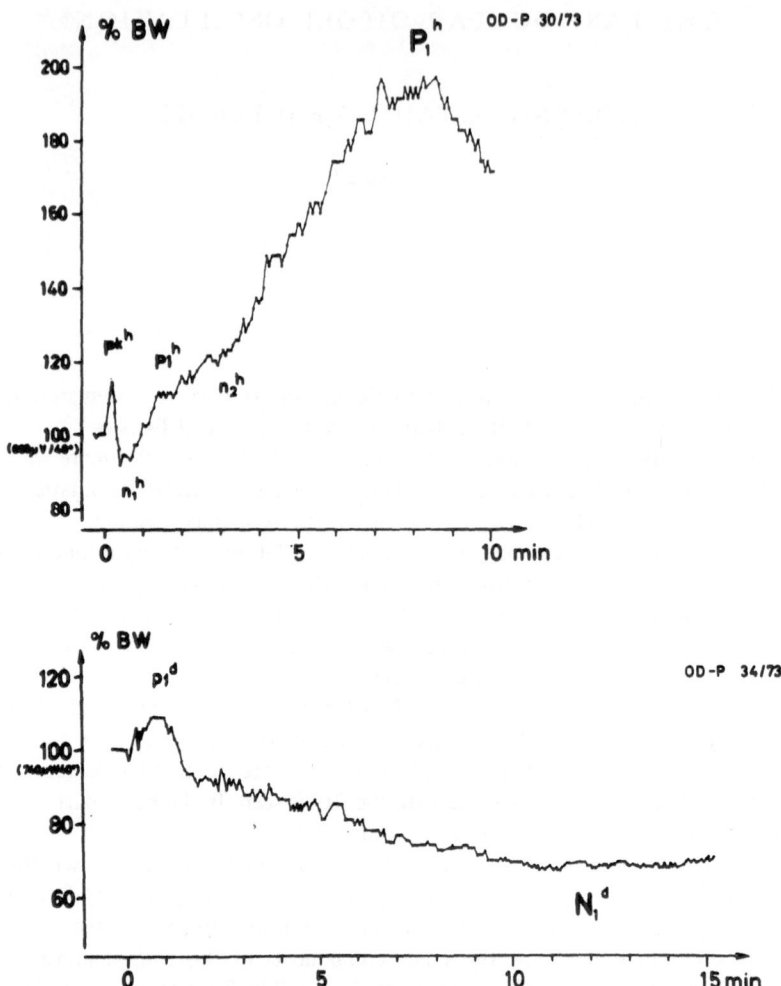

Fig. 1. The beginning part of the oscillation of the ODM following a luminance change: a. step increase in luminance from 0,2 to 2000 asb; b. step decrease in luminance from 2000 to 0,2 asb.

the ODM, and causes the two minimum n_1^h and n_2^h in Fig. 1, and probably also p_1^d.

But this fast wave could not be responsible for the on-peak (pk^h). According to its steep rising and decreasing, you could assume a further faster oscillation. But stimulating with a sinus form at frequencies which should be suitable to get resonance (faster than 1/min), no evidence of resonance was found.

We than have stimulated the system with square waves around the expected period time. Fig. 4 shows the result. With dark and light periods of 20 sec (period-time of 40 sec) the on-peak has developed well. Longer periods (60 sec)

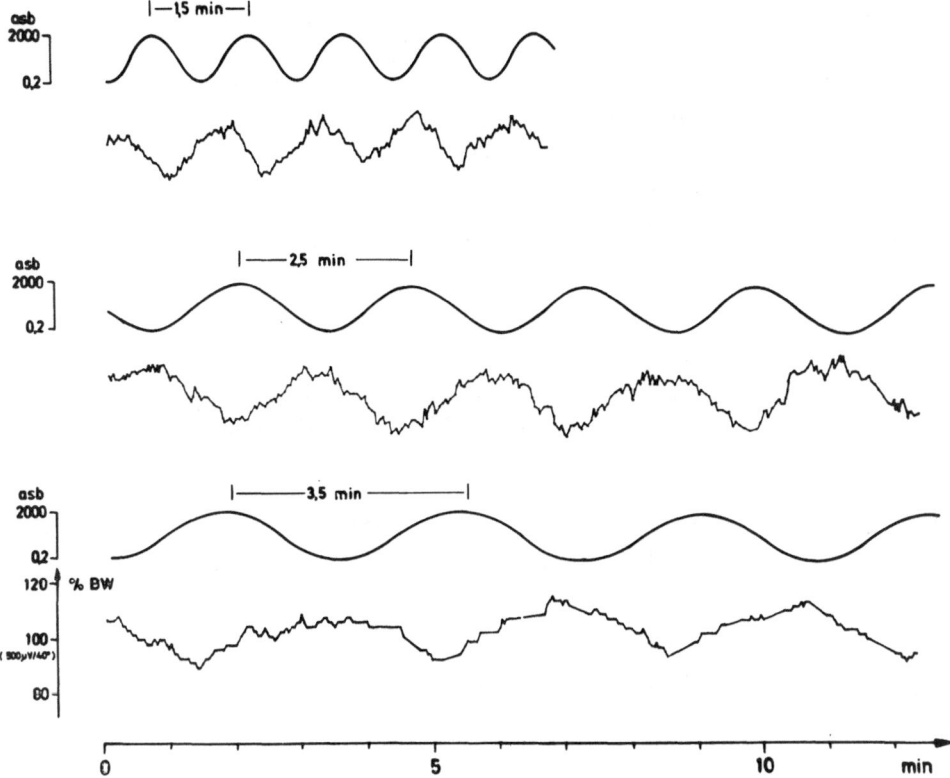

Fig. 2. Stimulation of the ODM with sinus of frequencies near the resonance point of 2,5 min.

show no further increase of the peak amplitude above the value seen in the single step answer. The single peaks are separated by intervals which equal the BL. In shorter periods (20 sec) a well-pronounced response is seen, but with less amplitude.

Yet, if we look more precisely no resonance will occur. The on-peak increases to the amplitude of the single step response and stays constant. It doesn't decline with longer period times as we would expect in case of resonance. So, we conclude that the on-peak of the light response is an yes- or no- answer with no further influence. The time relation to the light step doesn't change. The maximum of the peak always occurs at the 15th sec after the step.

Fig. 5 shows the answer to square waves of period times of 80 sec, 2.5 and 4 min. In all these curves we recognize the on-peaks of usual amplitude following each step to light. In addition, the square wave excites the fast wave. In the case of resonance of 2.5 min, this underlying fast wave has the largest amplitude.

We found three components of the light-stimulated ODM oscillation. In a first approximation the sum of these components will give the response of the ocular dipole to a luminance step. The components are: Fig. 6.

451

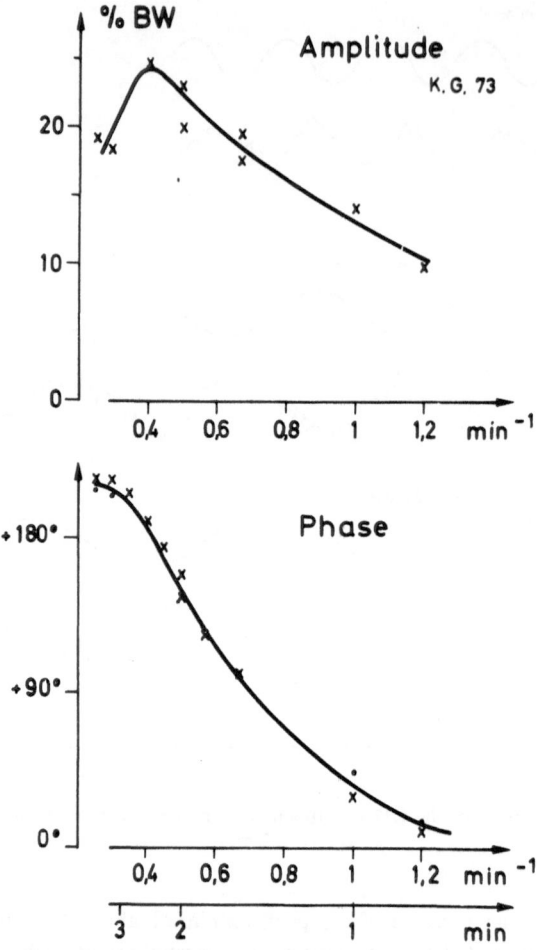

Fig. 3. Dependence of the amplitude and the phase of the ODM–fast wave from the period–time of the stimulating sinus.

1. a sinus with a period time of 26 min
2. a sinus with a period time of 2.5 min and beginning with a phase lag of about 180°
3. the on-peak evoked by the step increase of the luminance.

Both oscillations are highly damped. The constants K will differ by a factor of 4 (K_0 about 4 K_1). The approximation of the main oscillation by a sinus is not precise. Especially the comparison of the light and dark step shows that the system looks more like an oscillator swinging in a medium with higher resistance at lower values. (TÄUMER et al., 1974).

452

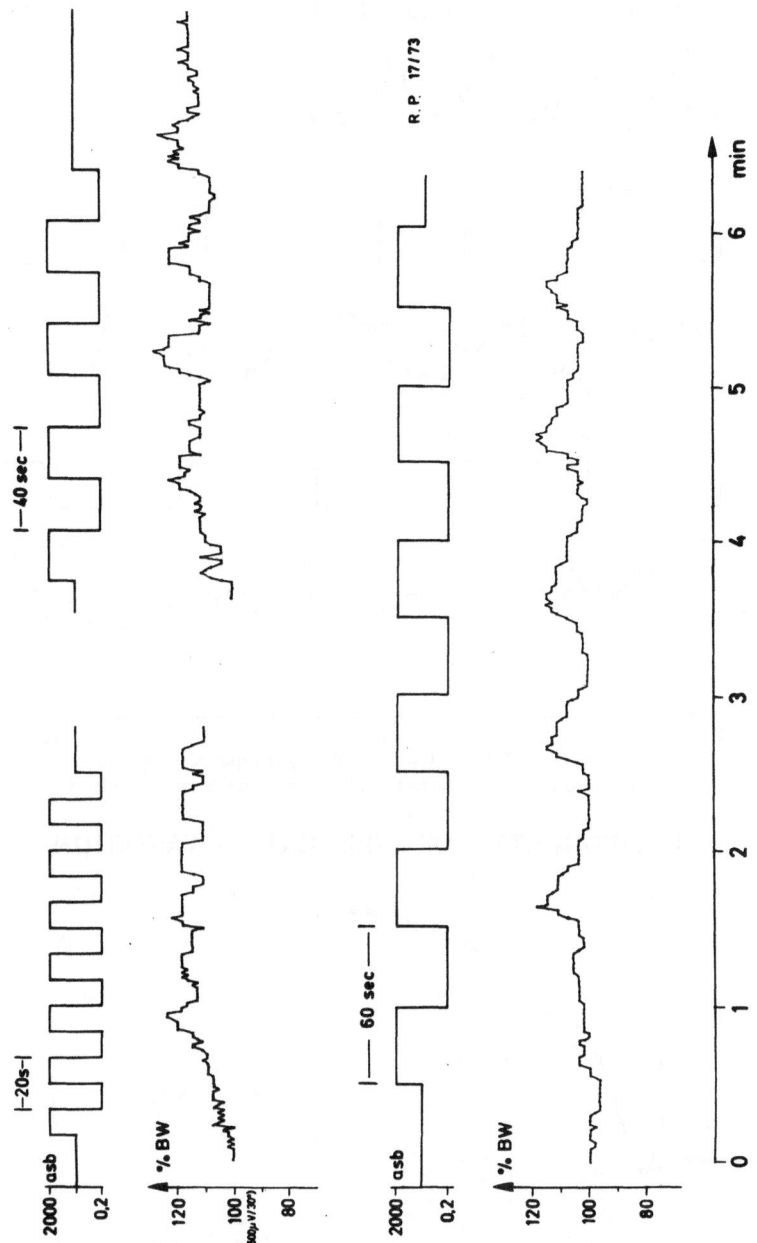

Fig. 4. Excitation of the on-peak by stimulation with square waves.

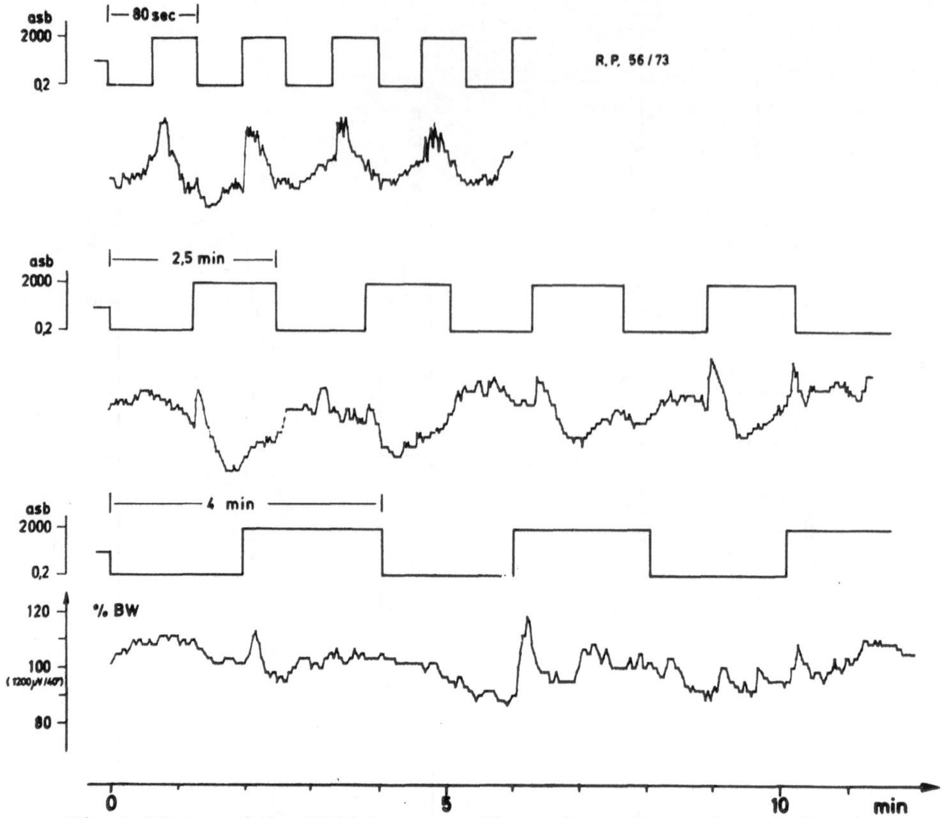

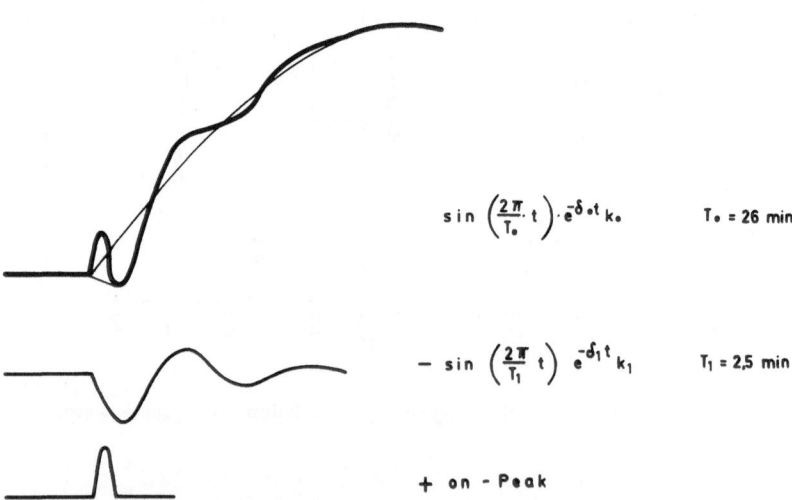

Fig. 5. Mixture of the ODM–fast wave with superimposed on-peaks excited by stimulation with square waves of period–times near 2,5 min.

COMPONENTS OF THE ODM - VARIATION

$$\sin\left(\frac{2\pi}{T_o} \cdot t\right) \cdot e^{-\delta_o t} k_o \qquad T_o = 26 \text{ min}$$

$$-\sin\left(\frac{2\pi}{T_1}t\right) e^{-\delta_1 t} k_1 \qquad T_1 = 2,5 \text{ min}$$

$$+ \text{ on - Peak}$$

Fig. 6. Summation of the single components of the ODM-variation to the light step response. On the dark step response the on-peak will be absent.

454

REFERENCES

ARDEN, G. B. & KELSEY, J. H. Changes Produced by Light in the Standing Potential of the Human Eye. *J. Physiol.* 161: *189-204* (1962).

ASERINSKY, E. Effects of Illumination and Sleep Upon Amplitude of Electro-Oculogram. *Arch. Ophthal.* 53: *542-546* (1955).

KOLDER, H. Spontane und experimentelle Änderungen des Bestandpotentials des menschlichen Auges. *Pflüg. Arch. Physiol.* 268: *258-272* (1959).

KOLDER, H. & BRECHER, G. A. Fast Oscillations of the Corneoretinal Potential in Man. *Arch. Ophthal.* 75: *232-237* (1966).

KOLDER, H. & NORTH, A. W. Oscillations of the Corneo-Retinal Potential in Animals. *Ophthalmologica* 152: *149-160* (1966).

KRIS, CH. Corneofundal Potential Variations During Light and Dark Adaptation. *Nature* 182: *1027-1028* (1958).

TÄUMER, R., HENNIG, J. & PERNICE, D. The Ocular Dipole – a Damped Oscillator Stimulated by the Speed of Change in Illumination. *Vision Res.* vol. 14 (1974).

Authors' address:

Department of Ophthalmology
University of Freiburg,
Germany

A FIRST ELECTRICAL ANALOG MODEL
OF THE ODM – OSCILLATIONS*

R. TÄUMER, H. KAPP, J. HENNIG & N. ROHDE

(Freiburg)

Summing up the results of our first two lectures we show in Fig. 1 the frequency characteristic response curve over the whole range investigated by us. We think that many wrong interpretations in the EOG experiments resulted from experiments performed with an experimental time too short to explore a damped oscillator with the extremely long period-time of half an hour. Regarding this we developed a model with an economic period-time (about 1 sec) and put in it all known results. Our model should show us immediately if the results of a recent experiment are in accordance with the properties of the ODM known by us from earlier studies. If there should be differences, we should see in this experiment new properties of the ocular dipole.

We can look at this device as an analogue computer. The advantage of an analogue model compared with a digital computer is the velocity of getting the results for new experimental conditions.

The outstanding points in constructing our model are:

1. a damped oscillator with a period-time of about 3,1 cps (main oscillation)
2. a damped oscillator with a period-time of one tenth of the first, of a smaller amplitude (about 25 % of the amplitude of the main oscillation) and inverse phase
3. an on-peak
4. a stronger damping of the system at lower levels

In Fig. 2, the realization of these points on our model is shown. The main parts are two parallel oscillating circuits (3,1 and 32 cps). In addition, there is a differentiator with a low pass filter which is responsible for the on-peak. The magnitude of the damping of the main oscillator will be controlled by the inverse of the current. We know that the two oscillations are quite different. They react in a different way with anaesthesia. Further there is a wide variation of the frequencies of the main oscillation in animals (KOLDER 1966). But in rabbits and dogs KOLDER found a resonance point at 2,2 min. Beside this, on a light step the main oscillation begins by increasing; whereas the fast oscillation starts by decreasing. Putting these facts in the model, it was necessary to take two parallel uninfluenced circuits.

Since all the components of the model can be separately modified, we have a

* Supported by the Deutsche Forschungsgemeinschaft SFB 70

457

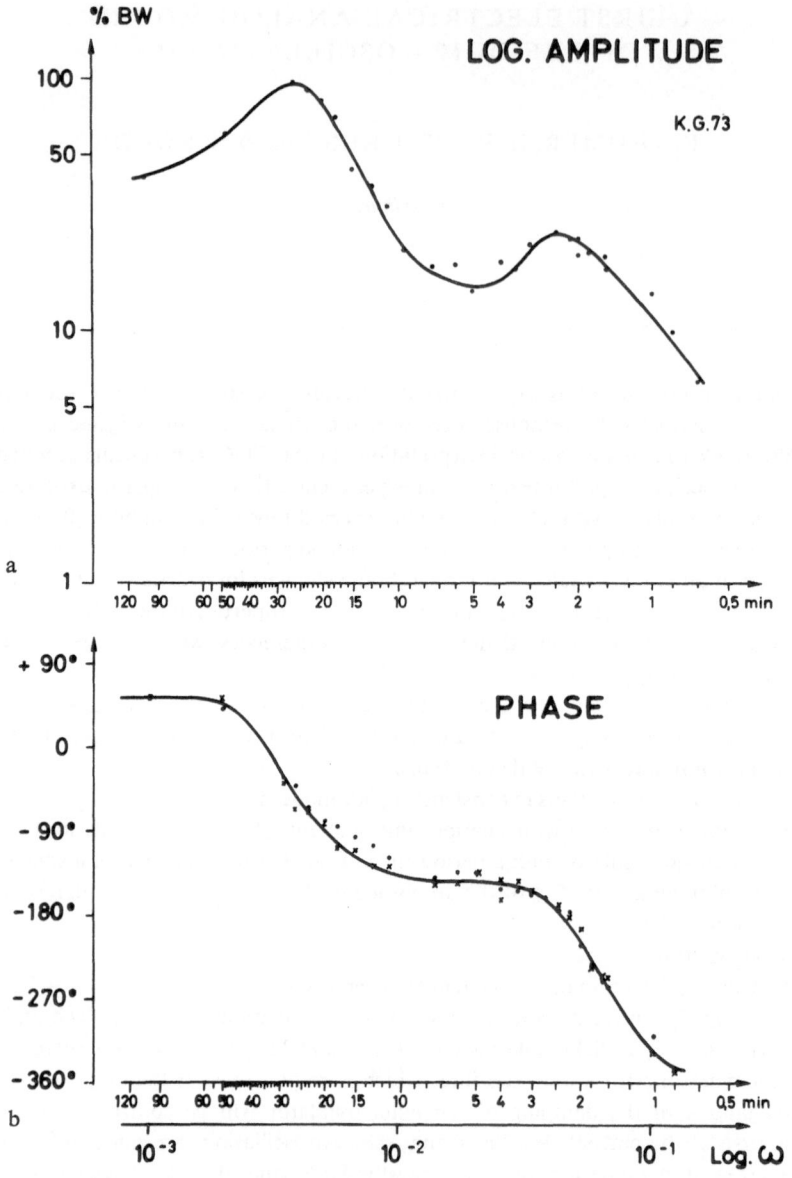

Fig. 1a. Bode-plot of the ODM-oscillation (log. amplitude and phase in dependence of log. frequency). Two resonance maxima of the amplitude at 23 and 2.5 min. Near the two resonance points the phase slides round about 180 deg down. b. Bode-plot of the model.

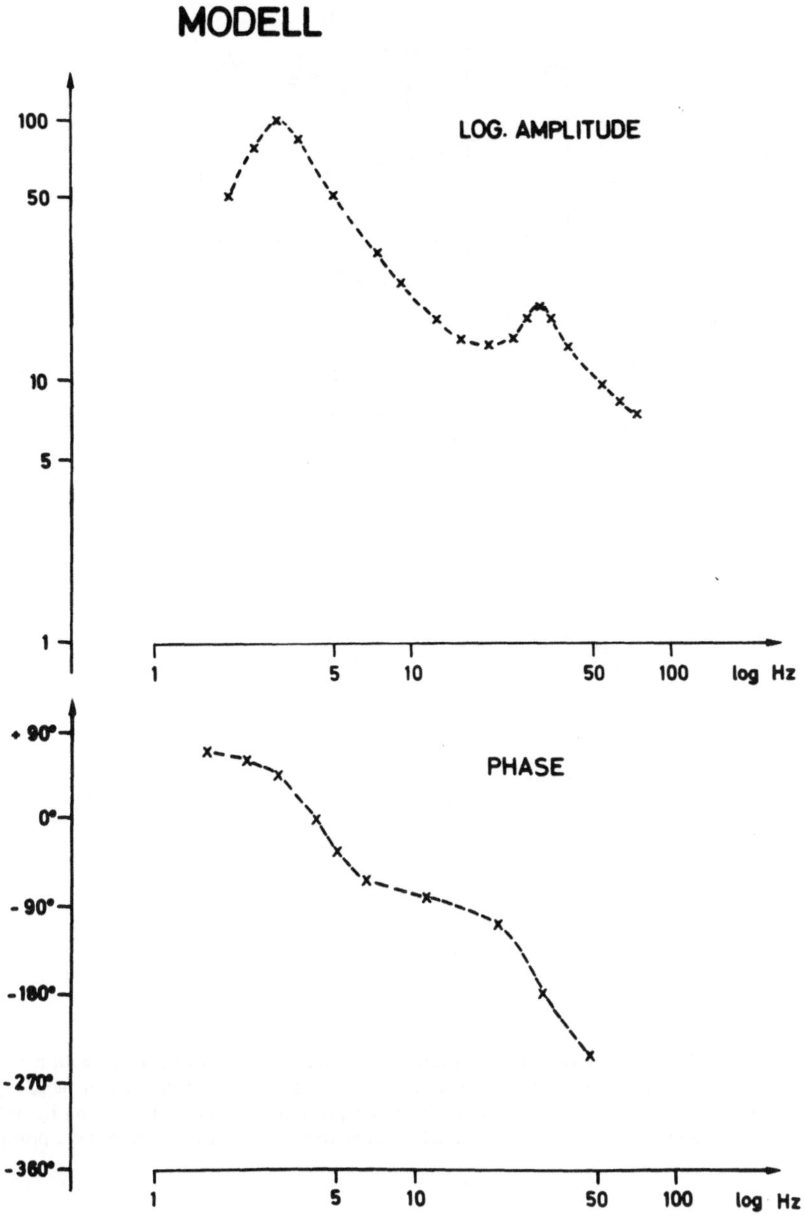

MODELL

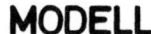

LOG. AMPLITUDE

PHASE

Fig. 2a.

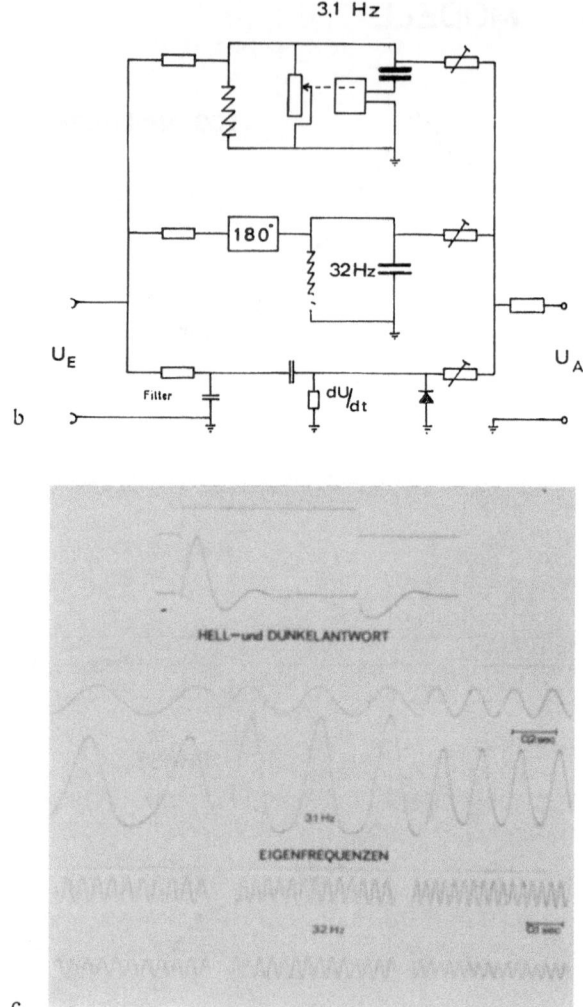

Fig. 2a. Model of the ODM-oscillation (one oscillating circuit of 3,1 cps with a level dependent variation of the resistance in the circuit; one oscillating circuit of 32 cps with an inverting input, a differentiator with a preceding filter); b. Excitation by light and dark step; c. Response of the model to sinus function near the two resonance points.

better understanding of the influence of one part of the system to the others.

Fig. 2b shows the different answer to 'light-' and 'dark-steps'. The higher damping at lower levels produces the flat minima at the main oscillation (Fig. 2c). The square wave (Fig. 3a) excites the fast oscillation. Superimposed on this at every 'light step', a peak occurs. Continuously increasing light will produce a small elevation of the ODM level (Fig. 3b). Fig. 4 shows the superimposition of the three single components (4b) and the comparison of the step response with

460

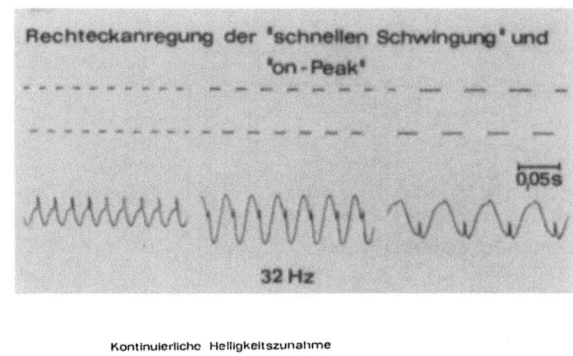

a

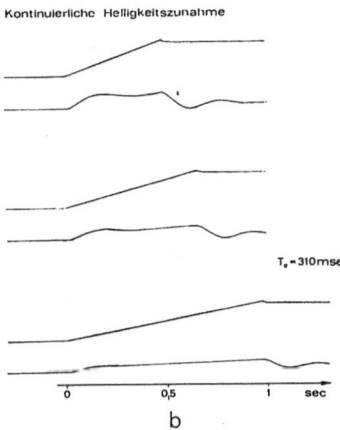

b

Fig. 3. Response of the model to: a. square waves; b. continuously increasing luminance.

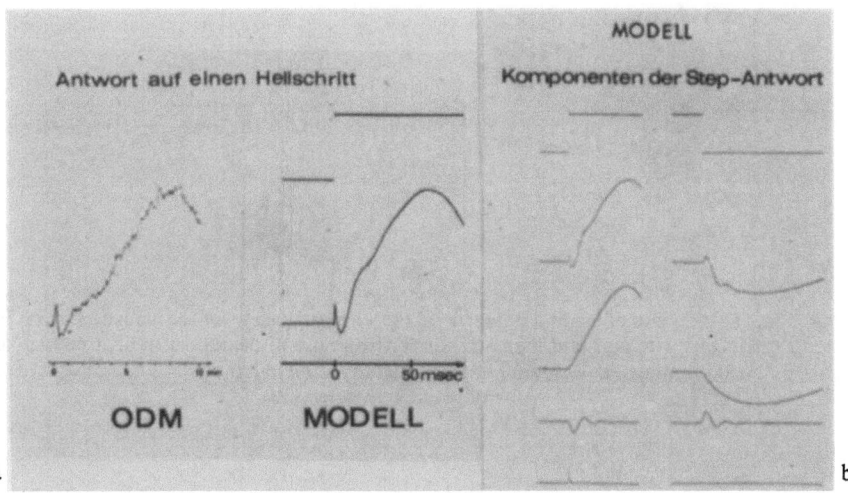

a

b

Fig. 4a. Comparison of the light step answer of the ODM with the model; b. The
single components of the model.

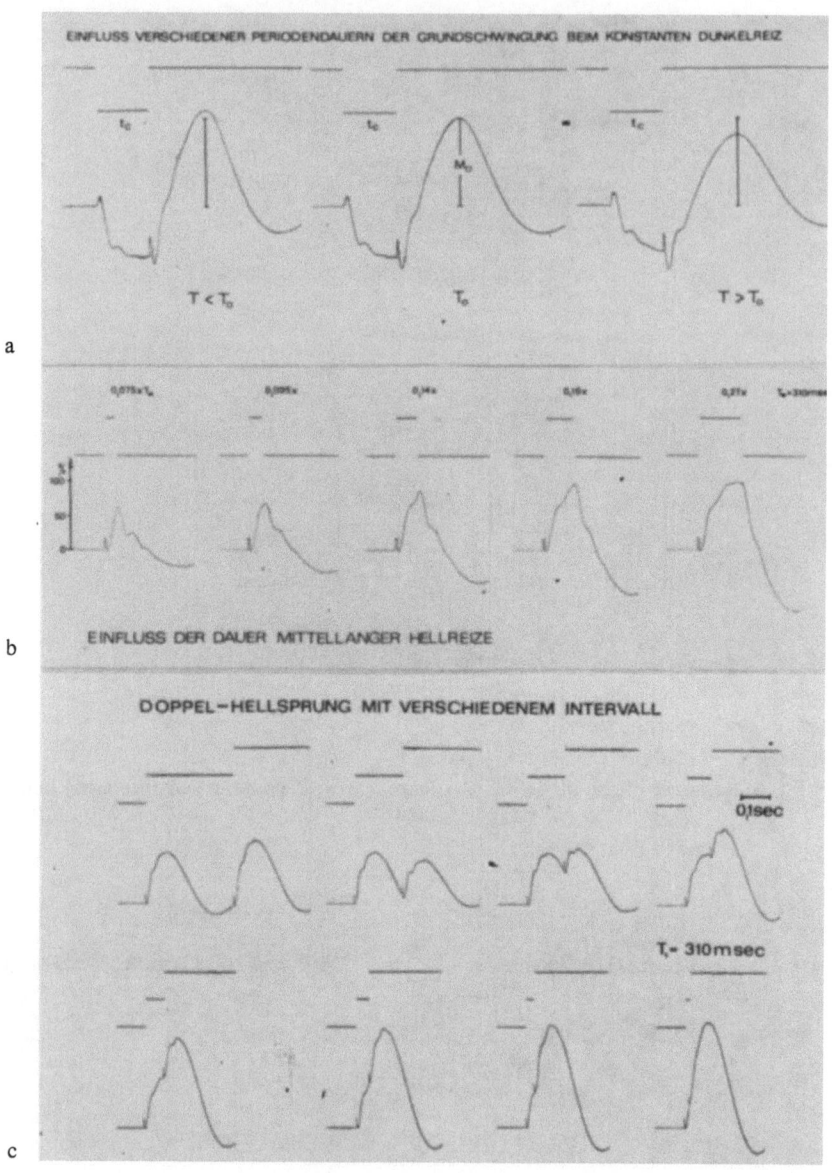

Fig. 5a. Influence of small differencies in the 'eigenfrequency' of the main oscillation in experiments with constant dark periods; b. Response of the model to light periods of different durations; c. Response of the model to a double-jump of luminance separated by different time intervals.

the step response of the original ODM. The importance of the onset of a second step put to the system at different points of the phase is seen in Fig. 5.

462

REFERENCES

KOLDER, H. & NORTH, A. W. Oscillations of the Corneo-Retinal Potential in Animals. *Ophthalmologica* 152: *149-160* (1966).

Authors' address:

Department of Ophthalmology
University of Freiburg
Germany

SLOW OCULAR DIPOLE MOMENT (ODM)
VARIATION – A DAMPED OSCILLATION*

R. TÄUMER, J. HENNIG & D. PERNICE

(Freiburg)

Physically the human eye is an electrical dipole. It has a negative pole at the fundus and a positive pole at the cornea. These two loads are separated by the diameter of the eye which is constant. The characteristic properties of such a dipole are the amount of the loads and the distance between them. The adequate description of a dipole is the dipole moment, which is the product of the loads and the separating distance. This ocular dipole causes an electric field which includes the surrounding tissues. The strength at the field is proportional to the dipole moment. If we compare the electrical effects of identical eye movements on a recorder for electro-nystagmography, we get an analogue function of this dipole (indirectly). Consequently, we speak of the ocular dipole moment (ODM). We prefer this expression because it is more exact then others used (Bestandpotential, Standing potential, Corneoretinal potential).

Following a light step the ODM will change like a damped oscillator (KRIS, KOLDER, ARDEN, TÄUMER) as the Fig. 1 shows. We will show that the damped oscillation is one of the most important properties of this system and must be carefully taken in consideration in all experiments involving this system.

Fig. 2 shows the stimulation of the system with repetitive dark and light steps

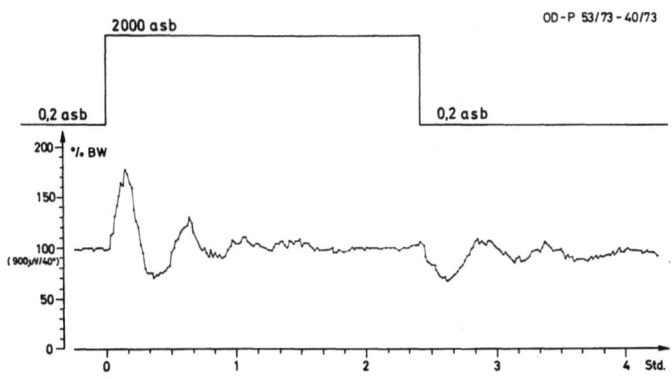

Fig. 1. The variation of the ODM following a step increase and decrease of 4 decimal logarithmical luminance units. Before the light step an adaptation of 1 hour with 0,2 asb was used until a steady base level (BL) was reached.

* Supported by the Deutsche Forschungsgemeinschaft SFB 70.

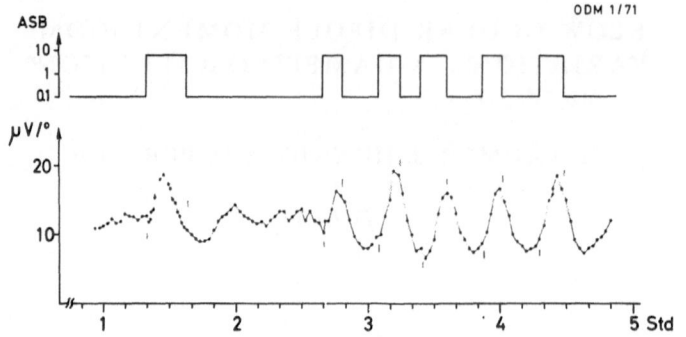

Fig. 2. Steady oscillation of the ODM excited by a sequence of light and dark steps.

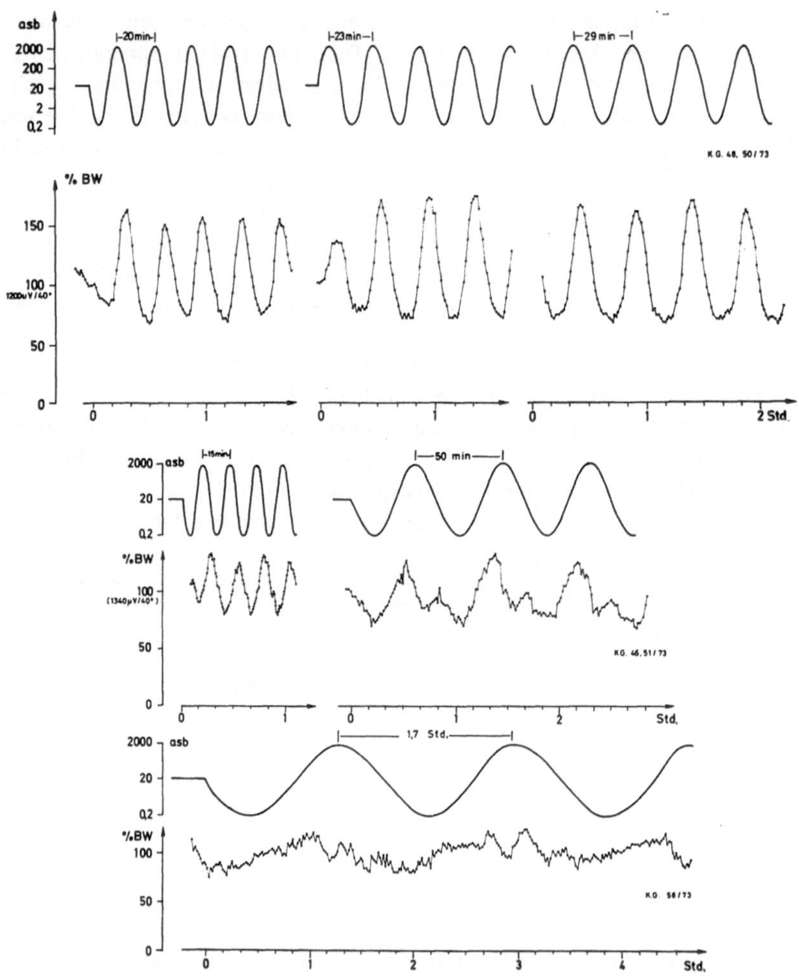

Fig. 3a. Stimulation of the ODM with sinus functions of frequencies near the resonance point. b. Stimulation of the ODM with sinus functions of frequencies far away from the resonance point.

466

of 2 log units. A steady oscillation of the ODM will appear. If we look more precisely, we notice differences in the amplitude of the oscillations. Since all luminance steps are the same, only the variable intervals between the steps can be responsible. We recognize that the time relation is of great importance in our problem.

The most effective stimulation for a damped oscillation is a sinus function. Because of the sensitivity of the human visual system to the logarithm of the luminance, we used an exponential sinus. Fig. 3 shows the result of the ODM to sinus of 4 log units amplitude and of different period-times. The maximal amplitude of the ODM oscillation we found at a period-time of 23 min. The system will also be stimulated by longer and shorter periods of the exciting sinus, but with smaller amplitudes. At a certain period-time of the sinus, the amplitude of the ODM is linearly correlated with the logarithm of the amplitude of the sinus.

In Fig. 4 the amplitude and the phase behaviour in relation to the period-time of the stimulating sinus is shown. This diagram is characteristic of a damped oscillator. With a period time of 23 min, a resonance maximum of the amplitude occurs. In the region between 60 and 15 min, the ODM oscillation comes down from + 60° to −100°. In case of resonance there is only a small phase difference. As the pendulum is a typical oscillator there is a phase difference of −90° between the force and the position.

From this phase behaviour we conclude that there must be a differentiating

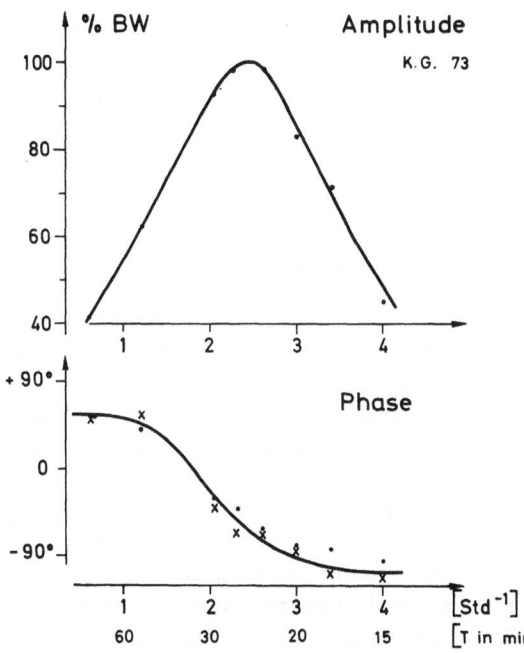

Fig. 4. Dependence of the amplitude and the phase of the ODM-oscillation on the period-time of the stimulating sinus.

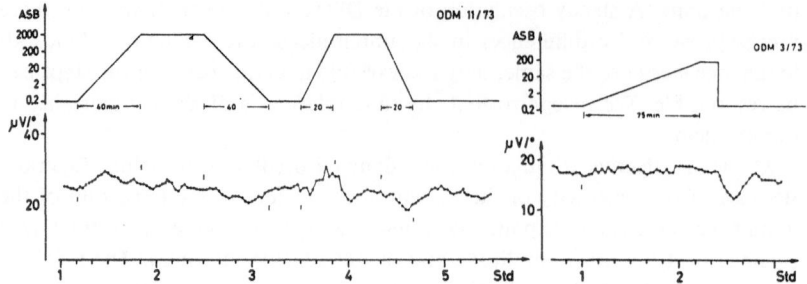

Fig. 5. Stimulation of the ODM with continuously increasing and decreasing light intensity.

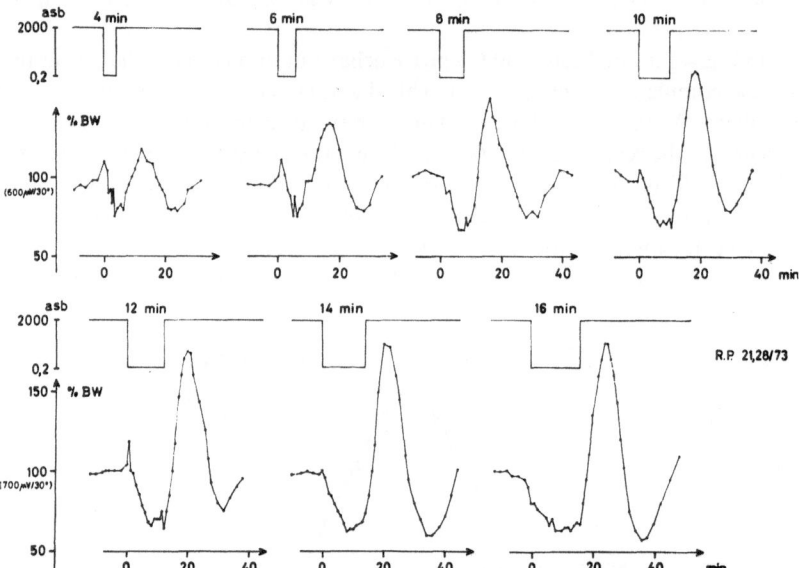

Fig. 6. Influence of dark stimuli of different duration on the variation of the ODM.

process at the input. Therefore, we stimulated the ocular dipole with a slowly increasing and decreasing light (Fig. 5). If the luminance is increased 3 log units in 75 min, or 4 log units in 40 min, you don't see a significant variation of the ODM. A change of 4 log units in 20 min will produce a discernible response. That means that a rate of change of 4 log units in 40 min (1 log unit/10 min) is the limit for any provable effect, if the ODM is measured by skin electrodes.

If we apply step stimuli to this oscillating system, we must look carefully to the phase relation. In the first approximation the ODM system reacts in a linear way. This means the first step will excite an oscillation, and also the second one. The summation of these two waves will give the resulting oscillation. Fig. 6 shows the effect of a dark step followed by a light step. The two steps are separated by different time intervals. At small intervals the light step excites a wave in the inverse phase to the dark wave. With longer intervals (14 and 16 min) the light wave comes more and more in phase with the dark wave. These two waves sum up to larger amplitudes.

REFERENCES

ARDEN, G. B. & KELSEY, J. H. Changes Produced by Light in the Standing Potential of the Human Eye. *J. Physiol.* 161: *189-204* (1962).

KOLDER, H. Spontane und experimentelle Änderungen des Bestandpotentials des menschlichen Auges. *Pflüg. Arch. Physiol.* 268: *258-272* (1959).

KRIS, CH. Corneo-fundal Potential Variations during Light and Dark Adaptation. *Nature* 182: *1027-1028* (1958).

TÄUMER, R., HENNIG. J. & PERNICE, D. The Ocular Dipole – a Damped Oscillator Stimulated by the Speed of Change in Illumination. *Vision Res.* vol. 14 (1974).

TÄUMER, R., MACKENSEN, G., HARTMANN, H., MOSER, U., STEHLE, R., WERNER, W. & WOLF, D. Änderung des 'Bestandpotentials' des menschlichen Auges nach Belichtungsänderungen. *Graefes Arch. klin. exp. Ophthal.* 189: *81-97* (1974).

Authors' address:

Department of Ophthalmology
University of Freiburg
Germany

THRESHOLDS OF THE OSCILLATORY POTENTIALS IN MICE.

I. WATANABE & K. A. HELLNER

(Hamburg)

ABSTRACT

The spectral sensitivity curve of the b-wave and the oscillatory potentials reveals no photopic activity. This finding is confirmed by evaluation of the increment thresholds of the b-wave and the oscillatory potentials. Using coloured lights no Purkinje-shift was observed. The increment thresholds of the b-wave obey the WEBER's law.

The oscillatory potentials show no increase of their sensitivity with increasing adaptive illumination. On the contrary, the thresholds fall with moderate light adaptation. The amplitudes of the oscillatory potentials gain voltage and reach their maximum after 4-5 repeated stimuli. These facts demonstrate that the oscillatory potentials show an independant behaviour towards retinal sensitivity; they are facilitated by repeated stimuli. Most probably they represent rebound phenomena in the retina.

Our investigations are concerned with the elaboration and description of phenomena which should demonstrate the independance of the b-wave and the oscillatory potentials (o.p.). Such differences in their behaviour have been already described in clinical study in man (ALGVERE, 1968; KURACHI, HIROSE & YONEMURA; JACOBSON, HIROSE & POPKIN, 1967 and YONEMURA, TSUZULI & AOKI, 1962). However, in the literature up to the present time only a few quantitative reports have been published on this phenomenon (ALGVERE & WESTBECK, 1972 and ALGVERE, WACHTHEIMER & WESTBECK, 1972).

Our present experiments are concerned with mice. These animals do not possess photopic activity (HELLNER, 1966 and WATANABE, RICKERS & HELLNER, 1972). Previous observations regarding the spectral sensitivity of the b-wave are confirmed through studies on the spectral behaviour of the o.p. (WATANABE, RICKERS & HELLNER, 1972). Therefore, these animals seem to be especially suitable for studying differentiations in the b-wave and the o.p. using the method of measurement of the increment threshold. This classical method for measurement of visual sensitivity has been extended from DODT et al. (DODT & JESSEN, 1960) to the ERG. According to DODT et al. in nocturnal animals like rats the threshold of the ERG in cygloplegic pupil increases parallel to the ratio of the adaptive illumination.

20 albinotic and 10 pigmented mice were used in these experiments, and were dark-adapted over night. Operative and ERG recording procedures have already been described (HELLNER, 1966; WATANABE, RICKERS & HELLNER, 1972). The ERG recordings were carried out starting always with weak stimuli (log −8.0 to log 0.0; the 0.0 log unit relative light energy corresponds to 1 × 10^3 cd/m²). The background illumination amounts to 1.7 × 10^2cd/m², while no neutral filters were employed in the optic pathway. For constant maintenance of the retinal adaptive state, before each ERG recording, 5 min light adaptation period was introduced using the light energy of the next higher adaptive level. Per minute 6 light stimuli of each 40 ms were repeated.

FINDINGS

Firstly, the amplitude of the b-wave and the o.p. are plotted against the relative energy of the light stimulus (Fig. 1). With background illumination stronger than log −3.0, the curves representing the amplitude to log light energy relationship became flatter when compared with those of the dark adapted state as well as in the range of log adaptive illumination of −7.0 to −4.0. However, energy measurements at the threshold criterion of 15 μV are little affected by the decrease of the maximum voltage of the potentials.

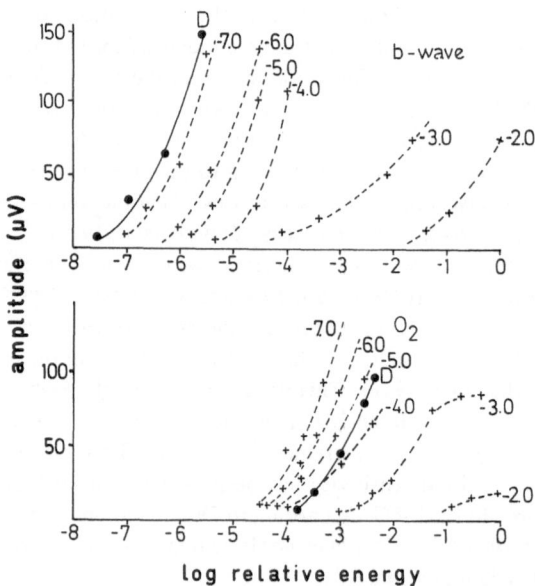

Fig. 1. Curves relating amplitude of the b-wave and the oscillatory potentials to light energy. (D = dark adaptation; each curve refers to a given light adaptation level (log −7,0 to log 0,0)).

If we plot the constant ERG response against the log adaptive illumination, the threshold of the b-wave increases fairly with WEBER's law ($\triangle$ I/I = constant), except for very high adaptive illumination (log -2.0). This result at high illumination most probably is caused from the flat course of the amplitude/light energy relationship curve.

As previously described, the o.p. in mice appear in the sequence of O_3, O_2 and O_1. The light energy necessary to evoke O_3 is in the same range as to produce the a-wave. The light necessary to record O_1 is 1.0 log unit higher than required for O_3 and O_2. These thresholds differences vanished when background illumination above log -5.0 was employed. The values of the increment thresholds of the o.p. are fairly constant. Thus, WEBER's law is not obeyed. On the contrary the thresholds fall during moderate light adaptations. At high illumination the threshold of O_2 lies only 1-2 log units higher than that of the dark adapted eye.

Under these conditions the determination of the threshold criterion becomes more difficult due to the flattening of amplitude/light energy relationship curve.

Using coloured lights, instead of the white the increment thresholds of the b-wave also show fair constant curves. A 0.5-0.7 log unit difference of threshold is measured between the light of 460 nm and 600 nm. There is a parallel rise of the thresholds for blue and red lights. A PURKINJE-shift is being missed indicating a shift of the sensitivity curve towards longer wavelength as compared to the spectral sensitivity curve during dark adaptation.

The o.p. show no significant changes of their thresholds with test lights of 500 nm and 600 nm. With blue test lights the increment thresholds seem to increase steadily in a small range. The differences of the thresholds between the measurements with blue and red amounts to 0.5-0.7 log units light energy. However, a PURKINJE-shift is absent.

As shown in the experiment with white test lights (Fig. 2) the thresholds of the o.p. decreased under dim background illumination. To verify this result following experiments were carried out:

a. repeated measurements of the ERG at near of b-wave threshold (Fig. 3).

The amplitudes were measured using log -7.0 and log -6.3 relative light energy. The first recording was conducted after a dark adaptation of 24 h and more (black dots); after a period of 10 s the next measurement was taken (circles). Repeated stimuli of constant energy do not yield constant amplitudes. After prolonged dark adaptation the higher stimulus (log -6.3) yields higher amplitudes. This behaviour does not coincide with the usual experience, that following light adaptation the b-wave amplitude decrease. However, an opposite behaviour towards light adaptation of low degree has been reported elsewhere (ALGVERE, 1968).

b. measurements at o.p. threshold (Fig. 4):

Primarily the o.p. are recognized at relative light energy levels of log -3.6. However, on repetition of the light stimuli they are recordable at the low stimuli of only log -4.3. These changes of O_1, O_2 and O_3 are demonstrated graphically in Fig. 5. It is clear from this figure that the amplitudes of the o.p. in-

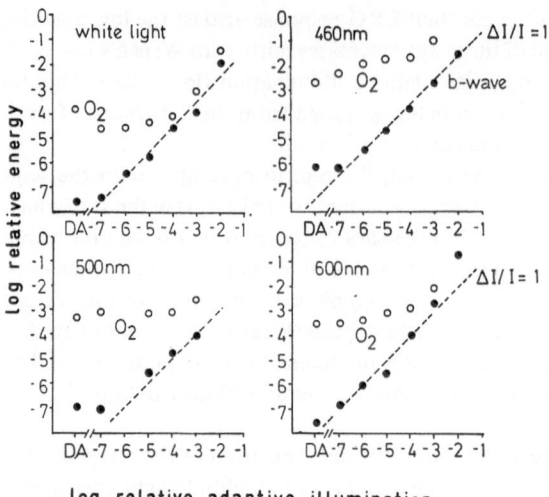

Fig. 2. White and coloured light in test beam required for constant ERG response at various adaptation levels. (Black dots = b-wave; circles = oscillatory potentials: DA = dark adaptation).

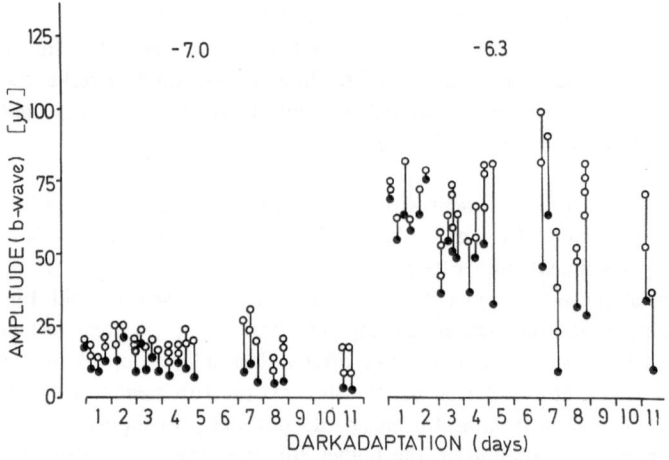

Fig. 3. Amplitudes of the b-wave, repeated stimulated with light energy at near of threshold (log –7.0; log –6.3; black dots = after dark adaptation, circles = repeated stimuli, frequency: 6 c/min; stimulus duration 40 ms).

creased till 3rd and 4th recording. Subsequently, at further stimuli they remained practically unchanged. Present results clearly prove that while using stimuli at near of the thresholds the relative enlargement of the o.p. is greater than that of the b-wave.

474

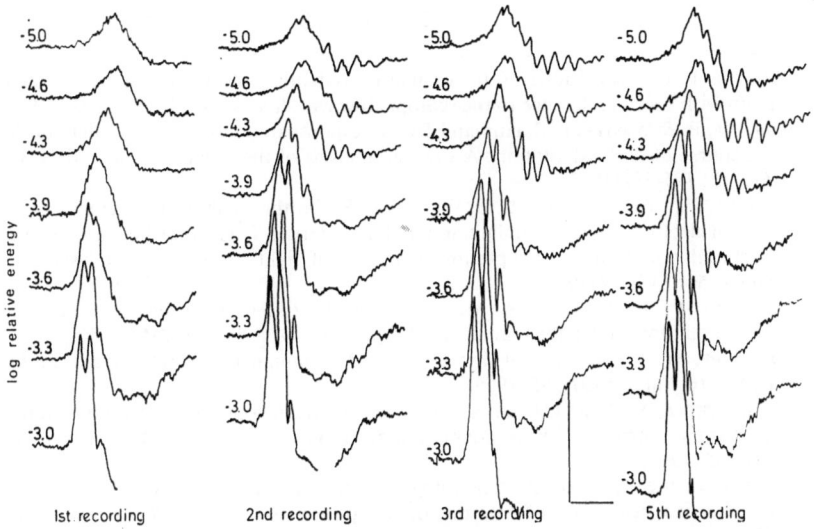

Fig. 4. Thresholds of the oscillatory potentials. Per minute 6 light stimuli of each 40 ms were repeated.

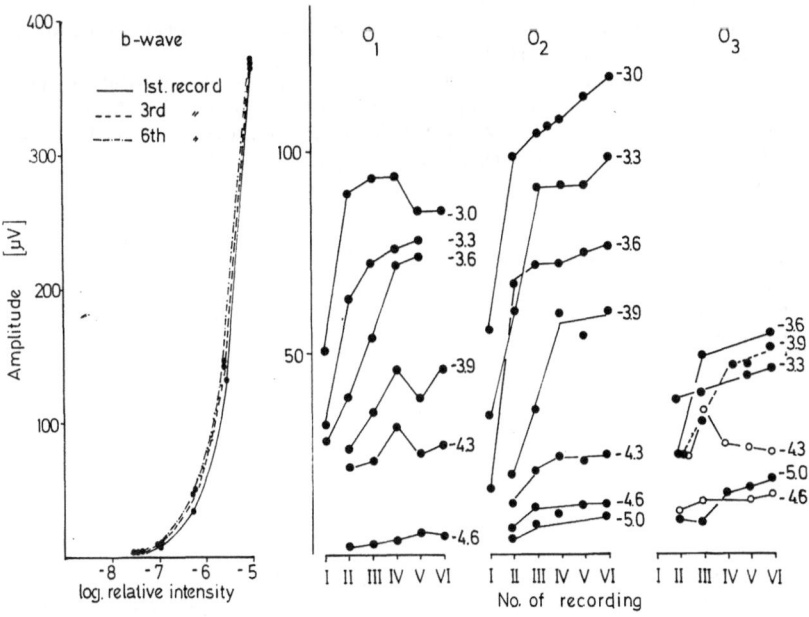

Fig. 5. Graphica representation of the amplitudes of the oscillatory potentials during repeated stimulation.

475

REFERENCES

ALGVERE, P. Clinical studies on the oscillatory potentials of the human electroretino-gram with special reference to the scotopic b-wave. *Acta Ophth.* 46: *993-1025* (1968).

ALGVERE, P. & WESTBECK, S. Human ERG in response to double flashes of light during the course of dark adaptation: A Fourier analysis of the oscillatory potentials. *Vis. Res.* 12: *195-214* (1972).

ALGVERE, P., WACHTHEIMER, L. & WESTBECK, S. On the oscillatory potentials of the human electroretinogram in light and dark adaptation. I. The threshold and relation to stimulus intensity on adaptation to flashes of light. A Fourier analysis. *Acta Ophth.* 50: *737-759* (1972).

BIERSDORF, W. R., GRANDA, A. M. & LOWSON, H. F. Electrical measurement of in-cremental threshold in the human eye. *J. Opt. Soc. Amer.* 55: *454-455* (1965).

BIERSDORF, W. R. Incremental threshold and the human Electroretinogram. *J. Jap. Ophth.* 10, Suppl.: *191-197* (1966).

DE MOLFETTA, V., SPINELLI, D. & POLENGHI, F. Behaviour of electroretinographic oscillatory potentials during adaptation to darkness. *A. M. A. Arch. Ophth.* 79: *531-535* (1968).

DODT, E. & JESSEN, K. H. Elektroretinographische Messung der Unterschiedsschwelle (increment threshold) bei Steigerung der adaptiven Beleuchtung. *Ber. Dtsch. Ophth. Ges.* 63: *319-322* (1960).

JACOBSON, J. H., HIROSE, T. & POPKIN, A. B. Oscillatory potentials of the electro-retinogram: Relationship to photopic b-wave in human. *A. M. A. Arch. Ophth.* 78: *58-68* (1967).

HELLNER, K. A. Das adaptive Verhalten der Mäusenetzhaut. *v. Graefes Arch. klin. exp. Ophth.* 169: *166-175* (1966).

KURACHI, Y., HIROSE, T. & YONEMURA, D. ERG in pulseless (Takayasu's) disease. *J. Jap. Ophth.* 10 (suppl.): H1-H7.

WATANABE, I., RICKERS, J. & HELLNER, K. A. Spectral sensitivity of oscillatory poten-tials in mice, rats, guinea pigs and rabbits. ISCERG Symposium, Los Angeles (1972).

YONEMURA, D., TSUZUKI, K. & AOKI, T. Clinical importance of the oscillatory poten-tial in the human ERG. *Acta Ophth. Suppl.* 70: *115-123* (1962).

Authors' address:

Universitäts-Krankenhaus Eppendorf
Universitäts-Augenklinik und -Poliklinik
Elektrophysiologische Abteilung
Hamburg
DBR

THRESHOLDS OF THE OSCILLATORY POTENTIALS
OF THE HUMAN ERG

L. WACHTMEISTER

(Stockholm)

Little is known of the light stimulus necessary for eliciting the oscillatory potentials of the human ERG at threshold. It has been stated that the oscillatory potentials are augmentated with an increase of light stimulus intensity (YONEMURA, TSUZUKI & AOKI, 1962; TSUCHIDA, KAWASAKI & JACOBSON, 1971). The frequency of the oscillatory potentials was reported to be around 140 Hz (BORNSCHEIN & GOODMAN, 1957) and unaltered despite the fact that stimulus intensity was varied (YONEMURA, TSUZUKI & AOKI, 1962).

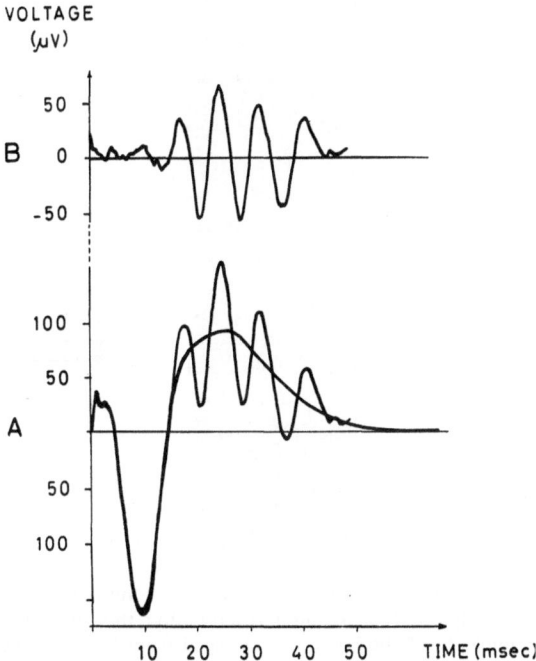

Fig. 1. Method of computer calculation of the residual function i.e. the oscillatory potential by means of a combined impulse response analysis. A. Total ERG and the curve approximating the biphasic slow response (a- and b-waves). B. Isolated oscillatory potentials including base-line noise, as the residual function after substraction of the approximating curve (shown in A) from the total ERG.

At the Department of ophthalmology,/Karolinska Hospital, Stockholm, Sweden we have studied the oscillatory potentials of the human ERG after adaptation to short flashes of light and then in response to varying stimulus intensity. Besides this study, the effect of adaptation to a continuous background illumination and the incremental thresholds have also been investigated. Unfortunately, time does not allow further presentation than the first mentioned study which was performed in colloboration with ALGVERE and WESTBECK.

The ERG was recorded after dark adaptation of 30 minutes in 4 healthy and young subjects. This apparatus previously described by ALGVERE (1968) was used.

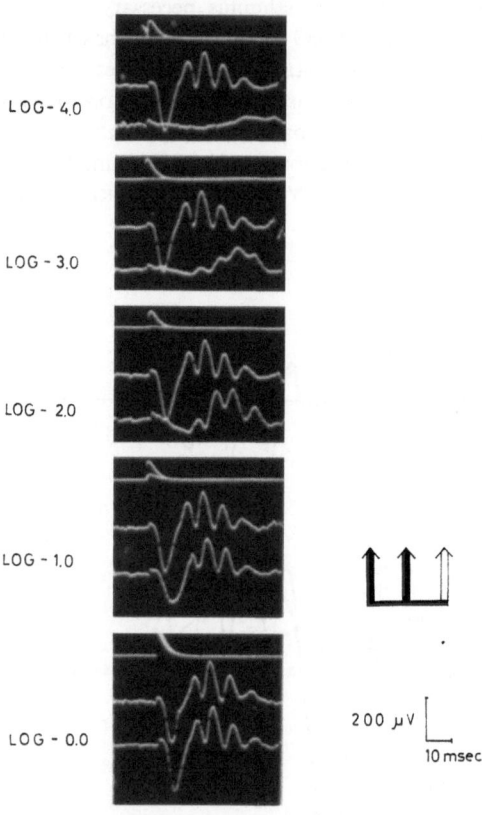

I.M.   STIMULUS LIGHT INTENSITY

LOG- 4.0

LOG - 3.0

LOG - 2.0

LOG - 1.0

LOG - 0.0

200 μV

10 msec

Fig. 2. Oscillatory potentials after adaptation to two (conditioning) flashes of constant and maximal intensity (log I_s = 0) and in response to a third (stimulus) flash of varied intensity. The intensity of the latter was changed from log I_s = 5,0 to log I_s = 0. The flashes were given every 30 sec. throughout this experiment. Oscillatory potentials first appeared at a stimulation intensity of log I_s = -3,0. Each picture shows the ERG in response to the second conditioning flash and the third stimulus flash. Stimulation pattern is symbolized by vertical arrows (flashes), connected by horizontal bar (time interval between flashes). Black symbols denote a constant condition, white symbol is a variable.

478

Traces of a scotopic b-wave were recorded by a stimulus intensity of log I = -8.0. On repetitive light stimulation with intervals of 5 minutes between the flashes a scotopic b-wave of about 20 μV was not recorded until the intensity of the stimulus light was log I = -6.0. A photopic b-wave appeared at a stimulus intensity of log I = -4.0. An a-wave of about 50 μV amplitude was elicited by a stimulus intensity of log I = -3.3.

To study the threshold of the oscillatory potentials, three consecutive flashes were given at an interval of 30 seconds and the ERG in response to the third flash was evaluated.

A mathematical evaluation of the amplitude and frequency of the oscillatory potentials was made possible by a combined impulse response and Fourier analysis (see ALGVERE & WESTBECK 1972). To each ERG-response an approximate function was sought by the aid of an analysing program of a computer. This approximate function was subtracted from our recorded ERG. The residual function then represented the isolated oscillatory potentials. (Fig. 1). Using Fourier analysis the energy density spectrum of the isolated oscillations was obtained. The energy and dominant frequency were then calculated.

In one experiment the threshold of the oscillations was studied after two conditioning flashes of maximal intensity (5×10^4 phot cd/m²). The intensity of the latter was varied and thereby increased by steps of one log unit. The oscillatory potentials appeared at a stimulation intensity of log I = -3.0. (Fig. 2). The peak latency for each individual oscillation showed a fairly uniform diminution with increasing intensity. (Fig. 3). The dominant frequency of the oscillations did

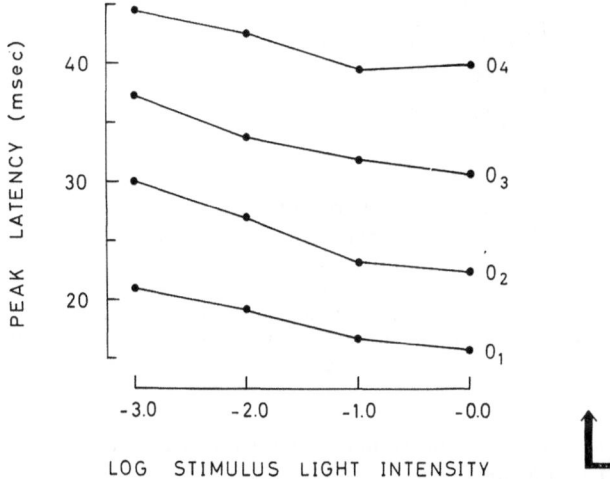

Fig. 3. Peak latencies of individual oscillatory peaks (0_1, 0_2, 0_3, 0_4) as plotted against log intensity of the third (stimulus) flash from ERGs shown in Fig. 2. The conditioning flashes were of constant and maximal intensity and that of the third (stimulus) flash, was varied. There was a fairly uniform decrease of peak latencies for all four oscillations. The average error of repetitive calliper-squale readings was less than 0,5 msec. symbols of stimulation pattern, as in Fig. 2.

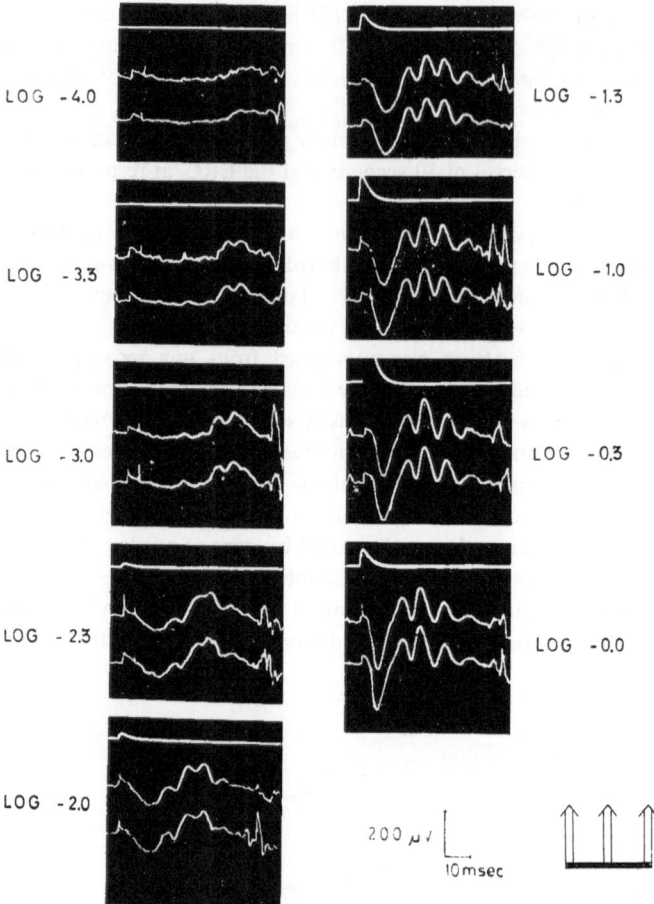

LOG -4.0

LOG -3.3

LOG -3.0

LOG -2.3

LOG -2.0

LOG -1.3

LOG -1.0

LOG -0.3

LOG -0.0

200 μv

10 msec

Fig. 4. Oscillatory potentials recorded after adaptation two (conditioning) flashes of the same intensity as the third (stimulus) flash. The intensity of all three flashes was succeedingly increased from log - 5 to log 0. The interval between the three flashes in each series was 30 seconds, and five minutes elapsed before a following series of stronger flashes was given. Symbols of stimulation pattern as in Fig. 2. Each picture shows the ERG in response to the second (conditioning) flash and the (third) stimulus flash.

not change significantly as the stimulus intensity increased. It was calculated to be 121-126 Hz. (Fig. 6).

In another study, the two conditioning flashes and the third stimulus flash were of the same intensity, which was varied for all three over 5 log units. The oscillatory potentials appeared at a stimulation intensity of $\log I = -3.3$. (Fig. 4). The time intervals between individual peaks were comparatively short when recorded in response to weak stimulation. As the stimulus intensity increased the

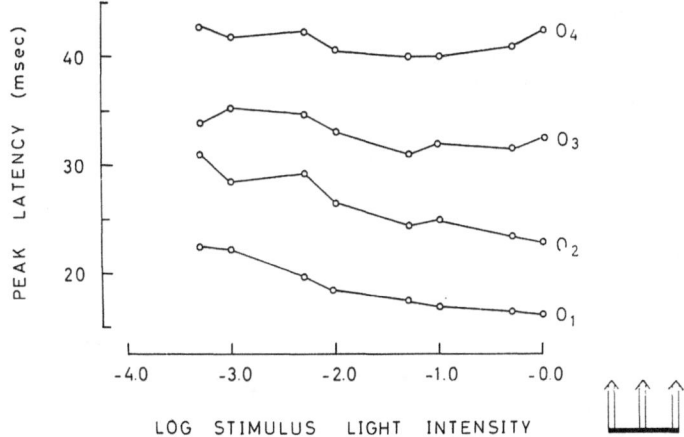

Fig. 5. Peak latencies of individual oscillatory peaks (O_1, O_2, O_3, O_4) as plotted against log intensity of the third (stimulus) flash from ERGs shown in Fig. 4. The two conditioning flashes and the third (stimulus) flash had the same intensity. Peak latencies for the first two oscillations (O_1, O_2) declined an increasing stimulus intensity. Peak latencies for O_3 and O_4 showed no distinct change. The same error of measurements as in Fig. 3. Symbols of stimulation pattern as in Fig. 2.

time interval between each individual peak prolonged. (Fig. 5). The dominant frequency of the oscillations was around 155 Hz at threshold stimulation intensity (log $= I -3.3$). There was a subsequent decline in frequency with an increase of stimulation intensity. With the strongest stimuli used the dominant frequency decreased to about 110 Hz. (Fig. 6). This was also clearly demonstrated on the isolated oscillations.

The energy of the oscillatory potentials was found to increase linearly with augmentation of light stimulus intensity over a range of 3 log units.

In summary, traces of oscillations were recorded at approximately the same stimulation intensity as the a-wave. In another study the incremental threshold curves of the a-wave and the oscillatory potentials were also found to be similar. This similarity in sensitivity of the a-wave and the oscillations indicate that the a-wave (reflecting activity of the receptor cells) must stimulate the regeneration of the oscillatory potentials.

The oscillations evoked at threshold differed in frequency from the high intensity oscillatory response. When the state of adaptation was kept constant, this frequency was not fundamentally changed. Thus, the dominant frequency varies with the retinal adaptation caused by short flashes of light. Later experiments have also shown that bleaching photopigments by using steady background light did not decrease the high frequency of the oscillatory potentials at threshold. Thus, the alteration in frequency must be based on other events of the retina – probably changes in neural organization.

481

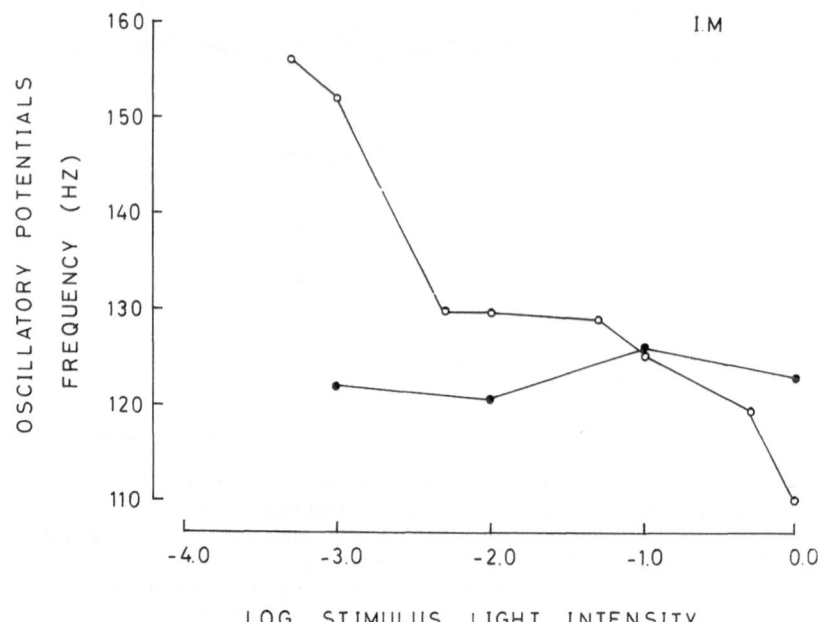

LOG STIMULUS LIGHT INTENSITY

Fig. 6. Dominant frequency of oscillatory potentials plotted against log stimulus light intensity of the third (stimulus) flash, eliciting ERGs shown in Fig. 2 and 4. Black circles: The two conditioning flashes were of constant and maximal intensity and the luminance of the third (stimulus) flash was succeedingly increased. Open circles: The conditioning flashes and the third (stimulus) flash were of the same intensity, which for all three flashes, was succeedingly increased. When the conditioning light adaptation was kept constant there was no significant change in oscillatory frequency (black circles). When the conditioning flashes and the third (stimulus) flash were of the same intensity (white circles) the dominant frequency of oscillatory potentials decreased on succeeding stronger light adaptation and increasing stimulus intensity.

REFERENCES

ALGVERE, P. Clinical studies on the oscillatory potentials of the human electroretinogram with special reference to the scotopic b-wave. *Acta Ophthal. (Kbh)* 46: *993-1025* (1968).

ALGVERE, P. & WESTBECK, S. Human ERG in response to double flashes of light during the course of dark adaptation: A Fourier analysis of the oscillatory potentials. *Vision Res.* 12: *195-214* (1972).

BORNSCHEIN, H. & GOODMAN, G. Studies of the a-wave in the human electroretinogram A.M.A. *Arch. Ophthal.* 58: *431-437* (1957).

TSUCHIDA, S., KAWASAKI, K. & JACOBSON, J. Rhythmic wavelets of the positive off-effect in human electroretinogram. *Amer. J. Ophthal.* 72: *60-69* (1971).

YONEMURA, D. TSUZYKI, K. & AOKI, T. Clinical importance of the oscillatory potential in the human ERG. *Acta Ophthal. (kbh)* Suppl. 70: *115-122* (1962).

Authors' address:

Dept. of Ophthalmology
Karolinska Hospital
104 01 Stockholm 60
Sweden

482

THE ELECTRORETINOGRAM OF ALBINO
AND PIGMENTED RABBITS

J. H. REUTER*

(Rotterdam)

ABSTRACT

ERG parameters of albino and pigmented rabbits were compared on the assumption that differences had been caused by the greater amount of stimulus light reaching the receptor cells in the albino due to lack of melanin. A further assumption was that no other difference between the retina's existed than the lack of melanin in the albino and equal ERG's thus meant equal stimulus conditions. These 'equal-stimulating-conditions' for the receptors were obtained by shifting the albino response curve along the intensity axis, so that the a-wave response curves overlapped. In this situation both b-wave response curves at lower intensities overlapped, but no overlap was seen at higher intensities. The c-wave response curve did not overlap either. It is concluded that only the differences of the parameters of the a-wave and the b-wave at lower intensities between albino and pigmented rabbits can be explained by the hypothesis tested.

In a number of comparative studies (DODT & ECHTE, 1961; KRILL & LEE, 1964; ALI & KOBAYASHI, 1968) it has been shown that differences in several parameters of the flash-evoked ERG can be found in albino and pigmented animals of the same species. One explanation offered for these differences is the absence of screening pigment in the eye of the albino.

This lack of pigment will consequently result in more light energy impinging on the visual pigment cells in albino than in pigmented animals at a given flash energy. If one assumes that the differences in the parameters of the ERG are caused by the lack of screening pigment only and if one assumes further that the a-wave amplitude (as a measure of receptor activity) is dependant on the light energy reaching the visual pigment cells (a.o. BRINDLEY, 1970; BROWN, 1968) and not on the light energy impinging on the eye, one should obtain comparable results for albino and pigmented eyes if one would use lower intensities to stimulate the albino eye. The aim of our experiments was to test this hypothesis in albino and pigmented rabbits. Our experiments show that this explanation is only partly correct.

* The author is indebted to Mrs. W. H. DE VOS-KORTHALS for her valuable help in the time consuming experiments.

Dutch belted rabbits (1,5-2 kg body weight) were used as the pigmented animals and New Zealand whites (2-2,5 kg body weight) as the albino's. The animals were anaesthetised with urethane (1500 mg/kg body weight, i.p.) the pupils were dilated with atropine (1 %). The eyelids were retracted with adhesive tape and the head fixed in a holder. The animal was placed in a light proof cabin with one eye viewing the bulb of a Grass P.S. 2 photic stimulator at a distance of 10 cm. Non-polarising cotton wick electrodes were placed on the cornea and on an area nasal to the eye of which the skin had been removed. The temperature in the cabin was kept constant by circulating hot water and air moisture was kept high by bubbling air through water of the same temperature. In each instance the animals were dark adapted for one hour after being placed in the holder.

One experimental group, 16 albino's and 16 pigmented animals, were dark adapted for 24 hours before the experiment. These animals were handled in dim red light and, in addition, were dark adapted for one hour. A second group of 16 albino's and 16 pigmented rabbits were not dark adapted for a long period before the experiment. These animals were dark adapted for one hour only.

A number of gray filters with a transmission of 35 % were used to reduce the lowest intensity of the P.S. 2 (Table 1). The responses to flashes were amplified with a Grass E.E.G. amplifier (A.C., model 7PSA) or a 1A7 Tektronix differential amplifier (DC-3 KHz) and averaged with a PAR Waveform Eductor (model THD-9). The averaged responses were recorded with a Servogor (model RE 511). Fig. 1 gives the parameters we compared and the way they were measured. The flash frequency was 1 c.p.s. in case of the a- and b-wave registrations and 0,2 c.p.s. in case of the c-wave registrations. The experiments were always started with a flash intensity far below threshold, and increased stepwise.

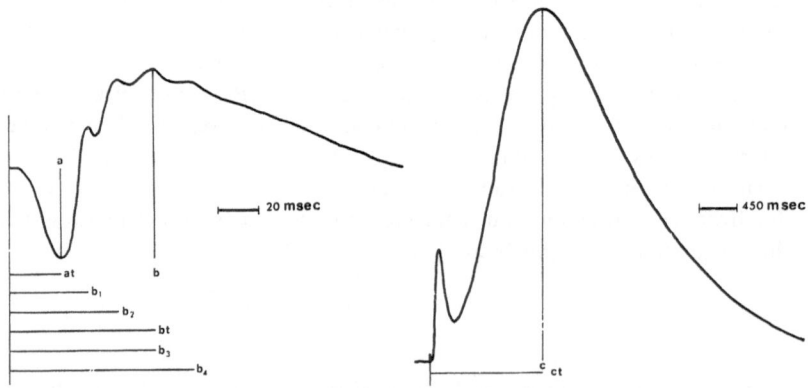

Fig. 1. Averaged ERG's and parameters measured.

Fig. 2 shows the result of the 24 hours dark adapted pigmented animals and
Fig. 3 those of the albino's. Both a- and b-wave curves look alike but those of
the albino seem to be shifted to the left on the intensity axis. This has also been

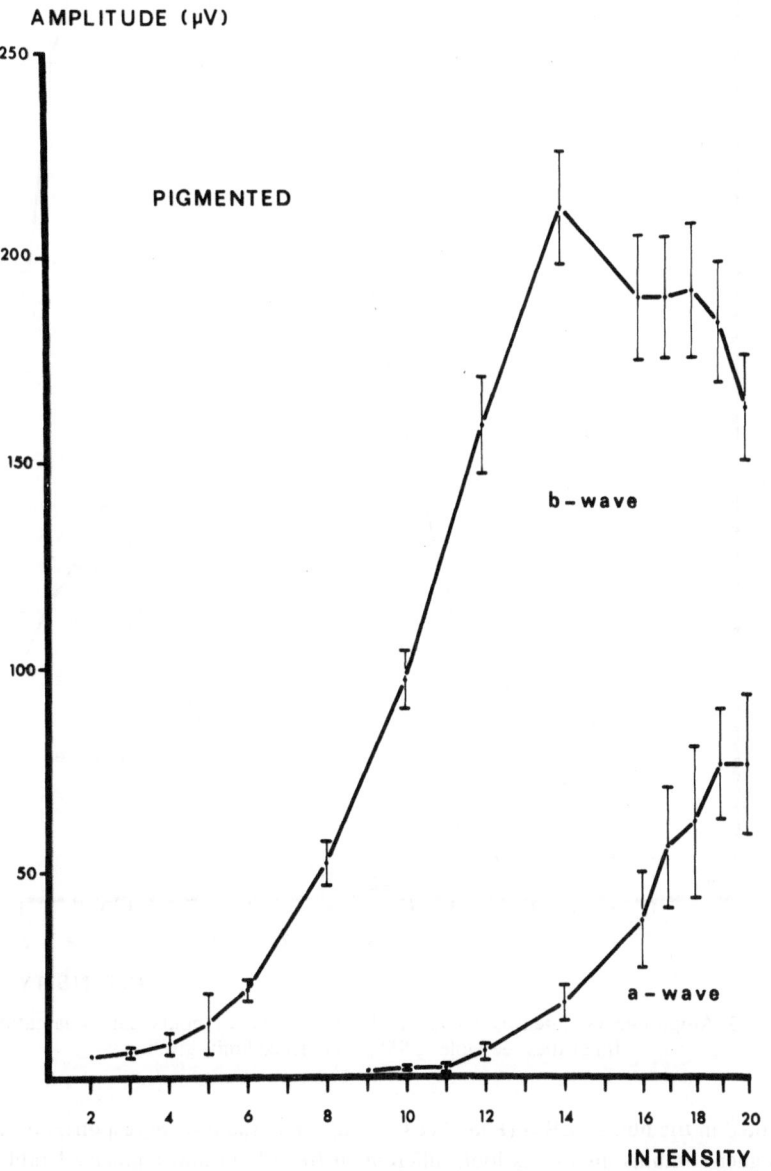

Fig. 2. Amplitude vs. intensity curve of pigmented rabbits. 24 hours dark adaptation.
Intensities see table 1, 95% confidence limits given.

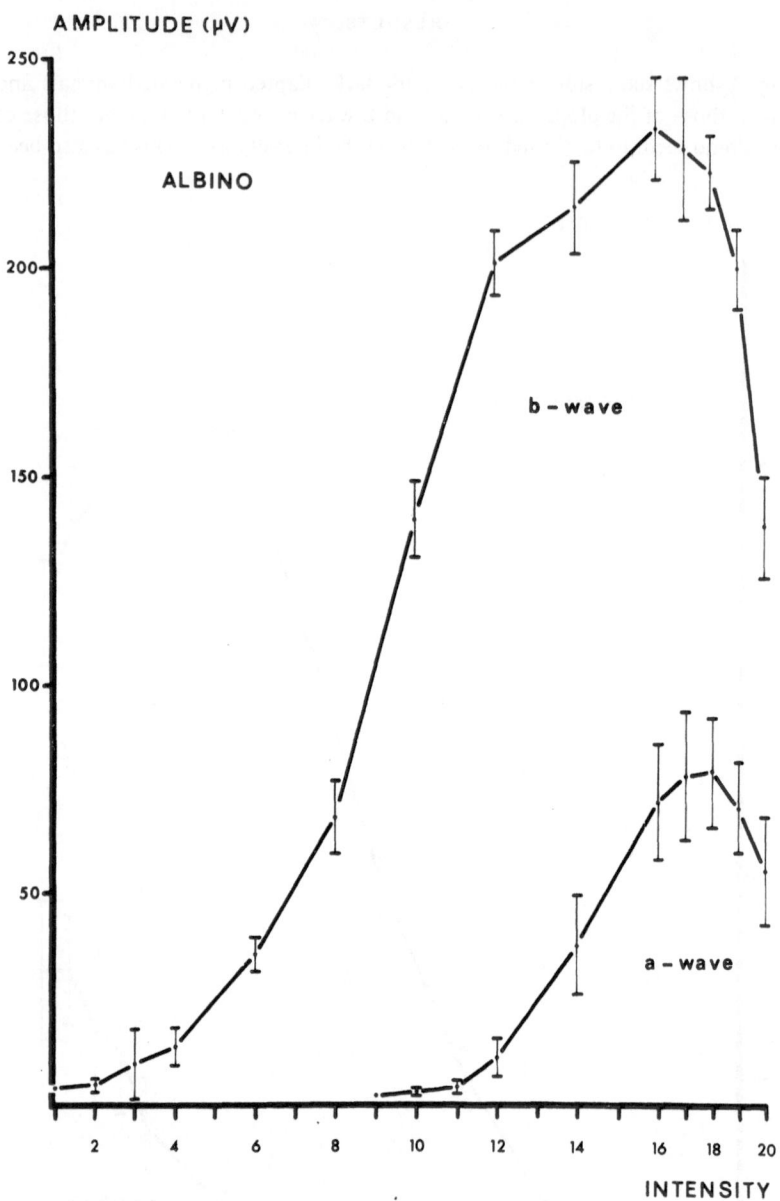

Fig. 3. Amplitude vs. intensity curve of albino rabbits. 24 hours dark adaptation. Intensities see table 1, 95% confidence limits given.

noted in the human ERG (KRILL & LEE l.c.). Only the b-wave responses to the higher stimulus intensities look different in the albino and pigmented rabbit. The a- and b-waves in the albino are larger than in the pigmented animals. These findings agree with those in trout (ALI & KOBAYASHI l.c.) and humans

486

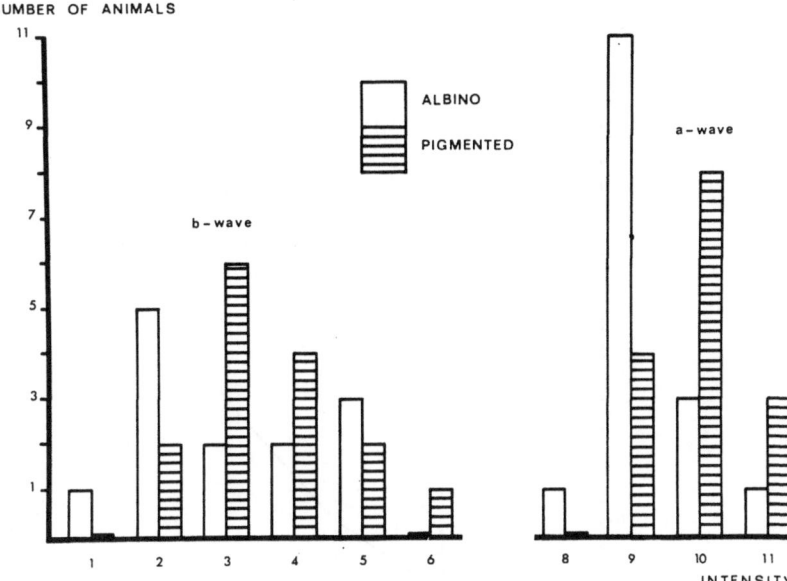

Fig. 4. A- and b-wave threshold.

(KRILL & LEE l.c.) but not with those in rats (DODT & ECHTE l.c.). In Fig. 4 the number of animals and the intensity at which their a- and b-wave were first noticeable (defined as threshold) is shown. For both the a- and b-wave the thresholds seems to be at a lower intensity in the albino's as compared with the pigmented animals. These findings also agree with those in humans (KRILL & LEE l.c.). The c-wave parameters were measured in the one hour dark adapted group only (Fig. 5). Because of the time consuming measuring procedure and the indirectness of the c-wave producing mechanisms to the path of the visual input to the brain a comparison of the c-waves in both groups was planned for a later date. The amplitude of the c-wave in the albino is greater than in the pigmented animals. Unlike the a- and b-wave amplitude it increases continuously in amplitude with increasing stimulus intensity in the intensity range used. With the lowest intensity used (intensity 16, Table I) a small c-wave could be detected in three pigmented animals only, whereas in the albino a clear, well developed c-wave was seen in all cases with this intensity.

Fig. 6 gives the latency times of the a-, b- and c-waves. Although not as clear as in the amplitude curves, the latency curves of the albino's also appear to be shifted to the left along the intensity axis. As has been found in other animals the latency time of the albino a- and b-waves are generally shorter than those of the pigmented animals. In contrast to these findings the latency time of the albino c-wave is longer than in the pigmented animals. Also, in contrast to the findings in a- and b-waves the latency of the c-wave increases with increasing stimulus intensity (see also HAMASAKI, 1967).

The latency time of the first four wavelets on the b-wave measured at the two

487

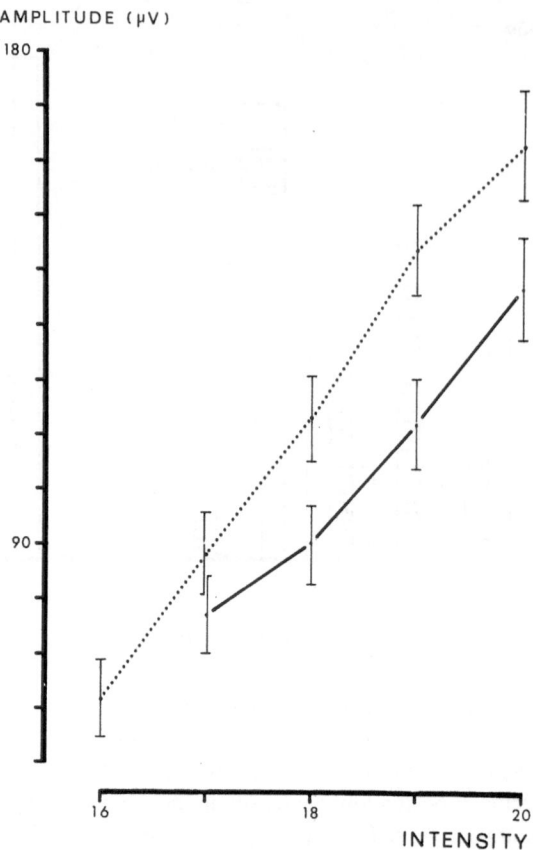

AMPLITUDE (μV)

INTENSITY

Fig. 5. C-wave amplitude vs. intensity curve. Drawn line pigmented, dotted line albino rabbits. 1 hour dark adaptation 95% confidence limits given.

highest stimulus intensities showed no difference in this parameter of the ERG in albino's and pigmented rabbits. As these results do not differ in any way from those published previously for normal and light deprived animals of different ages (REUTER et al. 1971), these results are not shown here.

DISCUSSION

We wanted to test the hypothesis as to whether the differences in the ERG parameters of the albino and pigmented animal can be explained solely on the basis of the greater amount of light energy reaching the receptor cells in the albino. This would mean that by adjusting the amount of light impinging on the albino eye, stimulus conditions could be obtained which would produce equal responses in albino and pigmented animals indicating equal stimulation of the receptor cells. As we have been unable to find evidence in the literature that in mammals, apart from the lack of melanin, the retina of albino's are different

488

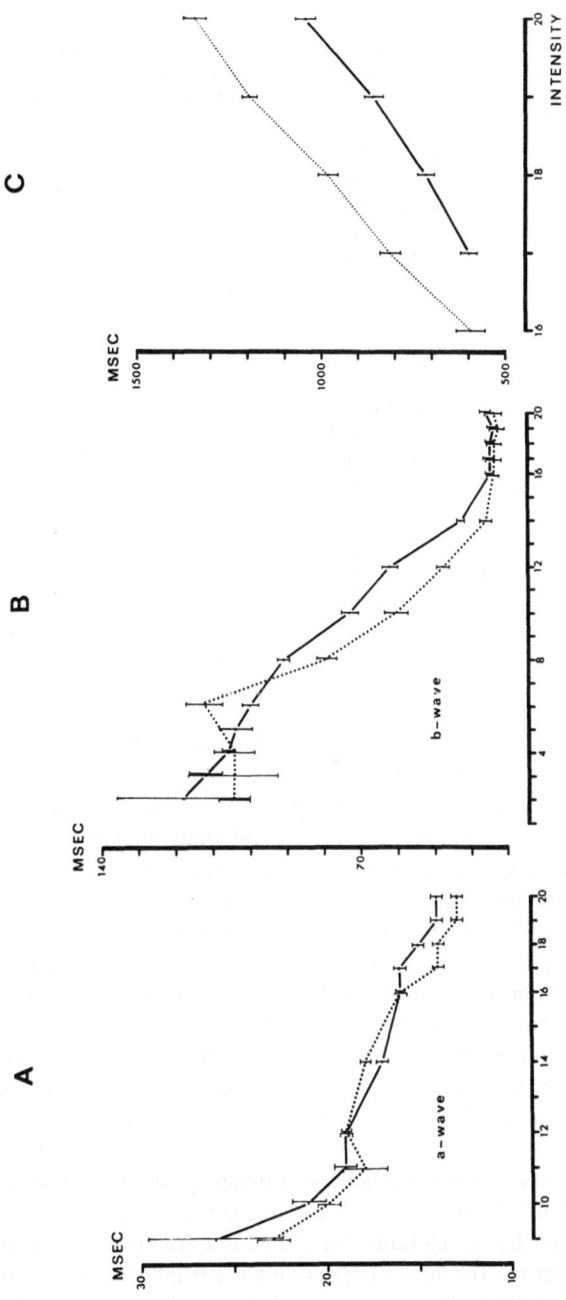

Fig. 6. A-, b- and c-wave latency vs. intensity curves. Dotted lines albino's, drawn lines pigmented rabbits. A and B 24 hours dark adapted and C 1 hour dark adapted animals. 95% confidence limits given.

TABLE I

intensity (used in the graphs)	candle power	number of filters used	intensity of PS 2
1	$1{,}36 \times 10^{-2}$	15	1
2	$3{,}88 \times 10^{-2}$	14	1
3	$1{,}11 \times 10^{-1}$	13	1
4	$3{,}17 \times 10^{-1}$	12	1
5	$9{,}05 \times 10^{-1}$	11	1
6	$2{,}59 \times 10^{0}$	10	1
7	$7{,}39 \times 10^{0}$	9	1
8	$2{,}11 \times 10^{1}$	8	1
9	$6{,}03 \times 10^{1}$	7	1
10	$1{,}72 \times 10^{2}$	6	1
11	$4{,}92 \times 10^{2}$	5	1
12	$1{,}41 \times 10^{3}$	4	1
13	$4{,}02 \times 10^{3}$	3	1
14	$1{,}15 \times 10^{4}$	2	1
15	$3{,}28 \times 10^{4}$	1	1
16	$9{,}38 \times 10^{4}$	0	1
17	$1{,}88 \times 10^{5}$	0	2
18	$3{,}75 \times 10^{5}$	0	4
19	$7{,}50 \times 10^{5}$	0	8
20	$1{,}50 \times 10^{6}$	0	16

from the retina of pigmented animals, the assumption was made that equal ERG's mean equal amount of stimulation of the retina. The overall finding is that the a- and b-wave amplitude is greater and that the latency time is shorter in albino's. This is in accordance with findings in trout and humans, but not completely with those in rats. The a-wave amplitude curves in Fig. 2 and 3 (the 24 hours dark adapted group) look very much alike, but the albino curve is shifted to the left along the intensity scale. Shifting the albino curve to the right results in overlap of the a-wave curves of both the albino and pigmented animals as shown in Fig. 7. The shift has been arbitrarily made in units given on the intensity scale and resulted in intensity 16 in the albino being equaled with intensity 18 in the pigmented animals. This would indicate that nearly 4 $\times$ as much stimulus intensity is needed in the pigmented rabbits to produce an ERG equal to one in the albino. This shift results also in an overlap of the left part of both b-wave amplitude response curves. At stimulus intensities higher than intensity 14 in the pigmented animals (intensity scale for the albino: between intensity 12 and 13) the curves do not overlap after this intensity 'correction'. This indicates that in the rabbit for the a-wave and the lower intensity b-wave responses, but not for higher intensity b-wave responses, the differences in the ERG parameters of albino and pigmented animals could be explained by the hypothesis we wanted to test. The same amount of shifting the albino results in the figures given by ALI & KOBAYASHI (l.c.) and KRILL & LEE (l.c.) results also in a reasonable overlap of albino and pigmented a- and b-wave response curves. The results given in Fig. 4 indicate that the a- and b-wave threshold in

AMPLITUDE (µV)

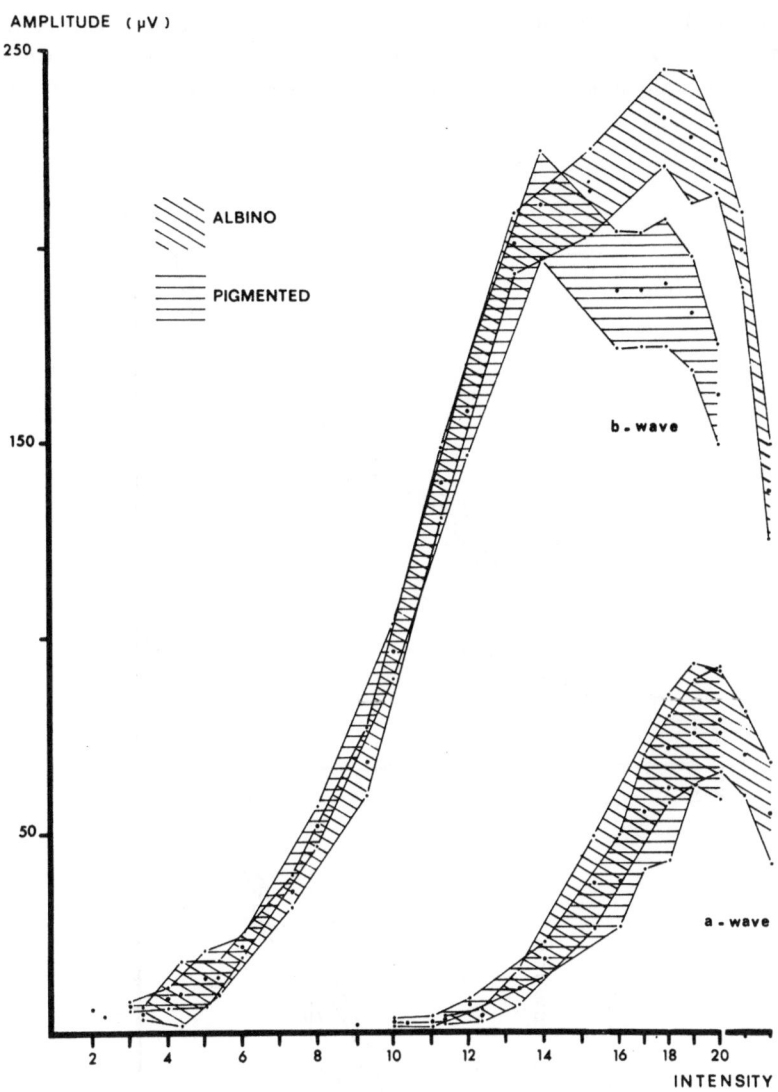

Fig. 7. Amplitude vs. intensity curves of albino and pigmented animals. Albino curves shifted along the intensity axis to the right. Intensity units given for the pigmented animals. Striped area is enclosed by 95 % confidence limit points.

the albino is also shifted approximately over the same amount of stimulus light intensity to the left along the intensity scale as was expected on the basis of the amplitude results. In Fig. 8 the a- and b-wave latency times are given after the same shift along the intensity axis as above. The differences are still evident.

In conclusion, we can say that the differences in a-wave parameters between albino and pigmented rabbits can be explained by the difference in light energy reaching the receptor cells due to the lack of melanin. This also holds true for the b-wave parameters up to a certain stimulus intensity range but that at higher intensities the b- and c-wave parameter differences cannot be explained this way.

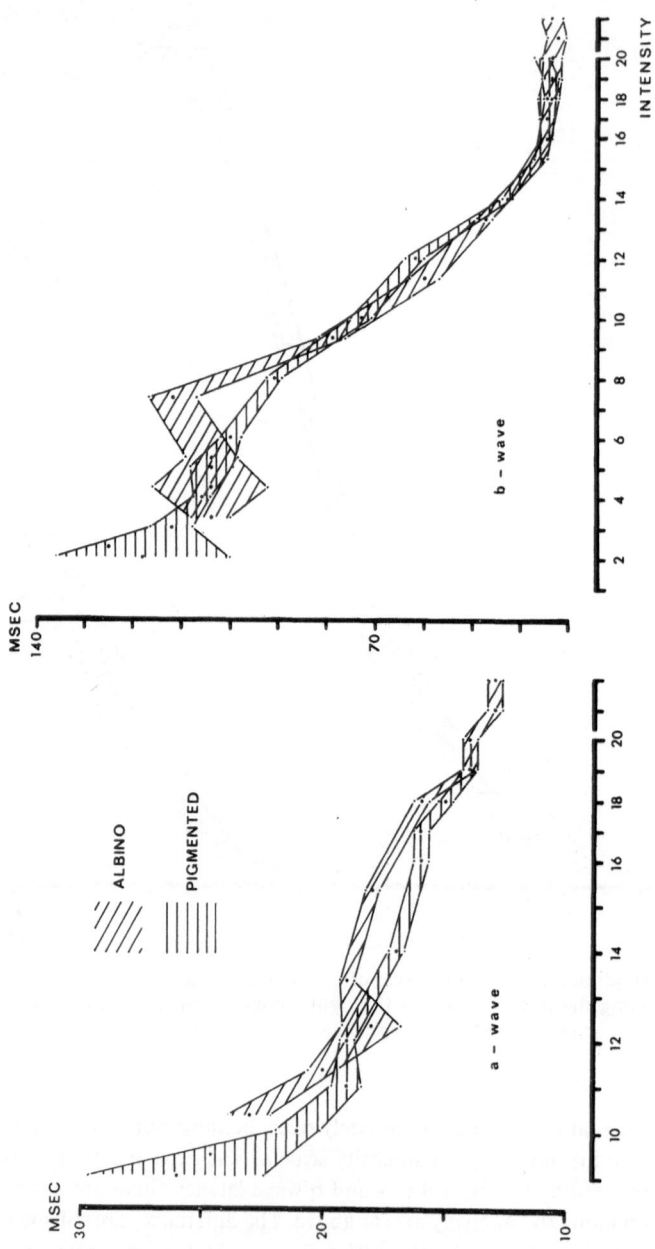

Fig. 8. Latency vs. intensity curves of albino and pigmented rabbits. Explanation as given in fig. 7.

REFERENCES

ALI, M. A. & KOBAYASHI, H. Electroretinogram of albino and pigmented brook trout Salvelinus fontinalis (Mitchell) *Rev. Can. Biol.* 27: *145-161* (1968).

BROWN, K. T. The electroretinogram: its components and their origins. *Vision Res.* 8: *633-678* (1968).

BRINDLEY, G. S. Physiology of the retina and visual pathway. Edward Arnold (publ.) Ltd. London (1970).

DODT, E. & ECHTE, K. Dark and light adaptation in pigmented and white rat as measured by electroretinogram threshold. *J. Neurophysiol.* 24: *427-445* (1961).

HAMASAKI, D. J. An anatomical and electrophysiological study of the retina of the owl monkey, Aotes trivirgatus. *J. Comp. Neur.* 130: *163-174* (1967).

KRILL, A. E. LEE, G. B. The electroretinogram in albino's and carriers of the ocular albino trait. *Arch. Ophthal.* 69: *32-38* (1963).

REUTER, J. H., LEGEIN, C. P. J. J. M. M., V. D. MARK, F., VAN HOF, M. W. The electroretinogram in normal and light deprived rabbits. *Doc. Ophthal.* 30: *349-361* (1971).

Authors' address:

Dept. of Physiology
Medical Faculty
Erasmus University
Rotterdam
The Netherlands

RETINAL INPUT AND EARLY DEVELOPMENT
OF THE VISUAL SYSTEM

M. W. VAN HOF

(Rotterdam)

The effect of retinal input restriction or modification has been studied in several species: binocular or monocular pattern deprivation, selective exposure to horizontal lines, artificial squint, etc. have been applied. Since animals reared under those conditions may develop visual defects it is often concluded that, to a certain extent, the interneuronal connections in the visual system are not genetically coded but develop under the organizational influence of the retinal input. However, this statement does not elucidate the nature of the disturbances found in the visual system of those animals.

Fig. 1A represents an extremely simplified neuronal network at a certain level in the visual system. Neuron 2 sends axonal branches to neurons 1, 4, 5, 7 and 9, neuron 3 to neurons 2, 5, 6, 7 and 8. Action potentials arrive from some

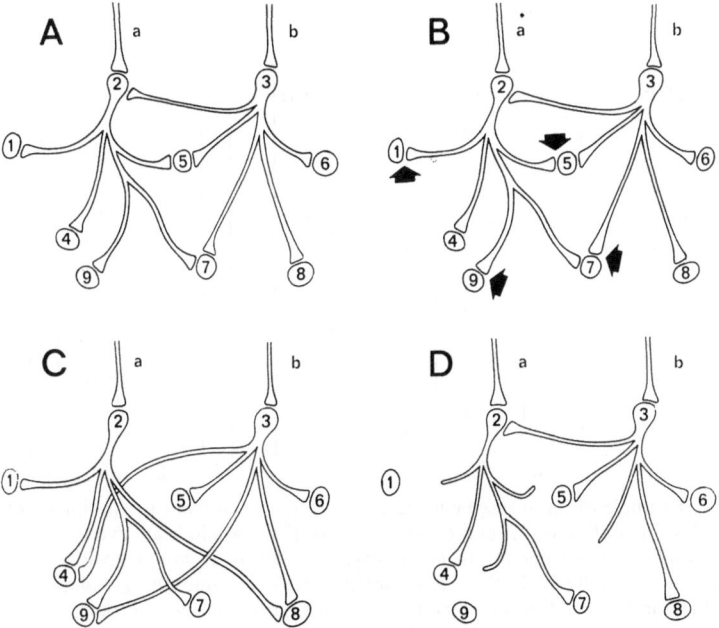

Fig. 1. Schematic representation of four neuronal networks.

other level by way of axon branches 'a' and 'b'. The response of the network will depend on the properties of the nervous elements and on the topology of the interneuronal connections.

Therefore, the electrophysiological response of this network to a given input can be changed in two fundamentally different ways. The first one is illustrated in Fig. 1B. Here the transmission characteristics in the synapses indicated by arrows are supposed to be altered, for instance by a reduction of the production of transmitter substance. In Fig. 1C and 1D the wiring diagrams have been changed: in 1C part of the connections are altered, in 1D the number of connections is reduced.

Which of the possibilities shown in Fig. 1 do apply to the visual system of animals raised under the conditions mentioned above?

The situation indicated in Fig. 1B is likely to be present in the experiment shown in Fig. 2. Essentially this experiment (Kobayashi & Van Hof, 1972) on visual evoked responses, recorded between an electrode implanted over the visual cortex and another one attached to the ear, is the same as that described by Bonaventura et al. (1971), but carried out in a more quantitative way. Four groups of rabbits were studied (7 animals per group):

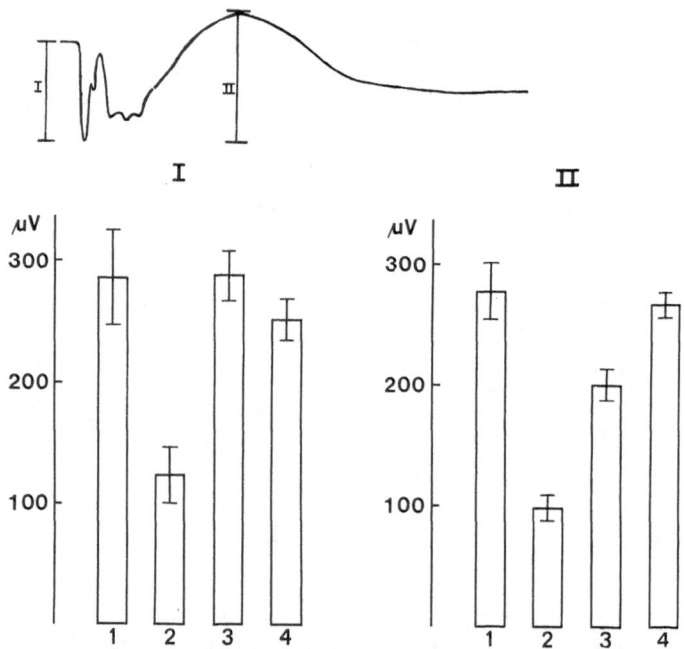

Fig. 2. Example of an average evoked response recorded from the occipital cortex of the rabbit. Duration of the curve: 500 msec. Vertical bars indicate average amplitudes and standard errors per group (7 animals per group). I: initial positive deflection, II: positive-negative deflection. 1. normally raised; 2. 7-month light deprived; 3. 7-month light deprived followed by one month of exposure to normal room illumination; 4. 7-month light deprived followed by two months of exposure to normal room illumination.

1. normally raised.
2. 7-month light deprived after birth.
3. 7-month light deprived followed by one month of exposure to normal room illumination.
4. 7-month light deprived followed by two months of exposure to normal room illumination.

The electrodes in group 2 were implanted with the eyes covered. All animals remained in complete darkness for 24 hours before recordings were made.

The maximal positive deflection (I) and the maximal positive-negative deflection (II) were measured in the averaged curves from all animals. Both deflections are reduced considerably in the dark-reared rabbits, but recovery occurs after additional light exposure. It was found by VRENSEN (personal communication) that by counting the synapses in the visual cortex (VRENSEN & DE GROOT, 1973) no differences were found between group 1 and 2. Since it is known that evoked responses consist mainly of summated post-synaptic potentials, the amplitude decrease is likely to be due to temporary synaptic inactivity (Fig. 1B).

On the other hand, examples of changes in the wiring diagram (Fig. 1C) can be found in the literature. FIFKOVA (1972) reported that the ratio between various types of connections in the inner plexiform layer of the retina of the albino rat changes after eyelid suturing. A strong increase of the percentage of amacrine-amacrine connections was found. This result receives support from a study by SOLULA & GLOW (1971) who found an increase of the total number of synapses in the inner plexiform layer of light deprived hooded rats. However, this phenomenon is not likely to be present in all species. Recording from ganglion cells, SHERMAN & STONE (1973) found the receptive field properties and the percentages of X, Y and W cells to be normal in the retina of cats raised with eyelids sutured till the age of 12-18 months.

Several studies have shown that in the visual cortex of kittens reared under conditions in which the eyes were exposed selectively to lines of one particular orientation, most cells react to that particular orientation (BLAKEMORE & COOPER, 1970, HIRSCH & SPINELLI, 1970, 1971). PETTIGREW et al (1973) found the density of responsive units to be the same as that in normal cats. In other words the dominance of the cells reacting to the orientation to which the eye had been exposed during development was due to an abnormal topology of the network in the sense of Fig. 1C.

An important question has not yet been answered. An abnormal topology could mean that:
a. the network is partially precoded and in the presence of a restricted visual input the uncoded connections, which under normal conditions develop under the organizational influence of the visual input, grow out randomly (as in the occluded eye of the albino rat) or adapt to the modified visual input (exposure to horizontal lines, e.g.)
b. the network is genetically prewired but an abnormal retinal input overrules the read-out of this information and induces a modification in the network.

An incomplete network as shown in Fig. 2D may arise under the influence of input restriction. LUND & LUND (1972a) studied the relative numbers of synaptic contact types in the superior colliculus of the rat. Three different stages of development could be distinguished. The third one (from 25 days to 30-40 days of age) is marked by a proliferation of synapse formation by intrinsic neurons. This process is disturbed by eyelid closure (LUND & LUND, 1972b).

In case of an incomplete network several possibilities emerge:

a. The genetic instructions are incomplete. Under normal circumstances part of the connections develop under the organizational influence of retinal stimuli.
b. The blueprint of the wiring diagram is genetically complete but retinal stimuli are required to trigger the read-out of the genetic information.
c. Initially the genetically precoded network grows out but degenerates secondarily due to disuse.

Both a and b could explain the findings by LUND & LUND. An example of c may be found in the study of CHOW et al. (1957) who described that the effects of dark rearing were reversible when chimpanzees were kept in darkness from birth to seven months of age. If this period lasted longer than 16 months, an almost complete degeneration of the ganglion cell layer occurred.

The examples given above show that input restriction or modification leads to a diversity of effects which, from the developmental point of view, cannot yet be reduced to the same denominator.

The system responsible for pattern recognition encompasses a larger part of the brain than the classical geniculocortical pathway. There is plenty of evidence that the tectum (colliculus superior and pretectal nucleï) plays an important role in this process (SPRAGUE et al., 1972, INGLE & SCHNEIDER, 1970). SCHNEIDER's experiments (1969) in the golden hamster have shown that lesions in the superior colliculus abolish the ability to orient toward an object without interference with the ability to identify it. Lesions in the visual cortex have the opposite effect. The importance of this trend in visual physiology for light deprivation studies may be illustrated by a paper presented at the 1973 meeting of the European Brain and Behaviour Society by VAN HOF-VAN DUIN.

A number of visuomotor tests were applied to kittens in which one eye was sutured after birth. At the age of 8-10 months the visually naïve eye was opened and the non-deprived eye sutured. The same tests were studied again over a period of about 12 months. The optokinetic nystagmus, tracking of small objects, visual placing reactions (both visually triggered stretching and visually guided reaching, as described by HEIN & HELD, 1967), visual cliff and jumping behavior were included in the program. Also, perimetry tests were carried out. Partial recovery was seen, be it that the recovery periods differed strongly between various tests. In several of them no recovery occurred at all. Besides these visuomotor tests, the ability to discriminate patterns of different orientation was studied in a way similar to that in the rabbit (VAN HOF, 1966, 1972). It was found that in most cats the 'blind' eye did equally well as the normal eye before reverse closure. It is of importance to note that in the training box used in those studies no decision alley was present; the animals were sitting right in front of the targets and no visuomotor behavior of any complexity was involved in the discrimination process. This means that the disturbances in the

498

open field situation were mainly due to a visuomotor disturbance, rather than to an inability to identify patterns.

Unfortunately, these extra-geniculate channels are still ill-defined and the relative contributions of various channels to different visual tasks are not yet conclusively established. With respect to the described effects of monocular light deprivation this means that as long as the topographical analysis is not completed, it is difficult to ascertain the topological nature of the neuronal defects underlying the behavioral deficits.

Since it can be expected that during the next few years great progress will be made in the functional analysis of the extra-geniculate pathways, it might be worthwhile anticipating on this by designing suitable visuomotor tests which can be applied in amblyopic human subjects. In this way it would be possible to bridge the gap between observations made in humans and conceptions based on animal experiments.

REFERENCES

BONAVENTURE, N., GOSWAMY, S. & KARLI, P. Electroretinogram and visual evoked response in rabbits reared in total darkness or continuous illumination. *Doc. Ophthal.* 30: *339-347* (1971).

BLAKEMORE, C. & COOPER, G. F. Development of the brain depends on visual experience. *Nature* 228: *477-478* (1970).

CHOW, K. L., RIESEN, A. H. & NEWELL, F. W. Degeneration of retinal ganglion cells in infant chimpanzees reared in darkness. *J. Comp. Neurol.* 107: *27-42* (1957).

FIFKOVA, E. Effect of visual deprivation and light on synapses of the inner plexiform layer. *Exp. Neurol.* 35: *458-469* (1972).

HEIN, A. & HELD, R. Dissociation of the visual placing response into elicited and guided components. *Science* 158: *390-392* (1967).

HIRSCH, H. V. B. & SPINELLI, D. N. Visual experience modifies distribution of horizontally and vertically oriented receptive fields in cats. *Science* 168: *869-871* (1970).

HIRSCH, H. V. B. & SPINELLI, D. N. Modification of the distribution of receptive field orientation in cats by selective visual exposure during development. *Exp. Brain Res.* 13: *509-527* (1971).

INGLE, D. & SCHNEIDER, G. E. (Eds.). Subcortical visual systems. Karger (1970).

KOBAYASHI, K. & VAN HOF, M. W. Visual evoked responses in rabbits deprived of light for seven months after birth. *Acta Soc. Ophthal. Jap.* 76: *257-259* (1972).

LUND, R. D. & LUND, J. S. Development of synaptic patterns in the superior colliculus of the rat. *Brain Res.* 42: *1-20* (1972).

LUND, R. D. & LUND, J. S. The effects of varying periods of visual deprivation on synaptogenesis in the superior colliculus of the rat. *Brain Res.* 42: *21-32* (1972).

PETTIGREW, J. D., OLSON, C. & HIRSCH, H. V. B. Cortical effect of selective visual experience: degeneration or reorganization? *Brain Res.* 51: *345-351* (1973).

SCHNEIDER, G. E. Two visual systems. *Science* 163: *895-902* (1969).

SHERMAN, S. M. & STONE, J. Physiological normality of the retina in visually deprived cats. *Brain Res.* 60: *224-230* (1973).

SOSULA, L. & GLOW, P. H. Increase in number of synapses in the inner plexiform layer in light deprived rat retinae: Quantitative electron microscopy. *J. Comp. Neurol.* 141: *427-452* (1971).

SPRAGUE, J. M., BERLUCCHI, G. & RIZOLATTI, G. The role of the superior colliculus and pretectum in vision and visually guided behavior. Handbook of Sensory Physiology VII/3B, 27-102 (1973). Springer Verlag. R. Jung (Ed.).

VAN HOF, M. W. Discrimination between striated patterns of different orientation in the rabbit *Vision Res.* 6: *89-94* (1966).

VAN HOF, M. W. & KOBAYASHI, K. Pattern discrimination in rabbits deprived of light for 7 months after birth. *Exp. Neurol.* 35: *551-557* (1972).

VAN HOF-VAN DUIN, J. Pattern discrimination and visuomotor behaviour after monocular visual deprivation in cats. Abstr. 5th Annual meeting of the EBBS. To be published in *Brain Res.*

VRENSEN, G. & DE GROOT, D. Quantitative stereology of synapses: a critical investigation. *Brain Res.* 58: *25-35* (1973).

Authors' address:

Department of Physiology, Medical Faculty
Erasmus University
Rotterdam
The Netherlands

ERG CHANGES IN THE CHICKEN REARED IN CONTINUOUS ILLUMINATION POSSIBLE INVOLVEMENT OF TAURINE

N. BONAVENTURE, H. PASANTES-MORALES, F. MEYER, N. WIOLAND & P. KARLI

(Strasbourg)

Within the scope of an experimental analysis of the effects of environmental factors on the functional maturation of the retina, we have recorded the ERG at various times between hatching and adult age in chickens brought up in conditions of continuous illumination. In parallel to the study of the electrophysiological effects of such a condition, we searched for possible ultrastructural as well as neurochemical correlates. As it came out that an altered taurine level might well be one of the latter correlates, we made intravitreal injections of taurine in adult control chickens (reared under natural conditions of illumination) in order to investigate some aspects of the possible involvement of taurine in intraretinal synaptic transmission.

METHODS

The developmental study was carried out on Hubbard chickens brought up from hatching in a continuous illumination of either 4000-5000 or 400-500 lux. As regards anesthesia, stimulation parameters, recording of the ERG, intravitreal injection of labelled taurine and measurement of its radioactivity in separate layers of the retina, previously described techniques were used (PASANTES-MORALES et al., 1973).

In the taurine-injected chickens, light-evoked potentials were also recorded from the optic tectum without opening the meninges. The active electrode consisted of a small chlorided silver ball; the indifferent one was inserted underneath the skin of the neck. The tectal potentials were recorded on magnetic tape in order to allow summation and analysis on a Didac 800 Intertechnique.

RESULTS

I. *ERG in chickens reared in continuous illumination*

In the control animal brought up in the natural light-dark alternation, the ERG has an adult-type morphology right from hatching; this is in agreement with the data reported by BLOZOVSKI & BLOZOVSKI (1968) and by OOKAWA (1971). The b-wave amplitude increases only slightly until 25 days after hatching and its culmination time decreases from 70 ms at 5 days to 42 ms at 30 days. There is

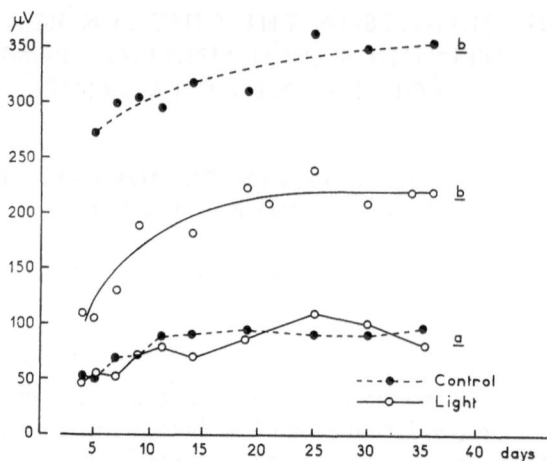

Fig. 1. *a* and *b* wave amplitude as a function of posthatching age. Solid line: animals reared in continuous illumination. Dotted line: control animals.

hardly any change of the a-wave after hatching (Fig. 1).

In the experimental animals (continuous illumination of 4000-5000 lux) the amplitude of the a-wave never differs from control values. But as soon as the third day after hatching and during the entire course of development, the amplitude of the b-wave is markedly reduced (about 40 per cent) (Fig. 1). This electrophysiological alteration is entirely reversible: the b-wave amplitude is no longer below control-values once the chicken has been kept in the natural environment for 48 hours after having been brought up for 40 days under the experimental conditions. If the continuous illumination is of 400-500 lux only, no ERG alteration is ever observed. If chickens are exposed to a continuous illumination of high intensity not right from hatching but from the age of 25 days, the ERG remains unaltered, whatever the duration of the exposure (durations tested: 1, 5, 10, 15 and 25 days).

II. *Retinal ultrastructure in chickens reared in continuous illumination*

The ultrastructure of the retina was studied in chickens exposed to the continuous 4000-5000 lux illumination for 5, 26 or 50 days following hatching. No morphological alteration was ever observed in any of the retinal layers. The visual cells and in particular the outer segments, look perfectly normal (Fig. 2). Entirely negative results were also obtained in 25-days old chickens exposed for 5-days to the same experimental conditions.

III. *Retinal free amino acids in chickens reared in continuous illumination*

The level of 17 retinal free amino acids were measured at various times after hatching in animals reared in continuous illumination as well as in control

502

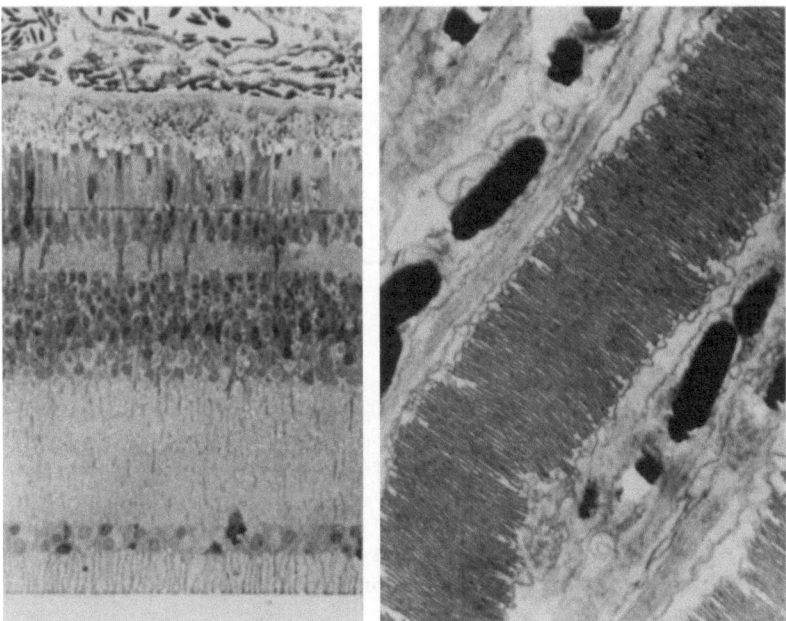

Fig. 2. Retina of chicken exposed to light (6000 Lux) for 50 days from hatching. A: whole retina; B: visual cell outer segments; G: 18000.

animals. The only alteration to be observed (in illumination of high intensity only) consisted in a reduced level of taurine (about 30 per cent below control levels in 3-week old animals) suggesting an increased utilization of this amino-acid. The light-induced alteration is readily reversible.

Taurine has been shown to amount to 40 per cent of the total free amino acid content of the adult chicken retina (PASANTES-MORALES et al., 1972). On the other hand, light stimulation induces a release of taurine in the isolated chicken retina (PASANTES-MORALES et al., 1973). Taken together, these facts lead us to study the effects of intravitreal injections of taurine on the ERG and the tectal potentials in chickens reared under natural conditions of illumination.

IV. *Effects of intravitreal injections of taurine on ERG and tectal evoked potentials*

A. *ERG*

The effects of intravitreal injections of taurine on the ERG have been published in detail elsewhere (PASANTES-MORALES et al., 1973). A few major points may be briefly recalled. The injection of taurine provokes a progressive reduction of the b-wave amplitude, whereas the a-wave amplitude remains unchanged (Fig. 3). The effect is maximal 5 to 7 hours following injection; the b-wave recovers its initial amplitude about 6 hours later. The depressant effect of taurine increases with increasing intensity of the photic stimulation. At the

503

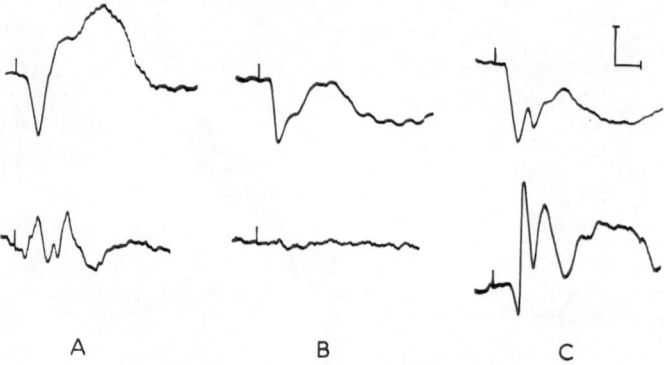

Fig. 3. ERG (upper tracings) and TER (lower tracings) before (A), one hour (B) and three hours (C) following intravitreal injection of taurine (calibration: 25 ms as regards time, 100 μV as regards amplitude).

peak of b-wave inhibition, the injected taurine is concentrated in the inner synaptic layer and in the innermost part of inner nuclear layer.

B. *Tectal potentials* (TER)

The intravitreal injection of taurine entails a decrease of the amplitude of the TER which parallels the b-wave depression. In some cases, a regular 8-cycle spontaneous activity appears on the tectum when the TER are no longer recorded. Some time later (the time depending on the concentration of the injected taurine), the TER recover and their amplitude may even exceed control values at a time when the b-wave amplitude is still maximally depressed (fig. 3).

DISCUSSION

In chickens reared from hatching in continuous illumination, a b-wave of reduced amplitude and a reduced taurine level in the retina were obtained only with illuminations of high intensity. These alterations are entirely reversible: they disappear once the animal has been kept for 3 days in normal environmental conditions. Furthermore, no morphological change was ever found in the retina of the experimental animals.

The reversibility of the b-wave depression observed in the chicken contrasts with the lasting character of the same ERG change found in rabbits reared in continuous illumination (BONAVENTURE et al., 1971). This difference most probably results from the different stage of structural and functional maturation reached at birth in the two species. In spite of its higher degree of maturity, the retina of the newly hatched chicken appears to keep some plasticity, as evidenced by the effect of continuous illumination which are no longer induced in 25-day old chickens.

504

The absence of any morphological or functional alteration in the retina of the adult chicken exposed to a continuous illumination of high intensity contrasts with the gross alterations found in the rat (NOELL et al., 1966; GORN et al., 1967; O'STEEN et al., 1972), in the rabbit (LAWWILL, 1973) and in the pigeon (MARSHALL, 1972). This discrepancy can hardly result from a differential sensitivity of the retina in the species taken into consideration, as we found in adult albino rats exposed to lights of high intensity (6000 lux) for a week no more than a mild degree of vesicles in the rod outer segments.

An early exposure of the chicken retina to continuous illumination seems to entail an increased utilization of taurine, an amino-acid which proved to have a depressant action on the b-wave of the ERG in vitro (PASANTES-MORALES et al., 1972) and in vivo (PASANTES-MORALES et al., 1973 and the present paper), as well as on the ganglion cell discharge (KISHIDA & NAKA, 1967). This suggests that the reduced b-wave amplitude found in the light-exposed animals may result from an excessive activation of intraretinal inhibitory mechanisms.

As regards the possible role of taurine as a retinal neurotransmitter, its biphasic effect on the TER, similar to that found by TRUBATCH et al. (1973) following intravitreal injection of glutamate, clearly points to a complex action of taurine in the retina. Further investigations will have to explain not only the concomitant depression of the b-wave of the ERG and of the TER, but also the recovery (even beyond control value) of the latter at a time when the b-wave is still maximally depressed.

REFERENCES

PASANTES-MORALES, H., BONAVENTURE, N., WIOLAND, N. & MANDEL, P. Effect of intravitreal injections of taurine and Gaba on chicken electroretinogram. *J. Neurosciences*, 5: 235-241 (1973).

BLOZOVSKI, D. & BLOZOVSKI, M. Développement comparé de l'ERG et des P.E.V. du toit optique du cervelet et du télencéphale chez le Poussin. *J. Physiol.* (Paris) 60: 33-50 (1968).

OOKAWA, T. On the ontogenetic study of the chicken ERG. *J. Physiol. Soc. Japan.* 33: 317-318 (1971).

PASANTES-MORALES, H., KLETHI, J., LEDIG, M. & MANDEL, P. Free amino acids of chicken and rat retina. *Brain Research* 41: 494-497 (1972).

PASANTES-MORALES, H., URBAN, P. F., KLETHI, J. & MANDEL, P. Light stimulated release of (35 S) taurine from chicken retina. *Brain Research* 51: 375-378 (1973).

BONAVENTURE, N., GOSWAMY, S. & KARLI, P. Electroretinogram and visual evoked response in rabbits reared in total darkness or continuous illumination *Doc. Ophthal.* 30: 339-347 (1971).

NOELL, W. K., WALKER, V. S., KANG, B. S. & BERMAN, S. Retinal damage by light in rats. *Investigative Ophthalmology* 5: 450-473 (1966).

GORN, R. A. & KUWABARA, T. Retinal damage by visible light. A physiological study. *Arch. Ophthal.* 77: 115-118 (1967).

O'STEEN, W. K. & ANDERSON, K. V. Photoreceptor degeneration after exposure of rats to incandescent illumination. *Zeitsch. Zellforsch. und mikrosc. Anat.* 127: 306-313 (1972).

LAWWILL, T. Effects of prolonged exposure of rabbit retina to low intensity light. *Investigative Ophthal.* 12: 45-51 (1973).

MARSCHALL, J., MELLENIO, J. & PALMER, D. A. Damage to pigeon retinae by moderate illumination from fluorescent lamps. *Exp. Eye Research* 14: *164-169* (1972).

PASANTES-MORALES, H., URBAN, P. F., KLETHI, J. & MANDEL, P. Etude de l'effect de la taurine sur l'électrorétinogramme de la rétine en perfusion. *C.R. Acad. sci.*, Série D, 275: *699-702* (1972).

KISHIDA, K. & NAKA, K. I. Amino acids and the spikes from the retinal ganglion cells. *Science* 156: *648-650* (1967).

TRUBATCH, J., VERHULST, F. C. & VAN HARREVELD, A. Glutamate as a transmitter: comparison between the crustacean neuromuscular junction and the chicken retina. *Comp. Biochem. Physiol.* 45A: *183-193* (1973).

Authors' address:

Laboratoire de Neurophysiologie
Centre de Neurochimie du C.N.R.S.
Strasbourg
France

THE AUTOMATED ELECTRO-OCULOGRAM
AND ITS CLINICAL USES.

C. BARBER & N. R. GALLOWAY

(Nottingham)

ABSTRACT

An instrument is described which performs electro-oculography and automatically calculates the Arden index. Experience with a series of normal subjects and some patients indicate that the method has certain advantages over techniques employed previously.

Measurement of the effect of a prolonged light stimulus on the standing potential of the eye has become recognised as a useful clinical test. The standard technique suggested by ARDEN and co-workers in 1962 has now become widely practiced. (ARDEN, BARRADA & KELSEY 1962; KELSEY 1966). However, the test has two disadvantages in that it takes time to complete and it requires skill in operation. When the test was originally performed the eye movements were recorded using a penwriter and individual movements were measured on the trace to assess the value of the standing potential.

A semi-automatic method has been introduced which reduces the operator participation required and gives good results in many cases. (HENKES et al., 1968). An alternative method has also been described (DORNE & ESPIARD, 1971) which uses maximal rather than controlled eye movements and gives good results when the patient is unable to maintain fixation; it does however require more operator involvement.

The method to be described here is fully automatic and demands no particular skill from the operator. The result is displayed as the Arden coefficient at the end of the test.

METHOD

The overall system is shown in Figure 1. A modified stimulus is used to control the eye movements which has certain advantages over the use of alternating fixation lights. It consists of a row of 49 light emitting diodes which are lit sequentially to give an impression of movement similar to that of a pendulum. This is achieved by driving the lamps by a voltage to frequency converter which is fed by a rectified 0.5 Hz sine wave. The row of lamps subtends an angle of 60 degrees at the eye and completes one horizontal sweep in 2 seconds. The

507

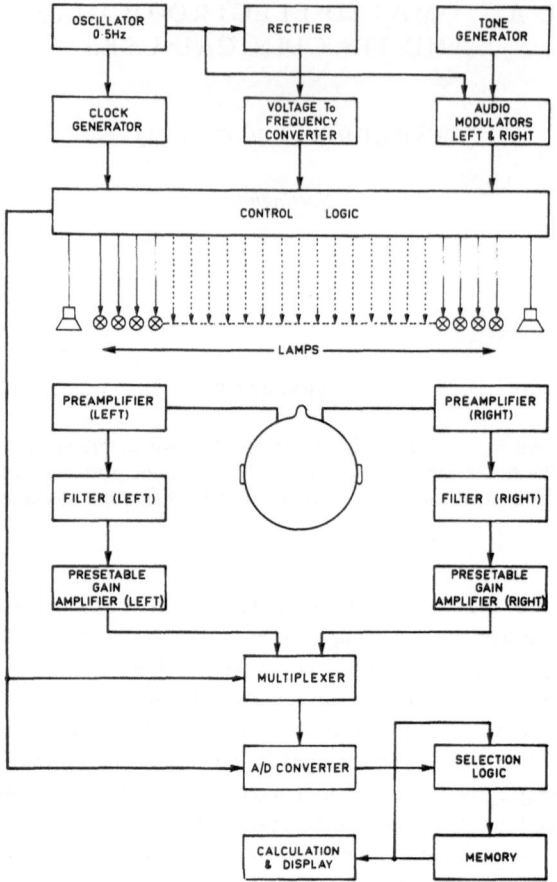

Fig. 1. Block diagram of automated system.

resulting eye movements produce a signal which is quite a good approximation to a sine wave, with some evidence of saccadic movement usually visible. Filtering this gives a pure sine waveform with well defined peaks which are easy to measure. For patients who have difficulty in fixation a pair of loudspeakers, located at the ends of the row of stimulus lamps, are fed with impulses which simulate a sound source moving in the same manner as the visual stimulus.

Elema-Schönander ECG electrodes are used and these are fixed to the skin at each lateral canthus and in the centre of the forehead. An ear electrode is used for ground. Dispensing with the electrodes at the medial canthi eliminates problems caused by lacrimation which tends to occur when the dark adapted eye is reilluminated. The central electrode carries a miniature pre-amplifier which has a separate channel for each eye with an amplification of 500 and a common mode rejection ratio of 90 dB. This produces quite a clean signal which

508

is passed through a bandpass filter of centre frequency 0.5 Hz and quality factor, Q, of 12 to give an almost pure sine waveform. This is available as an output from the instrument for display on an oscilloscope or pen recorder if required.

The stimulus light normally runs for 12 seconds every minute. The signals from the first two eye movements are ignored to allow the patient time to become accustomed to the motion, then the peak values of the next four are sampled and digitised. The signals from the two eyes are arranged so that they are 180° out of phase and the instrument takes measurements on each eye alternately. Because the size of the input signal varies considerably from subject to subject, the instrument uses the measurements taken in the first minute to set the gain of the amplifiers to a suitable value for the rest of the test. As each reading is taken it is compared with the previous set of readings for that eye and if it is grossly different it is rejected. We reject for a signal greater than twice or less than half the amplitude of the previous signal and so far this has been satisfactory. The stimulus lights continue to run until four acceptable readings have been taken and the average of these is stored in the memory. This is repeated each minute for twelve minutes in the dark and the minimum value recorded during that period is retained. When the twelve minutes have elapsed the instrument switches on a bank of fluorescent tubes giving a retinal illumination of about 3000 trolands. The stimulus and measurement procedure is repeated for twelve minutes of light adaptation and this time the maximum value recorded in the light is stored in the memory. This figure is then divided by the minimum value stored previously and the result which is the Arden coefficient is displayed on the instrument panel at the end of the test. (see Figure 2). The instrument will also display the measured values of the dark trough and light

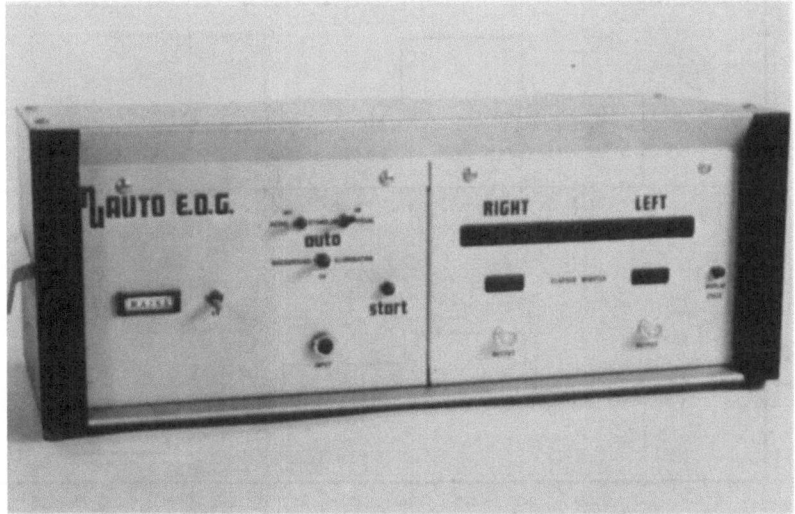

Fig. 2. The front panel of the instrument. The Arden coefficient is displayed immediately beneath the headings 'RIGHT' and 'LEFT'.

peak potentials together with the time in minutes of dark adaptation and light adaptation which was required to reach these levels.

So far we have examined a series of normal subjects as well as several patients selected at random from those attending the electrodiagnostic clinic. When the normal subjects were examined the input signals were analysed in three different ways;
1. They were displayed by a penwriter and the trace was measured and calculated by the standard method.
2. A semi-automatic method similar to that described by Henkes was used. (HENKES et al., 1966)
3. Readings from the fully automated instrument were used.

The results (Figure 3) show good agreement among themselves and with those

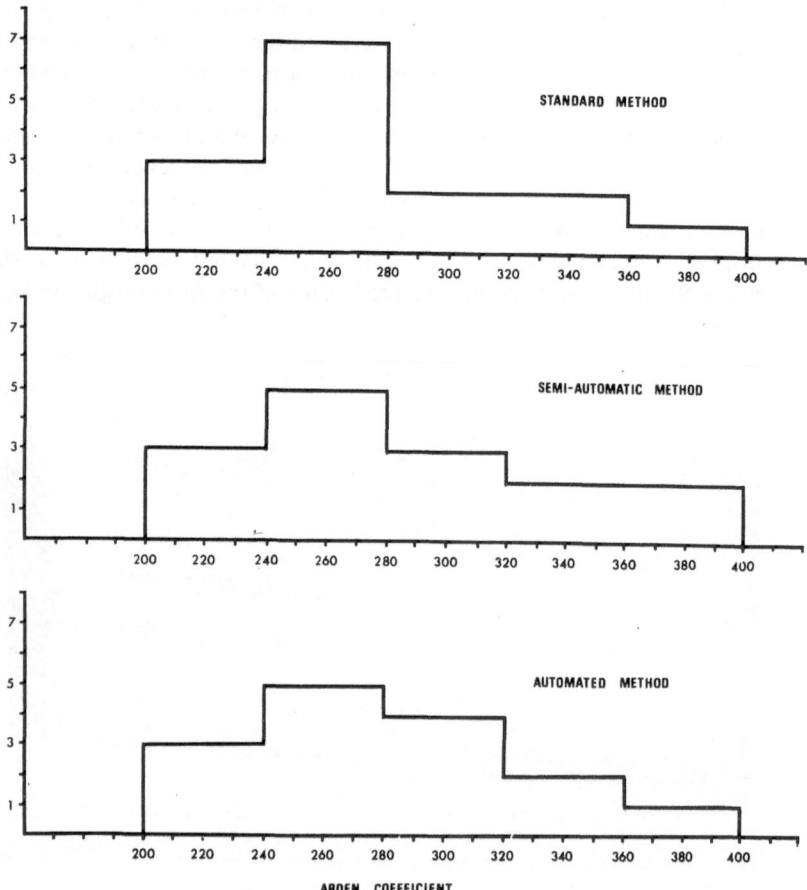

Fig. 3. Distribution of the normal values for the three methods described.

of ARDEN & BARRADA (1962). The difference between the three values obtained is not significant. In cases of poor-co-operation normal results were achieved by this method when the bar diagram of the semi-automatic method was extremely difficult to interpret.

ACKNOWLEDGEMENTS

We would like to express our thanks to the Sheffield Regional Hospital Board for financial assistance and to Mr. W. BETTS for his technical help.

REFERENCES

ARDEN, G. B. & BARRADA, A. *Brit. J. Ophthal.* 46: *468* (1962).
ARDEN. G. B., BARRADA, A. & KELSEY, J. H. *Brit. J. Ophthal.* 46: *449* (1962).
DORNE, P. A. & ESPIARD, J. F. *Arch. Ophthal.* (Paris) 31: *217* (1971).
HENKES, H. E., DENIER VAN DER GON, J. J., VAN MARLE, G. W. & SCHREINEMACHERS, H. P. *Brit. J. Ophthal.* 52: *122* (1968).
KELSEY, J. H. *Brit. J. Ophthal.* 50: *438* (1966).

Authors' address:

Medical Physics Dept.
General Hospital and
Eye Hospital
Nottingham
England

UNILATERAL RETINOPATHIA PIGMENTOSA

J. RICKERS & D. v. DOMARUS

(Hamburg)

The first description of unilateral retinopathia pigmentosa dates back to 1865 (PEDRAGLIA). Nearly 100 cases have been described since. Formerly the diagnosis was established by means of the ophthalmoscopic findings together with a decrease of the visual acuity, visual field defects and disturbance of the dark adaptation. The criteria up to date to establish the diagnosis of an unilateral retinopathia pigmentosa (u.r.p.) (after the exclusion of an inflammatory or traumatic aetiology) are:

1. Reduction or abolishment of the ERG-response
2. Decreased EOG-ratio
3. Diminished dark adaptation together with the other clinical criteria given above.

After critical consideration of the sources mentioned above, the diagnosis of an u.r.p. could be verified only in about 20 cases. A histological correlation of a case proven by electro-physiological examination has not been published, to our knowledge, up to now.

CASE HISTORY

G.S. female, 35 years. History: the patient was suffering from myasthenic reactions since the age of 13. With exception of the usual diseases in childhood, there were no other viral infections. There was no history of injury to the skull. Rough pigmentations of the right fundus were detected by the ophthalmologist of the patient on a screening test 1969.

In 1971, we had the opportunity to examine the patient.

Findings

Visual acuity OD 0,7 (−0,75 sph), OS 1,0 (−0,75 sph); anterior segments of the eyes within normal limits, especially no traumatic changes of the chamber angle.

The fundus of the right eye (Fig. 1) exhibits waxy yellow atrophy of the optic disc with sharp borders. The arteries are narrowed. In the intermediate zone, bone corpuscle-like pigmentations are pronounced. The whole fundus shows a mottled appearance. The fundus of the left eye (Fig. 2) shows no abnormalities.

513

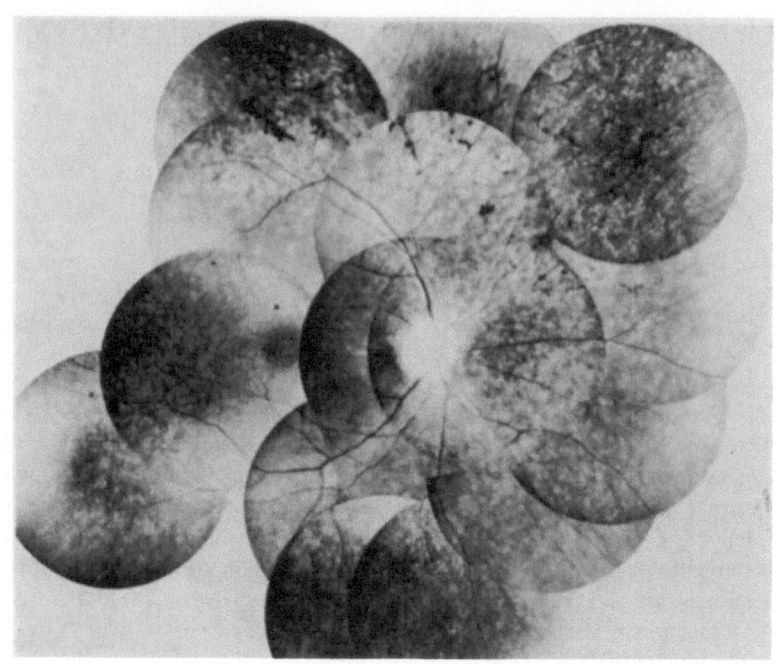

Fig. 1. Fundus OD

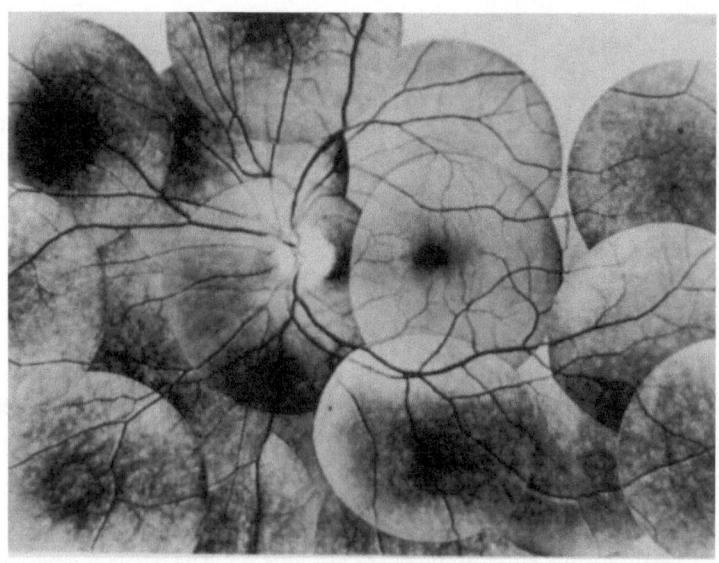

Fig. 2. Fundus OS

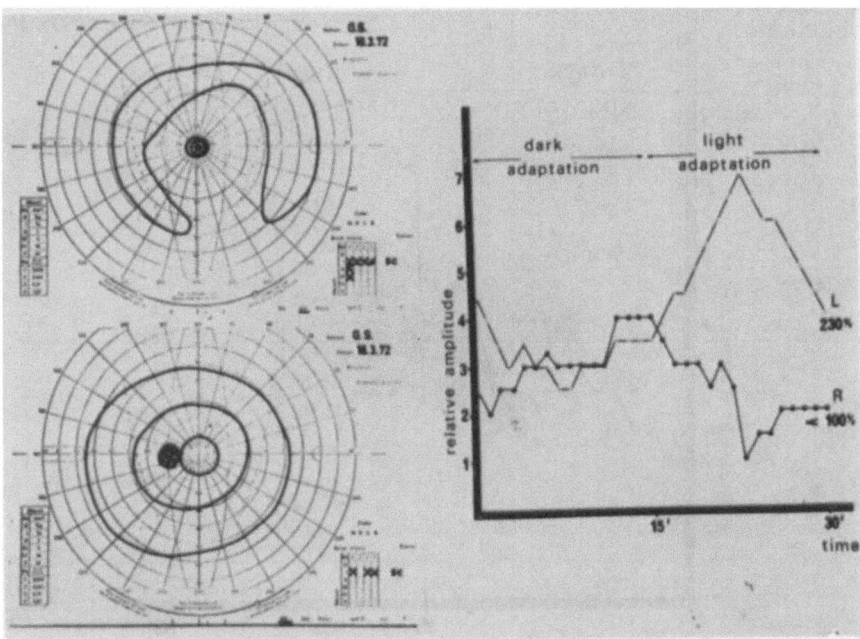

Fig. 3. Left side: Visual fields above OD, below OS. Right side: EOG, OD, OS.

The visual field of the right eye (Fig. 3) performed with the Goldmann-perimeter shows an annular scotoma with a break through and a central island within ten degrees for the target one four, and a normal visual field for the left eye. (Fig. 3).

The ERG response of the right eye is extinguished, in spite of a high intensity stimulus (Fig. 4). The potentials of the left eye reach a peak of 300 microvolt. EOG ratio (Fig. 3) OD less than 100%, OS 230%. Dark adaptation performed with the Goldmann-Weekers adaptometer OD showed a monophasic hemeralopic course, OS normal course, 5 log units.

Based on these findings, the clinical diagnosis of the unilateral retinopathia pigmentosa was established.

In 1972, the patient was admitted to the neurological ward of the university hospital because of a sudden onset of a palsy of the upper limbs. Three months later she developed a tetraplegia. A tentative diagnosis could not be established. The patient died 37 years old on a sudden heart failure following embolism to the lungs.

Both globes were enucleated 40 hours after death. On section we found the rough pigmentations in the area of the equator, which correlated to the funduscopic alterations. The further segments of the eye showed no pathologic findings with the exception of autolysis. The left eye showed no pathologic changes but autolysis.

The retinal pigmentation present allows for the following pathological differential diagnosis:

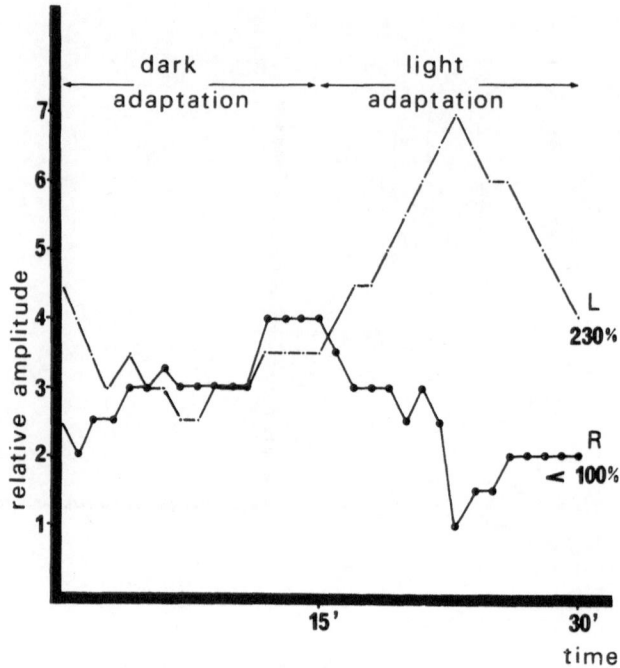

Fig. 4. Dark adaptation OD, OS

1. retinopathia sclopetaria
2. tapetoretinal degeneration
3. different forms of pseudoretinitis pigmentosa

As the retinopathia sclopetaria represents a circumscript entity which can be diagnosed histologically in specific alternations, it is impossible for the pathologist to draw a line between the tapetoretinal degenerations and the pseudoretinitis pigmentosa.

Histological findings

Left eye: (Fig. 5): The left eye shows, besides autolytic changes, a regular structure of the retina with intact rods and cones, normal pigment epithelium and unremarkable vessels.

Right eye: (Fig. 6): Rough perivascular pigmentations are remarkable together with the disorganisation of the different retinal layers, the atrophy of the layer of the ganglion cells and the layer of the granular cells. There is a nearly complete loss of rods and cones, however, it is not possible to tell whether artificial changes are responsible. In the outer retinal layers roughly granulated pigmentations are to be seen with some pigment laden macrophages. Furthermore, a hyalinization of the wall of the vessels is seen with a pronounced narrowing of the diameters. There is a disturbance of the pigment epithelium,

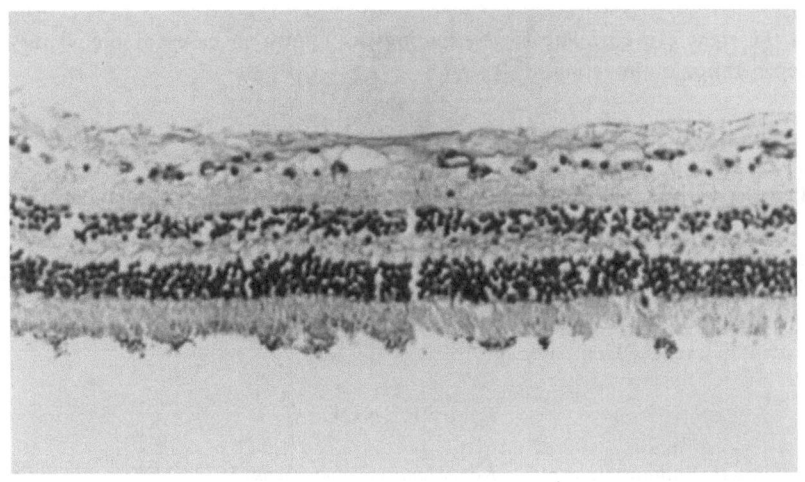

Fig. 5. Retina Os

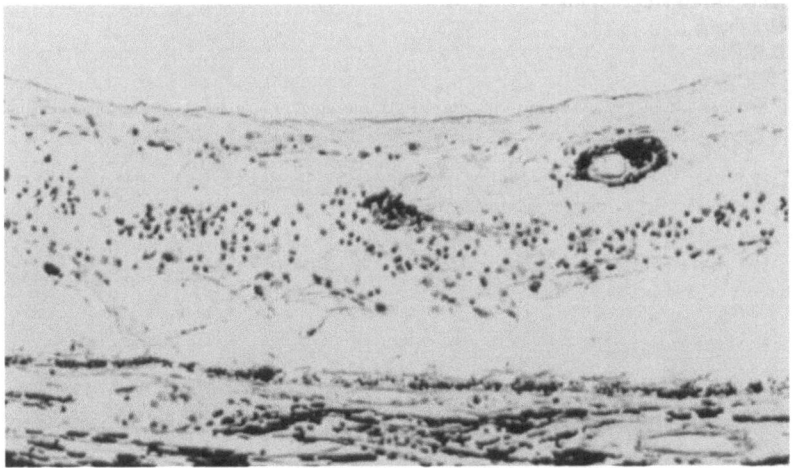

Fig. 6. Retina OD

characterized by aggregations of pigment and degeneration. Bruch's membrane is unremarkable, the structure of the chorioid is normal, without scars.

There is a difference in the histological sections of the optic nerve, as well. Contrary to the regular structure of the left optic nerve, we found an increase of the microglia and several vacuoles in the right optic nerve. With regard to the vacuoles, it is not possible to clarify whether we are dealing with a vacuolic degeneration or a fatty degeneration.

The described alterations have been localized only in the right eye without any alterations in the left eye except autolysis. The histological changes found in the right eye correlate to the findings as known in cases of pigmentary degeneration of the retina.

CONCLUSION

The disease presents as a strictly unilateral case of pigmentary retinal degeneration in the 37 years old patient. There is no evidence to indicate the involvement of the other eye. This speaks for the possibility that unilateral retinopathia pigmentosa is a definite entity. Nevertheless, the possibility can not be excluded that the disease would have ended with bilateral involvement if the patient had reached a greater age.

REFERENCE

PEDRAGLIA. Retinitis pigmentosa. *Klin. Monatsbl. Augenheilk.* 3: *114-117* (1865).

Authors' address:

Universitäts Krankenhaus Eppendorf
Universitäts Augenklinik
Hamburg
B.R.D.